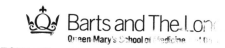

Illustrated Manual of
Pediatric
Dermatology

Illustrated Manual of
Pediatric Dermatology
Diagnosis and Management

Susan Bayliss Mallory MD
Professor of Internal Medicine/Division of Dermatology
and Department of Pediatrics
Washington University School of Medicine
Director, Pediatric Dermatology
St. Louis Children's Hospital
St. Louis, Missouri, USA

Alanna Bree MD
St. Louis University
Director, Pediatric Dermatology
Cardinal Glennon Children's Hospital
St. Louis, Missouri, USA

Peggy Chern MD
Department of Internal Medicine/Division of Dermatology
and Department of Pediatrics
Washington University School of Medicine
St. Louis, Missouri, USA

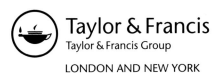

Taylor & Francis
Taylor & Francis Group

LONDON AND NEW YORK

© 2005 Taylor & Francis, an imprint of the Taylor & Francis Group

First published in the United Kingdom in 2005
by Taylor & Francis,
an imprint of the Taylor & Francis Group,
2 Park Square, Milton Park
Abingdon, Oxon OX14 4RN, UK

Tel: +44 (0) 20 7017 6000
Fax: +44 (0) 20 7017 6699
Website: www.tandf.co.uk

Although every effort has been made to ensure that all owners of copyright material have been acknowledged in this publication, we would be glad to acknowledge in subsequent reprints or editions any omissions brought to our attention.

British Library Cataloguing in Publication Data

Data available on application

Library of Congress Cataloging-in-Publication Data

Data available on application

ISBN 1-85070-753-7

Distributed in North and South America by

Taylor & Francis
2000 NW Corporate Blvd
Boca Raton, FL 33431, USA

Within Continental USA
Tel: 800 272 7737; Fax: 800 374 3401
Outside Continental USA
Tel: 561 994 0555; Fax: 561 361 6018
E-mail: orders@crcpress.com

Distributed in the rest of the world by
Thomson Publishing Services
Cheriton House
North Way
Andover, Hampshire SP10 5BE, UK
Tel: +44 (0) 1264 332424
E-mail: salesorder.tandf@thomsonpublishingservices.co.uk

Composition by Parthenon Publishing
Printed and bound by T.G. Hostench S.A., Spain

CONTENTS

PREFACE

Pediatric dermatology is an exciting area of medicine. When children are young, they cannot give a history. In fact, pediatrics is said to be much like veterinary medicine! The practitioner must use sharp observational skills to assess a problem. For example, rather than asking a 1 year old if they scratch or if a rash itches, merely observing the child scratching in the office or seeing excoriations on the skin will lead a physician to the correct conclusion. Thus, looking for clues further sharpens one's visual skills.

This book is a synopsis of basic pediatric dermatology. The approaches that we use are practical ones which we have found to be simple basic approaches to problems that pediatricians and dermatologists see in their practices. This book is aimed at the common problems seen in medical offices with some added information about unique conditions in pediatric dermatology.

Teaching at a pediatric tertiary care hospital, we find that pediatric and family practice residents ask us frequently which book they might purchase for their library. Mainly, they are interested in a book that has good photographs so that they can visually recognize skin diseases combined with a practical, concise text.

Our purpose in writing this book was to produce a manual of high-quality photographs which can easily aid the pediatric house officer and primary care physician in the diagnosis of pediatric skin diseases. In addition, we have tried to provide a pertinent, easy to read outline with easily applied suggestions on treatment. Realistic criteria for referring patients are also outlined and a few pertinent references are given.

We hope that you enjoy this text and that it can be of benefit to all who read it.

Susan Bayliss Mallory MD
Alanna Bree MD
Peggy Chern MD

DEDICATION

We would like to dedicate this book to our children and patients who have been a great source of learning not only about pediatrics but also about pediatric dermatology.

For Susan Bayliss Mallory, my children, Elizabeth and Meredith, have been a source of joy and encouragement as well as keeping me grounded. My parents, Milward William Bayliss MD and Jeanette Roedell Bayliss were always encouraging me to study and learn. God has been an ever-loving omniscient presence in my life and has been my source of inspiration.

For Alanna Bree, to all of my many teachers, especially my first teachers – my parents, Al and Shirley Flath. Most importantly, to my husband, Doug, and children Sam and Kendyl for their unconditional love and constant support.

For Peggy Chern, to my parents, Henry and Myra Chern, and to Matt Shaw for their support and encouragement.

Others who have been a major source of help and inspiration have been: General Elbert DeCoursey MD, Esther DeCoursey, Jere Guin MD, Arthur Eisen MD and Lynn Cornelius MD.

Special thanks to the following physicians who helped review the manuscript: Chan-Ho Lai, Pam Weinfeld, Jason Fung, Tony Hsu, Angela Spray, D. Russell Johnson, Alison Klenk, Margaret Mann and Yadira Hurley.

1

PRINCIPLES OF CLINICAL DIAGNOSIS

GENERAL

- Diagnosis of cutaneous disorders in infants and children requires careful inspection of skin, hair and nails
- Skin disorders of infants are different from skin disorders in adults
  1. For example, erythema toxicum neonatorum is only seen in newborns
  2. Skin of a young child tends to form blisters more easily (e.g. insect bites or mastocytomas)
- Determining morphology of skin lesions, their color and distribution will help generate a differential diagnosis

HISTORY

- Take a thorough history of events surrounding the skin disorder (Table 1.1)

1. This includes the patient's age, race, sex, details of previous treatments and duration of the problem
2. Focus attention on the particular morphology
3. Physicians should be sensitive to the anxieties that parents might have and address these issues appropriately
   a. While taking a family history, note whether a family member has a similar but more severe disorder that may cause concern (e.g. psoriasis). Talking about these issues will let the parent know that you understand their concerns
4. Developmental aspects, previous illnesses and previous surgery are important points in the history
5. Newborn history should include the prenatal period, pregnancy and delivery

---

Table 1.1 Interviewing and treating pediatric dermatology patients

1. Children are different from adults. Learn the differences.
2. Approach patients cautiously. Sit across the room and talk to the parents before examining the child. This gives them time to 'size you up'.
3. Speak directly to the child as if he/she understands what you are saying. Make eye contact with the child.
4. Keep the parent in the room for procedures as much as possible unless it interferes with the procedure or the parent wishes to step out of the room.
5. Conservative management is best. Try to use the lowest effective dose of medication for the shortest time.
6. Avoid new therapies which do not have a proven track record in pediatrics until adequate clinical trials are performed.
7. Do not use treatments which may decrease growth or mental development.
8. Anticipatory guidance and emotional support are helpful especially in chronic disorders (e.g. alopecia areata, atopic dermatitis).

Adapted from Honig PJ. Potential clinical management risks in pediatric dermatology. Risk Management in Dermatology, Part II. AM Medica Communications LTS: New York, 1988: 6

a. Maternal history may quickly lead to a diagnosis in some cases (e.g. maternal HIV or systemic lupus erythematosus)

6. Evaluation of young children requires a modified approach, depending upon the age of the child
   a. Establish a positive relationship with not only the parent but also the child
   b. Gain eye contact with the child at his own level. This is less threatening than standing over him in an intimidating manner
   c. Sit and talk to the parents without making any movements toward the young child. This allows time for him/her to observe your actions ('size you up') before speaking with them directly
   d. Refrain from using a loud voice or touching the child until he feels comfortable. These are techniques which pediatricians know very well
   e. Allow the child to play with small toys in the room. This is a way to distract him and allows one to observe his interactions, which could help with developmental history
   f. Obviously, young children cannot always answer specific questions. However, carefully observing the child may reveal answers to questions not even asked (e.g. observing scratch marks on a 6-month-old child obviates the necessity of asking whether the child is scratching)

7. School age children (5–10 years) can answer questions directly and are sometimes very informative
   a. Engaging them in conversation about school or an interest, such as a pet, may put the child at ease quickly

8. Adolescents can give a history and should be given instructions, giving the adolescent the ability to take care of his own skin, demonstrating his maturity and ability to care for his own health

PHYSICAL EXAMINATION

- Include the entire skin surface including hair, nails and oral mucosa
- Adequate lighting is important, preferably natural lighting through a window

1. Additional lighting with high-intensity examination lights
2. Side-lighting may demonstrate subtle elevations or depressions

- A magnifying glass may enlarge tiny variations of the skin
- Examination of the genitalia should not be overlooked; have an assistant or parent in the room, not only for the comfort of the patient but also for legal purposes
- Mucous membranes should also be examined, specifically looking for ulcers, white spots or pigmented lesions that may reflect a primary skin disorder
- Teeth should be examined for evidence of enamel dysplasia (pitting), infection or general hygiene

TERMINOLOGY

- The description of lesions is important to help determine whether lesions are primary (initial) lesions or secondary lesions
- Primary lesions are *de novo* lesions which are most representative of the disorder (Table 1.2)
- Secondary lesions occur with time and demonstrate other changes (Table 1.3)
- Configuration describes the pattern of lesions on the skin (Table 1.4)
- Distribution describes where the lesions are found. Examples: localized, generalized, patchy, symmetric, asymmetric, segmental, dermatomal, or following Blaschko lines
- Number of lesions: single, grouped or multiple
- Color of lesions: red, pink, blue, brown, black, white, yellow or a variation of these colors (Table 1.5)
- Regional patterns if lesions are found primarily in a certain distribution (Table 1.6). Examples: photosensitive eruptions are seen on the face and arms with sun exposure; tinea versicolor tends to be on the upper chest and back

DISEASES

- In a pediatric dermatological practice, 35 diseases account for more than 90% of the diagnoses seen in patients (Table 1.7)

Table 1.2   Primary lesions

Primary (initial) lesions	Description
Macule	Flat; any change in color of the skin < 1 cm in size
Patch	Flat lesion > 1 cm in size
Papule	Solid elevated lesion < 1 cm diameter; greatest mass above skin surface
Nodule	Solid elevated lesion > 1 cm diameter; greatest mass below skin surface
Tumor	Solid elevated lesion > 2 cm diameter; greatest mass below skin surface
Plaque	Raised, flat, solid lesion > 1 cm; may show epidermal changes
Wheal	Raised, solid, edematous papule or plaque without epidermal change
Vesicle	Fluid-filled (clear) < 1 cm diameter, usually < 0.5 cm
Bulla	Fluid-filled (clear) > 1 cm diameter
Pustule	Vesicle or bulla with purulent fluid
Cyst	Cavity lined with epithelium containing fluid, pus, or keratin
Comedone	Plugged sebaceous follicle containing sebum, cellular debris and anaerobic bacteria
Petechiae	Extravasated blood into superficial dermis appearing as tiny red macules
Purpura	Extravasated blood into dermis and/or subcutaneous tissues associated with inflammation; may or may not be palpable

Table 1.3   Secondary lesions

Secondary lesions	Description
Crust	Collection of dried serum, blood, pus and damaged epithelial cells
Exudate	Moist serum, blood or pus from either an erosion, blister or pustule
Eschar	Dark or black plaque overlying an ulcer; seen in tissue necrosis
Scale	Dry, flaky surface with normal/abnormal keratin; present in proliferative or retention disorders
Lichenification	Accentuation of normal skin lines caused by thickening, primarily of the epidermis, due to scratching or rubbing
Excoriation	Localized damage to skin secondary to scratching
Erosion	Superficial depression from loss of surface epidermis
Ulcer	Full-thickness loss of epidermis, some dermis and subcutaneous fat, which results in a scar when healed
Fissure	Linear crack in the skin, down to the dermis
Atrophy	Thinning or loss of epidermis and/or dermis Epidermal atrophy may be very subtle, showing only fine wrinkling of the skin with increased underlying vascular prominence Dermal atrophy shows little if any epidermal change but shows depressions, reflecting loss of dermis or subcutaneous tissue
Scar	Healed dermal lesion caused by trauma, surgery, infection
Papillomatous	Surface with minute finger-like projections
Friable	Skin bleeds easily after minor trauma
Pedunculated	Papule or nodule on a stalk with a base usually smaller than the papule or nodule
Filiform	Finger-like, usually associated with warts on the face

Table 1.4   Configuration of skin lesions

Configuration	Description
Annular	Round lesion with an active margin and a clear center (e.g. granuloma annulare, tinea corporis)
Linear	Lesion occurring in a line (e.g. poison ivy dermatitis, excoriations)
Grouped	Lesions of any morphology located close together (e.g. molluscum)
Target	Dark, dusky center with erythematous border and lighter area in between (e.g. erythema multiforme)
Arciform	Semicircular
Gyrate/polycyclic	Lesions which were annular and/or arched and have moved and become joined
Serpiginous	Snake-like margins (e.g. urticaria, creeping eruption)
Herpetiform	Appearing like an eruption of herpes simplex virus with tightly grouped vesicles or pustules (e.g. dermatitis herpetiformis)
Zosteriform/ dermatomal	Following a dermatome (e.g. herpes zoster)
Segmental	Following a body segment (e.g. hemangioma)
Reticulated	Net-like pattern (e.g. livedo reticularis)
Umbilicated	Surface has round depression in center (e.g. molluscum contagiosum)

Table 1.5   Other descriptive terms

Characteristic	Examples
Color	Pink – caused by increase in blood flow or interstitial fluid Red – caused by increased blood or dilated blood vessels Purple – caused by increased blood or dilated blood vessels Violaceous – lavender, bluish pink Depigmented – complete loss of pigment Hypopigmented – partial loss of pigment Brown – increase in melanin in epidermis Gray/blue – increase in melanin in dermis or subcutaneous tissue Black – intensely concentrated melanin Yellow – associated with lipids or sebaceous glands
Border	Circumscribed – limited in space by something drawn around or confining an area Diffuse – spreading, scattered
Palpation	Smooth – surface not different from surrounding skin Uneven – felt in scaly or verrucous lesions Rough – feels like sandpaper

- Reaction patterns help group disorders together (Table 1.8)
  1. Examples are eczematous eruptions: atopic dermatitis, allergic contact dermatitis
  2. Examples are papulosquamous disorders: psoriasis, seborrheic dermatitis

DIAGNOSTIC TESTS

Potassium hydroxide examination

Potassium hydroxide (KOH) examination is used for suspected fungal infections of skin, hair and nails

Table 1.6   Regional patterns and diagnosis

Scalp
Seborrheic dermatitis
Tinea capitis
Alopecia areata
Psoriasis
Nevus sebaceus
Aplasia cutis congenita

Face
Contact dermatitis
Perioral dermatitis
Pityriasis alba
Acne
Milia
Photosensitivity disorders

Trunk
Tinea corporis
Tinea versicolor
Pityriasis rosea
Psoriasis

Extremities
Psoriasis (also scalp and nails)
Scabies (also groin and waistline)
Granuloma annulare
Erythema nodosum
Erythema multiforme
Dyshidrotic eczema
Gianotti–Crosti syndrome
Cutis marmorata

Nails
Psoriasis
Alopecia areata
Twenty nail dystrophy
Lichen planus
Ingrown toenail

Oral
Lichen planus
Mucocele
Geographic tongue
Stevens–Johnson syndrome

Genital/groin
Lichen sclerosus
Condyloma acuminata
Acrodermatitis enteropathica
Intertrigo

Table 1.7   Most common dermatoses in children

Acne
Alopecia areata
Atopic dermatitis (eczema)
Café au lait macules
Capillary malformation (port wine stain)
Condyloma acuminata
Contact dermatitis
Drug eruption
Epidermal cyst
Folliculitis
Granuloma annulare
Hemangioma
Herpes simplex
Ichthyosis
Impetigo
Keloid
Keratosis pilaris
Mastocytosis
Milia
Molluscum
Nevi
Pityriasis alba
Postinflammatory hyperpigmentation
Postinflammatory hypopigmentation
Psoriasis
Pyogenic granuloma
Scabies
Seborrhea
Telangiectasias
Tinea capitis
Tinea corporis
Tinea versicolor
Urticaria
Viral exanthem
Vitiligo
Warts

- Scrapings (using a scalpel blade) from a scaly lesion are placed on a clean glass slide
- Nail scrapings can be obtained by scraping with a scalpel blade or small dermal curette underneath the nail for keratinous subungual debris
- Place scrapings on a glass slide
- Apply a few drops of 10–20% KOH
- Apply a cover slip
- Heat the slide to facilitate dissolution of the cell walls or allow the slide to sit for 15–20 min without heating
- If 20% KOH in dimethylsulfoxide (DMSO) is used, heating is unnecessary
- KOH can also be formulated in ink-based preparations which darken the hyphae for easier identification (examples: Chlorazole fungal stain from Delasco Dermatologic Lab and Supplies, Inc (www.delasco.com), or Swartz–Lampkin solution)
- Examine microscopically at 10× or 20× power with the condenser in the lowest position

Table 1.8   Common dermatologic diagnoses by reaction pattern

Eczematous	**Infiltrative pattern**	Erythema multiforme
Atopic dermatitis (eczema)	Nodular	Erythema annulare centrifugum
Infantile eczema	Erythema nodosum	
Nummular eczema	Pyogenic granuloma	**Acneiform**
Allergic contact dermatitis	Juvenile xanthogranuloma	Acne vulgaris
Dermatophytosis	Cyst	Steroid-induced acne
Diaper dermatitis	Papular	Perioral dermatitis
Scabies	Granuloma annulare	Rosacea
	Mastocytosis	
Papulosquamous	Xanthomas	**Verrucous**
Psoriasis	Molluscum contagiosum	Warts
Seborrheic dermatitis		Nevus sebaceus
Pityriasis rosea	**Atrophy and/or sclerosis**	Epidermal nevus
Syphilis	Scleroderma	
Lichen planus	Morphea	**Erosive**
	Lichen sclerosus	Acrodermatitis enteropathica
Vesiculobullous	Lipoatrophy	Epidermolysis bullosa
Impetigo	Aplasia cutis congenita	
Herpes simplex virus		
Varicella-zoster virus	**Vascular reactions/erythema**	
Epidermolysis bullosa	Urticaria	
Miliaria	Vasculitis	
Scabies	Viral exanthem	

- Demonstration of hyphae or spores confirms the diagnosis of tinea
- Oral lesions suspected of *Candida* can be scraped in a similar fashion to demonstrate the typical pseudohyphae or budding yeast forms

Scabies preparation

Scrape a burrow or unexcoriated papule, and apply KOH or mineral oil to the slide before microscopic examination

- Best areas to find mites: wrists, in between fingers, or along sides of feet of infants
- Examine at 4× power to demonstrate mites, eggs or scybala (feces)

Pediculosis

This can be confirmed by finding a live louse on the skin or scalp, or by demonstrating nits on the hair shafts

- Affected hairs can be cut with scissors, placed on a glass slide and covered with immersion oil or KOH to demonstrate nits

Fungal cultures

Fungal cultures confirm a diagnosis of tinea capitis, tinea corporis or onychomycosis

- Using appropriate fungal culture media (Sabouraud's agar, Mycosel agar) allows for identification of fungal species
- Dermatophyte Test Media (DTM) can be used in the office for easy identification of dermatophytes, but does not speciate fungi

Tzanck smear

This is used for diagnosis of herpes simplex or varicella-zoster virus

- Remove vesicle roof with a scalpel blade and place on a glass slide
- The base of the lesion is gently scraped and transferred to a slide, then stained with a Giemsa or Wright stain
- Multinucleated giant epithelial cells under 40× microscopy are diagnostic for herpes virus or varicella-zoster infections

Wood's lamp examination

A Wood's lamp emits long-wave ultraviolet light
- Screening for fungal scalp infections caused by *Microsporum* species shows green fluorescence of affected hair shafts
  1. It is important to verify that the actual hair shaft is causing fluorescence, which can easily be seen with a magnifying lens
  2. Lint, scales and other debris on the scalp also fluoresce and should not be confused with tinea
- Hypopigmentation or depigmentation can be accentuated (e.g. tuberous sclerosis patches) and delineated, particularly in light-skinned patients
- *Corynebacterium minutissimum*, which causes erythrasma, fluoresces a coral red color
- Urine of patients with certain types of porphyria fluoresces pink

Bacterial cultures

- Purulent material from representative lesions are swabbed with a soft sterile swab, inserted into the appropriate tube and sent to the laboratory

Viral culture

This requires a special transport medium, which is available at most large hospitals
- Blister fluid and the base of the lesion should be swabbed or aspirated and then inoculated into the appropriate media

Skin biopsy

Skin biopsy is carried out for routine histopathologic or immunofluorescence examination
- Topical anesthetic can be applied to the skin prior to biopsy to reduce the pain of the needle stick for local anesthesia
- Punch biopsies or elliptical biopsies should demonstrate all three levels of the cutis (epidermis, dermis and subcutaneous fat)
- Shave biopsies (saucerization) may be indicated for more superficial lesions
- Biopsy is best done by a physician who is trained in the knowledge of which areas are best biopsied and what histology is expected
- Immunofluorescence may be indicated for certain connective tissue disorders or bullous diseases and requires special transport media

Diascopy

Diascopy is performed by placing a glass slide over the skin lesions with light pressure
- Vascular lesions typically show characteristic blanching with refilling once the slide has been removed
- Granulomatous disorders such as sarcoidosis may demonstrate an apple jelly color

References

Brodkin RH, Janniger CK. Common clinical concerns in pediatric dermatology. Cutis 1997; 60: 279–30

Eichenfield LF, Frieden IJ, Esterly NB, eds. Textbook of Neonatal Dermatology. WB Saunders: Philadelphia, 2001

Eichenfield LF, Funk A, Fallon-Friedlander S, Cunningham BB. A clinical study to evaluate the efficacy of ELA Max (4% liposomal lidocaine) as compared with eutectic mixture of local anesthetics cream for pain reduction of venipuncture in children. Pediatrics 2002; 109: 1093–9

Freedberg IM, Eisen AZ, Wolff K, et al., eds. Fitzpatrick's Dermatology in General Medicine, 6th edn. McGraw Hill: New York, 2003

Harper J, Oranje A, Prose N, eds. Textbook of Pediatric Dermatology. Blackwell Science Oxford: UK, 2000

Lewis EJ, Dahl MV, Lewis CA. On standard definitions: 33 years hence. Arch Dermatol 1997; 133: 1169

Renzi C, Abeni D, Picardi A, et al. Factors associated with patient satisfaction with care among dermatological outpatients. Br J Dermatol 2001; 145: 617–23

Schachner LA, Hansen RC, eds. Pediatric Dermatology, 3rd edn. Mosby (Elsevier): New York, 2003

Sybert VP. Genetic Skin Disorders. Oxford University Press: New York, 1997

2

NEONATAL DERMATOLOGY

COMMON CUTANEOUS FINDINGS

Vernix caseosa

Major points

- Common finding in the neonatal period
- Characteristic white to gray, greasy covering on the skin surface of the newborn (Figure 2.1)
- Thickness increases with gestational age
- Considered a protective covering and mechanical barrier to bacteria
- Lipid composition is variable depending on gestational age
- Discoloration and odor can indicate fetal distress and/or intrauterine infection

Pathogenesis

- Composed of shed epidermal cells, sebum and lanugo hairs
- Variable lipid composition of cholesterol, free fatty acids and ceramide

Diagnosis

- Clinical diagnosis

Differential diagnosis

- Ichthyoses (disorders of keratinization) if atypical

Treatment

- None needed

Prognosis

- Sheds without therapy during the first week of life

References

Hoeger PH, Schreiner V, Klaassen IA, et al. Epidermal barrier lipids in human vernix caseosa: corresponding ceramide pattern in vernix and fetal skin. Br J Dermatol 2002; 146: 194–201

Joglekar VM. Barrier properties of vernix caseosa. Arch Dis Child 1980; 55: 817

Cutis marmorata

Major points

- Transient mottling of the skin in the newborn period
- Normal physiologic response to ambient temperature changes; accentuates with decreased temperatures and improves with rewarming
- Symmetrical, blanchable, red–blue reticulated mottling of trunk and extremities. (Figure 2.2)
- More common in premature infants, but also affects full-term newborns

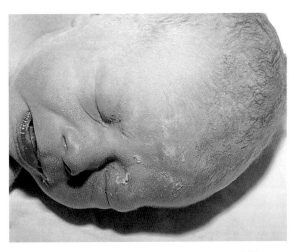

Figure 2.1 Vernix caseosa – cheesy white material in a newborn

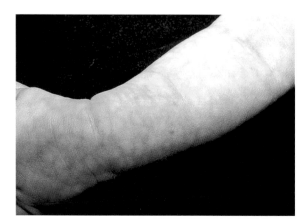

Figure 2.2 Cutis marmorata – reticulated vascular normal pattern in an infant

- Improves with increasing age; typically resolves by 1 year

Pathogenesis

- Physiologic vascular reaction based on immature autonomic control of the vascular plexus in response to temperature changes
- Postulated to be caused by increased sympathetic tone with delayed vasodilatation in response to a flux in temperature resulting in dilatation of capillaries and small venules
- Persistent cases associated with Down syndrome, trisomy 18, hypothyroidism, Cornelia de Lange syndrome, congenital heart disease

Diagnosis

- Clinical findings

Differential diagnosis

- Cutis marmorata telangiectatica congenita
- Livedo reticularis caused by collagen vascular disorder

Treatment

- Maintain even temperature of infant and surroundings

Prognosis

- Generally resolves spontaneously as vasomotor responses mature
- May require further evaluation for underlying disorder if persistent beyond 6 months of age and does not respond to warming (e.g. thyroid disorder, heart disease)

References

Devillers ACA, De Waard-Van der Spek, Oranje AP. Cutis marmarota telangiectatica congenita. Clinical features in 35 cases. Arch Dermatol 1999; 134: 34–8

Ercis M, Balci S, Atakan N. Dermatological manifestations in 71 Down syndrome children admitted to a clinical genetics unit. Clin Genet 1996; 50: 317–20

Treadwell PA. Dermatoses in newborns. Am Fam Physician 1997; 56: 443–50

Sebaceous gland hyperplasia

Major points

- Prominent sebaceous glands present in the newborn period
- Affects up to 50% of term infants; less common in premature infants
- Characteristic pinpoint yellow papules with no surrounding erythema (Figure 2.3)
- Location: nose, cheeks, upper lip and forehead

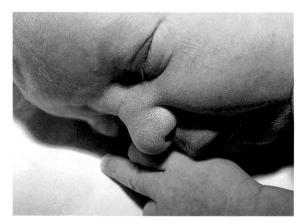

Figure 2.3 Sebaceous gland hyperplasia seen in a newborn

Pathogenesis

- Caused by maternal androgen stimulation of sebaceous glands that occurs in the final month of gestation

Diagnosis

- Clinical findings
- Histology: enlarged sebaceous gland with a widened sebaceous duct

Differential diagnosis

- Milia
- Neonatal acne

Treatment

- None required or recommended

Prognosis

- Spontaneous resolution during the first few months of life

Reference

Rivers JK, Friederikesn PC, Dibin C. A prevalence survey of dermatoses in the Australian neonate. J Am Acad Dermatol 1990; 23: 77–81

Milia

Major points

- Occurs in up to 40% of infants, most commonly on the face
- Known as Epstein's pearls when they occur in the oral cavity; affect up to 85% of newborns
- 1–2 mm white, firm papules on the face, but can also occur on the trunk, extremities, genitalia and oral mucosa (Figure 2.4)
- Can occur at sites of scars

Pathogenesis

- Keratinous cyst originating from vellus hair follicle
- Results from retention of keratin within the lowest portion of the infundibulum of the pilosebaceous unit at the level of the sebaceous duct

Diagnosis

- Clinical findings
- Histology: identical to epidermal cysts except for smaller size; lined by stratified epithelium; contains laminated keratin

Differential diagnosis

- Neonatal acne
- Sebaceous hyperplasia
- Molluscum contagiosum

Treatment

- No intervention required
- Incision and expression rarely required

Prognosis

- Typically resolves within weeks to months
- Can be associated with syndromes: type I oral–facial–digital syndrome, hereditary trichodysplasia, pachyonychia congenita

References

Akinduro OM, Burge SM. Congenital milia in the nasal groove. Br J Dermatol 1994; 130: 800

Bridges AG, Lucky AW, Haney G, Mutasim DF. Milia en plaque of the eyelids in childhood: case report and review of the literature. Pediatr Dermatol 1998; 15: 282–4

Langley RG, Walsh NM, Ross JB. Multiple eruptive milia: report of a case, review of the literature, and a classification. J Am Acad Dermatol 1997; 37: 353–6

Larralde de Luna M, Paspa ML, Ibargoyen J. Oral–facial–digital type I syndrome of Papillon-Leage and Psaume. Pediatr Dermatol 1992; 9: 52–6

Stefanidou MP, Panayotides JG, Tosca AD. Milia en plaque: a case report and review of the literature. Dermatol Surg 2002; 28: 291–5

Erythema toxicum neonatorum

Synonym: toxic erythema of the newborn

Major points

- Occurs in 40–70% of full-term infants

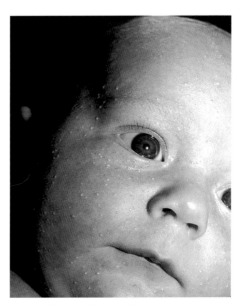

Figure 2.4 Milia – multiple white papules on the face

- Rarely affects preterm infants or infants weighing <2500 g
- Characteristic eruption with macular erythema and discrete, scattered yellow papules and pustules with surrounding erythematous wheals (Figure 2.5)
- Location: primarily face, trunk and extremities with sparing of the palms and soles
- Typically occurs on day 1–2 of life; not present at birth
- Waxing/waning course over 1 month and can occur in crops
- Can be associated with a peripheral eosinophilia

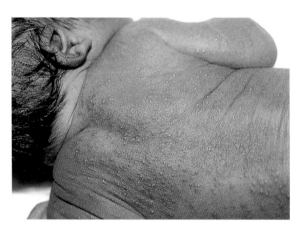

Figure 2.5 Erythema toxicum neonatorum – erythematous papules and pustules on the back

Pathogenesis

- Unknown but several unproven hypotheses, including a transient graft-versus-host reaction against maternal lymphocytes

Diagnosis

- Clinical findings
- Scrape a pustule; Wright stain of contents reveals numerous eosinophils and rare neutrophils
- Histology: subcorneal or intracorneal pustules filled with numerous eosinophils and some neutrophils within the follicle; exocytosis of eosinophils in the follicular epithelium; eosinophils and edema of the perifollicular papillary dermis

Differential diagnosis

- Transient neonatal pustular melanosis
- Congenital candidiasis

- Staphylococcal impetigo
- Neonatal herpes simplex
- Scabies

Treatment

- No treatment necessary

Prognosis

- Self-limited course typically over 1–4 weeks

References

Bassukas ID. Is erythema toxicum neonatorum a mild self-limited acute cutaneous graft-versus-host reaction from maternal-to-fetal lymphocyte transfer? Med Hypoth 1992; 38: 334

Marchini G, Stabi B, Kankes K, et al. AQP1 and AQP3, psoriasin, and nitric oxide synthases 1–3 are inflammatory mediators in erythema toxicum neonatorum. Pediatr Dermatol 2003; 20: 377–84

Mengesha YM, Bennett ML. Pustular skin disorders: diagnosis and treatment. Am J Clin Dermatol 2002; 3: 389–400

Nanda S, Reddy BSN, Ramji S, Pandhi D. Analytical study of pustular eruptions in neonates. Pediatr Dermatol 2002; 19: 210–15

Schwartz RA, Janniger CK. Erythema toxicum neonatorum. Cutis 1996; 58: 153–5

VanPraag MC, VanRooij RW, Folkers E, et al. Diagnosis and treatment of pustular disorders in the neonate. Pediatr Dermatol 1997; 14: 131–43

Wagner A. Distinguishing vesicular and pustular disorders in the neonate. Curr Opin Pediatr 1997; 9: 396–405

Transient neonatal pustular melanosis

Major points

- Self-limited, benign dermatosis of the newborn
- Occurs in 0.2–4% of all term infants; 4.4% of Black infants affected, 0.6% of White infants affected
- Lesions may be present *in utero* and are almost always present at birth
- Location: distributed diffusely on trunk, face, extremities and palms and soles
- Three stages:
    1. 1–5 mm, fragile pustules present at birth; may not be evident at birth due to rupture with birth trauma or initial cleaning (Figure 2.6)

2. Resolution of pustules with surrounding fine white collarettes of scale
3. Hyperpigmented macules represent postinflammatory hyperpigmentation (Figure 2.7); this stage may not be present in light-skinned infants
- All three lesion types can be present at any stage of presentation

Pathogenesis

- Unknown; possible variant of erythema toxicum

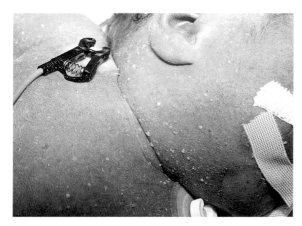

Figure 2.6 Transient neonatal pustular melanosis – pustular phase at birth

Diagnosis

- Clinical findings
- Scrape pustule and stain with Wright stain; reveals many neutrophils and rare eosinophils
- Histology
  1. Hyperpigmented macules: basilar hyperpigmentation; no dermal melanin
  2. Pustules: intracorneal or subcorneal collections of neutrophils with a few eosinophils

Differential diagnosis

- Erythema toxicum neonatorum
- Miliaria
- Acropustulosis of infancy
- Staphylococcal impetigo
- Candidiasis

Treatment

- No treatment necessary

Figure 2.7 Transient neonatal pustular melanosis – hyperpigmented phase

Prognosis

- Pustules resolve over a few days
- Hyperpigmented macules resolve over several weeks to months
- No systemic associations

References

Ramamurthy RS, Reveri M, Esterly NB, et al. Transient neonatal pustular melanosis. J Pediatr 1976; 88: 831–5

Van Praag MC, Van Rooij RW, Folkers E, et al. Diagnosis and treatment of pustular disorders in the neonate. Pediatr Dermatol 1997; 14: 131–43

Wagner A. Distinguishing vesicular and pustular disorders in the neonate. Curr Opin Pediatr 1997; 9: 396–405

Neonatal cephalic pustulosis

Major points

- Presents with monomorphic inflammatory papules and pustules on the face, scalp and neck during the first month of life
- Comedones are absent
- Lesions are not follicular
- Male/female ratio is 1 : 1

Pathogenesis

- Lesions may be induced by inflammatory reaction to *Malassezia furfur* or *M. sympodialis*

Diagnosis

- Potassium hydroxide preparation shows *Malassezia* sp.
- Histology: neutrophilic inflammation and yeast

Differential diagnosis

- Infantile acne
- Erythema toxicum neonatorum
- Transient neonatal pustular melanosis
- Eosinophilic pustulosis

Treatment

- Resolves spontaneously without treatment
- Ketoconazole or miconazole cream twice a day for 1–2 weeks

Prognosis

- Transient and resolves without residual scarring

References

Bernier V, Weill FX, Hirigoyen V, et al. Skin colonization by *Malassezia* species in neonates: a prospective study and relationship with neonatal cephalic pustulosis. Arch Dermatol 2002; 138: 215–18

Niamba P, Weill FX, Sarlangue J, et al. Is common neonatal cephalic pustulosis (neonatal acne) triggered by *Malassezia sympodialis?* Arch Dermatol 1998; 134: 995–8

Rapelanoro R, Mortureux P, Couprie B, et al. Neonatal *Malassezia furfur* pustulosis. Arch Dermatol 1996; 132: 190–3

Umbilical granuloma

Major points

- Pink papule or nodule within the umbilical stump that bleeds easily (Figure 2.8)
- Develops at the site of the umbilical cord remnant after it falls off
- Clinically resembles a pyogenic granuloma

Pathogenesis

- Inadequate healing at umbilical stump with subsequent endothelial cell proliferation and inflammation (granulation tissue)
- Not true granuloma

Diagnosis

- Clinical findings
- Histology: endothelial cell proliferation without atypia

Differential diagnosis

- Omphalomesenteric duct cyst/umbilical polyp
- Patent urachus

Treatment

- Silver nitrate application
- Cryocautery, ligature and excision have been reported to be successful

Prognosis

- Can resolve spontaneously but usually requires treatment
- Persistence indicates the presence of an umbilical remnant

References

Campbell J, Beasley SW, McMullin N, Hutson JM. Clinical diagnosis of umbilical swellings and discharges in children. Med J Aust 1986; 145: 450–3

Donlon CR, Furdon SA. Assessment of the umbilical cord outside of the delivery room. Part 2. Adv Neonatal Care 2002; 2: 187–97

OTHER CUTANEOUS DISORDERS

Neonatal lupus erythematosus

Major points

- Cutaneous findings seen in 50% with two variants: papulosquamous (most common) and annular (See Chapter 15)
- Location most common on the face and scalp with characteristic patterns:
  1. 'Raccoon eyes' or 'owl-like' periocular involvement
  2. 'Headband' distribution with lesions on the forehead and bilateral temporal areas (Figure 2.9)
- Skin lesions rarely present at birth and usually develop in the first few weeks of life after light exposure
- New lesions can continue to appear for up to 6 months and then fade with waning of the maternal autoantibodies
- Congenital heart abnormalities (most common is congenital heart block) occur in up to 30% of affected infants and have up to 20% mortality rate; appropriate work-up mandatory if diagnosis suspected

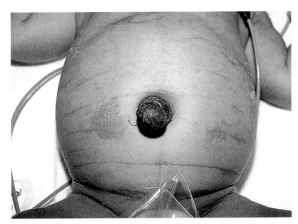

Figure 2.8 Umbilical granuloma – vascular nodule on the umbilicus

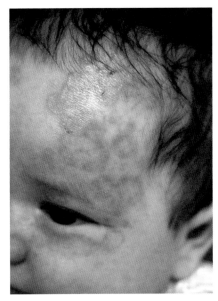

Figure 2.9 Neonatal lupus erythematosus – typical annular lesions on the face

- Other findings: thrombocytopenia, cholestatic liver enzyme elevation, anticardiolipin antibodies, thrombosis, hypocalcemia, pneumonia
- Transient brain computerized tomography (CT) abnormalities, spastic paraparesis, myasthenia gravis, and neurologic symptoms caused by vasculopathy of the central nervous system (CNS)

Pathogenesis

- 95% of mothers have anti-Ro (SS-A) autoantibodies and 60–80% have anti-La (SS-B)

autoantibodies, and occasionally anti-RNP autoantibodies
  1. The majority of mothers are asymptomatic
  2. Mothers are affected by mild systemic lupus erythematosus or Sjögren syndrome
- IgG autoantibodies are transplacentally passed to the fetus and bind to autoantigens, causing cellular cytotoxicity and inflammation
- Skin lesions resolve with waning maternal autoantibodies
- Cardiac inflammation causes permanent scarring in conduction system of the heart

Diagnosis

- Clinical findings confirmed by blood tests
- Serologic studies: anti-Ro (SS-A), anti-La (SS-B), anti-RNP, anti-DNA, anticardiolipin antibodies, antinuclear antibodies and rheumatoid factor may be positive
- Histology: epidermal atrophy, basal vacuolar changes, dermal edema and superficial mucin with minimal lymphocytic inflammation
- Direct immunofluorescence: linear IgG, IgM and C3 along the basement membrane zone in up to 60% of cases

Differential diagnosis

- Erythema multiforme
- Tinea corporis
- Urticaria
- Bullous pemphigoid
- Annular erythema of infancy
- Erythema annulare centrifugum

Treatment

- Broad-spectrum sunblock daily
- Topical steroids: low- or high-potency depending on severity
- Oral corticosteroids (rarely needed)
- Pulsed dye laser for residual telangiectasias after antibodies undetectable
- Congenital heart block: cardiology consultation intravenous immunoglobulins (IVIG), pacemaker as indicated

Prognosis

- Skin lesions resolve in 1–2 years with occasional residual dyspigmentation, telangiectasias and mild scarring

- Transient liver and brain CT abnormalities
- Congenital heart block: 50% require a pacemaker; 15% mortality
- Recurrent pancytopenia has been reported in the neonatal period, and may be related to ribonuclear protein and Smith autoantibodies
- Small increased risk of associated disorders later: juvenile rheumatoid arthritis, Hashimoto thyroiditis, congenital hypothyroidism, diabetes mellitus, psoriasis, nephritic syndrome and iritis

References

Arkachaisri T, Lehman TJ. Systemic lupus erythematosus and related disorders of childhood. Curr Opin Rheumatol 1999; 11: 384–92

Brucato A, Cimaz R, Stramba-Badiale M. Neonatal lupus. Clin Rev Allergy Immunol 2002; 23: 279–99

Buyon JP, Clancy RM. Neonatal lupus: review of proposed pathogenesis and clinical data from the US-based Research Registry for Neonatal Lupus. Autoimmunity 2003; 36: 41–50

Buyon JP, Clancy RM. Neonatal lupus syndromes. Curr Opin Rheumatol 2003; 15: 535–41

Cimaz R, Spence DL, Homberger L, Siverman FD. Incidence and spectrum of neonatal lupus erythematosus: a prospective study of infants born to mothers with anti-Ro autoantibodies. J Pediatr 2003; 142: 678–83

High WA, Costner MI. Persistent scarring, atrophy, and dyspigmentation in a preteen girl with neonatal lupus erythematosus. J Am Acad Dermatol 2003; 48: 626–8

Prendiville JS, Cabral DA, Poskitt KJ, Au S, Sargent MA. Central nervous system involvement in neonatal lupus erythematosus. Pediatr Dermatol 2003; 20: 60–7

Sandborg CI. Childhood systemic lupus erythematosus and neonatal lupus syndrome. Curr Opin Rheum 1998; 10: 481–7

Silverman ED, Laxer RM. Neonatal lupus erythematosus. Rheum Dis Clin 1997; 23: 599–618

Subcutaneous fat necrosis

Major points

- Presents with asymptomatic subcutaneous nodules or erythematous plaques in otherwise healthy full-term and post-term infants at 1–6 weeks of life (Figure 2.10)
- Often follows a difficult delivery with perinatal complications such as hypothermia and asphyxia
- Location: typically involves the cheeks, shoulders, buttocks, thighs and legs
- Can develop calcification, fluctuance or ulceration

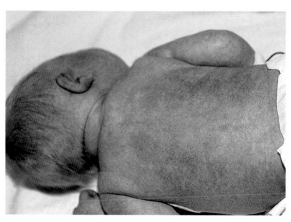

Figure 2.10 Subcutaneous fat necrosis – erythematous firm patches on the back

- Can develop hypercalcemia with symptoms of irritability, vomiting, failure to thrive and seizures as well as nephrocalcinosis up to 5 months after initial presentation

Pathogenesis

- Unknown with several hypotheses
  1. Localized hypoxic injury to fat secondary to trauma
  2. Increased saturated fatty acid : unsaturated fatty acid ratio in newborn that predisposes to crystallization with hypothermia
  3. Hypothermia

Diagnosis

- Clinical findings
- Histology: lobular panniculitis with patchy areas of fat necrosis and fat cyst formation, polymorphous inflammation and typical needle-shaped clefts

Differential diagnosis

- Traumatic panniculitis
- Post-steroid panniculitis
- Sclerema neonatorum

Treatment

- Treatment usually unnecessary
- Aspiration of fluctuant lesions

- Hypercalcemia requires appropriate treatment and may include hydration, furosemide, intravenous corticosteroids and etidronate

Prognosis

- Most infants have resolution of lesions within 1–2 months
- Subcutaneous atrophy can occur
- Monitor for hypercalcemia for 6 months after initial presentation of skin lesions (can be fatal), especially if lesions are extensive

References

Bachrach LK, Lum CK. Etidronate in subcutaneous fat necrosis of the newborn. J Pediatr 1999; 135: 530

Burden AD, Krafchik BR. Subcutaneous fat necrosis of the newborn: a review of 11 cases. Pediatr Dermatol 1999; 16: 384–7

Cook JS, Stone MS, Hansen JR. Hypercalcemia in association with subcutaneous fat necrosis of the newborn: studies of calcium-regulating hormones. Pediatrics 1992; 90: 3

Hicks MJ, Levy ML, Alexander J, Flaitz CM. Subcutaneous fat necrosis of the newborn and hypercalcemia: a case report and review of the literature. Pediatr Dermatol 1993; 10: 271–6

Mather MK, Sperling LC, Sau P. Subcutaneous fat necrosis of the newborn. Int J Dermatol 1997; 36: 435–52

Sclerema neonatorum

Major points

- Characteristic widespread thickening and induration of the skin in critically ill newborns (e.g. sepsis, hypoglycemia and metabolic acidosis)
- May occur up to 4 months of age
- Presents with sudden onset of rapid hardening of the skin that starts distally and progresses to involve the skin diffusely but with sparing of the palms, soles and genitalia
- No pitting of the skin is noted with pressure
- Skin becomes bound-down with mask-like facies and immobile joints

Pathogenesis

- Etiology unknown; hypothesis of cold injury and secondary solidification of the tissue due to enzymatic dysfunction

Diagnosis

- Clinical findings in typical setting
- Histology: identical to subcutaneous fat necrosis

Differential diagnosis

- Subcutaneous fat necrosis of newborn
- Restrictive dermopathy
- Systemic sclerosis
- Stiff skin syndrome

Treatment

- Supportive measures to reverse the underlying disorder: temperature control, hydration, electrolyte balance and aggressive antibiotic therapy
- Systemic corticosteroid use is controversial
- Exchange transfusions

Prognosis

- High infant mortality related to the underlying condition
- Skin changes can resolve with treatment of the underlying disorder
- Worse prognosis with thrombocytopenia, neutropenia, and progressive acidosis

References

Battin M, Harding J, Gunn A. Sclerema neonatorum following hypothermia. J Paediatr Child Health. 2002; 38: 533–4

Burden AD, Krafchik BR. Subcutaneous fat necrosis of the newborn: a review of 11 cases. Pediatr Dermatol 1999; 16: 384–7

Requena L, Sanchez Yus E, Panniculitis. Part II. Mostly lobular panniculitis. J Am Acad Dermatol 2001; 45: 325–61, quiz 362–4

Aplasia cutis congenita

Major points

- Occurs in approximately 1 : 5000 births
- Characterized by the absence of skin (i.e. epidermis, dermis and/or subcutaneous tissues) in localized or widespread areas at birth
- Location: most common on the scalp (Figure 2.11)
- May be an isolated finding, associated with underlying defects or seen with other isolated anomalies, syndromes and chromosomal disorders
- Lesion types:
  1. Membranous

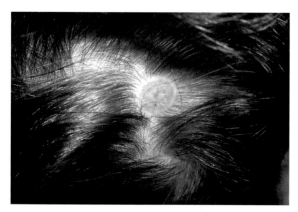

Figure 2.11 Aplasia cutis congenita – typical location on the vertex of the scalp

   a. Most common presentation
   b. Typically well-circumscribed, atrophic, 1–5 cm defects
   c. Can be solitary (75%) or multiple (25%) in a linear distribution
   d. Can be bullous, eroded, ulcerated or scar-like
   e. May have an associated 'hair collar sign,' suggestive of associated cranial dysraphism
   f. Location: vertex of the scalp or face
2. Stellate
   a. Midline scalp with associated underlying bony defects and vascular malformations
   b. Can also be seen as large defects on the face or trunk with associated disorders and multiple extracutaneous findings
- Proposed classification system:
1. Group 1: aplasia cutis congenita (ACC) of scalp without multiple anomalies
2. Group 2: ACC of scalp with associated limb anomalies (shortening, club feet) called Adams–Oliver syndrome
3. Group 3: ACC of scalp with associated epidermal and sebaceous nevi
4. Group 4: ACC overlying embryologic malformations
5. Group 5: ACC associated with fetus papyraceus or placental infarcts
6. Group 6: ACC associated with epidermolysis bullosa (Figure 2.12)
7. Group 7: ACC of the extremities without epidermolysis bullosa
8. Group 8: ACC due to teratogens
9. Group 9: ACC associated with syndromes or malformations

Pathogenesis

- Unknown
- Proposed etiologies include: developmental, genetic, vascular insufficiency, trauma, teratogens, infection
- Most cases are sporadic; some show autosomal dominant or autosomal recessive inheritance patterns

Diagnosis

- Clinical findings
- Histology: thinned or absent epidermis; thinned dermis with loose connective tissue and collagen disarray; thinned subcutis; small or absent appendages

Differential diagnosis

- Trauma
- Neonatal herpes simplex infection
- Encephalocele
- Dermoid cyst
- Goltz syndrome (focal dermal hypoplasia)
- Incontinentia pigmenti
- Amniotic band syndrome

Treatment

- Daily cleansing and topical antibiotic application if ulcerated
- Surgical excision, grafting, hair transplantation if indicated
- Genetic counseling recommended

Prognosis

- Excellent if isolated lesion
- Most small skin lesions heal completely without treatment, as do small underlying bony defects; asymptomatic scars persist for life
- Risk of infection high with exposed dura
- Hemorrhage and death can occur from associated intracranial anomalies (rare)
- Associated syndromes and defects with variable prognosis

References

Benjamin LT, Trowers AB, Schachner LA. Giant aplasia cutis congenita without associated anomalies. Pediatr Dermatol 2004; 21: 150–3

Casanova D, Amar E, Bardot J, Magalon G. Aplasia cutis congenita. Report on 5 family cases involving the scalp. Eur J Pediatr Surg 2001; 11: 280–4

Colon-Fontanez F, Fallon Friedlander S, Newbury R, Eichenfield LF. Bullous aplasia cutis congenita. J Am Acad Dermatol 2003; 48: S95–8

Drolet B, Prendiville J, Golden J, et al. 'Membranous aplasia cutis' with hair collars. Congenital abscence of skin or neuroectodermal defect? Arch Dermatol 1995; 131: 1427–31

Frieden IJ. Aplasia cutis congenita: a clinical review and proposal for classification. J Am Acad Dermatol 1986; 14: 646

Koshy CE, Waterhouse N, Peterson D. Large scalp and skull defect in aplasia cutis congenita. Br J Plast Surg 2000; 53: 619–22

Maman E, Maor E, Kachko L, Carmi R. Epidermolysis bullosa, pyloric atresia, aplasia cutis congenita: histopathological delineation of an autosomal recessive disease. Am J Med Genet 1998; 78: 127–33

Mempel M, Abeck D, Lange I, Strom K, et al. The wide spectrum of clinical expression in Adams–Oliver syndrome: a report of two cases. Br J Dermatol 1999; 140: 1157–60

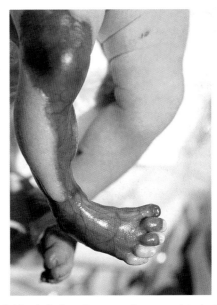

Figure 2.12 Aplasia cutis congenita – associated with dystrophic epidermolysis bullosa on the leg

Nevus sebaceus of Jadassohn

Major points

- Characteristic yellowish hairless plaque on the scalp (Figure 2.13)
- More prominent in the newborn period because of maternal hormone influence, becoming less obvious during childhood, but then more apparent and papillomatous with pubertal hormonal influences
- Location: head and neck
- Usually isolated but can be associated with other syndromes and anomalies
- Occurs in 0.3% of newborns

Pathogenesis

- Localized developmental anomaly of appendageal structures

Diagnosis

- Clinical findings
- Histology: mild acanthosis and papillomatosis with immature and malformed pilosebaceous units

Differential diagnosis

- Epidermal nevus
- Aplasia cutis congenita
- Encephalocele
- Juvenile xanthogranuloma
- Verruca vulgaris

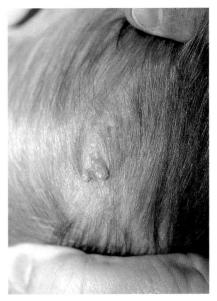

Figure 2.13 Nevus sebaceous of Jadassohn – yellow papules in a hairless patch

Treatment

- Observe for clinical change, since there is a low risk of malignant tumors
- Elective surgical excision, usually recommended around puberty when lesions become more apparent and annoying

Prognosis

- Lesions persist throughout life
- Potential for secondary tumors within these lesions: syringocystadenoma papilliferum, basal cell carcinoma. Variably reported risk, up to 30%, of benign and malignant neoplastic growths, but probably very low risk for malignant growths

References

Beer GM, Widder W, Cierpka K, et al. Malignant tumors associated with nevus sebaceous: therapeutic consequences. Aesthetic Plast Surg 1999; 23: 224–7

Chun K, Vazquez M, Sanchez JL. Nevus sebaceus: clinical outcome and considerations for prophylactic excision. Int J Dermatol 1995; 34: 538–41

Cribier B, Scrivener Y, Grosshans E. Tumors arising in nevus sebaceus: a study of 596 cases. J Am Acad Dermatol 2000; 42: 263–8

Dunkin CS, Abouzeid M, Sarangapani K. Malignant transformation in congenital sebaceous naevi in childhood. J R Coll Surg Edinb 2001; 46: 303–6

Santibanez-Gallerani A, Marshall D, Duarte AM, et al. Should nevus sebaceus of Jadassohn in children be excised? A study of 757 cases, and literature review. J Craniofac Surg 2003; 14: 658–60

Neonatal scars

Major points

- The number of neonatal scars is related to gestational age and length of time spent in an intensive care unit
- Scarring can occur with amniocentesis, chorionic villus sampling, fetal monitoring, arterial or venous punctures, catheter insertions, heel sticks, chest tubes, adhesives and extravasated intravenous fluids (Figure 2.14)
- Amniocentesis scars occur in <1% of neonates whose mothers underwent amniocentesis; risk decreases during second trimester; scars are usually not apparent for weeks to months after birth
- If less than 29 weeks' gestational age at birth, anetoderma can develop at sites of monitors and adhesives; presents as atrophic scars on the anterior trunk and proximal extremities

Pathogenesis

- Caused by multiple procedures performed *in utero* or in the neonatal intensive care unit

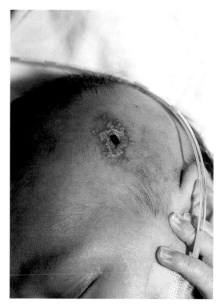

Figure 2.14   Neonatal scar caused by intravenous fluid extravasation

Diagnosis

- Consistent clinical history
- Clinical findings

Differential diagnosis

- Congenital dimples
- Congenital sinus tracts
- Aplasia cutis congenita
- Focal dermal hypoplasia (Goltz syndrome)

Treatment

- None effective
- Red lesions (vascular component) can be treated with vascular laser with variable results

Prognosis

- Most commonly small and inconspicuous, but can be large with underlying fibrosis
- Can develop secondary calcified papules and hypertrophic scars
- Puncture sites can rarely become secondarily infected with abscess or gangrene

References

Cambiaghi S, Restano L, Cavalli R, Gellmetti C. Skin dimpling as a consequence of amniocentesis. J Am Acad Dermatol 1998; 39: 888–90

Cartlidge PHT, Fox PE, Rutter N. The scars of newborn intensive care. Early Hum Dev 1990; 21: 1–10

Prizant TL, Lucky AW, Frieden IJ, et al. Spontaneous atrophic patches in extremely premature infants. Arch Dermatol 1996; 132: 671–4

Todd DJ. Anetoderma of prematurity. Arch Dermatol 1997; 133: 789

Dermal erythropoiesis

Synonyms: extramedullary hematopoiesis, blueberry muffin baby

Major points

- Hematopoiesis occurs in the skin during embryonic development
- Persistence of this process in the neonate can be seen in healthy newborns but typically results from intrauterine infection or hematologic dyscrasias
- Characteristically produces a generalized eruption with purpuric infiltrative papules primarily on the head, neck and trunk (Figure 2.15)

Pathogenesis

- Causes: intrauterine infections such as rubella, cytomegalovirus (CMV), coxsackievirus, parvovirus, toxoplasmosis, varicella virus, HIV
- Hematologic dyscrasias: hemolytic disease of the newborn (Rh incompatibility or ABO incompatibility), spherocytosis, twin to twin transfusion

Diagnosis

- Clinical findings
- Histology: superficial and deep dermal perivascular infiltration with myeloid and erythroid cells
- Work-up for underlying cause: complete blood count, TORCH serologies, viral cultures and Coombs test

Differential diagnosis

- Diffuse neonatal hemangiomatosis
- Congenital leukemia
- Metastatic infiltration: neuroblastoma, rhabdomyosarcoma, Langerhans cell histiocytosis
- Coagulation/platelet defects

Treatment

- None needed for skin involvement

Prognosis

- Skin lesions resolve spontaneously over several weeks
- Overall prognosis dependent on the underlying cause

References

Baselga E, Drolet BA, Esterly NB. Purpura in infants and children. J Am Acad Dermatol 1997; 37: 673–705

Epps RE, Pittelkow MR, Su WP. TORCH syndrome. Semin Dermatol 1995; 14: 179–86

Evole-Buselli M, Hernandez-Marti MJ, Gasco-Lacalle B, et al. Neonatal dermal hematopoiesis associated with diffuse neonatal hemangiomatosis. Pediatr Dermatol 1997; 14: 383–6

NEONATAL INFECTIONS

Herpes neonatorum

Major points

- Presentation is variable and depends on route and time of exposure, virulence and maternal immunity (Chapter 8)
- Primary congenital (intrauterine) infection:
  1. 5% of herpes simplex virus (HSV) infections in the newborn period
  2. Acquired *in utero*
  3. Exposure via ascending infection or viremia
  4. Can lead to intrauterine fetal death

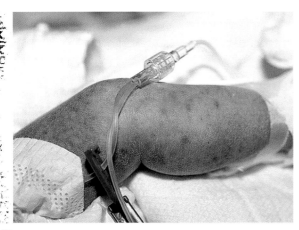

Figure 2.15   Dermal erythropoiesis caused by neonatal infection

5. Newborn will have specific cell-mediated immunity (i.e. lymphocyte transformation) to HSV at birth, as opposed to infants who are infected at the time of labor and delivery
6. 70% have vesicles and 30% have scars at birth
7. CNS involvement: >50% have microcephaly, 60% have chorioretinitis
- Primary neonatal infection:
  1. 95% of HSV infections in newborn period
  2. HSV is acquired perinatally (85%) or postnatally (10%)
  3. Risk of perinatal infection is 50% with primary maternal infection but only 5% with recurrent maternal infection
  4. Postnatal exposure can be from maternal infection (e.g. genital or extragenital), other family members or health-care workers
  5. Incubation period highly variable: 30% have symptoms at birth; the rest appear in the first 6 weeks of life
  6. Characteristic patterns:
     a. Skin, mouth and eye lesions – vesicles, erosions or ulcers typically on scalp or presenting part; oral vesicles, erosions or ulcers; conjunctivitis or keratitis; CNS involvement symptoms are often delayed or absent (Figures 2.16 and 2.17)

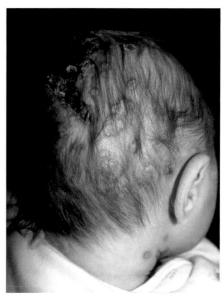

Figure 2.17 Herpes neonatorum with a positive culture for herpes simplex virus-1

     b. CNS disease – cutaneous lesions present in 60%; focal encephalitis or meningoencephalitis with irritability, lethargy, fever or seizures
     c. Disseminated disease – cutaneous lesions in 77%; affects liver, adrenals, lung and brain with symptoms suggestive of neonatal sepsis

Pathogenesis

- Caused by HSV type 1 or 2; most often transmitted from an infected mother
- Intrauterine, perinatal (during delivery) or postnatal (after delivery) transmission; or by postnatal contact with those with viral shedding or active lesions
- Recurrent maternal infection confers some degree of passive immunity to the neonate

Diagnosis

- Viral cultures from skin and oral mucosal lesions, nasopharynx, conjunctivae, urine, plasma and cerebrospinal fluid (CSF)
- Tzanck smear of vesicles: multinucleated epithelial giant cells
- Direct fluorescent antibody for HSV-1 or -2
- Serology for HSV antibodies: rising IgG titers are sensitive and specific for infection, whereas IgM titers are not sensitive in the newborn

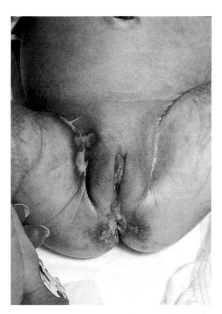

Figure 2.16 Herpes neonatorum in a 28-day-old neonate

- Polymerase chain reaction for HSV is highly sensitive
- CSF: lymphocytic pleocytosis, elevated protein and red blood cell count indicative of CNS involvement
- Imaging: CT or magnetic resonance imaging (MRI) of the brain if indicated
- Histology: intraepidermal vesicles, ballooning and reticular degeneration with secondary acantholysis and eosinophilic intranuclear inclusion bodies

Differential diagnosis

- Congenital infections: varicella, syphilis, enterovirus, parainfluenza, adenovirus, toxoplasmosis, CMV, bacterial sepsis
- Bullous impetigo
- Erythema toxicum neonatorum
- Transient neonatal pustular melanosis
- Sucking blister
- Incontinentia pigmenti
- Langerhans cell histiocytosis

Treatment

- Systemic antiviral therapy:
  1. Acyclovir 30 mg/kg per day intravenously every 8 h for cutaneous-only disease; adjust for renal disease
  2. Acyclovir 60 mg/kg per day intravenously every 8 h for congenital disease, CNS or disseminated disease; adjust for renal disease
  3. Vidarabine 30 mg/kg per day intravenously every 12 h or foscarnet 40 mg/kg per day intravenously every 12 h
- Prevent secondary bacterial infection of the eroded lesions with topical mupirocin or antibiotic ointments

Prognosis

- Intrauterine infection can result in fetal demise; nearly 100% of congenital HSV survivors have significant neurologic delay
- Cutaneous-only disease has nearly 100% survival; 40% will have ocular sequelae
- CNS infection is more severe with HSV-2 infection; 50% mortality rate if untreated, 15% mortality rate if treated; approximately 75% have permanent neurologic disease and 20% have persistent ocular disease

- Neonatal disseminated infection: 75% mortality rate if untreated and 50% mortality rate if treated; 40% will have CNS sequelae

References

Enright AM. Prober CG. Neonatal herpes infection: diagnosis, treatment and prevention. Semin Neonatol, 2002; 7: 283–91

Jacobs RF. Neonatal herpes simplex virus infections. Semin Perinatol 1998; 22: 64–71

Kimberlin DW. Neonatal herpes simplex infection. Clin Microbiol Rev 2004; 17: 1–13

Kohl S. The diagnosis and treatment of neonatal herpes simplex virus infection. Pediatr Ann 2002; 31: 726–32

Trizna Z, Tyring SK. Antiviral treatment of diseases in pediatric dermatology. Dermatol Clin 1998; 16: 539–52

Congenital varicella and infantile herpes zoster

Major points

- Most infants exposed to varicella *in utero* (i.e. mother had varicella during pregnancy) are normal with no sequelae (Chapter 8)
- Disease manifestations depend on the time of exposure and maternal immune response
- Congenital varicella syndrome (fetal varicella syndrome or varicella embryopathy):
  1. Fetal exposure before 20 weeks of gestation with greatest risk from 13 to 20 weeks
  2. 9% reported risk of developing disease with exposure
  3. Presents with dermatomal lesions: denuded or scarred with associated underlying tissue hypoplasia
  4. Additional findings: low birth weight, neurologic (e.g. hydrocephalus, retardation, seizures), ophthalmologic (e.g. chorioretinitis, cataracts, nystagmus), musculoskeletal (e.g. extremity hypoplasia and paresis), gastrointestinal and genitourinary anomalies
- Neonatal varicella:
  1. Due to fetal exposure near the time of delivery with maternal infection between 5 days prior to and 2 days following delivery
  2. 23–62% risk of developing disease with exposure
  3. Cutaneous findings from 1 to 16 days postpartum: papulovesicular lesions which can become hemorrhagic or necrotic

4. High risk for disseminated disease: pneumonitis, hepatitis, encephalitis
- Infantile herpes zoster:
  1. Develops during first year of life after *in utero* varicella exposure
  2. 2% of infants exposed to intrauterine varicella will develop infantile herpes zoster
  3. Clinical findings: papulovesicles in dermatomal pattern, typically thoracic area

Pathogenesis

- Maternal varicella infection with viremia leads to fetal exposure to the varicella zoster virus (VZV)
- Infantile herpes zoster is caused by reactivation of dormant virus in the sensory dorsal root ganglia

Diagnosis

- Consistent maternal history
- Clinical findings
- Congenital:
  1. Viral culture of amniotic fluid or fetal blood for VZV
  2. Prenatal serology and cultures are neither sensitive nor specific for diagnosing fetal infection
- Neonatal:
  1. Tzanck smear of vesicle shows multinucleated epithelial giant cells
  2. Direct fluorescent antibody for VZV
  3. Viral culture

Differential diagnosis

- Aplasia cutis congenita
- Epidermolysis bullosa
- Neonatal infections: HSV, candidiasis, *Staphylococcus aureus*
- Erythema toxicum neonatorum
- Transient neonatal pustular melanosis

Treatment

- Intrauterine exposure
  1. Varicella zoster immunoglobulin (VZIG) given within 5 days to nonimmune mothers with recent VZV exposure
  2. Acyclovir is considered safe for pregnant women who are infected and may minimize the risk of disease in the newborn
- Congenital varicella
  1. Supportive

2. Ultrasound anomalies include fetal hydrops, polyhydramnios, microcephaly and limb hypoplasia
- Neonatal varicella
  1. VZIG
  2. Acyclovir
  3. Isolation
- Infantile herpes zoster
  1. No specific therapy needed if immunocompetent
  2. Consider systemic acyclovir, especially if there are hemorrhagic or disseminated lesions

Prognosis

- Most exposures during pregnancy result in no fetal sequelae
- Intrauterine infection may lead to fetal demise
- Neonatal varicella – 10–30% mortality

References

Enders G, Miller E, Cradock-Watson J, et al. Consequences of varicella and herpes zoster in pregnancy: prospective study of 1739 cases. Lancet 1994; 343: 1548–51

Harger JH, Ernest JM, Thurnau GR, et al. Frequency of congenital varicella syndrome in a prospective cohort of 347 pregnant women. Obstet Gynecol 2002; 100: 260–5

Nathwani D, Maclean A, Conway S, Carrington D. Varicella infections in pregnancy and the newborn. A review prepared for the UK Advisory Group on Chickenpox on behalf of the British Society for the Study of Infection. J Infect 1998; 36 (Suppl 1): 59–71

Sauerbrei A, Wutzler P. Neonatal varicella. J Perinatol 2001; 21: 545–9

Sauerbrei A, Wutzler P. The congenital varicella syndrome. J Perinatol 2000; 20: 548–54

Tseng HW, Liu CC, Wang SM, et al. Complications of varicella in children: emphasis on skin and central nervous system disorders. J Microbiol Immunol Infect 2000; 33: 248–52

Candidiasis

Major points

- Congenital candidiasis
  1. Caused by ascending vaginal infection of *Candida albicans* with *in utero* exposure or direct inoculation during labor and delivery
  2. Cervical sutures and retained intrauterine devices are risk factors for infection

3. Lesions typically appear on the first day of life, presenting with generalized erythematous papulovesicular eruption leading to desquamation (Figures 2.18 and 2.19)
4. Often involves palms, soles and oral mucosa (thrush)
5. Can have respiratory and gastrointestinal involvement from aspiration of infected amniotic fluid
6. Rare development of systemic disease

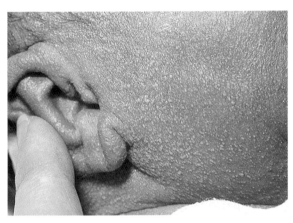

Figure 2.18 Congenital candidiasis – close-up of pustules, associated with candida septicemia

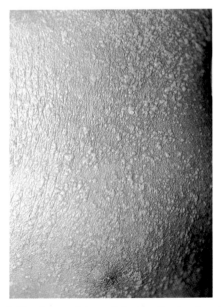

Figure 2.19 Congenital candidiasis – sheets of pustules in a 3-day-old with only cutaneous involvement

- Neonatal candidiasis
  1. Caused by postnatal colonization of *Candida albicans*
  2. More common in low-birth-weight infants (<1500 g)
  3. Develop classic mucocutaneous eruption with satellite lesions and diaper area involvement
  4. Dissemination to the lungs, meninges and urinary tract with sepsis more common in low-birth-weight infants

Pathogenesis

- Caused by vertical transmission with intrauterine chorioamnionitis or direct inoculation of *Candidia albicans*, typically from the mother

Diagnosis

- Potassium hydroxide preparation from skin scrapings reveals budding yeasts and pseudo-hyphae (Chapter 9)

Differential diagnosis

- Neonatal herpes infection
- Erythema toxicum neonatorum
- Transient neonatal pustular melanosis
- Miliaria
- Staphylococcal scalded skin syndrome

Treatment

- Topical: nystatin cream or imidazole cream BID for cutaneous disease is typically sufficient
- Fluconazole 3–6 mg/kg per day PO for severe skin involvement
- Disseminated disease:
  1. Amphotericin B 0.5–1.0 mg/kg per day IV or
  2. Fluconazole 5 mg/kg per day IV or
  3. 5-fluorocytosine 50–150 mg/kg per day PO
- Intravenous fluconazole for preterm, low-birth-weight infants at risk for systemic candidiasis

Prognosis

- Excellent for only cutaneous disease with rapid resolution over 1 week with topical therapy alone
- Disseminated disease carries a worse prognosis with increased risk of renal and CNS involvement, as well as sepsis and death

References

Darmstadt GL, Dinulos JG, Miller Z. Congenital cutaneous candidiasis: clinical presentation, pathogenesis, and management guidelines. Pediatrics 2000; 105: 438–44

Kaufman D. Strategies for prevention of neonatal invasive candidiasis. Semin Perinatol 2003; 27: 414–24

Pradeepkumar VK, Rajadurai VS, Tan KW. Congenital candidiasis: varied presentations. J Perinatol 1998; 18: 311–16

Congenital syphilis

Major points

- 50–60% of infants are asymptomatic at birth
- 2–6 weeks after birth is the most common age of onset for those infants infected in the third trimester
- Early congenital syphilis is clinically similar to presentation of exaggerated secondary syphilis in an adult (Chapter 7)
- Early disease
  1. Usually apparent by 3 months of age but can be up to 2 years
  2. Presenting signs:
     a. Syphilitic rhinitis (snuffles)
     b. 'Barber' pole umbilical cord (red and blue with white streaks)
     c. Cutaneous lesions: condyloma lata, mucous patches, petechiae, hemorrhagic vesicles/bullae on palms and soles (Figure 2.20), or diffuse papulosquamous eruption involving the palms/soles and resembling that of secondary syphilis (Figure 7.29)
     d. Other systemic findings: meningioencephalitis, chorioretinitis, hepatosplenomegaly, lymphadenopathy (especially epitrochlear), low birth weight, prematurity, anemia, thrombocytopenia, respiratory distress and osteochondritis
- Late disease (very rare)
  1. Develops >2 years of age
  2. Cutaneous findings: rhagades, gummata
  3. Extracutaneous findings:
     a. Neurosyphilis
     b. Interstitial keratitis
     c. Sensorineural hearing loss
     d. Bony changes (saddle nose, frontal bossing, saber shins, syphilitic arthritis, Clutton joints (effusions of the knees),

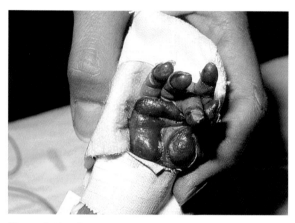

Figure 2.20 Congenital syphilis – acquired early in pregnancy; with hepatosplenomegaly, respiratory distress and erosions of palms and soles (previously published in Pediatric Dermatology 1989; 6: 51–2)

  Higoumenaki sign (thickening of the inner third of the clavicle)
     e. Oral deformities: mulberry molars and Hutchinson pegged central incisors
     f. Paroxysmal cold hemoglobinuria
  4. Hutchinson triad includes: interstitial keratitis, Hutchinson incisors, cranial nerve VIII deafness

Pathogenesis

- Infection with spirochete *Treponema pallidum* during gestation
- Invades via placenta to infect multiple fetal organs
- Adheres to endothelial cells and causes vasculitis

Diagnosis

- Consistent maternal history
- Clinical findings
- Spirochete identification from placenta, umbilical cord or a mucocutaneous lesion: dark field microscopy or direct fluorescent antibody
- Maternal and infant serology: infant nontreponemal titer >4 times maternal titer indicates true neonatal infection; treponemal serologies are more specific, especially IgM FTA-ABS or VDRL on CSF
- Long-bone radiologic evaluation for osteochondritis
- Histology: swelling of vascular endothelium and lymphoplasmocytic perivascular inflammation

Differential diagnosis

- Congenital candidiasis
- Scabies
- Psoriasis
- Epidermolysis bullosa

Treatment

- Establish status of CNS involvement by examining CSF
- Aqueous crystalline penicillin G 50 000 units/kg per dose intravenously every 12 h for first 7 days of life, then every 8 h thereafter to complete a 10-day course; infants and children are dosed at 200 000–300 000 units/kg per day divided every 4–6 h for 10 days

Prognosis

- 25–40% intrauterine fetal death
- High risk for preterm birth and neurologic sequelae
- Skin lesions typically resolve with postinflammatory hypo- and hyperpigmentation

References

Evans HE, Frenkel LD. Congenital syphilis. Clin Perinatol 1994; 21: 149–62

Hollier LM, Cox SM. Syphilis. Semin Perinatol 1998; 22: 323–31

Parish JL. Treponemal infections in the pediatric population. Clin Dermatol 2000; 18: 687–700

van Voorst Vader PC. Syphilis management and treatment. Dermatol Clin 1998; 16: 699–711

Wicher V, Wicher K. Pathogenesis of maternal–fetal syphilis revisited. Clin Infect Dis 2001; 33: 354–63

NEONATAL DEFECTS

Nasal glioma

Major points

- Typically presents at birth
- Firm bluish or red swelling on the nasal root with overlying telangiectasias (Figure 2.21)
- Composed of ectopic neural tissue
- Regarded as a variant of encephalocele; intracranial connection not always present
- Does not increase in size with crying or Valsalva maneuver

- Majority are external; 30% can be intranasal or with oropharyngeal extension

Pathogenesis

- Evagination of neuroectodermal tissue via a developmental abnormality of the nasofrontal fontanelle
- Failure of complete retraction during formation of dura leads to isolation of this tissue upon suture closure; a stalk may connect to the underlying brain through the foramen caecum

Diagnosis

- Imaging: CT or MRI recommended prior to biopsy
- Histology: collections of astrocytes embedded in dense connective tissue trabeculae with occasional striated muscle

Differential diagnosis

- Encephalocele
- Hemangioma
- Nasal dermoid cyst
- Lacrimal duct cyst
- Neuroblastoma
- Rhabdomyosarcoma

Treatment

- Evaluate with MRI
- Treatment is surgical by experienced pediatric surgeons in collaboration with neurosurgeons as needed

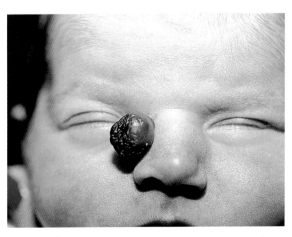

Figure 2.21 Nasal glioma resembling a hemangioma but with a connection through the cranium in a newborn

Prognosis

- Excellent with appropriate resection
- Recurrences occasional

References

El Shabrawi-Caelen L, White WL, Soyer HP, et al. Rudimentary meningocele: remnant of a neural tube defect? Arch Dermatol 2001; 137: 45–50

Paller AS, Pensler JM, Tomita T. Nasal midline masses in infants and children. Arch Dermatol 1991; 127: 362–6

Rahbar R, Resto VA, Robson CD, et al. Nasal glioma and encephalocele: diagnosis and management. Laryngoscope 2003; 113: 2069–77

Encephalocele

Major points

- Cystic structure on the midline face
- Presents in the neonatal period with nasal broadening (67%) or as a soft, blue pulsatile mass that transilluminates on the nasal bridge
- Increases in size with crying, Valsalva maneuver, or external compression of the jugular veins
- Associated with facial clefting and other midline defects

Pathogenesis

- Herniation of brain tissue through the skull with connection to the underlying brain

Diagnosis

- Image with MRI
- Biopsy of the skin lesion not recommended, owing to the connection with the subarachnoid space which could lead to CSF rhinorrhea and infection
- Histology: similar to nasal glioma

Differential diagnosis

- Hemangioma
- Nasal glioma
- Dermoid cyst
- Hypertelorism

Treatment

- Evaluation with MRI or CT scan is essential
- Surgical excision is recommended by a skilled pediatric neurosurgeon and otolaryngologist

Prognosis

- Lesions persist if not surgically corrected and may become infected

References

Brown MS, Sheridan-Pereira M. Outlook for the child with a cephalocele. Pediatrics 1992; 90: 914–19

Davis DA, Cohen PR, George RE. Cutaneous stigmata of occult spinal dysraphism. J Am Acad Dermatol 1994; 31: 892–6

El Shabrawi-Caelen L, White WL, Soyer HP, et al. Rudimentary meningocele: remnant of a neural tube defect? Arch Dermatol 2001; 137: 45–50

Hoving EW. Nasal encephaloceles. Childs Nerv Syst 2000; 16: 702–6

Hunt JA, Hobar PC. Common craniofacial anomalies: facial clefts and encephaloceles. Plast Reconstruct Surg 2003; 112: 606–15

Paller AS, Pensler JM, Tomita T. Nasal midline masses in infants and children. Arch Dermatol 1991; 127: 362–6

Congenital dermal sinus

Major points

- Cutaneous sign of potential spinal dysraphism
- Midline epithelium-lined tract most common in occipital or lumbar area
- Typically associated with a dermoid or epidermal cyst
- Presents as a dimple with an opening visible on the skin
- Tuft of hair may arise from the sinus tract
- A cord may be extend from the dimple to the bony defect

Pathogenesis

- Occurs as a result of a developmental abnormality in the separation of the neuroectoderm and the cutaneous ectoderm

Diagnosis

- Characteristic skin findings
- Imaging studies: MRI

Differential diagnosis

- Pilonidal sinus

Treatment

- Excision of area only after appropriate imaging

Prognosis

- 30% of patients are asymptomatic
- Complications: repeated meningitis or space-occupying symptoms
- In the absence of complications, surgical removal leads to resolution of symptoms and minimizes the risk of meningitis

References

Pacheco-Jacome E, Ballesteros MC, Jayakar P, et al. Occult spinal dysraphism: evidence-based diagnosis and treatment. Neuroimag Clin North Am 2003; 13: 327–34, xii

Saito H, Ogonuki R, Yanadori A, et al. Congenital dermal sinus with intracranial dermoid cyst. Br J Dermatol 1994; 130: 235–7

Schijman E. Split spinal cord malformations: report of 22 cases and review of the literature. Childs Nerv Syst 2003; 19: 96–103

Branchial cleft cyst/sinus

Major points

- Cysts or sinus tracts on the lateral aspect of the neck which are deep to sternocleidomastoid muscle (Figure 2.22)
- May be unilateral or bilateral
- Usually present at birth or become obvious in early childhood
- Can be apparent on the cutaneous surface or drain into the pharynx
- Most cases are sporadic, but familial cases have been reported

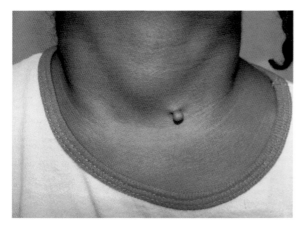

Figure 2.22 Branchial cleft with skin tag

Pathogenesis

- Branchial cysts are epithelial cysts arising from incomplete closure of the branchial clefts in embryologic development, most commonly the second or third branchial clefts
- Branchial sinuses are remnants of branchial clefts with depressions

Diagnosis

- Histology: cyst lined by stratified squamous epithelium and ciliated columnar epithelium on deeper portions; wall of cyst can be surrounded by heavy lymphoid infiltrate

Differential diagnosis

See Table 17.2

Treatment

- Preoperative imaging to assess for a fistulous connection to the posterior pharynx
- Surgical excision

Prognosis

- If untreated, cyst may have persistent mucoid discharge or become infected

References

Eastlack JP, Howard RM, Frieden IJ. Congenital midline cervical cleft: case report and review of the English language literature. Pediatr Dermatol 2000; 17: 118–22

Glosser JW, Pires CA, Feinberg SE. Branchial cleft or cervical lymphoepithelial cysts: etiology and management. J Am Dent Assoc 2003; 134: 81–6

Mukherji SK, Fatterpekar G, Castillo M, et al. Imaging of congenital anomalies of the branchial apparatus. Neuroimag Clin North Am 2000; 10: 75–93, viii

Vaughan TK, Sperling LC. Diagnosis and surgical treatment of congenital cartilaginous rests of the neck. Arch Dermatol 1991; 127: 1309–10

Preauricular cyst/sinus

Synonyms: ear pits, congenital auricular fistula

Major points

- An epithelial cyst, sinus, or swelling in preauricular region
- Common, occurs in 1% of the population
- Autosomal dominant or sporadic

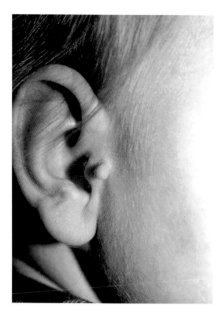

Figure 2.23   Accessory tragus

- Most cases are bilateral and asymptomatic
- May become infected and drain purulent material
- Associated defects include deafness and renal abnormalities

Pathogenesis

- Due to incomplete fusion of the first two branchial arches with epithelial entrapment

Diagnosis

- Imaging, preferably CT, defines the lesion
- Histology: cysts and sinus tracts are lined by stratified squamous epithelium

Differential diagnosis

- Epidermal cyst

See Table 17.2

Treatment

- Most lesions are asymptomatic and do not require treatment
- Secondarily infected cysts can be treated with antibiotics
- Excision is indicated if there is chronic inflammation, drainage or infection

Prognosis

- Lesion persists throughout life

References

Leung AK, Robson WL. Association of preauricular sinuses and renal anomalies. Urology 1992; 40: 259–61

Marres HA, Cremers CW. Congenital conductive or mixed deafness, preauricular sinus, external ear anomaly, and commissural lip pits: an autosomal dominant inherited syndrome. Ann Otol Rhinol Laryngol 1991; 100: 928–32

Moreland RF, Elston DM. Photo quiz. Preauricular pit. Cutis 2001; 68: 324, 353–4

O'Mara W, Guarisco L. Management of the preauricular sinus. J LA State Med Soc 1999; 151: 447–50

Accessory tragus

Major points

- Presents with round, pedunculated, skin-colored papule, occurring anywhere along the line from the tragus to the lateral commissure of the mouth (Figure 2.23)
- Can be unilateral or bilateral; single or multiple
- Familial cases have been reported

Pathogenesis

- Anomalous migration of the dorsal portion of the first branchial arch

Diagnosis

- Clinical findings
- Histology: polypoid lesion with numerous hair follicles, small sebaceous glands and often cartilaginous core; eccrine glands, nerve fibers and Pacinian corpuscles may also be present

Differential diagnosis

- Skin tag
- Preauricular cyst/sinus
- Goldenhar syndrome (oculoauriculovertebral syndrome)

Treatment

- Surgical excision

Prognosis

- Usually asymptomatic, may need surgery

References

Ban M, Kamiya H, Yamada T, Kitajima Y. Hair follicle nevi and accessory tragi: variable quantity of adipose tissue in connective tissue framework. Pediatr Dermatol 1997; 14: 433–6

Jansen T. Romiti R. Altmeyer P. Accessory tragus: report of two cases and review of the literature. Pediatr Dermatol 2000; 17: 391–4

Resnick KI, Soltani K, Berstein JE, Fathizadeh A. Accessory tragus and associated syndromes involving the first branchial arch. J Dermatol Surg Oncol 1981; 7: 39–41

Tadini G, Cambiaghi S, Scarabelli G, et al. Familial occurrence of isolated accessory tragi. Pediatr Dermatol 1993; 10: 26

3

PAPULAR AND PAPULOSQUAMOUS DISORDERS

Psoriasis

Major points

- Affects approximately 1–3% of the population
- <1% of all cases develop in infancy with reports of congenital presentation; 37% develop lesions prior to 20 years of age; peak age of onset is 15–25 years
- Variable course triggered or exacerbated by drugs (e.g. antimalarials, withdrawal of steroids), trauma (e.g. surgery, physical, sunburn) or infections (e.g. streptococcal, HIV)
- Classic lesions are well-circumscribed erythematous plaques with overlying silvery scale that produces pinpoint bleeding when removed (Auspitz sign) (Figure 3.1)
- Koebner or isomorphic phenomenon can develop in sites of trauma, often producing linear lesions

- Infantile psoriasis
  1. Most common in the diaper area; sharply demarcated and involves skin folds (Figure 3.2)
  2. Can also affect face, scalp, palms and soles
  3. Periumbilical involvement common
  4. Can progress quickly to erythroderma
- Guttate psoriasis
  1. Common presentation in children and adolescents
  2. Abrupt development of numerous small plaques on the trunk and proximal extremities; can have follicular accentuation (Figure 3.3)

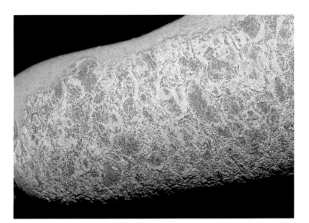

Figure 3.1   Psoriasis – classic erythematous plaque with silvery scale

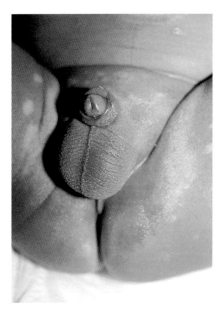

Figure 3.2   Psoriasis – diaper area involved with mild scaling and erythematous plaques

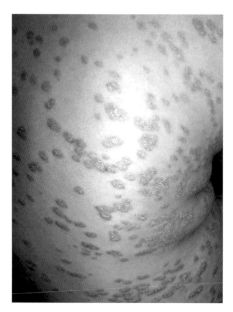

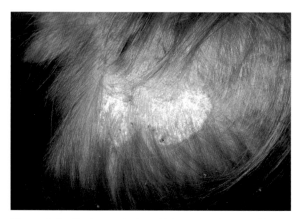

Figure 3.4   Scalp psoriasis – thick, scaly plaques without significant hair loss

Figure 3.3   Guttate psoriasis – numerous drop-like erythematous scaly papules

3. Can be initial presentation of psoriasis vulgaris; increased likelihood of developing typical psoriasis within 5 years
- Plaque psoriasis (psoriasis vulgaris)
  1. Typical silvery-scaled pink plaques; children often have finer scale than adults; may be pruritic
  2. Plaque-type variants: annular, figurate, follicular, linear
  3. Scalp involvement (common): frontal hairline and retroauricular crease involvement; can have thick scale surrounding clumps of matted hair (pityriasis amiantacea) (Figure 3.4)
  4. Flexural involvement occurs in 44% of pediatric cases: axillae, umbilicus, gluteal cleft, inguinal creases, perineum, labia and penis
  5. Facial involvement common
- Pustular/erythrodermic psoriasis
  1. Very rare in the pediatric age group; more common in males <2 years old
  2. Localized variants:
     a. Palmoplantar pustulosis: pustules on palms and soles turn to brown macules, then desquamate (Figure 3.5)
     b. Digital acropustulosis (acrodermatitis continua of Hallopeau): swelling of the nail folds with glazed erythema, pustules and

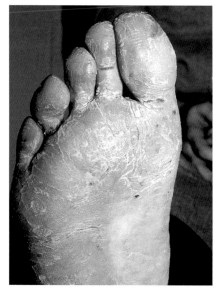

Figure 3.5   Psoriasis of the palms and soles with marked thickening and fissuring

desquamation of the fingertips with nail dystrophy
  3. Generalized variants:
     a. Acute generalized pustular psoriasis (von Zumbusch): diffuse erythroderma with overlying pustules and lakes of pus which later form sheets of desquamation; often accompanied by fever and constitutional symptoms
     b. Annular pustular psoriasis: erythematous, annular plaques with pustules and desquamation at the periphery

c. Generalized pustular variant has been associated with lytic bone lesions and capillary leak syndrome/acute respiratory distress syndrome

4. Associated findings: alopecia, geographic tongue, nail dystrophy, arthritis, lytic bone lesions, osteomyelitis, renal failure and jaundice

- Nail psoriasis (Chapter 19)
  1. Occurs in 15–79% of children with cutaneous signs of psoriasis
  2. Rarely the initial presentation of childhood psoriasis
  3. Pitting of the nail plate is most common; rarely can involve all 20 nails (Figure 3.6)
  4. Other findings: discoloration, onycholysis, distal subungual debris and oil spotting
  5. Periungual psoriasis can lead to marked nail dystrophy with hyperkeratosis and crumbling of the nail plate
  6. Psoriatic nail changes are seen in 80% of children with psoriatic arthritis

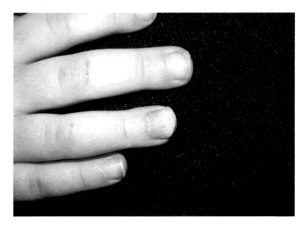

Figure 3.6 Nail psoriasis with pitting

- Psoriatic arthritis
  1. Develops in 1% of children with psoriasis; represents 8–20% of all childhood arthritis; peak age of onset is 9–12 years old
  2. 50% will have only one joint involved at initial presentation
  3. Subgroups:
     a. Oligoarthritis of the interphalangeal joints is the most common presentation in childhood
     b. Asymmetric distal interphalangeal joint involvement
     c. Arthritis mutilans with sacroileitis
     d. Symmetric arthritis
     e. Ankylosing spondylitis
  4. Can have associated eye inflammation (e.g. conjunctivitis, uveitis, episcleritis)

Pathogenesis

- Etiology not known; probably complex interactions of the vasculature, immune system and epidermis
- Genetic susceptibility
  1. HLA Cw6, B57, DR7 with early-onset type
  2. HLA B27 with pustular variant
  3. HLA B13 or B17 with guttate and erythrodermic type
  4. HLA B8, Bw35, Cw7, DR3 with palmoplantar psoriasis
  5. Increased risk if first-degree relative affected; increased in monozygotic twins
- Immune system activation
  1. Antigen presentation by Langerhans cells leading to T-cell activation
  2. Role of activated CD4+ T-helper cells in initiation
  3. Role of activated CD8+ T-helper cells in establishment and maintenance
  4. Th1 cytokine profile: interferon-γ, interleukin-2, tumor necrosis factor (TNF)-α
  5. Neutrophil accumulation
  6. Lesional increase in antimicrobial peptides (β-defensins)
  7. Often precipitated by a pharyngeal or perianal streptococcal infection; caused by superantigen stimulation of T lymphocytes
- Keratinocyte proliferation
  1. May be T-cell activated, cytokine-mediated or a primary defect of keratinocyte proliferation
  2. Reduced keratinocyte cell-cycle time
  3. Reduced apoptosis: increased Bcl-2
  4. Leads to hyperproliferation and keratinocyte hyperplasia: increased keratins 6, 16 and 17 plus reduced keratins 1, 2 and 10

Diagnosis

- Clinical diagnosis
- Histology: regular epidermal hyperplasia, parakeratosis, intracorneal neutrophils (Munro

microabscesses), diminished granular layer, keratinocyte mitoses, intraepidermal neutrophils (spongiform pustules of Kugoj), thinned suprapapillary plate, dilated vessels in the dermal papillae, perivascular lymphocytic infiltrate, mild erythrocyte extravasation

Treatment

- Avoid triggering factors
- Topical treatments
  1. Liberal emollients
  2. Topical corticosteroids (moderate to ultrapotent)
  3. Calcipotriene
  4. Exfoliants
  5. Anthralin
  6. Coal tar preparations
  7. Topical retinoids
  8. Topical immunomodulators: tacrolimus, pimecrolimus
- Phototherapy
  1. Ultraviolet B (UVB)
  2. Oral psoralen and ultraviolet A (PUVA, not recommended for those <11 years of age) or topical PUVA
- Systemic therapy for severe disease: methotrexate, cyclosporine, oral retinoids, immunomodulators (anti-TNF agents)

Differential diagnosis

- Eczema
- Seborrheic dermatitis
- Pityriasis rosea
- Drug eruption
- Tinea
- Secondary syphilis
- Candidiasis
- Acute generalized pustular dermatosis
- Staphylococcal scalded skin syndrome

Prognosis

- Chronic skin condition with intermittent exacerbations and remissions
- Typically partially responsive to topical therapy alone
- Unpredictable; may spontaneously resolve or persist into adulthood
- Systemically treated psoriasis can lead to side-effects associated with the medications

References

Cassandra M, Conte E, Cortez B. Childhood pustular psoriasis elicited by the streptococcal antigen: a case report and review of the literature. Pediatr Dermatol 2003; 20: 506–10

Leman J, Burden D. Psoriasis in children: a guide to its diagnosis and management. Paediatr Drugs 2001; 3: 673–80

Liao PB, Robinson R, Howard R, et al. Annular pustular psoriasis – most common form of pustular psoriasis in children: report of three cases and review of the literature. Pediatr Dermatol 2002; 19: 19–25

Morris A, Rogers M, Fischer G, Williams K. Childhood psoriasis: a clinical review of 1262 cases. Pediatr Dermatol 2001; 18: 188–98

Rogers M. Childhood psoriasis. Curr Opin Pediatr 2002; 14: 404–9

Pityriasis rubra pilaris

Major points

- Chronic skin disorder with variable clinical spectrum
- Most cases are sporadic; familial cases with autosomal dominant pattern
- Characterized by salmon-orange plaques with classic 'islands of sparing' and perifollicular 'nutmeg grater' papules with palmoplantar keratoderma
- Clinically defined classification
  1. Type I: Classic type, adult onset
  2. Type II: Atypical type, adult onset
  3. Type III: Classic type, juvenile onset
     a. Accounts for 10% of all reported cases
     b. Usually develops within first decade
     c. Typically begins on scalp, face and neck with palmoplantar keratoderma followed by development of characteristic coalescent plaques on trunk and extremities (Figure 3.7)
     d. Facial skin taut with ectropion
     e. Nails thickened and dystrophic
  4. Type IV: Localized or circumscribed juvenile onset
     a. Accounts for 25% of all reported cases; 60% of all childhood cases
     b. Typically prepubertal children
     c. Presents with hyperkeratotic follicular papules coalescent to plaques over the elbows and knees (Figure 3.8)
     d. May have palmoplantar keratoderma

5. Type V: Atypical type, juvenile onset
   a. Accounts for 5% of all cases
   b. Typically develops in the first 2 years of life; may be seen at birth; often familial
   c. Presents with widespread erythema and folliculocentric papules
   d. Variable palmoplantar keratoderma
   e. May have associated arthropathy
- May be associated with underlying HIV

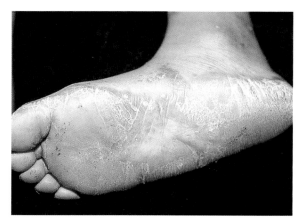

Figure 3.7   Pityriasis rubra pilaris – palmar keratoderma with typical yellow, waxy appearance

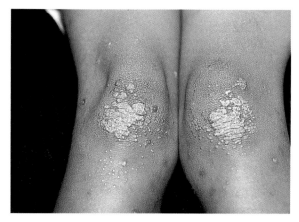

Figure 3.8   Pityriasis rubra pilaris – juvenile type with keratotic plaques on the knees

Pathogenesis

- Unknown etiology
- Increased epidermal cell proliferation
- Reduced levels of retinol-binding protein that is a specific carrier of vitamin A

Diagnosis

- Characteristic clinical findings
- Histology: alternating ortho- and parakeratosis in a 'geometric' pattern, superficial follicular plugging, acanthosis, hypergranulosis, variable spongiosis, perinuclear vacuolation and mild superficial lymphohistiocytic infiltrate

Differential diagnosis

- Psoriasis
- Atopic dermatitis
- Lichen planus
- Lichen nitidus
- Viral exanthem
- Kawasaki disease
- Nonbullous congenital ichthyosiform erythroderma

Treatment

- Treatment is often difficult
- Topical treatments
  1. Emollients
  2. Exfoliants
  3. Topical corticosteroids
  4. Calcipotriene
- Systemic therapy
  1. Systemic retinoids
  2. Methotrexate
  3. Cyclosporine

Prognosis

- Type III and IV disease may resolve spontaneously within 3 years of onset
- Type V persists throughout life

References

Albert MR, Mackool BT. Pityrisis rubra pilaris. Int J Dermatol 1999; 38: 1–11

Allison DS, El-Azhary RA, Calobrisi SD, Dicken CH. Pityriasis rubra pilaris in children. J Am Acad Dermatol 2002; 47: 386–9

Griffith WA. Pityriasis rubra pilaris. J Am Acad Dermatol 1984; 10: 1086–8

Menni S, Brancaleone W, Grimalt R. Pityriasis rubra pilaris in a child seropositive for the human immunodeficiency virus. J Am Acad Dermatol 1992; 27: 1009

Terasaki K, Kanekura T, Saruwatari H, Kanzaki T. Classical juvenile pityriasis rubra pilaris in a patient with Down syndrome. Clin Exp Dermatol 2004; 29: 49–51

Pityriasis rosea

Major points

- Acute, transient papulosquamous disorder of unknown etiology
- Peak incidence: 20–24 years old; 45% of cases in patients <19 years old, 4% <4 years old; rare reports in patients <2 years old
- Preceding viral prodrome in some cases
- Presents with 'herald patch' as the initial lesion: oval pink macule which becomes an annular plaque developing a collarette of scale (Figures 3.9 and 3.10)
- Similar lesions then develop on the trunk and proximal extremities over 1–3 weeks
- May be pruritic
- Lesions oriented parallel to skin lines and show a 'school of minnows' pattern in the flank area and a 'Christmas-tree' pattern on the back
- May have oral lesions
- Variant lesion types: vesicular, pustular, purpuric and erythema multiforme-like
- Variant patterns: inverse, atypical (inverse with acrofacial lesions) and localized

Pathogenesis

- Unknown etiology
- Epidemiologic data support a viral etiology, possibly human herpes virus-6 (HHV-6) and -7 (HHV-7), cytomegalovirus (CMV), Epstein–Barr virus (EBV) or parvovirus B19 virus

Diagnosis

- Clinical findings
- Histopathology: mounding parakeratosis, focal spongiosis, exocytosis of lymphocytes, dyskeratosis, papillary dermal edema, upper dermal erythrocyte extravasation, lymphocytic infiltrate in upper dermis

Treatment

- None usually required
- Symptomatic therapy
  1. Topical steroids
  2. Erythromycin
  3. UVB phototherapy
  4. Oral steroids (short course)

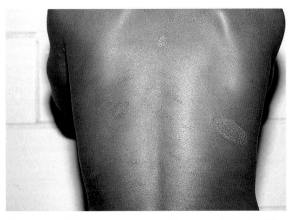

Figure 3.9   Pityriasis rosea – herald patch with typical 'fir tree' distribution of secondary lesions

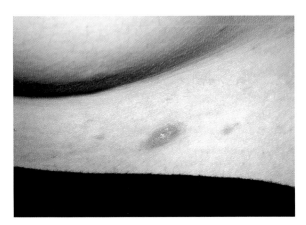

Figure 3.10   Pityriasis rosea – typical oval lesion with trailing collarette of scale

Differential diagnosis

- Tinea
- Secondary syphilis
- Psoriasis
- Nummular eczema
- Drug eruption
- Graft-versus-host disease

Prognosis

- Self-limited
- Resolves with or without therapy over 4–12 weeks
- May result in postinflammatory hypo- or hyperpigmentation

References

Chuh AA. The association of pityriasis rosea with cytomegalovirus, Epstein–Barr virus and parvovirus B19 infections – a prospective case control study by polymerase chain reaction and serology. Eur J Dermatol 2003; 13: 25–8

Imamura S, Ozaki M, Oguchi M, et al. Atypical pityriasis rosea. Dermatologica 1985; 171: 474–7

Sharma PK, Yadav TP, Gautam RM, et al. Erythromycin in pityriasis rosea: a double-blind, placebo-controlled clinical trial. J Am Acad Dermatol 2000; 42: 241–4

Watanabe T, Kawamura T, Jacob SE, et al. Pityriasis rosea is associated with systemic active infection with both human herpesvirus-7 and human herpesvirus-6. J Invest Dermatol 2002; 119: 793–7

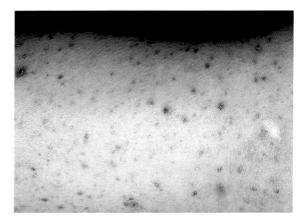

Figure 3.11 Pityriasis lichenoides et varioliformis acuta with generalized erythematous and necrotic papules

Pityriasis lichenoides

Major points

- Disease entity encompasses pityriasis lichenoides et varioliformis acuta (PLEVA) and pityriasis lichenoides chronica (PLC), which are thought to be on a clinicopathological spectrum
- Variable clinical presentation
- Typically occurs in children and young adults
- Pityriasis lichenoides et varioliformis acuta (PLEVA) (synonym: Mucha–Habermann disease)
  1. Polymorphous eruption of diffuse reddish-brown macules, papules and varicella-like vesicles with abrupt onset (Figure 3.11)
  2. Lesions progress with ulceration, crusting, central petechiae and necrosis
  3. Usually involves the trunk and flexural surfaces of proximal extremities
  4. Crops of new lesions develop over weeks to months
  5. Can resolve with hyper- or hypopigmentation, and depressed scars
  6. May be accompanied by fever, malaise, lymphadenopathy and arthritis
  7. Papulonecrotic variant: rare, severe form; associated with high fever and constitutional symptoms; acute onset of large nodules with hemorrhagic necrosis and ulceration; may be fatal
- Pityriasis lichenoides chronica (PLC)
  1. Can arise *de novo* or may evolve from PLEVA
  2. Lesions are pink–brown macules and papules with thin centrally adherent scales (Figure 3.12)

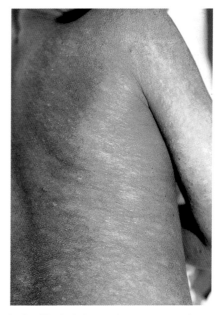

Figure 3.12 Pityriasis lichenoides chronica with hypopigmentation and scaling

  3. Resolves with postinflammatory hypo- or hyperpigmentation
  4. Indolent and persistent course

Pathogenesis

- Unknown etiology
- Hypotheses include:
  1. Response to foreign antigens: infectious agents and drugs
  2. Cutaneous T-cell lymphoproliferative disorder

Diagnosis

- Clinical findings
- Histology: lymphocytic vasculitis with lichenoid reaction pattern
  1. PLEVA: parakeratosis, variable erosion/ulceration, spongiosis, basal vacuolar change, exocytosis of lymphocytes and erythrocytes, epidermal necrosis, papillary dermal edema, dense perivascular wedge-shaped papillary dermal infiltrate of lymphocytes (mostly CD8+), endothelial swelling, extravasated erythrocytes
  2. PLC: Confluent parakeratosis, mild spongiosis, focal necrotic keratinocytes, mild lymphocytic (mostly CD4+) interface and perivascular inflammation, limited erythrocyte extravasation
- Recommend biopsy of persistent or clinically atypical lesions to rule out progression to malignancy (rare)

Differential diagnosis

- Pityriasis rosea
- Psoriasis
- Secondary syphilis
- Lichen planus
- Arthropod reaction
- Lymphomatoid papulosis
- Drug eruption
- Varicella
- Vasculitis
- Erythema multiforme

Treatment

- Topical treatments
  1. Topical low or mid-strength corticosteroids
  2. Coal tar preparations
- Phototherapy
  1. Ultraviolet B (UVB)
  2. Psoralen + ultraviolet A (PUVA) - not recommended <11 years old
- Systemic therapies
  1. Oral antihistamines
  2. Oral antibiotics: erythromycin, tetracycline
  3. Methotrexate (low dose)
  4. Systemic corticosteroids

Prognosis

- Most cases resolve over several months
- 25% of patients will have recurrences with a chronic relapsing course over years

- Rare subset progresses to lymphomatoid papulosis or T-cell lymphoma

References

Gelmetti C, Rigoni C, Alessi E, et al. Pityriasis lichenoides in children: a long-term follow-up of eighty-nine cases. J Am Acad Dermatol 1990; 23: 473–8

Ito N, Ohshima A, Hashizume H, et al. Febrile ulceronecrotic Mucha–Habermann's disease managed with methylprednisolone semipulse and subsequent methotrexate therapies. J Am Acad Dermatol 2003; 49: 1142–8

Margo C, Crowson AN, Kovatich A, Burns F. Pityriasis lichenoides: a clonal T-cell lymphoproliferative disorder. Hum Pathol 2002; 33: 788–95

Romani J, Puig L, Fernandez-Figueras MT, de Moragas JM. Pityriasis lichenoides in children: clinicopathologic review of 22 patients. Pediatr Dermatol 1998; 15: 11–16

Lymphomatoid papulosis

Major points

- Recurrent self-healing papulonodular eruption with risk of malignant transformation
- Rare in children
- Presents with recurrent crops of red–brown papules and nodules with variable crusting, ulceration and necrosis (Figure 3.13)
- Lesion variants: pustular and vesicular
- Occurs primarily on trunk and proximal extremities
- Lesions involute spontaneously over weeks to months
- May resolve with pigmentary change or scarring

Pathogenesis

- T-cell lymphoproliferative disorder
- Majority of cells are CD4+; a few cells may be CD30+
- 60% of lesions have clonal T-cell populations

Diagnosis

- Clinical diagnosis
- Histopathology important in establishing diagnosis
- Three histologic subtypes:
  1. Type A: mixed cellular, wedge-shaped infiltrate with large atypical lymphocytes
  2. Type B: band-like or perivascular inflammation with epidermotropism, lymphocytes with cerebriform nuclei

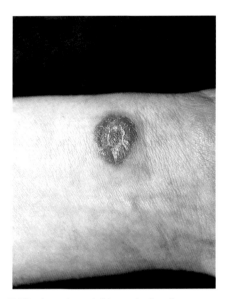

Figure 3.13 Lymphomatoid papulosis – 1 cm erythematous nodule on the wrist

3. Type C: single population of large atypical CD 30+ lymphocytes

Differential diagnosis

- Pityriasis lichenoides
- Arthropod reaction
- Pseudolymphoma
- Anaplastic large cell lymphoma

Treatment

- Potent topical or intralesional corticosteroids for individual lesions
- Phototherapy: UVB and PUVA (not recommended for <11 years of age)
- Oral antibiotics: erythromycin and tetracycline
- Systemic corticosteroids
- Methotrexate

Prognosis

- May spontaneously regress
- May persist with recurrences over many years
- 5–20% progress to an associated malignant form: cutaneous T-cell lymphoma anaplastic large cell lymphoma, Hodgkin disease
- Requires careful long-term follow-up

References

Paulli M, Berti E, Rosso R, et al. CD30/Ki-1-positive lymphoproliferative disorders of the skin clinicopathologic correlation and statistical analysis of 86 cases: a multicentric study from the European Organization for Research and Treatment of Cancer Cutaneous Lymphoma Project Group. J Clin Oncol 1995; 13: 1343–54

Rifkin S, Valderrama E, Lipton JM, Karayalcin G. Lymphomatoid papulosis and Ki-1+ anaplastic large cell lymphoma occurring concurrently in a pediatric patient. J Pediatr Hematol Oncol 2001; 23: 321–3

VanNeer FJ, Toonstra J, VanVoorstVader PC, et al. Lymphomatoid papulosis in children: a study of 10 children registered by the Dutch Cutaneous Lymphoma Working Group. Br J Dermatol 2001; 144: 351–4

Zackheim HS, Jones C, Leboit PE, et al. Lymphomatoid papulosis associated with mycosis fungoides: a study of 21 patients including analyses for clonality. J Am Acad Dermatol 2003; 49: 620–3

Zirbel GM, Gellis SE, Kadin ME, Esterly NB. Lymphomatoid papulosis in children. J Am Acad Dermatol 1995; 33: 741–8

Cutaneous T-cell lymphoma

Synonym: mycosis fungoides

Major points

- Cutaneous neoplasm with an indolent progression and late involvement of the lymph nodes, bone marrow and viscera
- Typically a disease of adults but reported with increasing frequency in childhood and adolesence
- Presents with a solitary or a few scaly pink patches and plaques on the lower trunk or buttocks; may have a surrounding hypopigmented halo; can progress with increased infiltration of the plaques and eventual development of pink nodules and tumors that can ulcerate (Figure 3.14)
- Hypopigmented variant (seen in up to 24% of childhood cases) presents with hypopigmented macules and patches on the trunk and extremities
- Can present with concurrent lymphomatoid papulosis, which is more common in childhood and seen in up to 18% of cases
- Variable progression through the clinical stages: patch, plaque, tumor
- Sezary syndrome (leukemic variant) with erythroderma and lymphadenopathy; rare in children
- TNMB staging: skin (T), lymph nodes (N), viscera (V) and peripheral blood (B)

1. Skin
   a. T1: <10% body surface area (BSA)
   b. T2: >10% BSA
   c. T3: tumors
   d. T4: erythroderma
2. Lymph nodes
   a. N0: no involvement
   b. N1: clinically palpable only
   c. N2: pathologic involvement only
   d. N3: both clinical and pathologic involvement

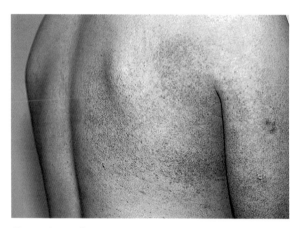

Figure 3.14 Cutaneous T-cell lymphoma – presenting as poikiloderma in a teenager

3. Viscera
   a. V0: not involved
   b. V1: involved
4. Blood
   a. B0: not involved
   b. B1: involved
   c. 'B' does not affect the staging
5. Stages
   a. Stage IA   T1, N0, M0
   b. Stage IB   T2, N0, M0
   c. Stage IIA   T1–2, N1, M0
   d. Stage IIB   T3, N0–1, M0
   e. Stage IIIA   T4, N0, M0
   f. Stage IIIB   T4, N1, M0
   g. Stage IVA   T1–4, N2–3, M0
   h. Stage IVB   T1–4, N0–3, M1

Pathogenesis

- Malignant neoplasm of T-helper cells with monoclonal proliferation of CD4+ cells most common, can also be CD8+ cell proliferation

- Cause of malignant transformation unknown; HTLV-1, HTLV-5 and HHV-8 have been implicated as possible causes

Diagnosis

- Clinical findings; diagnosis is often delayed for many years because of nonspecific cutaneous lesions
- Skin biopsy imperative: histology depends on stage of disease
  1. Patch stage
     a. Sparse infiltrate of lymphocytes tagging along the basal cell layer either in small groups or singly as 'a string of beads'
     b. Limited epidermotropism (i.e. lymphocytes ascending in the epidermis)
     c. Rare Pautrier microabscesses (i.e. clusters of closely apposed lymphocytes in the epidermis without spongiosis)
  2. Plaque stage
     a. More dense infiltration of lymphocytes along the epidermis and within the papillary dermis with aggregation around vessels and adnexae
     b. Increased numbers of atypical lymphocytes with classic cerebriform nuclei
     c. Conspicuous epidermotropism
     d. Increased number of Pautrier microabscesses
  3. Tumor stage
     a. Deep monomorphic infiltration of atypical lymphocytes throughout the dermis and into the subcutaneous tissue
     b. Increased number of mitoses
     c. Epidermotropism and Pautrier microabscesses are rare
- T-cell receptor rearrangements by polymerase chain reaction (PCR)
- Staging work-up should include complete blood count, serum chemistries including renal and liver functions, chest X-ray, lymph node biopsy if palpable lymphadenopathy

Differential diagnosis

- Eczema
- Psoriasis
- Tinea corporis
- Pityriasis lichenoides
- Lymphomatoid papulosis

Treatment

- Depends on symptoms, degree of cutaneous involvement, and presence of systemic involvement
- Main treatment goals are symptomatic relief and control of the disease
- Treatment has not been shown to prevent the progression of disease
  1. Topical antipruritics
  2. Potent or ultrapotent topical corticosteroids
  3. Topical retinoids (e.g. Targretin)
  4. PUVA
  5. Topical nitrogen mustard
  6. Oral RXR-receptor retinoids (e.g. Targretin)

Prognosis

- Typical slow progression from cutaneous to systemic involvement
- 95% disease-specific survival at 5 years
- 93% disease-specific survival at 10 years
- Complete remissions are rare but reported

References

Crowley JJ, Nikko A, Varghese A, et al. Mycosis fungoides in young patients: clinical characteristics and outcome. J Am Acad Dermatol 1998; 38: 696–701

Garzon MC. Cutaneous T cell lymphoma in children. Semin Cutan Med Surg 1999; 18: 226–32

Neuhaus IM, Ramos-Caro FA, Hassanein AM. Hypopigmented mycosis fungoides in childhood and adolescence. Pediatr Dermatol 2000; 17: 403–6

Quaglino P, Zaccagna A, Verrone A, et al. Mycosis fungoides in patients under 20 years of age: report of 7 cases, review of the literature and study of the clinical course. Dermatology 1999; 199: 8–14

Wain EM, Orchard GE, Whittaker SJ, et al. Outcome in 34 patients with juvenile-onset mycosis fungoides: a clinical, immunophenotypic, and molecular study. Cancer 2003; 98: 2282–90

Whittam LR, Calonje E, Orchard G, et al. CD8-positive juvenile onset mycosis fungoides: an immunohistochemical and genotypic analysis of six cases. Br J Dermatol 2000; 143: 1199–204

Lichen planus

Major points

- 2–3% of all cases occur in children

- Characterized by purple, polygonal, planar, pruritic papules (Figure 3.15)
- May have overlying Wickham striae (superficial white reticulate pattern)
- Commonly occurs on the volar wrists, sacral area and pretibial surfaces
- May display Koebner phenomenon (development at sites of trauma)
- Oral mucosa (uncommon in children): white reticulate pattern on buccal mucosa
- Nail involvement in children is uncommon; may present with trachyonychia or twenty-nail dystrophy
- Clinical variants: linear, hypertrophic, annular, follicular, erosive, bullous and actinic
- Typically resolves with prominent postinflammatory hyperpigmentation

Pathogenesis

- Unknown etiology
- Possible genetic susceptibility with familial cases reported
- Evidence for a cell-mediated immune response
- Increased prevalence in adults with hepatitis C; may cause presentation of viral antigens to antigen-presenting cells leading to the induction of effector T cells with cytotoxic activity

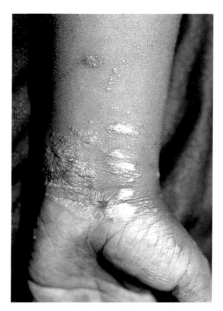

Figure 3.15 Lichen planus – violaceous flat-topped papules with white Wickham striae

Diagnosis

- Clinical diagnosis (usually)
- Histology: hyperkeratosis, wedge-shaped hypergranulosis, variable acanthosis with saw-toothing of the rete ridges, band-like lymphohistiocytic infiltrate at the dermal–epidermal junction, basal layer damage causing Caspary–Joseph spaces, Civatte bodies and colloid bodies, variable melanin incontinence

Differential diagnosis

- Lichenoid drug eruption
- Lichen nitidus
- Lichen simplex chronicus
- Psoriasis
- Granuloma annulare
- Sarcoidosis

Treatment

- Mid-strength or potent topical corticosteroids
- Oral antihistamines
- Oral corticosteroids
- Oral retinoids
- Phototherapy: UVB, PUVA (not recommended for <11 years of age)

Prognosis

- Typically resolves within 1–12 months
- 10–20% will have intermittent recurrences for many years
- Residual pigmentary changes can be disfiguring

References

Alam F, Hamburger J. Oral mucosal lichen planus in children. Int J Paediatr Dent 2001; 11: 209–14

Eisen D. The clinical manifestations and treatment of oral lichen planus. Dermatol Clin 2003; 21: 79–89

Kabbash C, Laude TA, Weinberg JM, Silverberg NB. Lichen planus in the lines of Blaschko. Pediatr Dermatol 2002; 19: 541–5

Nocente R, Ceccanti M, Bertazzoni G, et al. HCV infection and extrahepatic manifestations. Hepato-Gastroenterology 2003; 50: 1149–54

Peluso AM, Tosti A, Piraccini BM, Cameli N. Lichen planus limited to the nails in childhood: case report and literature review. Pediatr Dermatol 1993; 10: 36–9

Sharma R, Maheshwari V. Childhood lichen planus: a report of fifty cases. Pediatr Dermatol 1999; 16: 345–8

Lichen nitidus

Major points

- Uncommon, benign dermatosis of childhood
- Male/female ratio >1
- Discrete pinpoint, shiny, skin-colored or hypopigmented papules (Figure 3.16)
- Location: trunk and extremities, penis
- Typically asymptomatic but may be pruritic
- May display Koebner phenomenon: linear lesions in areas of trauma

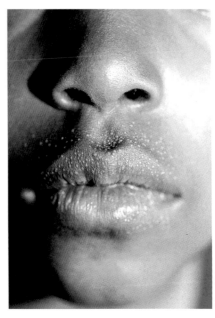

Figure 3.16   Lichen nitidus – hypopigmented tiny papules

- Rare associated oral and nail involvement
- Rarely lesions can be vesicular, hemorrhagic or purpuric

Pathogenesis

- Unknown etiology
- Considered a variant of lichen planus

Diagnosis

- Clinical findings
- Histology: 'ball and claw' circumscribed lymphohistiocytic infiltrate within 2–3 dermal papillae; can have thinning of the overlying epidermis; claw-like extension of the rete ridges;

multinucleate giant cells within inflammatory infiltrate

Differential diagnosis

- Papular eczema
- Molluscum contagiosum
- Planar warts
- Keratosis pilaris
- Eruptive vellus hair cysts
- Lichen planus

Treatment

- No therapy usually required
- Symptomatic relief with topical corticosteriods and topical/oral antihistamines
- For severe, persistent cases: PUVA (not recommended <11 years), systemic steroids or oral retinoids

Prognosis

- Variable course
- Spontaneous resolution occurs in 69% of patients within 1 year
- May be persistent and unresponsive to therapy for many years

References

Arizaga AT, Gaughan MD, Bang RH. Generalized lichen nitidus. Clin Exp Dermatol 2002; 27: 115–17

Kubota Y, Kiryu H, Nakayama J. Generalized lichen nitidus successfully treated with an antituberculous agent. Br J Dermatol 2002; 146: 1081–3

Lestringant GG, Piletta P, Feldmann R, et al. Coexistence of atopic dermatitis and lichen nitidus in three patients. Dermatology 1996; 192: 171–3

Sanders S, Collier de AH, Scott R, et al. Periappendageal lichen nitidus: report of a case. J Cutan Pathol 2002; 29: 125–8

Soroush V, Gurevitch AW, Peng SK. Generalized lichen nitidus: case report and literature review. Cutis 1999; 64: 135–6

Elastosis perforans serpiginosa

Synonym: perforating elastosis

Major points

- Male/female ratio >1
- Typically presents at >20 years of age
- Clinical presentation with asymptomatic, skin-colored to red keratotic papules in a linear, arcuate or serpiginous array; most common on neck but can involve upper extremities, face or trunk (Figure 3.17)
- Can demonstrate Koebner phenomenon
- 25% of cases associated with disorder: Down syndrome, Ehlers–Danlos syndrome, Marfan syndrome, pseudoxanthoma elasticum, osteogenesis imperfecta, cutis laxa, Rothmund–Thomson syndrome, systemic sclerosis, morphea, acrogeria, XYY syndrome and chronic renal disease
- Has been described associated with D-penicillamine therapy
- Familial cases reported with an autosomal dominant inheritance pattern suspected

Pathogenesis

- Unknown etiology
- Histologic transepidermal elimination of fragmented elastic fibers may be a common pathway for elimination of abnormal elastic fibers; keratinocytes with elastin receptors can be found surrounding eliminated elastic material

Diagnosis

- Clinical findings, especially in presence of associated disorders
- Histopathology: acanthosis of the epidermis; central channel through the epidermis with an overlying keratinous plug and elimination of fragmented eosinophilic elastic fibers and

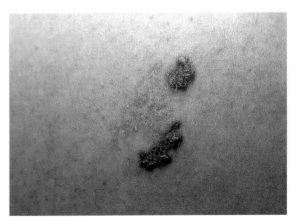

Figure 3.17 Elastosis perforans serpiginosa with typical keratotic, grouped papules

basophilic nuclear debris; papillary dermis contains increased coarse elastic fibers that are easily seen on elastic stains; variable amount of inflammation and foreign body giant cells

Differential diagnosis

- Porokeratosis of Mibelli
- Granuloma annulare
- Tinea corporis
- Sarcoidosis
- Lichen planus
- Cutaneous larva migrans

Treatment

- Typically not required; limited effectiveness
- Keratolytic agents
- Topical retinoids
- Cryotherapy
- Lasers

Prognosis

- Slowly enlarges
- Typically resolves spontaneously over 5–10 years
- With associated disorder, the overall prognosis is based on the specific disease entity

References

Mehta RK, Burrows NP, Payne CM, et al. Elastosis perforans serpiginosa and associated disorders. Clin Exp Dermatol 2001; 26: 521–4

Outland JD, Brown TS, Callen JP. Tazarotene is an effective therapy for elastosis perforans serpiginosa. Arch Dermatol 2002; 138: 169–71

Saxena M, Tope WD. Response of elastosis perforans serpiginosa to pulsed CO_2, Er:YAG, and dye lasers. Dermatol Surg 2003; 29: 677–8

Sehgal VN, Jain S, Thappa DM, et al. Perforating dermatoses: a review and report of four cases. J Dermatol 1993; 20: 329–40

Wu JJ, Wagner AM. A case of elastosis perforans serpiginosa. Cutis 2002; 69: 423–5

Porokeratosis

Major points

- Clinically variable disease of keratinization
- Classic lesion: papule or plaque with a thin, keratotic, thread-like border, resembling 'Great Wall of China' (Figure 3.18)

- Porokeratosis of Mibelli
  1. Male/female ratio >1
  2. Onset in infancy or adolescence
  3. Presents with solitary, localized annular plaque with a distinctive keratotic border
  4. Typically occurs on the legs
- Linear porokeratosis
  1. Presents in infancy or childhood; can be congenital
  2. Classic porokeratotic plaques distributed in the lines of Blaschko (Figure 3.19)
  3. Most common on an extremity
  4. Can coexist with disseminated superficial actinic porokeratosis
  5. Rare risk of malignant degeneration
- Punctate porokeratosis
  1. Noted during adolescence or adulthood
  2. Characterized by small discrete keratotic papules on the palms and soles in association with linear porokeratosis or porokeratosis of Mibelli
- Porokeratosis palmaris et plantaris disseminata
  1. Occurs during childhood or adolescence
  2. Develops multiple keratotic papules on the palms and soles initially, then spreads diffusely on the trunk and extremities with areas of confluence; male/female ratio >1, autosomal dominant
- Disseminated superficial actinic porokeratosis (DSAP)
  1. Most common type
  2. Develops in mid-adulthood typically
  3. Widespread small keratotic papules on sun-exposed areas, usually lower legs

Pathogenesis

- Unknown etiology
- Genetic susceptibility; autosomal dominant in some cases
- Hypothesis: proliferation of aberrant keratinocyte clone
- Overexpression of p53 tumor suppressor protein
- May be due to loss of heterozygosity

Diagnosis

- Clinical findings
- Histology: pathognomonic cornoid lamella (parakaratotic column) overlying a reduced or absent granular layer

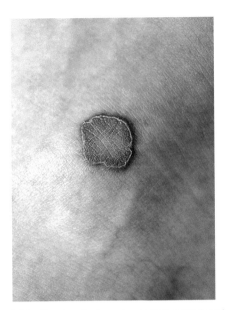

Figure 3.18   Porokeratosis – classic thin-edged scale resembling the 'Great Wall of China'

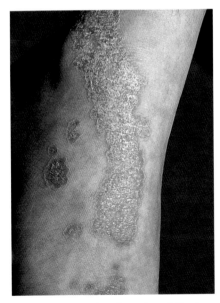

Figure 3.19   Porokeratosis – linear type following Blaschko lines

Differential diagnosis

- Elastosis perforans serpiginosa
- Tinea corporis
- Lichen striatus
- Lichen sclerosus
- Granuloma annulare

- Morphea
- Punctate keratoderma

Treatment

- Variable results with topical 5-fluorouracil, surgical excision, cryotherapy, CO_2 laser ablation, dermabrasion, exfoliants, topical and systemic retinoids

Prognosis

- Chronic and persistent course
- Linear variant has a small risk of malignant degeneration to squamous cell carcinoma in later life

References

Boente MC, López-Baró AM, Frontini MV, Asial RA. Linear porokeratosis associated with disseminated superficial actinic porokeratosis: a new example of type II segmental involvement. Pediatr Dermatol 2003; 20: 514–18

Fisher CA, LeBoit PE, Frieden IJ. Linear porokeratosis presenting as erosions in the newborn period. Pediatr Dermatol 1995; 12: 318–22

Flanagan N, Boyadjiev SA, Harper J, et al. Familial craniosynostosis, anal anomalies, and porokeratosis: CAP syndrome. J Med Genet 1998; 35: 763–6

Pierson D, Bandel C, Ehrig T, Cockerell C. Benign epidermal tumors and proliferations: porokeratosis. In Dermatology. Bolognia JL, Jorizzo JL, Rapini RP, et al. eds. Mosby: New York, 2003: 1707–9

Silver SG, Crawford RI. Fatal squamous cell carcinoma arising from transplant-associated porokeratosis. J Am Acad Dermatol 2003; 49: 931–3

Suh DH, Lee HS, Kim SD, et al. Coexistence of disseminated superficial porokeratosis in childhood with congenital linear porokeratosis. Pediatr Dermatol 2000; 17: 466–8

Keratolysis exfoliativa

Major points

- Chronic superficial desquamative dermatosis (Figure 3.20)
- Acral variant (synonym: lamellar dyshidrosis)
  1. Presents with recurrent peeling of the palms and soles with circinate or annular exfoliation
  2. No antecedent primary lesions
  3. No associated hyperhidrosis
- Diffuse variant (synonyms: keratolysis exfoliativa congenita, familial continual skin peeling)

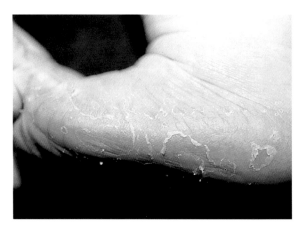

Figure 3.20   Keratolysis exfoliativa – nonerythematous chronic scaling on the feet, not associated with tinea

1. Can be noninflammatory or associated with congenital erythroderma
2. Sporadic, but has been described in families; autosomal recessive inheritance suspected
3. Presents with chronic, superficial peeling over large areas of the body, often sparing the palms and soles
4. Typically begins at birth or early childhood
5. Usually asymptomatic, although may have associated stinging and burning

Pathogenesis

- Unknown etiology

Diagnosis

- Consistent clinical history and examination
- Histopathology reveals hyperkeratosis and epidermal separation at the stratum corneum–granular layer interface

Differential diagnosis

- Juvenile plantar dermatosis
- Dyshidrotic eczema
- Atopic dermatitis
- Tinea
- Sunburn
- Virus-induced exfoliation
- Congenital ichthyosiform erythroderma
- Netherton syndrome

Treatment

- No effective treatment available
- Topical steroids, keratolytics and retinoids tend to be ineffective

Prognosis

- Typically lifelong with spontaneous, continual peeling
- Can worsen during the summer months

References

Hashimoto K, Hamzavi I, Tanaka K, Shwayder T. Acral peeling skin syndrome. J Am Acad Dermatol 2000; 43: 1112–19

Lee HJ, Ha SJ, Ahn WK, et al. Clinical evaluation of atopic hand-foot dermatitis. Pediatr Dermatol 2001; 18: 102–6

Mevorah B, Orion E, de Viragh P, et al. Peeling skin syndrome with hair changes. Dermatology 1998; 197: 373–6

Tastan HB, Akar A, Gur AR, Deveci S. Peeling skin syndrome. Int J Dermatol 1999; 38: 208–10

Tolat SN, Gharpuray MB. Skin peeling syndrome. Cutis 1994; 53: 255–7

4

ECZEMATOUS DERMATOSES

ECZEMATOUS DERMATITIS

General

- Eczema is a general term, often used interchangeably with dermatitis
- Results from inflammation of superficial dermis and epidermal spongiosis leading to crusting, oozing and sometimes cracking (fissures)

ATOPIC DERMATITIS

Major points

- One of the most common skin disorders of childhood
- Inherited disorder, presumably autosomal dominant
- Often associated with either a family or a personal history of other 'allergic' conditions (e.g. asthma or allergic rhinitis)
- The word 'atopy' comes from the Greek word meaning 'without place, unusual.' Described by Coca and Cooke in 1923
- Characteristics
  1. Diagnosis is made clinically by recognizing a combination of features. No single diagnostic criterion exists, but there is a constellation of features (Table 4.1)
  2. Crusty, oozing, eruption with frequent secondary changes from scratching (Figure 4.1)
  3. Pruritus is a hallmark and can be severe, often set off by certain environmental or psychological causes

Table 4.1   Criteria for the diagnosis of atopic dermatitis in children

Major features

1. Pruritus
2. Typical morphology and distribution
   Facial and extensor involvement during infancy and early childhood
   Flexural lichenification in childhood or adolescence
3. Chronic or chronically relapsing dermatitis
4. Personal or family history of atopy

Minor or less specific features

1. Xerosis
2. Periauricular fissures
3. Ichthyosis
4. Hyperlinear palms
5. Keratosis pilaris
6. IgE reactivity (increased serum IgE, RAST, or prick test positivity)
7. Hand or foot dermatitis
8. Cheilitis
9. Scalp dermatitis
10. Susceptibility to cutaneous infections (especially *Staphylococcus aureus* and herpes simplex)
11. Perifollicular accentuation (especially in darkly pigmented races)
12. Dennie's lines (Figure 4.12)
13. Pityriasis alba (Figure 4.13)

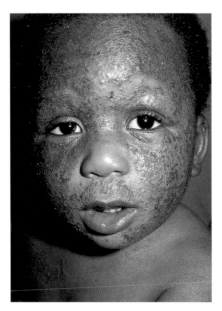

Figure 4.1   Infantile eczema – typical facial, oozing pruritic plaques

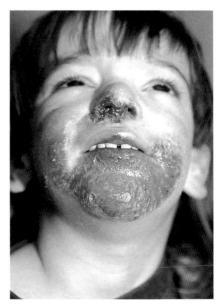

Figure 4.2   Secondarily – infected atopic dermatitis with *Staphylococcus aureus*

    a. Itching often intensifies in the evening and disrupts sleep patterns

    b. Threshold for itching is low and often prolonged

4. Distribution often depends on the age of the child (e.g. infants have significant facial involvement, older children have flexural involvement)

5. Lesions can be follicular and papular

6. More susceptible to viral infections (e.g. molluscum contagiosum, warts, herpes simplex) and staphylococcal infections (Figure 4.2)

7. Types of eczema

    a. Generalized – this can become erythrodermic, and usually denotes more severe involvement

    b. Infantile eczema (from infants to 2 years) – distribution primarily on cheeks, face, extensor surfaces of arms and legs; tends to spare diaper area

    c. Childhood eczema (from about 2 years to puberty) – tends to occur on flexural areas (antecubital fossae, popliteal fossae, hands and feet) (Figures 4.3 and 4.4)

    d. Adult/teenage eczema (puberty through adulthood) – occurs in flexural areas, hands

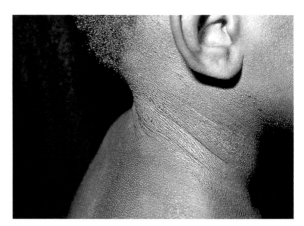

Figure 4.3   Childhood eczema – lichenified, pruritic plaque on the neck

and face, especially eyelids (Figure 4.5) Face has typical central pallor

    e. Nummular eczema

Coin-shaped, oozing plaques with minute papules and vesicles at the periphery (Figure 4.6); generally scattered over the body, but may be mainly localized to one area, such as the legs; plaques usually >1 cm; pruritus common but variable; staphylococcal infections commonly play a role

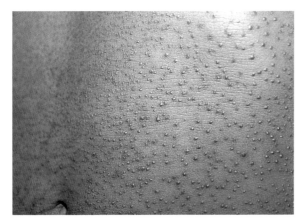

Figure 4.4 Follicular eczema – multiple keratotic, pruritic, follicular papules

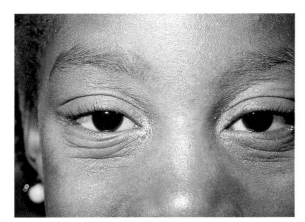

Figure 4.5 Eyelid eczema with accentuation of skin markings

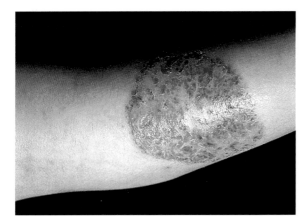

Figure 4.6 Nummular eczema – typical round, oozing plaque

f. Lichen simplex chronicus
    Thickened lichenified plaques with accentuated skin markings caused by chronic scratching (Figure 4.7); nodules are called prurigo nodularis

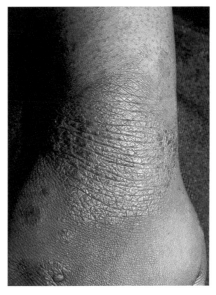

Figure 4.7 Lichen simplex chronicus with typical lichenification

g. Dyshidrotic eczema
    Bilateral hand and/or foot dermatitis with characteristic tiny vesicles along the sides of fingers or toes with intense itching (Figure 4.8); frequent relapses

h. Juvenile plantar dermatitis ('sweaty sock syndrome')
    Scaling, cracking, fissuring of both plantar feet, especially the big toe (Figure 4.9); spares toewebs

i. Frictional lichenoid dermatitis
    Papular eruption of elbows in patients aged ~4–12 years; discrete 1–2 mm lichenoid skin-colored papules (Figure 4.10); pruritus occasional; considered to be secondary to trauma

j. Autoeczematization ('id' reaction)
    Acute pruritic dermatitis that develops at a site distant from the primary inflammatory focus and is not caused by the primary inciting event; papulovesicular lesions

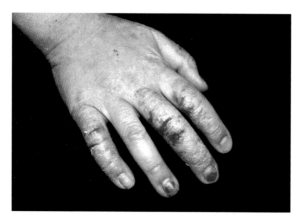

Figure 4.8 Dyshidrotic eczema affecting the hands with tiny, pruritic vesicles

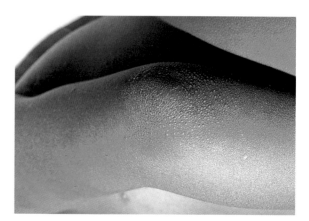

Figure 4.10 Frictional lichenoid dermatitis – lichenoid papules on elbows and knees

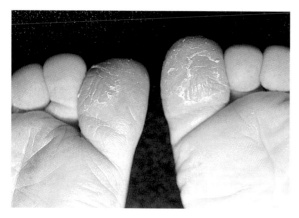

Figure 4.9 Juvenile plantar dermatosis – shiny, glazed toes with scaling

scattered over the body; can evolve into scaly oozing plaques; infection, wounding, or irritation can precipitate; diagnosis of exclusion; example: papular eruption with tinea capitis

Pathogenesis

- Etiology is multifactorial
- Clinical factors:
  1. Primary lesion is subclinical and may be papular or erythematous
  2. Xerosis (dry skin), which most atopic patients have, is caused by reduced water content of the stratum corneum, with decreased secretion of sebum and sweat
     a. Dry, ichthyotic skin may result in loss of epidermal barrier and a higher incidence of irritation from certain stimuli such as wool clothing, soaps, etc
     b. In winter months, in cool climates, or in dry climates, the skin is prone to increased dryness, often causing exacerbations
  3. Vasomotor responses
     a. Unusual reaction patterns such as a tendency to vasoconstriction
     b. White dermatographism is produced by stroking erythematous or normal-appearing skin in an atopic patient. Instead of the stroked area turning red (normal), it turns white, demonstrating vasoconstriction (Figure 4.11)
     c. Facial skin, particularly around the nose, may be pale

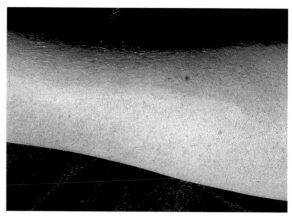

Figure 4.11 White dermatographism – reactive vasoconstriction after stroking the skin in an atopic patient

d. Distal extremities may have a lower skin temperature

4. Sensitivity
   a. Patients are more sensitive to irritation by wool, detergents and certain chemicals
   b. Localization of dermatitis may be a clue to certain irritants (e.g. hand dermatitis in a frequent hand washer)

5. Humoral immunity: elevated IgE levels

6. Cell-mediated immunity
   a. Increased susceptibility to viral infections (herpes simplex, vaccinia, molluscum contagiosum)
   b. Anergy can be demonstrated with increased frequency
   c. Numbers of T helper (Th) >T suppressor (Ts) cells
   d. Chemotactic defects of polymorphonuclear leukocytes and monocytes

- Molecular factors
   1. Keratinocytes primed to react to antigenic stimuli by producing preformed interleukin (IL)-1, followed by more IL-1 produced by endothelial cells and macrophages
   2. Secondary cytokines (tumor necrosis factor (TNF)-α, IL-6, IL-8) are then produced
   3. T lymphocytes bind to endothelial cells and migrate into the dermis and epidermis, producing damage to the epidermal barrier
   4. Antigens are presented to stimulated Langerhans cells
   5. Imbalance of Th2 > Th1 lymphocytes
      a. Th1 cells produce interferon-α, IL-1, IL-2, TNF-β
      b. Th2 cells produce IL-4, IL-5, IL-6, IL-10
   6. Cytokines of Th2 cells are self-amplifying and inhibit Th1 responses
   7. T cells in atopic dermatitis are responsive to IL-4, which suppresses IFN-γ, with subsequent promotion of B-cell proliferation and increased IgE production
   8. IL-4 stimulates mast cells to release histamine
   9. Vicious cycle caused by repeated stimulation, abnormal responses and cytokine release

Diagnosis

- Clinical diagnosis (see Table 4.1)
- Laboratory: no specific laboratory criteria
   1. Allergy testing (prick tests)

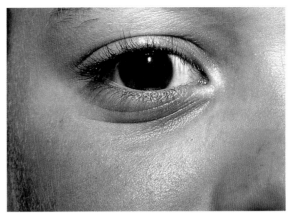

Figure 4.12   Dennie's lines – extra skin folds on lower lid

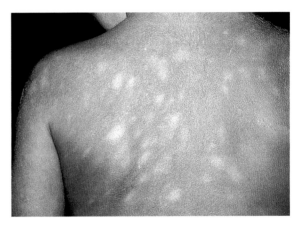

Figure 4.13   Pityriasis alba – hypopigmented slightly scaly patches

   a. Food allergies in minority of patients
   b. Inhalant allergies in some patients
   2. Blood tests
      a. Complete blood count – may see increase in numbers of eosinophils
      b. Serum IgE may be slightly or markedly elevated
      c. Radioallergosorbent test (RAST) may help define some allergies

- Histology: variable spongiosis and lymphocytic infiltration of the upper dermis and epidermis; acanthosis, hyperkeratosis; thick-walled blood vessels in papillary dermis

Differential diagnosis

- Scabies
- Seborrheic dermatitis

- Immunodeficiences
- Langerhans cell histiocytosis
- Acrodermatitis enteropathica
- Psoriasis
- Contact dermatitis
- Phenyketonuria

Treatment

- Eliminate precipitating factors
  1. Bathing can be performed once daily, but excessive bathing causes increased dryness
     a. Apply ointments immediately after patting skin dry
     b. Oils in bath are messy, and make children slippery to handle; may be useful for older children
     c. Tepid temperature is best; avoid very hot water; do not make the water too cool, causing the child to shiver
     d. Soap should be kept to a minimum, and applied only to excessively dirty areas
     e. Superfatted soaps (e.g. Dove®, Tone®) or soapless cleansers (e.g. Cetaphil®, Aquanil®) are best
  2. Excessive sweating, whether heat- or exercise-induced, can cause itching
  3. Temperature extremes (hot and humid, or cold and dry) can increase itching
  4. Avoid coarse or irritating clothing (e.g. wool)
- Emollients are necessary to decrease dryness (which can lead to itching)
- Topical corticosteroids reduce pruritus and inflammation
  1. Hydrocortisone 1% or 2.5% ointment (class 6–7 steroids) for mild inflammation
  2. Mid-strength steroids (class 3–5) (triamcinolone 0.1% ointment) only in isolated areas for young children
  3. High-potency steroids may be indicated for hand or foot dermatitis because of the thickness of the stratum corneum. Be careful to avoid dorsa of hands and feet with high-potency steroids
- Antipruritics
  1. Antihistamines (see Chapter 21)
- Topical tacrolimus 0.03% for children aged 2–15 years BID, or 0.1% for children aged >15 years BID or pimecrolimus 1% for children aged >2 years) BID
- Antibiotics
  1. Antistaphylococcal drugs
     a. Topical agents (e.g. mupirocin) may be helpful for the short term, but some topical antibiotics (e.g. neomycin, bacitracin) can sensitize the skin and cause further allergic contact dermatitis
     b. Oral antibiotics may be given in short courses to reduce staphylococcal infections of the skin
     c. Frequent use of antibiotics can lead to resistant bacteria
- Systemic corticosteroids
  1. Short courses for acute, severe exacerbations may be indicated
  2. Long-term oral steroids are not recommended
- Referral to a dermatologist is recommended for severe and moderately severe cases uncontrolled by standard measures
- Hospitalization is indicated only if not controlled by methods at home
- Consider psychological stresses and counseling if unresponsive to treatment
- For severe, recalcitrant cases consider phototherapy (PUVA, UVB), IFN-γ, or immunosuppressive drugs (e.g. cyclosporine, methotrexate)

Prognosis

- Half of the cases of typical atopic dermatitis improve by 2 years of age
- Most improve by teenage years
- Patients tend to have dry, sensitive skin throughout life
- <10% of patients have lifelong problems

References

Eichenfield LF, Hanifan JM, Luger TA, et al. Consensus conference on pediatric atopic dermatitis. J Am Acad Dermatol 2003; 49: 1088–95

Eichenfield LF, Lucky AW, Boguniewicx M, et al. Safety and efficacy of pimecrolimus (ASM 981) cream 1% in the treatment of mild and moderate atopic dermatitis in children and adolescents. J Am Acad Dermatol 2002; 46: 495–504

Feingold, S, Huang C, Kristol L, et al. Eczemas. Curr Probl Dermatol 1998; 10: 41–92

Hanifin JM, Cooper KD, Ho VC, et al. Guidelines of care for atopic dermatitis. J Am Acad Dermatol 2004; 50: 391–404

Nghiem P, Pearson G, Langley RG. Tacrolimus and pimecrolimus: from clever prokaryotes to inhibiting calcineurin and treating atopic dermatitis. J Am Acad Dermatol 2002; 46: 228–41

Ong PY, Ontake T, Brandt C, et al. Endogenous antimicrobial peptides and skin infections in atopic dermatitis. N Engl J Med 2002; 347: 1151–60

Patel RR, Vander Straten MR, Korman NJ. The safety and efficacy of tacrolimus therapy in patients younger than 2 years with atopic dermatitis. Arch Dermatol 2003; 139: 1184–6

Proceedings of an International Consensus Conference on Atopic Dermatitis. Understanding atopic dermatitis: pathophysiology and etiology. J Am Acad Dermatol 2001: S1–S68

Resnick SD, Hornung R, Konrad TR. A comparison of dermatologists and generalists, management of childhood atopic dermatitis. Arch Dermatol 1996; 132: 1047–52

Ricci G, Patrizi A, Neri I, et al. Frequency and clinical role of Staphylococcus aureus overinfection in atopic dermatitis in children. Pediatr Dermatol 2003; 20: 529–30

Rothe MJ, Grant-Kels JM. Atopic dermatitis, an update. J Am Acad Dermatol 1996; 35: 1–13

KERATOSIS PILARIS

Major points

- Common papular eruption of childhood which tends to continue into adulthood but may improve

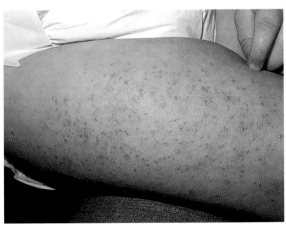

Figure 4.14   Keratosis pilaris – keratotic, follicular, slightly erythematous papules on upper legs

- Prominent follicular plugs over extensor surfaces of extremities, especially upper arms, upper legs, buttocks and cheeks (Figure 4.14)
- Erythema may be seen, especially if the areas have been rubbed or irritated
- Dryness aggravates the condition
- Associated with atopic disorders: atopic dermatitis, hay fever, asthma, allergic rhinitis
- Rarely extensive and generalized
- More common in people of northern European or Celtic ancestry

Pathogenesis

- Cause unknown
- Considered a disorder of keratinization because a keratinous plug is produced by abnormal follicular epithelium
- May be a response to dryness, and is seen more commonly in cold dry climates

Diagnosis

- Clinical presentation

Differential diagnosis

- Acne
- Folliculitis
- Molluscum contagiosum
- Warts
- Milia
- Lichen spinulosus
- Follicular mucinosis

Treatment

- Lubricants or emollients can improve dry skin, especially if applied after a bath or after wetting of the skin
- Topical keratolytics
  1. Lactic acid preparations such as ammonium lactate 5–12% (e.g. LacHydrin®)
  2. Urea creams (e.g. Carmol-20® OTC)
  3. Topical retinoids (e.g. adapalene cream) may be reserved for severe involvement in a patient who is very compliant, as it can actually aggravate dryness and irritation
- Treatment takes time and should be used twice daily for at least a month, except retinoids (used once daily, at bed time) before results can be expected

- Class 6–7 topical steroids may be indicated for inflammation; do not recommend long-term usage, but only for temporarily decreasing irritation

Prognosis

- Chronic condition which responds poorly to treatment. Parents should be educated on what to expect
- During adolescence, lesions on the face may improve
- Improvement may occur in more humid environments

References

Lateef A, Schwartz RA. Keratosis pilaris. Cutis 1999; 63: 205–7

Oranje AP, Van Osch LDM, Oosterwijk JC. Keratosis pilaris atrophicans. Arch Dermatol 1994; 130: 500–2

XEROSIS

Synonyms: winter eczema, erythema cracquele, asteatotic eczema

Major points

- Clinical characteristics
    1. Dryness, scaling (Figure 4.15)
    2. Cracking
    3. Hands or lower legs most frequently involved
    4. Pruritus if severe
    5. Frequently occurs in winter in cool climates
- Physical examination
    1. Superficial reticular cracks in skin appear like a 'dried river bed' (Figure 4.16)
    2. Fissures may be mildly erythematous

Pathogenesis

- Associated with dryness and dehydration of the epidermis
- Low humidity
- Mainly in atopic individuals

Diagnosis

- Clinical characteristics

Differential diagnosis

- Atopic dermatitis
- Contact dermatitis
- Irritant dermatitis
- Ichthyosis vulgaris

Treatment

- Avoid harsh, drying soaps
- Hydration of the stratum corneum with a daily bath with plain water only

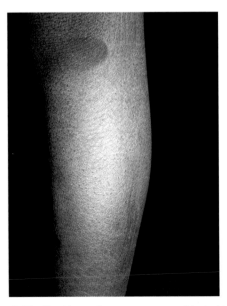

Figure 4.15   Xerosis – ashy appearance on black skin

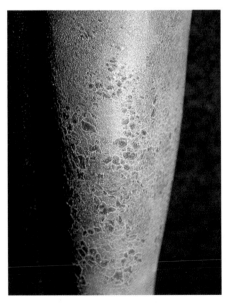

Figure 4.16   Eczema cracquele – extremely dry skin aggravated by soap and water

- Use mild soaps, superfatted soaps (e.g. Dove, Tone, etc.) or non-soaps (e.g. Cetaphil) only where needed (groin, axillae)
- Increase ambient humidity with humidifier in house or child's room
- Emollients should be liberally used (e.g. petroleum jelly, Eucerin®, Aquaphor®)
- Emollients best applied after bath when skin is moist as well as several times a day
- Unscented moisturizers are best in order to avoid contact sensitivity
- Mild topical corticosteroids (0.5–1% hydrocortisone) in ointment base for erythema only

Reference

Hara M, Kikuchi K, Watanabe M, et al. Senile xerosis: functional, morphological, and biochemical studies. J Geriatr Dermatol 1993; 3: 111–20

ECZEMATOUS DERMATITIS WITH IMMUNODEFICIENCIES

Major points

- Eczematous dermatitis associated with immunodeficiencies looks similar to atopic dermatitis, but is usually more severe and does not respond well to therapy
- Dermatitis can be the first sign of:
  1. Wiskott–Aldrich syndrome
  2. Severe combined immunodeficiency
  3. Hyperimmunoglobulin E syndrome
- Characteristics
  1. Generalized, eczematous dermatitis with scaling, erythema, pruritus
  2. Bacterial infections are common (Figure 4.17)
     a. Impetigo
     b. Furuncles
     c. Otitis media
     d. Pneumonia
  3. Fungal infections common
     a. Candidiasis
  4. Diarrhea
  5. Failure to thrive
  6. If a sibling has died after live viral vaccine, this may be a clue
  7. Petechiae – suggests Wiskott–Aldrich syndrome in a male

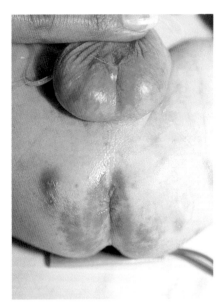

Figure 4.17 Eczematous dermatitis in chronic granulomatous disease with abscess formation

Pathogenesis

See Atopic dermatitis

Diagnosis

- Laboratory
  1. Wiskott–Aldrich syndrome
     a. Deficiency of sialophorin (glycoprotein) on the surface of lymphocytes and platelets
     b. Low or absent antibodies to blood group antigens A and B
     c. Increased IgA and IgE
     d. Decreased IgM
     e. Splenomegaly
     f. Hepatomegaly
     g. Adenopathy
     h. Thrombocytopenia with petechiae and purpura
     i. Defects in cell-mediated immunity
     j. Platelet dysfunction
     k. X-linked recessive
  2. Hyperimmunoglobulin E syndrome (Job syndrome)
     a. Marked elevated serum IgE levels (>10 times normal)
     b. Eosinophilia
     c. Neutrophil chemotaxis abnormal
     d. Sinopulmonary infections

e.   Coarse facial features in some patients

f.   Recurrent staphylococcal infections of skin, lungs, joints, etc.

3. Severe combined immunodeficiency syndrome

a.   Decreased levels of IgG, IgM, IgD, IgA, IgE

b.   Lymphopenia

c.   Defects in cell-mediated immunity

d.   Adenosine deaminase deficiency, and others

Treatment

- Usual treatment for atopic dermatitis with topical steroids, emollients, etc
- Infections should be treated with appropriate antibiotics
- Fresh frozen plasma or whole blood for severe life-threatening illnesses
- Bone marrow transplantation when indicated

References

Arbiser JL. Genetic immunodeficiencies: cutaneous manifestations and recent progress. J Am Acad Dermatol 1995; 33: 82–9

Badour K, Zhang J, Siminovitch KA. The Wiskott–Aldrich syndrome protein: forging the link between actin and cell activation. Immunol Rev 2003; 192: 98–112

Berron-Ruiz A, Berron-Perex R, Ruiz-Maldonado R. Cutaneous markers of primary immunodeficiency diseases in children. Pediatr Dermatol 2000; 17: 91–6

Bonilla FA, Geha RS. 12. Primary immunodeficiency diseases. J Allergy Clin Immunol 2003; 111(Suppl 2): S571–81

Buckley RH. The hyper-IgE syndrome. Clin Rev Allergy Immunol 2001; 20: 139–54

Dave S, Thappa DM, Karthikeyan K. Disseminated and disfiguring molluscum contagiosum in a child. Pediatr Dermatol 2003; 20: 436–9

Erlewyn-Lajeunesse MD. Hyperimmunoglobulin-E syndrome with recurrent infection: a review of current opinion and treatment. Pediatr Allergy Immunol 2000; 11: 133–41

Lindegren ML, Kobrynski L, Rasmussen SA, et al. Applying public health strategies to primary immunodeficiency diseases: a potential approach to genetic disorders. Morbid Mortal Weekly Rep 2004; 53: 1–29

Mueller BJ, Pizzo PA. Cancer in children with primary or secondary imunodeficiencies. J Pediatr 1995; 126: 1–10

Paller AS. Immunodeficiency syndromes. Dermatol Clin 1995; 13: 65–71

Ratko TA, Cummings JP, Blebea J, Matuszewski KA. Clinical gene therapy for nonmalignant disease. Am J Med 2003; 115: 560–9

Rosen FS, Cooper MD, Wedgwood RJP. The primary immunodeficiencies. N Engl J Med 1995; 333: 431–40

Schurman SH, Candotti F. Autoimmunity in Wiskott–Aldrich syndrome. Curr Opin Rheumatol 2003; 15: 446–53

Stewart DM, Tian L, Nelson DL. Linking cellular activation to cytoskeletal reorganization: Wiskott–Aldrich syndrome as a model. Curr Opin Allergy Clin Immunol 2001; 1: 525–33

Thrasher AJ, Burns S, Lorenzi R, Jones GE. The Wiskott–Aldrich syndrome: disordered actin dynamics in haematopoietic cells. Immunol Rev 2000; 178: 118–28

ALLERGIC CONTACT DERMATITIS

Major points

- Characteristics
  1. First exposure does not cause a reaction
  2. Reaction begins 12–96 h after subsequent exposure if already allergic
  3. Lesions can persist up to 3 weeks
  4. Pruritus may vary from mild to severe
- Clinical pattern and shape give clues to offending antigen (Table 4.2)
  1. Linear configuration with sharp borders (Figure 4.18)
  2. Individual lesions are pruritic, erythematous papules or papulovesicles which may become vesicular with oozing, weeping and crusting
  3. Erythema with scaling in chronic cases
  4. Edema may be prominent especially around the face and groin
  5. Urticaria-like eruption can occur
  6. Heat, sweating and friction accentuate the reaction
- Major causes in childhood
  1. *Toxicodendron* – poison ivy/oak/sumac (Figure 4.19)
     a.   Most common allergic contact dermatitis in the USA
     b.   Sensitizing substance is an oleoresin called urushiol
     c.   Typical lesions in spring, summer, fall
     d.   Pruritic, erythematous streaks with vesicles are typical
     e.   Erythematous patches, papules can occur

Table 4.2   Contact dermatitis history

1. Determine the onset – exact time and location of appearance of lesions
2. Course of dermatitis – progression, recurrence, remission
3. Topical medicines used
4. Previous therapy and response
5. Work exposure – relation to work, days off, vacation, duties
6. Other persons having similar dermatitis
7. Hobbies – chemical exposure
8. Topical cosmetics – perfumes, soaps, sunscreens, toothpaste, nail polish, hair dyes, etc.
9. Plant exposure – poison ivy, chrysanthemums, weeds, etc.
10. Chemical exposure – work and home
11. Water exposure – hand washing, job-related
12. Clothing history – underwear, jewelry, watches, earrings, belts, snaps
13. Atopic history – asthma, eczema, personal and/or family history
14. Immune status

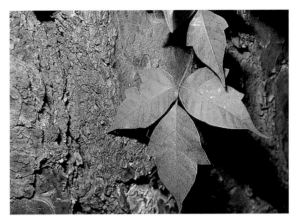

Figure 4.19   Poison ivy plant – leaves of three, let them be

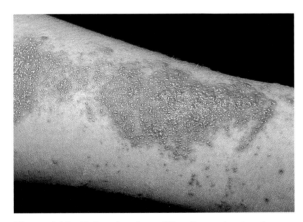

Figure 4.18   Poison ivy dermatitis – linear streaks of vesicles and erythema

2. Nickel
   a. Common in children who wear earrings for pierced ears, metal belt buckles, metal zippers, metal snaps, or metal buttons
   b. Erythema, scaling, crusting and pruritus on earlobes from earrings or around umbilicus

from snaps or belt buckles (Figure 4.20 and 4.21)
   c. Infants may have involvement from snaps on undershirts
3. Rubber/adhesives, causes:
   a. Antioxidants: paraphenylenediamine, hydroquinone
   b. Accelerators: mercaptobenzathiazole, thiuram, carbamate
4. Shoe dermatitis – acute or subacute dermatitis on dorsal feet (Figure 4.22); toewebs spared, causes:
   a. Rubber (most common)
   b. Chromates (in leather)
   c. Glutaraldehyde (in leather)
   d. Adhesives
   e. Dyes
5. Adhesive tape dermatitis caused by rubber or colophony: well-demarcated area where adhesive tape is applied
6. Cosmetics
   a. Acute or subacute (may require detective work)
   b. Parabens
   c. Perfumes – can be generalized or localized
   d. Deodorants – in axillae
   e. Nail lacquers – may see reaction around the eyes from zlacquer which was not completely dried and patient rubbed the eyelids
   f. Eye products
   g. Lipstick – rim of erythema around lips

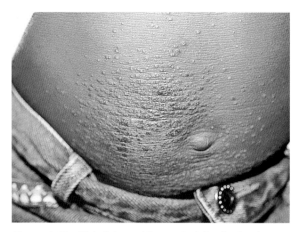

Figure 4.20 Nickel dermatitis – typical distribution from a snap on the pants or belt buckle

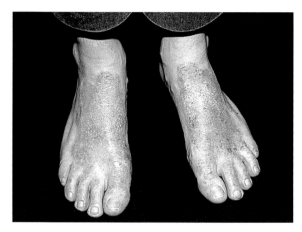

Figure 4.22 Shoe dermatitis – typical distribution on dorsal feet

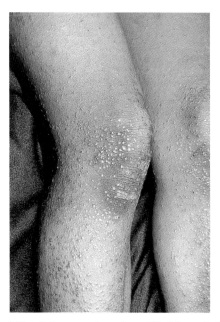

Figure 4.21 Autoeczematous dermatitis 'id reaction' – generalized eczematous changes from nickel dermatitis

7. Formaldehyde – used in clothing (permanent-press fabric finishes); periaxillary area
8. Benzocaine – over-the-counter (OTC) topical anesthetics
9. Caines/diphenhydramine (e.g. Benadryl®) – topical anesthetics
10. Neomycin – topical antibiotics; increased sensitivity if applied to broken skin
11. Mercury – e.g. Merthiolate®, Mercurochrome®

Pathogenesis

- Delayed-type hypersensitivity reaction (type IV)
  1. Afferent (induction) phase (5–25 days)
  2. First contact; allergen penetrates skin and acts as hapten, binding to skin proteins
  3. Helper T cells activated
  4. Langerhans cells recognize antigen as nonself and present it to T lymphocytes
  5. Langerhans cells with hapten move from epidermis to lymph nodes
  6. Naïve T cells differentiate into clones of effector cells directed at foreign antigen
  7. Results in committed sensitized T cells reactive to specific antigen
- Elicitation reaction (24–48 hours)
  1. Re-exposure results in accumulation of effector cells which produce numerous cytokines (e.g. IFN-γ, TNF, etc.) and mediators which result in dermatitis in areas limited to skin contact

Diagnosis

- Laboratory – not indicated. Refer to dermatologist for evaluation if diagnosis unclear
- Skin patch tests (T.R.U.E. tests) (Tables 4.3 and 4.4)
  1. Helpful for difficult cases
  2. Patches applied to normal nonhairy skin (back or upper arms) for 48 h; read at 72 h and 5 days
  3. False-positive reactions often seen in atopic patients

Table 4.3   Patch testing T.R.U.E. Test (Glaxo Dermatology)

Standard allergens	Found in:
1. Nickel sulfate	Jewelry, belt buckles, eyeglass frames, alloys, orthopedic appliances, money, scissors, eating utensils
2. Wool alcohols	Cosmetics, creams, lotions, ointments, soaps (cross-reacts with lanolin)
3. Neomycin sulfate	Topical antibiotics, first-aid creams, eardrops, nosedrops
4. Potassium dichromate	Tanning solutions for leather, cement, photography solutions, paints, glues, pigments and some detergents
5. Caine mix	Topical anesthetics
6. Fragrance mix	Toiletries, soaps, perfumes, shampoo, scented products, industrial cutting fluids
7. Colophony (rosin)	Used by violinists, ball players, bowlers; in cosmetics, adhesives, lacquers, varnishes, paper and industrial products
8. Epoxy resin	Uncured epoxy resin, nail products
9. Quinolone mix	Topical antimicrobial medicated creams, medicated bandages and veterinary products
10. Balsam of Peru	Perfumes, flavoring in drinks, tobacco, topical medications, dental agents
11. Ethylenediamine dihydrochloride	Stabilizer for some creams; found in rubber, color photography solutions, epoxy catalyst systems and some antifreeze solutions (cross-reacts with hydroxyzine, aminophylline)
12. Cobalt dichloride	Some paints, cement, metal, metal-plated objects
13. *Para-tert* butylphenol formaldehyde resin	Leather finishes (shoes), paper fabrics, furniture, glues
14. Paraben mix	Preservative in numerous creams, cosmetics, industrial oils, glues
15. Carba mix	Rubber, rubber glues, vinyl, pesticides
16. Black rubber mix	Rubber antioxidant, hair dyes
17. Cl+Me– Isothiazolinone	Preservative found in cosmetics, medications, household cleaning products, industrial fluids and greases
18. Quaternium 15	Stabilizer, formaldehyde releaser found in cosmetics, creams, lotions
19. Mercaptobenzothiazole	Shoes, rubber accelerator, antifreeze, cutting oils, flea and mosquito repellants
20. Paraphenylenediamine	Hair dyes, inks, photodevelopers, textile dyes
21. Formaldehyde	Clothes, textiles, preservatives, disinfectants, dental plastics, glues, nail polishes, adhesives, shampoo Formaldehyde releasers: Quaternium 15, imiadiazoyl urea, Bronopol
22. Mercapto mix	Rubber, glues, coolants, industrial products
23. Thimerosal	Preservative in vaccines, contact lens solutions, eye cosmetics, nose and ear drops
24. Thiuram mix	Rubber, disinfectant, lubricating oils, fungicide

Table 4.4   Patch test materials/nickel detection kits can be ordered

Glaxo Dermatology (T.R.U.E. Test)
5 Moore Drive
Research Triangle Park, NC 27709, USA
www.truetest.com/

Hermal Pharmaceutical Laboratories, Inc.
Route 145
Oak Hill, NY 12460, USA
(518) 475-0175
www.hermal.de/english/index.html

Allerderm Labs Inc.
28 Glen Drive
Mill Valley, CA 94941, USA
(415) 381-0106
www.allerderm.com

- Histology:
  1. Multilocular intraepidermal spongiotic vesicles
  2. Eosinophils in dermis and epidermis
  3. Langerhans cells in the epidermis associated with lymphocytes
  4. Immunohistochemical studies show primarily memory T-helper lymphocytes, although T-suppressor cells can be noted
- Nickel detection kit: dimethylglyoxime in a 10% aqueous solution of ammonia – turns pink on contact with nickel (see Table 4.4)

Differential diagnosis

- Atopic dermatitis
- Irritant contact dermatitis
- Autoeczematization

Treatment

- Avoidance of contactant
  1. Education
  2. Give patients a list of objects or products which contain allergens
  3. Wash skin with plain water if known allergen is contacted
- Acute dermatitis with oozing and weeping, vesicles or bullae
  1. Compresses with Burrow's solution (e.g. Domeboro®, Blurobor®) for 15 min
  2. Apply shaken lotion of calamine three times a day for drying effect

3. Avoid topical diphenhydramine or caines which are added to some products
4. Topical corticosteroids
   a. Medium to ultra-potent steroids (class 1–4) for about 5–7 days used two or three times a day then taper to lowest strength to keep erythema and itching under control
5. Oral antipruritics (see doses in Chapter 21), diphenhydramine (Benadryl), hydroxyzine (Atarax®), cetirizine (Zyrtec®), fexofenadine (Allegra®)
6. Systemic corticosteroids
   a. Oral prednisone 0.5–2 mg/kg per day tapered over 10–21 days for widespread or severe involvement
   b. Barrier creams: Stokogard® (OTC)–linoleic acid dimer, Hollister Moisture Barrier Ointment® (OTC by Hollister Inc., Libertyville® IL) and Theraseal®

Prognosis

- Most patients recover from acute hypersensitivity in 14–21 days
- Hyposensitization injections not effective and may be unsafe
- Oral hyposensitization used mainly for workers in forest industry who cannot avoid contact with toxicodendrons (of questionable value)
- Wash skin and clothes with water and soap immediately after contact
- Most contact allergens bind to the epidermis and set up response within 0.5–2 h of contact
- Chronic exposure to allergens such as rubber, perfumes, preservatives which are not obvious, would benefit from patch testing by a dermatologist skilled in this technique

References

Bourke J, Coulson I, English J. Guidelines for care of contact dermatitis. Br J Dermatol 2001; 145: 877–85

Drake LA, Dorner W, Goltz RW, et al. Guidelines of care for contact dermatitis. J Am Acad Dermatol 1995: 32: 109–13

Mallory SB. The pediatric patient. In Practical Contact Dermatitis. Guin JD, ed. McGraw-Hill, 1995: 603–21

Maouad M, Fleischer AB, Sherertz EF, Feldman SR. Significance–prevalence index number: a reinterpretation and enhancement of data from the North American Contact Dermatitis Group. J Am Acad Dermatol 1999; 41: 573–6

Sharma V, Beyer DJ, Paruthi S, Nopper AJ. Prominent pruritic periumbilical papules: allergic contact dermatitis to nickel. Pediatr Dermatol 2002; 19: 106–9

Silverberg NB, Licht J, Friedler S, et al. Nickel contact hypersensitivity in children. Pediatr Dermatol 2002; 19: 110–13

Wildemore JK, Junkins-Hopkins JM, James WD. Evaluation of the histologic characteristics of patch test confirmed allergic contact dermatitis. J Am Acad Dermatol 2003; 49: 243–8

IRRITANT CONTACT DERMATITIS

Major points

- In general, all people will react to an irritant if applied in a high enough concentration
  1. People with atopic dermatitis are more susceptible to irritant dermatitis, especially in dry climates
  2. Skin of infants can redden quickly when irritated
- Characteristic erythematous, pruritic patches and plaques with ill-defined borders
- Common causes:
  1. Hands repeatedly exposed to water, cleansers, or soaps show fissuring or a 'glazed' appearance (Figure 4.23)
  2. Bubble baths, bleaches, detergents, solvents, acids, alkalis
  3. Lip-licking habit – wetting and drying caused by saliva
  4. Thumb-suckers in toddlers
  5. Perioral area in babies – foods, dribbling saliva and rubbing the area
  6. Diaper area secondary to multiple factors such as wetting, maceration, urine, feces
- Severe forms: chemical burns (alkalis, acids) with vesiculation, necrosis, or ulceration
- Chronic irritant dermatitis usually lacks vesicles and is characterized by dryness and chapping

Pathogenesis

- Wetting and drying causes decreased lipids in the epidermis with a resultant break in the epidermal barrier
- Occurs more commonly in atopic patients

Diagnosis

- Clinical findings

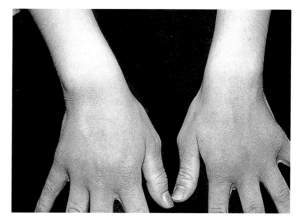

Figure 4.23   Irritant contact dermatitis – caused by excessive hand washing

- Histology: mild to moderate epidermal spongiosis; epidermal necrosis; usually does not contain eosinophils (as in allergic causes); perivascular lymphocytes and neutrophils

Differential diagnosis

- Atopic dermatitis
- Allergic contact dermatitis

Treatment

- Avoid offending agents
- Occlusive pastes (zinc oxide paste) or barrier creams (e.g. Desitin®)
- Emollients (e.g. petrolatum)
- Steroids of low to moderate potency

Prognosis

- Benign condition but usually reappears if same circumstances occur

References

Weedon D. Skin Pathology. Churchill Livingstone: New York, 1997: 88–9

DIAPER DERMATITIS

Major points

- Irritant diaper dermatitis (chafing dermatitis)
  1. Involves convex surfaces of buttocks, upper thighs, abdomen (Figure 4.24)

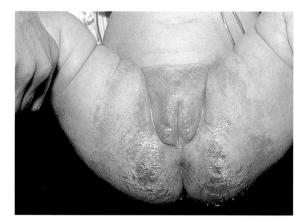

Figure 4.24 Diaper dermatitis (irritant) – caused by infrequent diaper changes

a. Spares inguinal folds
b. Common between 7 and 12 months of age
2. Ulcerative form
   a. Marked erythema
   b. Shallow or deep ulcers (Jacquet ulcers) (Figure 4.25)
   c. Most frequent around perianal area
   d. Commonly follows diarrhea
- *Candida albicans* dermatitis
  1. Beefy-red, confluent erythema (Figure 4.28)
  2. Involves inguinal creases

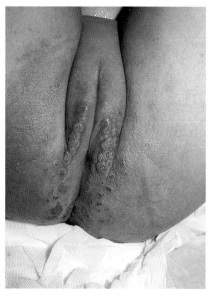

Figure 4.25 Jacquet ulcers – caused by chronic moisture in an incontinent child

3. Satellite red papules or pustules at the periphery are common
4. Frequently occurs after diaper dermatitis has lasted >72 h
5. KOH: budding yeast and pseudohyphae
6. Commonly seen with thrush (oral candidiasis)
- Seborrheic dermatitis
  1. Involves inguinal folds (Figure 4.26)
  2. Yellowish-pink scale
  3. Cradle cap can be prominent on scalp and a clue to correct diagnosis (Figure 4.27)
  4. Typical lesions present elsewhere

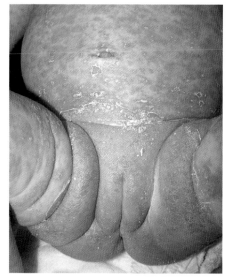

Figure 4.26 Seborrheic dermatitis – erythematous scaling in the diaper area

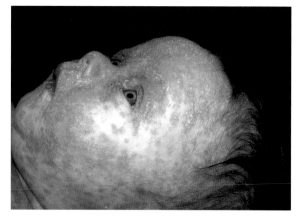

Figure 4.27 Seborrheic dermatitis – erythematous scaling on the face

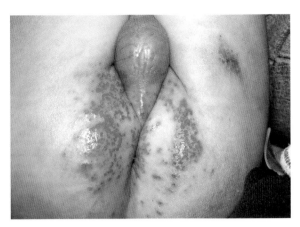

Figure 4.28 Candidal diaper dermatitis – satellite erythematous papules

Pathogenesis

- Moisture, maceration, occlusion and possibly *Candida* and bacteria play a role, causing damage to the epidermis
- Elevation in pH of skin allows fecal lipases and proteases to further irritate skin

Diagnosis

Clinical presentation

Differential diagnosis

- Langerhans cell histiocytosis
- Atopic dermatitis
- Immunodeficiencies
  1. HIV – uncommon presentation with granulomatous component
  2. Severe combined immunodeficiency – usually generalized, eczematous eruption
- Psoriasis
- Bullous impetigo
- Granuloma gluteale infantum

Treatment

- Remove contactants (urine and feces)
- Eliminate wetness and maceration
  1. Frequent diaper changes with absorptive gel disposable diapers
  2. Air dry if possible
  3. Change diapers in middle of night so baby does not sleep all night with wet diapers
- Protective maintenance with barrier creams can be used once dermatitis has cleared

- Minimize irritants
  1. Use water with or without mild soap
  2. Avoid diaper wipes which may contain alcohol, propylene glycol or perfumes
  3. Use soft washcloth or soft paper towel for cleaning
- Candidal infections
  1. Topical antifungal therapy (e.g. nystatin, miconazole, ketoconazole, clotrimazole) with every diaper change until clear
- Erythema
  1. Hydrocortisone cream or ointment 1%, 3–4 times a day until clear (usually <7 days)
  2. Avoid steroids stronger than class 7 in diaper area

References

Berg RW, Milligan MC, Sarbaugh FC. Association of skin wetness and pH with diaper dermatitis. Pediatr Dermatol 1994; 11: 18–20

Janniger CK, Thomas I. Diaper dermatitis: an approach to prevention employing effective diaper care. Cutis 1993; 52: 153–5

Jordan WE, Lawson KD, Berg RW, et al. Diaper dermatitis: frequency and severity among a general infant population. Pediatr Dermatol 1986; 3: 198–207

Singalavanija S, Frieden IJ. Diaper dermatitis. Pediatr Review 1995; 16: 142–7

Sires UI, Mallory SB. Diaper dermatitis. Postgraduate Med 1995; 98: 79–86

Wilson PA, Dallas MJ. Diaper performance: maintenance of healthy skin. Pediatr Dermatol 1990; 7: 179–84

SEBORRHEIC DERMATITIS

Major points

- Age:
  1. Infancy: usually begins 4–6 weeks of age with cradle cap (Figure 4.27)
  2. Adolescents: dry, fine, flaky desquamation of scalp, mid-face and eyebrows (Figure 4.29)
- Location:
  1. Scalp, mid-face, mid-chest, perineum
  2. Less common areas: forehead, anterior chest, axillae, umbilicus, intertriginous areas
  3. Facial involvement in adolescents along nasolabial folds

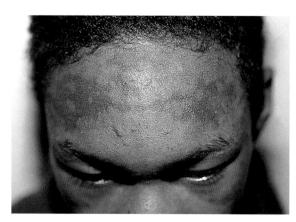

Figure 4.29 Seborrheic dermatitis – in a teenager, often seen on the central face

4. Lesions have greasy, yellowish scale with slightly salmon-colored, erythematous base which can be easily removed
5. Blepharitis – erythema and scaling along lid margins
6. Pruritus slight or absent
7. Persistent recalcitrant seborrhea may be early sign in HIV infection
8. Rare cause of erythroderma in infants

Pathogenesis

- Mechanism unknown
- Excess sebum accumulation
- Increased quantities of *Pityrosporum ovale* (*Malessezia furfur*) are seen in sites of seborrheic dermatitis and may contribute to the disorder

Diagnosis

- Clinical features are typical
- Histology: parakeratosis of the follicular infundibulum; perifollicular collections of neutrophils and lymphocytes in stratum corneum; acanthosis with mild to moderate spongiosis

Differential diagnosis

- Atopic dermatitis
- Contact dermatitis
- Psoriasis
- Dermatophyte infection
- Langerhans cell histiocytosis
- Scabies
- Immunodeficiency diseases (severe combined immunodeficiency, HIV infection)

- Tinea capitis
- Rosacea
- *Candida* infection
- Systemic lupus erythematosus

Treatment

- Low-potency topical steroid creams (class 5–7) twice a day, usually necessary for <7 days
- Shampoos
    1. Keratolytic tar shampoos – sulfur or salicylic acid (e.g. T-gel®)
    2. Zinc pyrithione (e.g. Head & Shoulders®)
    3. Selenium sulfide 2.5% shampoo (e.g. Selsun®)
    4. 2% ketoconazole shampoo (e.g. Nizoral®)
- Mineral oil in scalp for a few hours then shampoo and scrub with soft brush
- Blepharitis – warm compresses, non-irritating baby shampoo, mechanical removal of scales, topical sulfacetamide ointment (e.g. Sulamyd®)
- Topical antifungal agents BID (e.g. Micatin®, Lotrimin®)

Prognosis

- Usually clears with topical corticosteroids, but tends to recur

References

Heng MCY, Henderson CL, Barker DC, Haberfelde G. Correlation of Pityrosporum ovale density with clinical severity of seborrheic dermatitis as assessed by a simplified technique. J Am Acad Dermatol 1990; 23: 82–6

Mimouni K, Mukamel M, Zeharia A, Mimouni M. Prognosis of infantile seborrheic dermatitis. J Pediatr 1995; 127: 744–6

Tollesson A, Frithz A, Berg A, Karlman G. Essential fatty acids in infantile seborrheic dermatitis. J Am Acad Dermatol 1993; 28: 957–61

Williams ML. Differential diagnosis of seborrheic dermatitis. Pediatr Review 1986; 7: 204–11

INTERTRIGO

Major points

- Superficial inflammatory dermatitis which occurs in skin folds where there is apposition of the skin (e.g. folds of the neck of infants or axillae)
- Skin develops well-demarcated erythematous, macerated patches which are often secondarily

infected with *Candida* or bacteria (e.g. streptococci) (Figure 4.30)

- Obesity, diabetes, immunosuppression are predisposing factors

Pathogenesis

- Caused by friction, heat and moisture
- May be a form of seborrheic dermatitis

Diagnosis

- Clinical appearance is typical
- KOH prep shows budding yeast and pseudohyphae
- Culture may demonstrate *Candida*

Differential diagnosis

See Seborrheic dermatitis

Treatment

- Eliminate causes of maceration (e.g. obesity)
- Keep skin dry with air drying and dusting powders (not in infants because of inhalation)
- For inflammation, hydrocortisone 1% cream TID
- For secondary infection with *Candida*, a topical antifungal agent TID (e.g. clotrimazole, miconazole)
- For secondary bacterial infections: oral antibiotics or topical mupirocin

Prognosis

- Excellent if skin apposition decreases

References

Garcia Hidalgo L. Dermatological complications of obesity. Am J Clin Dermatol 2002; 3: 497–506

Honig PJ, Frieden IJ, Kim HJ, Yan AC. Streptococcal intertrigo: an underrecognized condition in children. Pediatrics 2003; 112: 1427–9

LICHEN STRIATUS

Major points

- Self-limited, unilateral, asymptomatic, linear dermatitis which is sudden in onset
- Linear, shiny, hypopigmented or erythematous papules which occur in streaks following lines of Blaschko (Figure 4.31)
- May have fine scale on surface or hypopigmented papules

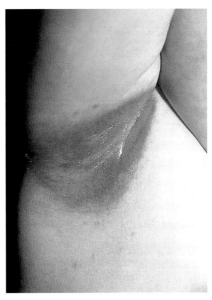

Figure 4.30   Intertrigo – erythema and maceration in the axilla

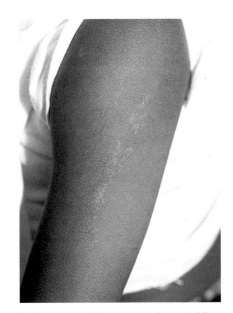

Figure 4.31   Lichen striatus – hypopigmented linear papules following Blaschko lines

- Usually limited to one extremity, but can affect the face
- Asymptomatic
- Common in ages 2–12 years; more common in girls
- Starts proximally and spreads distally in a linear fashion

- Lesions last 3 months to 3 years (mean 9 months), then flatten and resolve

Pathogenesis

- Unknown etiology

Diagnosis

- Clinical characteristics are typical
- Histology: lichenoid dermatitis limited to 3–4 dermal papillae with perieccrine lymphoctyic involvement
- Skin biopsy is rarely indicated

Differential diagnosis

- Epidermal nevus
- Lichen nitidus
- Contact dermatitis
- Lichen planus
- Psoriasis
- Gianotti–Crosti syndrome
- Porokeratosis
- Verruca plana

Therapy

- Treatment usually unnecessary
- Low-strength topical steroids (class 5–7) may be beneficial to hasten resolution
- Patient education as to course of the disease

Prognosis

- Spontaneous resolution

References

Kennedy D, Rogers M. Lichen striatus. Pediatr Dermatol 1996; 13: 95–99

Patrizi A, Neri I, Fiorentini C, et al. Simultaneous occurrence of lichen striatus in siblings. Pediatr Dermatol 1997; 14: 293–5

Tosti A, Peluso AM, Misciali C, Cameli N. Nail lichen striatus: clinical features and long-term follow-up of five patients. J Am Acad Dermatol 1997; 36: 908–13

ACROPUSTULOSIS OF INFANCY

Major points

- Seen most commonly in 15–18-month old Black male infants
- Presents as pustules or vesicles on palms and soles or along sides of hands and feet (Figure 4.32)
- May be present at birth but more common in infancy
- Occurs in recurrent crops until 2–3 years of age
- Extremely pruritic
- Pustules resolve with scale and hyperpigmentation
- Cultures of the pustules are sterile

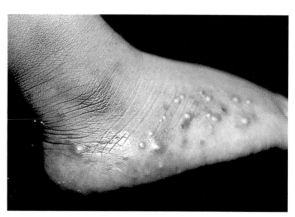

Figure 4.32 Acropustulosis of infancy – typical intensely pruritic papules and pustules along the sides of the feet

Pathogenesis

- Cause unknown

Diagnosis

- Clinical presentation, rule out other disorders (e.g. scabies)

Differential diagnosis

- Scabies
- Dyshidrotic eczema
- Contact dermatitis

Treatment

- Moderate potency topical steroids (class 3–6) two or three times a day during outbreaks
- Oral antihistamines: hydroxyzine, diphenhydramine
- If no relief from the above therapy, refer to a dermatologist

Prognosis

- Eruption lasts several months to several years, slowly becoming less symptomatic, then abates

References

Braun-Falco M, Stachowitz S, Schnopp C, et al. Infantile acropustulosis successfully controlled with topical corticosteroids under damp tubular retention bandages. Acta Dermato-Venereologica 2001; 81: 140–1

Dorton DW, Kaufmann M. Palmoplantar pustules in an infant. Acropustulosis of infancy. Arch Dermatol 1996; 132: 1365–6

Dromy R, Raz A, Metsker A. Infantile acropustulosis. Pediatr Dermatol 1991; 8: 284–7

Mancini AJ, Frieden IJ, Paller AS. Infantile acropustulosis revisited: history of scabies and response to topical corticosteroids. Pediatr Dermatol 1998; 15: 337–41

Prendiville JS. Infantile acropustulosis – how often is it a sequela of scabies? Pediatr Dermatol 1995; 12: 275–6

Wagner A. Distinguishing vesicular and pustular disorders in the neonate. Curr Opin Pediatr 1997; 9: 396–405

5

ACNE AND ACNEIFORM DISORDERS

Early-onset acne

Major points

- Neonatal acne (neonatal cephalic pustulosis)
  1. Inflammatory papules on cheeks, face and scalp in first 2–3 weeks of life (Figure 5.1)
  2. No associated comedones
- Infantile acne
  1. Onset prior to 2 years of age
  2. Male/female ratio >1
  3. Facial involvement only
  4. No identifiable underlying endocrine abnormality

5. Resolves without treatment
- Prepubertal acne
  1. Onset after 2 years of age
  2. Male/female ratio <1
  3. Facial, chest, back involvement (Figure 5.2)
  4. Uncommon underlying endocrinopathy; only noted when other signs of virilization are also present

Pathogenesis

- Considered to be caused by androgen excess or sensitivity to androgens
- An enlarged zona reticularis in the fetal adrenal gland produces increased levels of dehydroepiandrosterone (DHEA) and dehydroepiandrosterone sulfate (DHEAS) until 6 months of age
- Testosterone production from the male gonads is also increased until 12 months of age

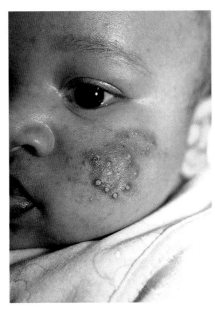

Figure 5.1 Neonatal acne – grouped papules, pustules and comedones at 2 months of age

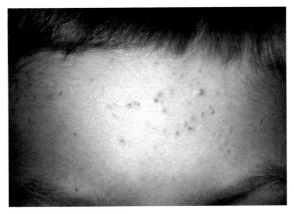

Figure 5.2 Childhood acne in a 6-year-old boy without evidence of androgen excess

Diagnosis

- Clinical examination
- If severe, signs of virilization or rapid growth, a work-up for an underlying endocrine disorder should be pursued
- Hand X-ray for bone age is a good screening evaluation

Differential diagnosis

- Miliaria rubra
- Neonatal cephalic pustulosis

Treatment

- Varies depending on the severity and risk for scarring
- Topical retinoids (e.g. adapalene)
- Topical antibiotics (e.g. benzoyl peroxide or erythromycin)
- Systemic antibiotics (e.g. erythromycin)
- Systemic isotretinoin (rarely needed)

Prognosis

- Neonatal and infantile types often resolve spontaneously without treatment
- Prepubertal subset has a higher risk of scarring and often requires treatment
- Higher incidence and increased severity of adolescent acne vulgaris
- Monitor for development of endocrine abnormality

References

Chew EW, Bingham A, Burrows D. Incidence of acne vulgaris in patients with infantile acne. Clin Exp Dermatol 1990; 15: 376–7

Cunliffe WJ, Baron SE, Coulson IH. A clinical and therapeutic study of 29 patients with infantile acne. Br J Dermatol 2001; 145: 463–6

Lucky AW. A review of infantile and pediatric acne. Dermatology 1998; 196: 95–7

Acne vulgaris

Major points

- Most prevalent skin disorder in pediatrics
  1. Affects 40% of children aged 8–10 years
  2. Affects 85% of adolescents aged 15–17 years
- Lesion types:
  1. Comedones: obstructive lesions
     a. Microcomedone: microscopic plugging of the hair follicle that is the precursor lesion to acne vulgaris
     b. Open comedone (blackhead): plugging at the follicular opening; cellular plug of stratum corneum with oxidized melanin within the follicle (Figure 5.3)

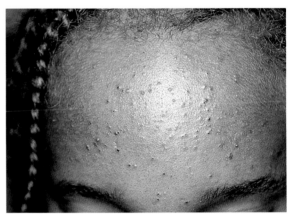

Figure 5.3   Comedonal acne – on forehead with open and closed comedones

     c. Closed comedone (whitehead): plugging of the pilosebaceous unit just below the follicular opening with cystic swelling of the duct; filled with cellular debris
  2. Inflamatory lesions: papules, pustules, cysts, sinus tracts (Figures 5.4–5.6)
  3. Scars: depressed, pitted, macular, papular, hypertrophic, keloidal
- Acne is one of the earliest stages of adrenarche
- Lesion type often correlates with pubertal stage
  1. Comedonal acne is predominant type in prepubertal children
  2. Inflammatory acne is more prevalent in adolescents
- Develops in areas with high numbers of pilosebaceous units: face, chest, back
- Increased severity often predicted by earlier onset and positive family history of scarring acne

Pathogenesis

- Acne development is a complex process that involves four main contributing factors

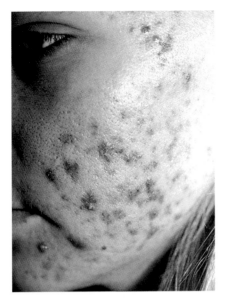

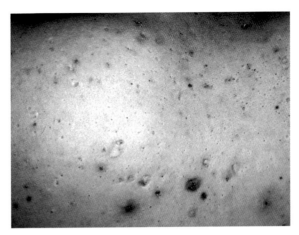

Figure 5.6 Inflammatory acne with comedones, erythematous papules and nodules on the back of a teenager

Figure 5.4 Papulopustular acne – numerous erythematous papules and pustules on the face

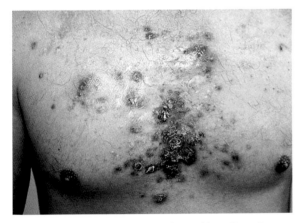

Figure 5.5 Cystic acne on the chest with erythematous nodules, crusts and scarring

1. Abnormal keratinization and obstruction of the pilosebaceous unit
   a. Initial lesion is a microcomedone; caused by obstruction of the follicular opening with the accumulation of cellular debris
   b. Obstruction is due to abnormal keratinization of the cells lining the follicle with delayed shedding and increased cohesiveness
2. Hormonal stimulation and increased sebum production

   a. Increased secretion and accumulation of sebum within the follicle which is stimulated by increased adrenal and gonadal androgens that occur with adrenache
   b. Polycystic ovary syndrome, a heterogeneous disorder with altered gonadotropin secretion, hyperandrogenism (acne, hirsutism and virilization), chronic anovulation, obesity and insulin resistance
3. Bacterial overgrowth
   a. *Propionibacterium acnes* overgrows within the dilated follicle
   b. Bacterial lipases convert accumulated sebum triglycerides into free fatty acids that cause inflammation
   c. *P. acnes* also releases other proteolytic enzymes and chemotactic factors that further stimulate inflammation and recruitment of polymorphonuclear cells (PMNs)
4. Inflammatory reaction
   a. Inflammatory cells including PMNs are recruited to the area
   b. Ingestion of bacteria by PMNs causes release of hydrolytic enzymes that causes rupture of the follicular wall
   c. This leads to intense inflammation and a surrounding foreign body reaction

Diagnosis

- Clinical findings

Differential diagnosis

- Drug-induced acne
- Chemical-induced acne
- Rosacea
- Gram-negative folliculitis
- Pityrosporum folliculitis

Treatment

- Topical retinoids: important for normalizing keratinization (e.g. tretinoin, adapalene)
- Topical keratolytics: salicylic acid, azelaic acid
- Topical benzoyl peroxide preparations
- Topical antibiotics: clindamycin, erythromycin
- Systemic antibiotics for inflammatory lesions
  1. Doxycycline, tetracycline and minocycline most commonly used in those >9 years of age
- Systemic retinoids for severe cystic acne or early scarring
- Oral contraceptives

Prognosis

- Can have significant impact on social interactions and self-esteem and can lead to depression in severe cases
- May produce significant scarring in inflammatory and cystic lesions
- Can rarely be associated with an underlying endocrine disorder

References

Cunliffe WJ, Holand DB, Clark SM, Stable GI. Comedogenesis: some new aetiological, clinical and therapeutic strategies. Br J Dermatol 2000; 142: 1084–91

Harper JC, Thiboutot DM. Pathogenesis of acne: recent research advances. Adv Dermatol 2003; 19: 1–10

Lee DJ, VanDyke GS, Kim J. Update on pathogenesis and treatment of acne. Curr Opin Pediatr 2003; 15: 405–10

Leyden JJ. A review of the use of combination therapies for the treatment of acne vulgaris. J Am Acad Dermatol 2003; 49: S200–10

Lucky AW, Biro FM, Simbartl LA, et al. Predictors of severity of acne vulgaris in young adolescent girls: results of a five-year longitudinal study. J Pediatr 1997; 130: 30–9

Weiss JS. Current options for topical treatment of acne vulgaris. Pediatr Dermatol 1997; 14: 480–8

Drug-induced acne

Major points

- Acneiform eruption precipitated by medication
- Associated drugs: adrenocorticotropic hormone, systemic corticosteroids (Figure 5.7), topical steroids under occlusion (Figure 5.8), androgens, anticonvulsants (e.g. phenytoin, phenobarbital), lithium, isoniazid, bromide and iodides

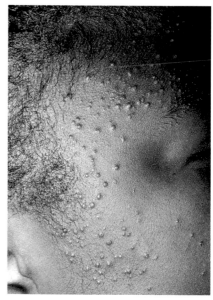

Figure 5.7   Acne aggravated by steroids with multiple pustules arising simultaneously

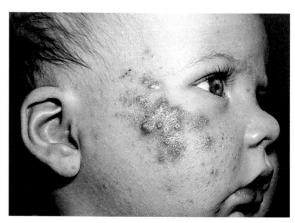

Figure 5.8   Acne in an infant caused by potent topical steroids on the face

- Medications can be the sole cause of an acneiform eruption or can exacerbate underlying acne vulgaris
- Drug-induced lesions are typically monomorphic, papulopustular and diffuse, involving the shoulders and upper arms
- Comedones are typically absent

Pathogenesis

- Variable, depending on drug; steroids affect keratinization, while androgens stimulate sebaceous gland activity

Diagnosis

- Clinical examination and history

Differential diagnosis

- Acne vulgaris
- Folliculitis

Treatment

- Discontinuation or tapering of offending agent if possible
- Topical agents (e.g. benzoyl peroxide, antibiotics)
- Oral antibiotics

Prognosis

- Typically resolves without residua after discontinuation of the causative agent

References

Guillot B. Adverse skin reactions to inhaled corticosteroids. Expert Opin Drug Saf 2002; 1: 325–9

Shaw JC. Acne: effect of hormones on pathogenesis and management. Am J Clin Dermatol 2002; 3: 571–8

Perioral dermatitis

Synonym: periorificial dermatitis

Major points

- Common acneiform eruption in children
- Presents with erythema, scaling, skin-colored papules and pinpoint pustules around the mouth with sparing of the vermillion border (Figures 5.9 and 5.10)
- Granulomatous lesions can involve the entire face, and be concentrated in perioral, perinasal,

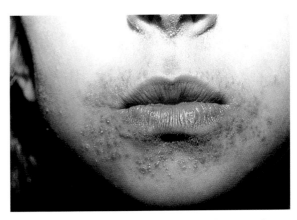

Figure 5.9 Perioral dermatitis – with acneiform papules around the mouth aggravated by topical steroids

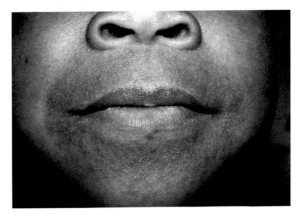

Figure 5.10 Perioral dermatitis – with tiny erythematous papules

periocular and possible genital areas with monomorphic coalescent papules
- Symptoms include stinging/burning and occasional pruritus

Pathogenesis

- Unknown etiology
- Known to be induced by use of topical steroids on the face
- Also exacerbated by fluorinated toothpaste and other substances

Diagnosis

- Clinical findings
- Histology: spongiosis of the follicular infundibulum with lymphocytic exocytosis and perivascular lymphohistiocytic inflammation

Differential diagnosis

- Atopic dermatitis
- Seborrheic dermatitis
- Contact/irritant dermatitis
- Rosacea
- Planar warts
- Sarcoidosis

Treatment

- Eliminate aggravating/precipitating topical agents, especially topical steroids
- Topical antibiotics (e.g. metronidazole, clindamycin)
- Systemic antibiotics (e.g. erythromycin) – may be needed for 2 months of continuous therapy

Prognosis

- Intermittent course
- Can worsen after withdrawal of precipitating agent
- Recurrences are not uncommon
- Responds well to therapy in 1–3 months

References

Knautz MA, Lesher JL. Childhood granulomatous periorifical dermatitis. Pediatr Dermatol 1996; 13: 131–4

Laude TA, Salvemini JN. Perioral dermatitis in children. Semin Cutan Med Surg 1999; 18: 206–9

Manders SM, Lucky AW. Perioral dermatitis in childhood. J Am Acad Dermatol 1992; 27: 688–92

Urbatsch AJ, Frieden I, Williams ML, et al. Extrafacial and generalized granulomatous periorificial dermatitis. Arch Dermatol 2002; 138: 1354–8

Rosacea

Major points

- Rare condition in childhood
- Can present with chronic and intermittent facial erythema, flushing, telangectasias and papulopustular eruption (Figure 5.11)
- Eye involvement including blepharitis, conjunctivitis and episcleritis may occur
- Comedones are absent
- Typically involves the cheeks and chin
- Most children have an associated family history of rosacea

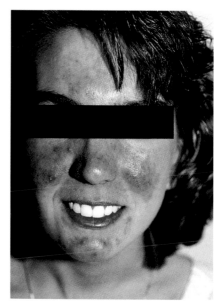

Figure 5.11 Rosacea associated with easy blushing in a teenage girl

Pathogenesis

- Unknown but probably multifactorial
- Questionable role of *Demodex folliculorum*
- Chronic topical steroid application can lead to rosacea-like eruption (steroid-induced acne)

Diagnosis

- Clinical features
- Histology variable; most common findings include vascular dilatation and perivascular and perifollicular lymphocytic infiltrates

Differential diagnosis

- Perioral dermatitis
- Acne vulgaris
- Folliculitis
- Sarcoidosis
- Discoid lupus erythematosus
- Papular granuloma annulare

Treatment

- Topical antibiotics (e.g. metronidazole, clindamycin)
- Systemic antibiotics (e.g. erythromycin, tetracycline, doxycycline, minocycline)
- Discontinuation of topical steroids

Prognosis

- Intermittent and chronic course

References

Drolet B, Paller AS. Childhood rosacea. Pediatr Dermatol 1992; 9: 22–6

Howard R, Tsuchiya A. Adult skin disease in the pediatric patient. Dermatol Clin 1998; 16: 593–608

Morras PG, Santos SP, Imedio IL, et al. Rosacea-like demodicidosis in an immunocompromised child. Pediatr Dermatol 2003; 20: 28–30

Weston WL, Morelli JG. Steroid rosacea in prepubertal children. Arch Pediatr Adolesc Med 2000; 154: 62–4

Hidradenitis suppurativa

Major points

- Chronic scarring disease of the apocrine glands that occurs after puberty
- Occurs in apocrine gland-bearing areas of the skin including the axillae, inframammary fold, inguinal area and anogenital region (Figure 5.12)
- More common in Blacks
- Male/female ratio <1
- Obesity is a predisposing factor
- Presents with tender, suppurative nodules and abscesses which heal with fibrosis leading to sinus tracts and bridging hypertrophic scars
- Associated with other follicular occlusion diseases: acne conglobata, dissecting cellulitis of the scalp, pilonidal cysts

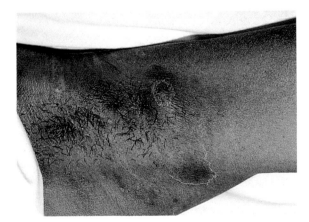

Figure 5.12 Hidradenitis suppurativa – with multiple draining cysts in the axilla

Pathogenesis

- Disrupted keratinization with follicular hyperkeratosis and plugging of the apocrine duct leading to dilatation of the duct with perifolliculitis, abscess formation, destruction of the pilosebaceous unit ending in fibrosis
- Secondary bacterial infection can occur with staphylococci, streptococci and Gram-negative organisms

Diagnosis

- Typical clinical presentation

Differential diagnosis

- Furunculosis
- Lymphadenitis
- Keratinaceous cysts
- Ulcerative colitis

Treatment

- Topical antibiotics
- Benzoyl peroxide preparations
- Systemic antibiotics
- Systemic retinoids
- Intralesional triamcinolone for inflamed lesions
- Excision of the affected area

Prognosis

- Disease severity is variable
- Mild disease can remit with age
- Severe disease can be chronic with relapses and significant morbidity

References

Adams DR, Gordon KB, Devenyi AG, Ioffreda MD. Severe hidradenitis suppurativa treated with infliximab infusion. Arch Dermatol 2003; 139: 1540–2

Mengesha YM, Holcombe TC, Hansen RC. Prepubertal hidradenitis suppurativa: two case reports and review of the literature. Pediatr Dermatol 1999; 16: 292–6

Palmer RA, Keefe M. Early-onset hidradenitis suppurativa. Clin Exp Dermatol 2001; 26: 501–3

Slade DE, Powell BW, Mortimer PS. Hidradenitis suppurativa: pathogenesis and management. Br J Plast Surg 2003; 56: 451–61

Wiseman MC. Hidradenitis suppurativa: a review. Dermatol Ther 2004; 17: 50–4

Miliaria

Major points

- Miliaria crytallina
  1. Presents as generalized small clear vesicles that are easily ruptured with no surrounding erythema (Figure 5.13)
  2. Accentuated in intertriginous areas
  3. Can be congenital or develop in the first few weeks of life
  4. Can follow sunburn

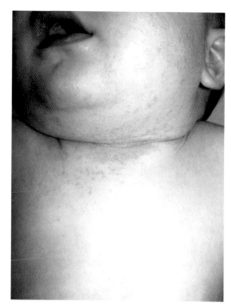

Figure 5.14   Miliaria rubra – typical 'prickly heat' around the neck of a child in the summer

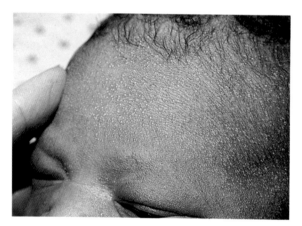

Figure 5.13   Miliaria crystallina in a newborn from overheating

- Miliaria rubra (prickly heat, heat rash)
  1. Common in febrile, overheated infants or in hot weather
  2. Presents with generalized 1–3 mm nonfollicular papules, vesicles and pustules with an erythematous base (Figures 5.14 and 5.15)
  3. Accentuated in intertriginous areas and in areas of occlusion
- Miliaria profunda
  1. Clinically appears as erythematous-based papules and pustules
  2. Can prevent adequate sweating leading to hyperthermia in older children

Pathogenesis

- Caused by obstruction of the eccrine ducts that leads to retention of sweat in the skin
- Level of obstruction of the eccrine duct determines the clinical presentation

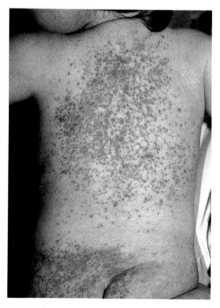

Figure 5.15   Miliaria rubra/pustulosa – caused by lying in bed for several days with a febrile illness

1. Miliaria crystallina: subcorneal or intracorneal (superficial)
2. Miliaria rubra: intraepidermal

3. Miliaria profunda: at the dermal–epidermal junction
- Secondary inflammatory response can develop if there is deeper obstruction
- Questionable role of extracellular polysaccharide substance of *Staphylococcus epidermidis* causing duct occlusion

Diagnosis

- Clinical findings
- Histologic findings:
  1. Miliaria crystallina: intra- or subcorneal vesicles that contain few neutrophils
  2. Miliaria rubra: spongiosis and spongiotic vesicles with surrounding lymphocytic infiltrate; variable papillary dermal edema; can have amorphous casts that are PAS-positive within the intraepidermal sweat duct
  3. Miliaria profunda: similar to miliaria rubra with subepidermal vesiculation and deeper inflammation involving the lower epidermis and upper dermis

Differental diagnosis

- Neonatal acne
- Neonatal infections: *Candida*, *Staphylococcus* and herpes simplex

Treatment

- Limit bundling of infants; recommend light-weight clothing
- Cooler ambient temperatures; air-conditioning
- Cool baths
- Avoidance of excessive heat and occlusion

Prognosis

- Lesions resolve spontaneously with avoidance of overheating
- Obstruction of sweat ducts in miliaria profunda can lead to hyperthermia and heat stroke

References

Feng E, Janniger CK. Miliaria. Cutis 1995; 55: 213–16

Gan VN, Hoang MP. Generalized vesicular eruption in a newborn. Pediatr Dermatol 2004; 21: 171–3

Mowad CM, McGinley KJ, Foglia A, Leyden JJ. The role of extracellular polysaccharide substance produced by Staphylococcus epidermidis in miliaria. J Am Acad Dermatol 1995; 33: 729–33

Sellheyer K, Medenica M, Stein SL. Vesicular eruption on the trunk and in intertiginous folds. Arch Dermatol 2004; 140: 231–6

Van Praag MC, Van Rooij RW, Folkers E, et al. Diagnosis and treatment of pustular disorders in the neonate. Pediatr Dermatol 1997; 14: 131–43

Wenzel FG, Horn TD. Nonneoplastic disorders of the eccrine glands. J Am Acad Dermatol 1998; 38: 1–17

Hyperhidrosis

Major points

- Sweating beyond what is necessary to maintain thermal regulation
- May be primary (idiopathic, essential) or secondary to diseases or drugs
- May be localized, regionalized or generalized
- Frequently socially embarrassing and occupationally disabling
- Generalized hyperhidrosis caused by febrile illnesses, neoplastic disease, neurologic diseases, metabolic disorders and drugs
- Localized hyperhidrosis includes primary or focal hyperhidrosis, unilateral circumscribed, intrathoracic neoplasms, olfactory hyperhidrosis, gustatory hyperhidrosis, spinal cord injuries, Frey syndrome and others

Pathogenesis

- Eccrine sweat glands assist in maintenance of body temperature in response to heat exposure or exercise as a function of the sympathetic nervous system
- Sweat glands are innervated by sympathetic postganglionic fibers mediated by acetylcholine
- Stimuli include thermal or emotional stimuli (more common on palms, soles and forehead)

Diagnosis

- Clinical findings

Differential diagnosis

- Miliaria

Treatment

- Aluminum chloride (Drysol® 20%)
- Anti-anxiety medications: diazepam (Valium®), fluoxatine (Prozac®)
- Systemic anticholinergic agents: Robinul®

- Iontophoresis
- Botulinum toxin (Botox®)
- Surgical excision of axilla eccrine/apocrine glands
- Sympathectomy

Prognosis

- Usually lifelong
- May improve in middle age

Reference

Stolman LP. Treatment of hyperhidrosis. J Drugs Dermatol 2003; 2: 521–7

6

BULLOUS DISORDERS

GENERAL

- Blisters in children are generally caused by:
  1. Acute eczematous dermatitis (e.g. contact dermatitis)
  2. Viral infections (e.g. herpes simplex)
  3. Bacterial infections (e.g. bullous impetigo)
  4. Mechanobullous genetic diseases (e.g. epidermolysis bullosa)
  5. Immunobullous disorders (e.g. chronic bullous dermatosis of childhood)
- When taking a history, it is important to determine whether trauma played a role in blister formation, and when the blisters began. This helps distinguish the mechanobullous disorders (genetic blistering disorders which usually start at birth) from acquired blistering disorders
- Although most blisters are fragile and break spontaneously, blisters on the palms and soles have a thick stratum corneum covering and may appear deeper and not rupture
- Blisters in the mouth are superficial and do not stay intact long, because of the lack of stratum corneum in the oral mucosa

IMMUNOBULLOUS DISORDERS

General

- Immunobullous diseases in childhood are uncommon but should be considered if the blistering condition has been persistent for longer than a month, particularly if unresponsive to antibiotic therapy

- Characterized by the presence of autoantibodies to components of the skin
- Diagnosis is made by correlating the histologic findings with the direct immunofluorescence (DIF)
- Blisters may appear flaccid, tense or may present as erosions

References

Fine J-D. Management of acquired bullous skin diseases. N Engl J Med 1995; 333: 1475–84

Weston WL, Morelli JG, Huff JC. Misdiagnosis, treatments, and outcomes in the immunobullous diseases in children. Pediatr Dermatol 1997; 14: 264–72

Pemphigus

General

- Autoimmune blistering disease of the skin and mucous membranes with intraepidermal blisters, acantholysis and circulating IgG directed against cell surfaces of keratinocytes
- Four major types: pemphigus vulgaris, pemphigus foliaceus, paraneoplastic pemphigus and fogo selvagem
- Very rare in childhood

Major points

- Pemphigus vulgaris (PV)
  1. Blisters occur in lower epidermis, just above the basal layer
  2. Painful fragile flaccid blisters occur anywhere on the body, and arise on normal or erythematous skin (Figure 6.1)
  3. Intact blisters are sparse; erosions are common

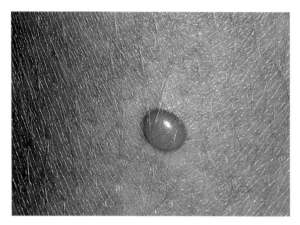

Figure 6.1 Pemphigus vulgaris – in an 11-year-old girl

4. Nikolsky sign is positive (application of lateral pressure to the periphery of an active lesion causing extension of the blister)
5. Excessive granulation tissue may be seen in intertriginous areas, on scalp or face
6. Mucous membrane lesions (particularly in the mouth) occur prior to skin involvement and affect the majority of patients (Figure 6.2)
7. Erosions may involve the pharynx or the larynx, causing hoarseness
8. Associations: myasthenia gravis and/or thymoma

9. Antigen is desmoglein 3
-   Neonatal pemphigus displays clinical, histologic, and immunopathologic signs of PV
    1. Neonatal PV occurs when maternal IgG crosses the placenta, causing disease in the neonate
    2. Remits when maternal antibodies decrease (~6–12 months)
    3. May be mild or severe
-   Pemphigus foliaceus (PF) (superficial pemphigus)
    1. Superficial blisters occur in granular layer
    2. Scaly, crusted erosions, often on an erythematous base, located in seborrheic distribution (face, scalp, upper trunk) (Figure 6.3)
    3. Primary lesions: small flaccid blisters which are painful or burn
    4. Disease may stay localized for years or progress rapidly to exfoliative erythroderma
    5. Sun and heat may exacerbate
    6. Oral lesions rare
    7. Antigen is desmoglein 1
-   Fogo selvagem (endemic pemphigus foliaceus)
    1. Endemic in rural Brazil
    2. Affects children <14 years in 25% of cases, two-thirds are <30 years old
    3. Occurs along inland river beds where black fly *Simulium nigrimanum* is endemic
-   Pemphigus erythematosus

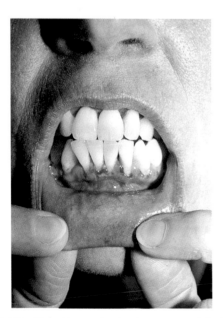

Figure 6.2 Pemphigus vulgaris – in a young adult with erosions in the mouth

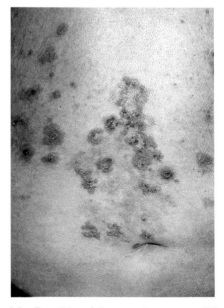

Figure 6.3 Pemphigus foliaceus – in a young adult

1. Localized variant of pemphigus foliaceus, usually on face, associated with lupus erythematosus
- Paraneoplastic pemphigus
  1. Very rare in childhood
  2. Associated with neoplasms mainly of lymphoid tissue (e.g. leukemia, lymphoma, thymoma, benign lymphoid tumors)
  3. DIF shows IgG and C3 in between keratinocytes and linear or granular pattern along the basement membrane zone (BMZ)
  4. Indirect immunofluorescence is positive in other desmosome-containing tissues
  5. Clinical:
     a. Severe oral and conjunctival erosions with erythematous blistering
     b. Polymorphic lesions with blisters and erosions, may resemble erythema multiforme (Figure 6.4)
- Drug-induced pemphigus can be caused by penicillamine or captopril, and resolves when medicine stopped; DIF positive; antigen is desmoglein 3

Pathogenesis

- IgG autoantibodies are directed against desmosomes in epidermis, interfering with calcium-sensitive adhesional function. Acantholysis is in areas of deposition of IgG (See Table 6.1)

Diagnosis

- DIF is positive for IgG on the cell surfaces of keratinocytes in perilesional skin
- In PV and pemphigus foliaceus (PF), 75% will have circulating antiepithelial cell surface IgG found on indirect immunofluorescence
- Correlation between titer of circulating anti-cell surface antibodies and disease activity
- Histology:
  1. PV shows suprabasilar blister with acantholysis, leaving a 'row of tombstones' where basal cells stay attached to the basement membrane by hemidesmosomes
  2. PF shows acantholysis in the granular layer
  3. Paraneoplastic pemphigus shows a combination of PV and erythema multiforme-like histology

Differential diagnosis

- Bullous pemphigoid
- Bullous insect bite reactions
- Chronic bullous disease of childhood
- Staphylococcal scalded skin syndrome
- Stevens–Johnson syndrome

Treatment

- Prednisone 1–2 mg/kg per day until activity is suppressed. Once under control, steroids should be tapered to avoid side-effects
- Steroid-sparing agents can be used as an adjunct: cyclophosphamide, azathioprine, cyclosporine, methotrexate, or gold
- High-potency topical steroids might be helpful for localized disease
- Intravenous immunoglobulins (IVIG) may be a promising therapy

Prognosis

- Pemphigus has significant morbidity and mortality
- Infection is often the cause of death in adults
- Prognosis without treatment is poor

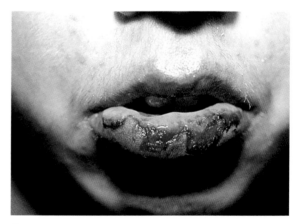

Figure 6.4 Paraneoplastic pemphigus – with extensive mouth involvement in an adult

References

Bystryn JC, Steinman NM. The adjuvant therapy of pemphigus. An update. Arch Dermatol 1996; 132: 203–12

Harman KE, Albert S, Black MM. Guidelines for the management of pemphigus vulgaris. Br J Dermatol 2003; 149: 926–37

Kanwar AJ, Dhar S, Kaur S. Further experience with pemphigus in children. Pediatr Dermatol 1994; 11: 107–11

Lyde CB, Cox SE, Cruz PD. Pemphigus erythematosus in a five-year-old child. J Am Acad Dermatol 1994; 31: 906–9

Table 6.1   Major immunobullous disorders

Disorder	Target antigen	Histology	DIF
Pemphigus vulgaris	In desmosomes: Desmoglein 3 (130 kDa)	Suprabasilar acantholysis	IgG, C3 or both along keratinocyte surfaces
Neonatal pemphigus	Desmoglein 3 (130 kDa) Maternal IgG	Suprabasilar acantholysis	IgG, C3 or both along keratinocyte surfaces
Pemphigus foliaceus	Desmoglein 1 (160 kDa)	Granular cell layer acantholysis	IgG, C3 or both along keratinocyte surfaces
Fogo selvagem	Desmoglein 1 (160 kDa)	Granular cell layer acantholysis	IgG, C3 or both along keratinocyte surfaces
Pemphigus erythematosus	Desmoglein 1 (160 kDa)	Granular cell layer acantholysis	IgG, C3 or both along keratinocyte surfaces
Bullous pemphigoid	In hemidesmosomes: BPAG-1 (230 kDa) BPAG-2 (180 kDa)	Subepidermal blister with eosinophils	Linear IgG/ C3, IgA, IgM at BMZ
Pemphigoid gestationis	BPAG-2 (180 kDa)	Subepidermal blister (in lamina lucida)	IgG, C3 or both in linear pattern at BMZ
Dermatitis herpetiformis	Gliadin Tissue transglutaminase	Dermal papillary neutrophils; with subepidermal blister in lamina lucida	Granular IgA in dermal papillae
Chronic bullous disease of childhood	LABD, 97 kDa, others	Subepidermal bullae in lamina lucida with neutrophils	Linear IgA along BMZ
Paraneoplastic pemphigus	Desmoplakin 1 (250 kDa) Envoplakin (190 kDa) Periplakin (170 kDa) Desmoplakin 2 (210 kDa) BP antigen (230 kDa) Others	Suprabasilar acantholysis and lichenoid dermatitis	Linear granular IgG, C3 or both along keratinocyte surfaces and in BMZ
EB acquisita	Type 7 collagen (290 kDa and 145 kDa)	Subepidermal blister with neutrophils or cell poor infiltrate	IgG, C3 or others in linear pattern along BMZ

BMZ, basement membrane zone; DIF, direct immunofluorescence; IF, immunofluorescence; EB, epidermolysis bullosa

Prendiville JS, Israel DM, Wood WS, Dimmick JE. Oral pemphigus vulgaris associated with inflammatory bowel disease and herpetic gingivostomatitis in an 11-year-old girl. Pediatr Dermatol 1994; 11: 145–50

Rybojad M, Leblanc T, Flageul B, et al. Paraneoplastic pemphigus in a child with a T-cell lymphoblastic lymphoma. Br J Dermatol 1993; 128: 418–22

Stanley JR. Pemphigus. In Fitzpatrick's Dermatology in General Medicine, 6th edn. Freedberg IM Eisen AZ, Wolff K, Austen KF, eds. McGraw-Hill: New York, 2003: 558–67

Tope WD, Kamino H, Briggaman RA, et al. Neonatal pemphigus vulgaris in a child born to a woman in remission. J Am Acad Dermatol 1993; 29: 480–5

Walker DC, Kolar KA, Hebert AA, Jordan RE. Neonatal pemphigus foliaceus. Arch Dermatol 1995; 131: 1308–11

Wanaukul S, Pongprasit P. Childhood pemphigus. Int J Dermatol 1999; 38: 29–35

Weston WL, Morelli JG, Huff JC. Misdiagnosis, treatments, and outcomes in the immunobullous diseases in children. Pediatr Dermatol 1997; 14: 264–72

Bullous pemphigoid

Major points

- Large, tense blisters arising on normal or erythematous skin
- Mucous membrane involvement in 10–35%
- Sites of predilection: lower abdomen, inner thighs, flexor forearms or generalized
- Bullae may have clear or hemorrhagic fluid (Figures 6.5 and 6.6)

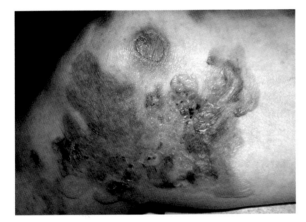

Figure 6.5   Bullous pemphigoid – large bullae on erythematous patches

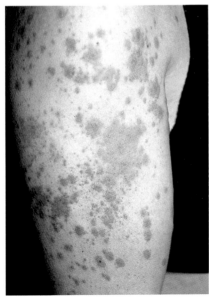

Figure 6.6   Pemphigoid gestationis – in a young pregnant woman. Her child was unaffected

- Erosions tend to re-epithelialize quickly
- Nikolsky sign is negative
- New vesicles may form at the edge of old blisters
- Blisters do not tend to scar but may be hyperpigmented
- Mild to moderate pruritus
- Early lesions tend to look urticarial
- Rare in childhood

Pathogenesis

- Bullous pemphigoid (BP) antigens are proteins in the hemidesmosomes (HDs). Autoantibody binds both inside the cell to plaques of HDs and outside cells to the extracellular section of HDs
- BP antibodies are directed against both BPAg-1 (230 kDa) component and also BPAg-2 (180 kDa) (also called type XVII collagen)
- BP IgG can activate complement by the classical pathway causing leukocyte adherence to the basement membrane, degranulation of polymorphonuclear leukocytes and subsequent dermal–epidermal separation

Diagnosis

- Histology: subepidermal blister without necrosis, and superficial dermal infiltrate with lymphocytes, histiocytes and eosinophils
- DIF: linear pattern of C3 and IgG at BMZ
- Indirect immunoflourescence: 70–80% of patients will have circulating IgG which binds to stratified squamous epithelium; titers do not correlate with disease extent or activity
- ~50% have elevated IgE, and sometimes eosinophilia, which correlates with pruritus

Differential diagnosis

- Bullous insect bite reactions
- Bullous impetigo
- Bullous erythema multiforme
- Chronic bullous disease of childhood

Treatment

- Prednisone 1–2 mg/kg per day until activity is suppressed. Once under control, steroids should be tapered to avoid side-effects
- Steroid-sparing agents can be used as an adjunct: cyclophosphamide, azathioprine, cyclosporine, methotrexate, or gold

- Localized BP can be treated with high-potency topical steroids
- Some patients respond to sulfones, tetracycline, or nicotinamide

Prognosis

- BP may be self-limited and can last several months to many years
- Prognosis is good. In adults, half of treated patients go into remission in 2.5–6 years

References

Chimanovitch I, Hamm H, Georgi M, et al. Bullous pemphigoid of childhood. Arch Dermatol 2000; 136: 527–32

Kuenzli S, Grimaitre M, Krischer J, et al. Childhood bullous pemphigoid: report of a case with life-threatening course during homeopathy treatment. Pediatr Dermatol 2004; 21: 160–3

Nagano T, Tani M, Adachi A, et al. Childhood bullous pemphigoid: immunohistochemical, immunoelectron microscopic, and Western blot analysis. J Am Acad Dermatol 1994; 30: 884–8

Nemeth AJ, Klein AD, Gould EW, Schachner LA. Childhood bullous pemphigoid: clinical and immunologic features, treatment and prognosis. Arch Dermatol 1991; 127: 378–86

Oranje AP, Vuzevski VD, van Joost T, et al. Bullous pemphigoid in children. Int J Dermatol 1991; 30: 339–42

Petronius D, Bergman R. Bullous pemphigoid in two young infants. Pediatr Dermatol 2002; 19: 119–21

Stanley JR. Bullous pemphigoid. In Fitzpatrick's Dermatology in General Medicine, 6th edn. Freedberg IM, Eisen AZ, Wolff K, Austen KF, eds. McGraw-Hill: New York, 2003: 574–81

Trüeb RM, Didierjean L, Fellas A, et al. Childhood bullous pemphigoid: report of a case with characterization of the targeted antigens. J Am Acad Dermatol 1999; 40:338–44

Vaillant L, Bernard P, Joly P, et al. Evaluation of clinical criteria for diagnosis of bullous pemphigoid. Arch Dermatol 1998; 134: 1075–80

Weston WL, Morelli JG, Huff JC. Misdiagnosis, treatments, and outcomes in the immunobullous diseases in children. Pediatr Dermatol 1997; 14: 264–72

Dermatitis herpetiformis

Major points

- Most common immunobullous disease in children
- Characterized by intensely pruritic chronic small papules and vesicles located symmetrically over extensor surfaces (elbows, knees, upper spine), scalp hairline and posterior nuchal area (Figure 6.7)

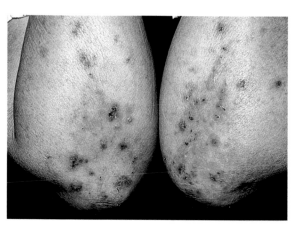

Figure 6.7   Dermatitis herpetiformis – typical excoriated lesions on extensor surfaces

- Primary lesions: erythematous papules, urticarial plaques or vesicles, but crusted lesions are frequently the only lesions seen. Large bullae infrequent
- Mucous membrane involvement is uncommon
- Onset is usually in adolescence or later
- Most have gastrointestinal (GI) abnormality similar to celiac disease (villous atrophy of the small intestine) but are asymptomatic
- About 80% of patients have HLA-B8 and DR3
- Lesions can be exacerbated by gluten or oral iodides
- Sometimes associated with GI lymphomas, or autoimmune disease (e.g. thyroid disease, diabetes, lupus erythematosus, Sjögren syndrome, or vitiligo)

Pathogenesis

- Gluten plays a critical role
- IgA deposits may be complexes of immunoglobulins and GI-derived antigens which react with an unidentified skin antigen
- IgA is found in all skin sites, not just lesional skin
- IgA activates complement, probably via the alternative pathway, causing chemotaxis of neutrophils which release enzymes causing blistering. Cytokines or proteases that induce basal keratinocytes to produce collagenases or stromelysin-1 contribute to blister formation

Diagnosis

- Histology: dermal papillary collections of neutrophils. Blood vessels are surrounded by lymphohistiocytic infiltrates with neutrophils and eosinophils
- Blister formation is within lamina lucida of the BMZ, and above lamina densa
- DIF shows granular IgA deposits (subclass IgA1) in dermal papillary tips in normal appearing skin; frequently, C3 is seen
- Antireticulin antibodies of IgA and IgG classes can be detected in the majority of patients
- Circulating IgA autoantibodies to endomysium (EMA), tissue transglutaminase (tTG) and gliadin are detected in both dermatitis herpetiformis and celiac disease

Differential diagnosis

- Scabies
- Eczema
- Impetigo
- Pityriasis lichenoides
- Erythema multiforme
- Bullous drug reaction
- Factitial excoriations
- Bullous pemphigoid
- Bullous insect bite reactions
- Chronic bullous disease of childhood
- Pemphigus vulgaris

Treatment

- Dapsone 2 mg/kg per day, adult dose 100–150 mg/day
- Sulfapyridine 1–4 g/day given four times a day for an adult
- Gluten-free diet may be effective; may take >5 months to 1 year to see an effect

Prognosis

- Lifelong disorder, persisting indefinitely with varying severity

References

Bardella MT, Fredella C, Trovato C, et al. Long-term remission in patients with dermatitis herpetiformis on a normal diet. Br J Dermatol 2003; 149: 968–71

Caproni M, Cardinali C, Renzi D, et al. Tissue transglutaminase antibody assessment in dermatitis herpetiformis [Letter]. Br J Dermatol 2001; 144: 196–7

Chorzelski TP, Rosinska D, Beutner EH, et al. Aggressive gluten challenge of dermatitis herpetiformis cases converts them from seronegative to seropositive for IgA-class endomysial antibodies. J Am Acad Dermatol 1988; 18: 672–8

Ermacora E, Prampolini L, Tribbia G, et al. Long-term follow-up of dermatitis herpetiformis in children. J Am Acad Dermatol 1986; 15: 24–30

Weston WL, Morelli JG, Huff JC. Misdiagnosis, treatments, and outcomes in the immunobullous diseases in children. Pediatr Dermatol 1997; 14: 264–72

Zone JJ, Meyer LJ, Petersen MJ. Deposition of granular IgA relative to clinical lesions in dermatitis herpetiformis. Arch Dermatol 1996; 132: 912–18

Chronic bullous disease of childhood (linear IgA dermatosis)

Major points

- Presents as blisters which resemble bullous impetigo unresponsive to antibiotics
- Second most common immunobullous disease in childhood
- Typically presents in children <5 years of age with large tense bullae or vesicles on an erythematous base in the diaper area, face and other areas (Figures 6.8–6.10)
- Lesions are symmetrical and pruritic
- Numerous crusted vesicles or a 'cluster of jewels' appearance with new lesions appearing around the periphery of previous lesions
- Mucous membranes involved in up to 70% of cases, ranging from asymptomatic oral ulcerations to severe disease

Pathogenesis

- Caused by linear deposition of IgA to 97-kDa antigen among others in lamina lucida of BMZ, which incites inflammation and destruction of the epidermal–dermal barrier
- Associations:
  1. Drugs: vancomycin, lithium, diclofenac
  2. Lymphoid and nonlymphoid malignancies

Diagnosis

- Diagnosis is usually overlooked initially, because of the rarity of this disease and its confusion with bullous impetigo

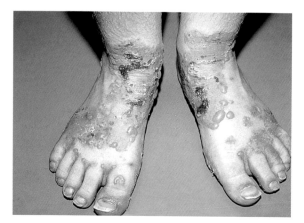

Figure 6.8 Chronic bullous dermatosis of childhood – typical ringed blisters on the feet

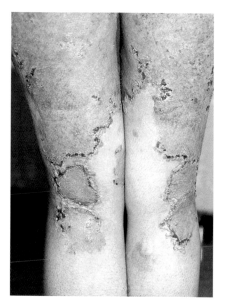

Figure 6.10 Linear IgA bullous dermatosis – typical blisters along the edge of healed blisters

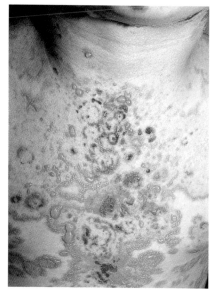

Figure 6.9 Chronic bullous dermatosis of childhood – extensive involvement of the trunk

- Histology:
  1. Biopsies should be taken in skin adjacent to a blister, not an old blister or crusted lesion
  2. Subepidermal bulla with neutrophils along the BMZ, often in papillary tips. Lymphocytic infiltrate may be present around superficial dermal blood vessels without vasculitis
- DIF: IgA in a homogeneous linear pattern along BMZ; occasional IgG and C3
  1. Three patterns of IgA deposition (found on electron microscopy): in lamina lucida (similar

to BP); at or below lamina densa (similar to epidermolysis bullosa acquisita); both above and below lamina densa
- Low titer IgA serum autoantibodies can sometimes be detected

Differential diagnosis

- Bullous impetigo
- Pemphigus
- Bullous pemphigoid
- Epidermolysis bullosa
- Erythema multiforme
- Bullous systemic lupus erythematosus

Treatment

- Dapsone 2 mg/kg per day
- Prednisone 1–2 mg/kg per day
- Most cases respond to combination of prednisone and dapsone
- Topical antibiotics and nonstick gauze covering if lesions are oozing or crusted
- Patients do not benefit from gluten-free diet
- Other drugs which may be beneficial: dicloxacillin, colchicine, sulfapyridine

Prognosis

- Usually lasts several years and then remits. Occasionally, persists into puberty but is less severe

- Oral medications can be tapered as child improves, and then discontinued when totally clear of lesions for 6 months

References

Legrain V, Taïeb A, Surlève-Bazeille J-E, et al. Linear IgA dermatosis of childhood: case report with an immunoelectron microscopic study. Pediatr Dermatol 1991; 8: 310–13

Powell J, Kirtschig G, Allen J, et al. Mixed immunobullous disease of childhood: a good response to antimicrobials. Br J Dermatol 2001; 144: 769–74

Rao CL, Hall RP. Linear IgA dermatosis and chronic bullous disease of childhood. In Fitzpatrick's Dermatology in General Medicine, 6th edn. Freedberg IM, Eisen AZ, Wolff K, Austen KF, eds. McGraw-Hill: New York, 2003: 587–92

Siegfried EC, Sirawan S. Chronic bullous disease of childhood: successful treatment with dicloxacillin. J Am Acad Dermatol 1998; 39: 797–800

Wojnarowska F. Chronic bullous disease of childhod. Semin Dermatol 1988; 7: 58–65

Zone JJ, Taylor TB, Kadunce DP, et al. IgA antibodies in chronic bullous disease of childhood react with a 97 kDa basement membrane zone protein. J Invest Dermatol 1996; 106: 1277–80

EPIDERMOLYSIS BULLOSA

General

- Epidermolysis bullosa (EB) is a group of genetic diseases where mild trauma induces blister formation

- At least 18 distinct types, based on identification of mutations in various genes encoding proteins and clinical symptoms (Table 6.2)

Major points

- In general, EB is divided into scarring (dystrophic) and nonscarring (simplex and junctional) types
- Nonscarring types demonstrate an intraepidermal separation (EB simplex) or a separation at the dermal–epidermal junction (junctional EB)
- Scarring types: subepidermal blisters are found in dystrophic EB
- Usually presents in newborn period with blisters and erosions. Extensive blistering may be potentially life-threatening to newborns

Pathogenesis

- Defects associated with anchoring complexes along the basal cell layer and dermal–epidermal BMZ determine the type of EB
- Gene mutations (See Table 6.2)

Diagnosis

- Diagnosis is established by clinical symptoms and skin biopsy. Electron microscopy is the gold standard. Gene mutation can be identified
- Biopsy of an infant may be difficult
  1. Induce a blister with gentle traction with a cotton-tipped applicator
  2. Shave biopsy, gentle punch biopsy or excisional biopsy should include both epidermis and dermis

Table 6.2 Common types of epidermolysis bullosa

Type gene	Mutations	Locations
Simplex		
Weber–Cockayne type	Keratins 5, 14	Hands, feet
Koebner type	Keratins 5, 14	Generalized
Dowling–Meara type	Keratins 5, 14	Generalized
Junctional		
Herlitz type	Laminin-5	Generalized, laryngeal
Generalized atrophic benign type	Type 17 collagen or Laminin A3, B3	Generalized
With pyloric atresia	$\alpha_6\beta_4$ integrin	Generalized, laryngeal, pylorus
Dystrophic		
Recessive type	Type 7 collagen	Generalized
Dominant types	Type 7 collagen	Generalized

3. Avoid old blisters because secondary changes occur with re-epithelization
4. Specimen should be sent for light and electron microscopic examination as well as immunofluorescence mapping

Epidermolysis bullosa simplex

Major points

- Weber–Cockayne type (localized EB simplex)
  1. Most common form of EB
  2. Localized to hands and feet (Figure 6.11)
  3. Aggravated by warm weather
  4. Begins in childhood or adolescence
  5. Hyperhidrosis common
- Generalized EB simplex (Koebner type)
  1. Presents with generalized blistering within first 12 months of life (Figures 6.12–6.14)
  2. Blisters tend to be more common on distal extremities, especially the feet, knees, elbows and hands
  3. Palmoplantar keratoses
- EB herpetiformis (Dowling–Meara type) (Figure 6.15)
  1. Generalized with pronounced oral mucosa involvement (Figure 6.11)

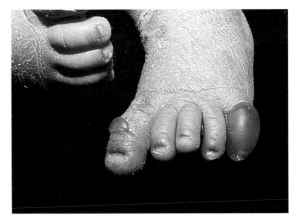

Figure 6.12 Epidermolysis bullosa simplex – typical tense blisters in a neonate

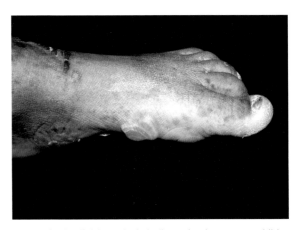

Figure 6.13 Epidermolysis bullosa simplex – same child as in Figure 6.12, age 6 years

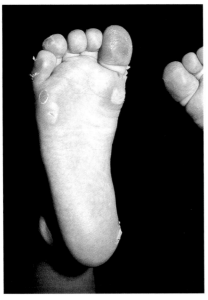

Figure 6.11 Epidermolysis bullosa simplex (Weber–Cockayne type) localized to hands and feet

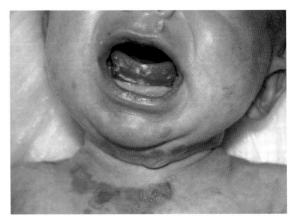

Figure 6.14 Epidermolysis bullosa simplex – mouth involvement causing difficulty feeding

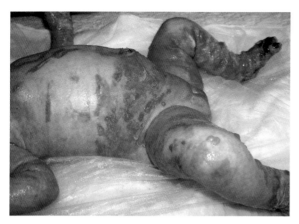

Figure 6.15 Epidermolysis bullosa simplex, Dowling–Meara type, severe generalized blistering in the neonatal period

2. Blisters are grouped
3. Nails may be shed and regrow
4. Hyperkeratosis of palms and soles

Junctional epidermolysis bullosa

Major points

- Two major forms of junctional EB, although other subtypes exist
- Herlitz type
  1. Severe form usually fatal before the age of 5 years
  2. Blisters appear in the neonatal period
  3. Oral mucosa is usually affected, causing failure to thrive from poor nutrition
  4. Laryngeal involvement is common; may present with hoarse cry
  5. Nonhealing granulation tissue (mid-face, neck, spine, ears and nail beds) is characteristic (Figures 6.16 and 6.17)
  6. Enamel dysplasia
  7. Bacterial infection occurs frequently
  8. Nails usually lost
  9. Respiratory, GI and genitourinary systems can be involved
  10. Growth retardation
  11. Anemia
- Mitis junctional EB
  1. Mild but chronic ulcerations with poor healing, which may improve with age
  2. Hoarseness mild or absent

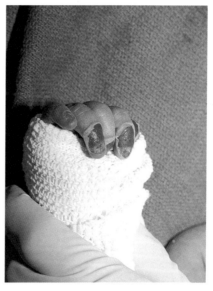

Figure 6.16 Junctional type epidermolysis bullosa – typical granulation tissue on the fingertips

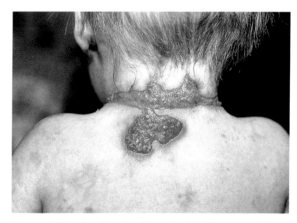

Figure 6.17 Junctional epidermolysis bullosa – typical chronic nonhealing granulation tissue around the neck

  3. Periorifical nonhealing erosions common
  4. Enamel dysplasia
  5. Scalp and nail lesions prominent
  6. Atrophic scarring
- Generalized atrophic benign EB
  1. Generalized involvement
  2. Bullae on extremities and fewer on trunk, scalp and face
  3. Alopecia
  4. Mucous membrane involvement mild
  5. Enamel defects
  6. Normal lifespan

Dystrophic epidermolysis bullosa

- Recessive dystrophic EB of Hallopeau–Siemens
  1. Lesions heal with scar formation and milia (tiny white cysts within the scars)
  2. Scarring results in loss of nails; webbing of fingers and toes leads to mitten-like appearance; flexion contractures common (Figures 6.18–6.20)
  3. Scarring in scalp causing alopecia
  4. Eyelid involvement can lead to blindness
  5. Bullae of oral mucosa can cause pain and severe restriction in eating
  6. Blisters of esophagus can cause esophageal strictures resulting in dysphagia
  7. Vagina, urethra and anus can be involved with blistering and stricture
  8. Although teeth are usually normal, they often become carious because of difficulty with oral hygiene
  9. Mixed anemia from chronic blood loss and malnutrition occur in childhood
  10. Failure to thrive is common with growth retardation
  11. Secondary bacterial infection frequent
  12. Aggressive squamous cell carcinoma commonly arises in poorly healed atrophic areas in adolescence or early adulthood – usually fatal
- Dominant dystrophic EB of Cockayne–Touraine type
  1. Blisters are similar to recessive dystrophic EB but generally not as severe, usually acral
  2. Babies may be born with erosions secondary to intrauterine blister formation
  3. Atrophic scars with milia (Figures 6.21 and 6.22)
  4. Loss of nails may occur, but no webbing of fingers and toes
  5. Failure to thrive and chronic anemia rare
  6. Oral lesions uncommon
  7. Teeth normal
- Dominant dystrophic EB of Pasini
  1. Hypopigmented atrophic lesions (called albopapuloid lesions) in symmetrical pattern
  2. Dystrophic nails common
  3. Mucous membranes and teeth normal

Pathogenesis

- Gene mutations of major structural proteins are known to cause the different types of EB (see Table 6.2)

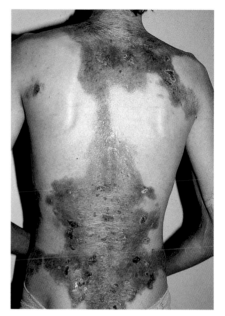

Figure 6.18   Recessive dystrophic type epidermolysis bullosa – scarring and chronic blistering in a teenager

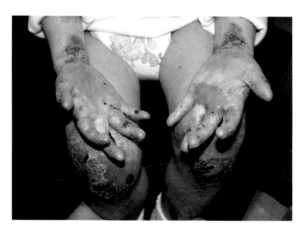

Figure 6.19   Recessive dystrophic epidermolysis bullosa with severe involvement on extremities

Diagnosis

- Skin biopsy (light microscopy, electron microscopy) as well as a molecular genetic analysis can differentiate the types of EB
- Electron microscopy: blister formation in EB simplex is found within epidermal cells above basal cell layer
- In junctional EB, blister formation occurs within the lamina lucida, just below the plasma

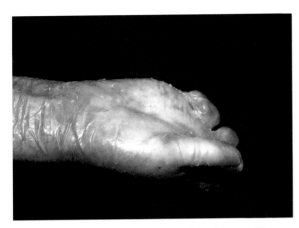

Figure 6.20 Dystrophic epidermolysis bullosa – mitten deformity of the hand

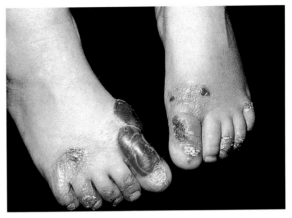

Figure 6.22 Dominant dystrophic type epidermolysis bullosa – blistering at the site of trauma

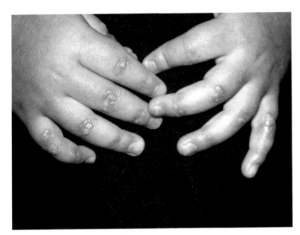

Figure 6.21 Dominant dystrophic epidermolysis bullosa with residual milia and scarring on the hands

membrane of basal cells and above the lamina densa
- Dystrophic EB demonstrates a separation within anchoring fibrils below the basal lamina within the dermis
- Genetic analysis may be required if combination of clinical signs and electron microscopy is not conclusive

Differential diagnosis

- Bacterial infections (e.g. bullous impetigo, staphylococcal, streptococcal)
- Fungal infections (e.g. *Candida* infection)
- Viral infections (e.g. herpes simplex)
- Epidermolytic hyperkeratosis
- Erythema multiforme
- Immunobullous diseases (e.g. pemphigus)

Treatment

- Supportive with avoidance of trauma and wound management
- Physician with knowledge of EB is the best source for a comprehensive care program including skilled nursing
- Nutritional support: frequent feedings with soft nipples; may require G-tube placement
- Gentle handling: avoid clothing or devices which might injure skin
- Sheep-skin pad in crib and car seat softens friction
- Blisters should be opened with a sterile needle or scissors and roof allowed to remain intact by gently pressing out of blister fluid, leaving a 'biologic bandage'
- Topical antibiotics (e.g. bacitracin or mupirocin) can help prevent secondary bacterial infection
- Most patients, especially young children, benefit from gauze wrapping
- Care should be given to wrap the fingers individually in recessive dystrophic EB in order to prevent webbing of fingers
- Physical therapy can help prevent contractures
- Cool ambient temperature may help decrease blistering
- Wound dressings such as hydrophilic dressings, occlusive dressings and hydrogel dressings (e.g. Exudry®, Omniderm®, Vigilon®, DuoDerm®, Mepitel®) may aid in healing and reduce pain. Be careful not to pull dressings off forcefully

- Protein and caloric requirements may be twice normal. Extra calories should be encouraged with nutritional supplements or even gastric buttons
- Anemia: vitamin supplements and iron
- Constipation: high-fiber foods, stool softeners or mineral oil may help prevent rectal blistering
- Genetic counseling: chorionic villus sampling sent for prenatal diagnosis if gene defect is known
- Surgical release of fused digits followed by grafting and splinting
- Support group: D.E.B.R.A. of America, Inc. Internet address: www.DEBRA.org

Prognosis

- Lifelong, chronic, blistering disorder
- EB simplex tends to improve with age, perhaps because older children and adults learn how to avoid blisters
- Recessive dystrophic EB tends to be slowly progressive, with further destruction of skin, including fingernails, web spaces and, in most severe cases, causing mitten deformities of hands

References

Eady RA, McGrath JA, McMillan JR. Ultrastructural clues to genetic disorders of skin: the dermal-epidermal junction. J Invest Dermatol 1994; 103: 13S–18S

Fine JD. Skin bioequivalents and their role in the treatment of inherited epidermolysis bullosa. Arch Dermatol 2000; 136: 1259–60

Livingston RJ, Sybert VP, Smith LT, et al. Expression of a truncated keratin 5 may contribute to severe palmar–plantar hyperkeratosis in epidermolysis bullosa simplex patients. J Invest Dermatol 2001; 116: 970–4

Marinkovich MP. The molecular genetics of basement membrane diseases. Arch Dermatol 1993; 129: 1557–65

Marinkovich MP, Khavari PA, Herron GS, Bauer EA. Inherited epidermolysis bullosa. In Fitzpatrick's Dermatology in General Medicine, 6th edn. Freedberg IM, Eisen AZ, Wolff K, Austen KF, eds. McGraw-Hill: New York, 2003: 596–609

Nakano A, Pulkkinen L, Murrell D, et al. Epidermolysis bullosa with congenital pyloric atresia: novel mutations in the beta-4 integrin gene (ITGB4) and genotype/phenotype correlations. Pediatr Res 2001; 49: 618–26

Parisi MA, Sybert VP. Molecular genetics in pediatric dermatology. Curr Opin Pediatr 2000; 12: 347–53

Pearson RW. Clinicopathologic types of epidermolysis bullosa and their nondermatological complications. Arch Dermatol 1988; 124: 718–25

Pfender E, Uitto J, Fine JD. Epidermolysis bullosa carrier frequencies in the US population [Letter]. J Invest Deramtol 2001; 116: 483–4

Uitto J, Christiano AM. Molecular genetics of the cutaneous basement membrane zone. J Clin Invest 1992; 90: 687–92

Uitto J, Pulkkinen L. Molecular genetics of heritable blistering disorders. Arch Dermatol 2001; 137: 1458–61

7

BACTERIAL AND SPIROCHETAL DISEASES

Impetigo

Major points

- Most common bacterial skin infection in children
- Occurs superficially with no scarring
- More common in hot, humid climates or in crowded environments
- Associated with regional lymphadenopathy
- Nonbullous impetigo (impetigo contagiosa)
  1. Presents with fragile vesicles and pustules that are easily ruptured forming characteristic 'honey-colored' crusts (Figure 7.1)
  2. Most common on face and around nose, but can also occur on the extremities
  3. Can be a primary infection or can be secondary with an underlying dermatosis, called 'impetiginization'
- Bullous impetigo
  1. Most common in infancy
  2. Typically affects the diaper area
  3. Presents with flaccid, transparent bullae with little surrounding erythema; leads to erosions with a rim of scale (Figure 7.2)
  4. Can present with constitutional symptoms

Pathogenesis

- Nonbullous impetigo
  1. *Staphylococcus aureus* causes in up to 85% of cases
  2. Group A streptococcus causes in up to 30% of cases with groups B, C, G and F rarely present
  3. Epidemics are caused by *Streptococcus pyogenes* M-serotypes (i.e. 2, 49, 53, 55–57, 60)

- Bullous impetigo
  1. *Staphylococcus aureus* is the causative organism with 80% from phage group 2
  2. *S. aureus* produces epidermolytic toxins A or B (exfoliatin) which interacts with desmoglein-1 to form bullae
- Causative organisms enter through breaks in the skin such as abrasions or insect bites
- Carriage of the organism in the nares can be a source of infection

Diagnosis

- Clinical findings
- Gram stain reveals Gram-positive cocci in clusters or chains
- Staphyloccoci or steptococci may be isolated from lesions
- KOH prep and Tzanck prep are both negative
- Histology
  1. Nonbullous lesions reveal an intraepidermal vesicopustule within the subcorneal or granular layer with numerous neutrophils
  2. Bullous lesions reveal a bulla with cleavage in the uppermost epidermis and limited inflammation

Differential diagnosis

- Nonbullous impetigo
  1. Nummular eczema
  2. Tinea corporis
  3. Herpes simplex
  4. Pemphigus foliaceus
- Bullous impetigo
  1. Arthropod reaction

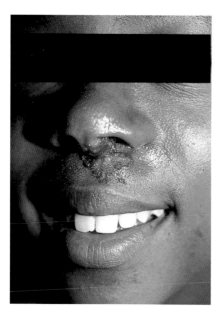

Figure 7.1   Impetigo contagiosa – typical crusted lesions on the face

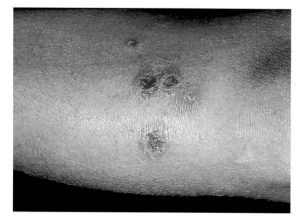

Figure 7.2   Bullous impetigo – with annular, crusted plaques

2. Fixed drug eruption
3. Erythema multiforme
4. Staphylococcal scalded skin syndrome
5. Chronic bullous disease of childhood

Treatment

- Topical mupirocin
- Topical mupirocin to the nares may be effective at reducing carriage in recurrent cases
- If widespread or associated with constitutional symptoms: oral antibiotics with Gram-positive coverage (e.g. dicloxacillin, cephalexin or erythromycin)
- Can resolve spontaneously over 2 weeks if left untreated in some cases

Prognosis

- Typically resolves without scarring
- Can be recurrent with nasal carriage of staphylococci
- 2–5% of cases of impetigo are associated with the development of acute glomerulonephritis; most commonly associated with *Streptococcus pyogenes* M-serotypes 2, 49, 55, 57 and 60; treatment does not reduce risk of development
- Development of cellulitis is uncommon
- Hematogenous spread is rare

References

George A, Rubin G. A systematic review and meta-analysis of treatments for impetigo. Br J Gen Pract 2003; 53: 480–7

Hedrick J. Acute bacterial skin infections in pediatric medicine: current issues in presentation and treatment. Paediatr Drugs 2003; 5 (Suppl 1): 35–46

Hirschmann JV. Impetigo: etiology and therapy. Curr Clin Top Infect Dis 2002; 22: 42–51

Mancini AJ. Bacterial skin infections in children: the common and the not so common. Pediatr Ann 2000; 29: 26–35

Folliculitis

Major points

- Infection of the hair follicle
- Variable clinical presentation depending on the infectious organism, depth of penetration and location
- Staphylococcal folliculitis
  1. Most common type
  2. Often related to maceration, occlusion or poor hygiene
  3. Presents with diffuse, discrete, erythematous-based, perifollicular papules and pustules on the scalp, face, buttocks and extremities (Figures 7.3 and 7.4)
  4. Can present concurrently with impetigo
  5. Patient or household members may be nasal carriers of *S. aureus*

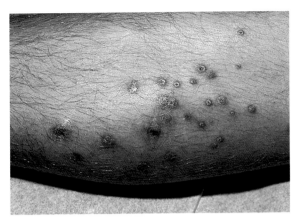

Figure 7.3   Folliculitis – caused by *Staphylococcus aureus*

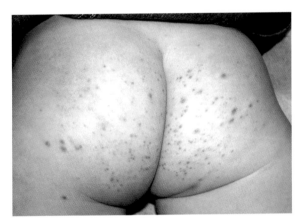

Figure 7.4   Folliculitis – common location on the buttocks

6. Rarely related to immunodeficiency, HIV, or diabetes mellitus
- Furunculosis
  1. Caused by *S. aureus*, especially phage type 80/81
  2. Develops from preceding superficial folliculitis with extension into the dermis and subcutaneous tissue
  3. Presents with tender, erythematous, perifollicular nodules with eventual central necrosis and rupture
  4. Often resolves with scarring
  5. Most common on the face, neck, axillae, or buttocks
  6. Carbuncle: two or more confluent furuncles
- Pityrosporum folliculitis
  1. Superficial infection of the hair follicle with *Malassezia furfur*

2. Presents with pinpoint perifollicular papules and pustules on the back, chest and upper arms
3. Can be pruritic
4. May be associated with tinea versicolor or seborrheic dermatitis
5. KOH reveals characteristic hyphae and spores
6. Responds to topical or systemic antifungal therapies
7. Typically chronic and recurrent
- Gram-negative folliculitis
  1. Infection of the hair follicles by *Escherichia coli* and species of *Enterobacter*, *Klebsiella* or *Proteus*
  2. Occurs in patients with acne who have been on long-term oral antibiotic therapy
  3. Presents as suddenly worsening acne with facial papules, pustules or nodules
  4. Responds well to isotretinoin as well as amoxicillin–clavulanic acid or trimethoprim–sulfamethoxazole
- Pseudomonas folliculitis (hot tub folliculitis)
  1. Caused by follicular infection with *Pseudomonas aeruginosa*
  2. Acquired in hot tubs, whirlpools, swimming pools and water slides or using body sponges that have not dried completely
  3. Presents with follicular papules and pustules accentuated in the bathing suit distribution (Figure 7.5)
  4. Can be associated with otitis externa, conjunctivitis, mild constitutional symptoms and rarely pneumonia and urinary tract infections
  5. Cutaneous disease resolves without treatment but can be recurrent

Pathogenesis

- Bacterial organism invades the follicular wall, leading to occlusion of the follicular orifice and causing inflammation
- Can be precipitated by occlusion with emollients, dressings or tar in hair-bearing areas

Diagnosis

- Clinical presentation
- Gram stain reveals organism
- Bacterial culture
- Histology rarely needed; reveals subcorneal pustules with surrounding neutrophilic infiltrate

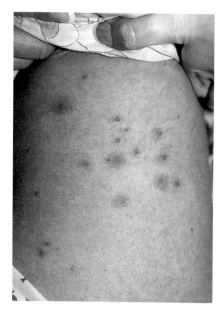

Figure 7.5 Hot tub folliculitis caused by *Pseudomonas*

Differential diagnosis

- Eosinophilic pustular folliculitis
- Candidiasis

Treatment

- Can improve with antibacterial cleansers and drying
- Topical antibiotics (e.g. mupirocin, clindamycin)
- Penicillinase-resistant systemic antibiotic may be needed if extensive
- Consider topical mupirocin ointment to the nares and perianal area of patient and household members if there are recurrent episodes

Prognosis

- Good, typically responds to therapy
- Can be recurrent if poor hygiene or nasal carriage of *S. aureus*
- Unresponsiveness, severe or systemic involvement warrants evaluation for an underlying immunodeficiency

References

Duarte AM, Kramer J, Yusk JW, et al. Eosinophilic pustular folliculitis in infancy and childhood. Am J Dis Child 1993; 147: 197–200

Fleischer AB Jr, Ling M, Eichenfield L, et al. Tacrolimus Ointment Study Group. Tacrolimus ointment for the treatment of atopic dermatitis is not associated with an increase in cutaneous infections. J Am Acad Dermatol 2002; 47: 562–70

Neubert U, Jansen T, Plewig G. Bacteriologic and immunologic aspects of gram-negative folliculitis: a study of 46 patients. Int J Dermatol 1999; 38: 270–4

Stahelin-Massik J, Gnehm HE, Itin PH. Pseudomonas folliculitis in a young child. Pediatr Infect Dis J 2000; 19: 362–3

Ecthyma

Major points

- Deep, punched out, ulcerative, painful, cutaneous infection (Figure 7.6)
- Typically develops on legs and buttocks at sites of minor trauma, insect bites or excoriations
- Often occurs in the setting of malnutrition or poor hygiene
- Develops as an erythematous-based vesiculopustule with progression to a crusted ulcer with overlying adherent crust and elevated peripheral rim
- Slow healing with resultant scarring
- Can be associated with fever and lymphadenopathy

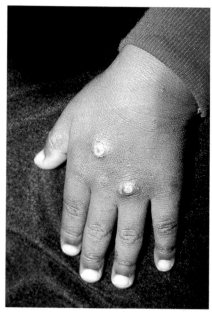

Figure 7.6 Ecthyma – typical punched out crusted papules and ulcers

Pathogenesis

- Caused by *Streptococcus pyogenes* most commonly, or *Staphylococcus aureus*

Diagnosis

- Clinical appearance
- Can be confirmed with Gram stain and bacterial culture

Differential diagnosis

- Anthrax
- Cutaneous diphtheria
- Ecthyma gangrenosum caused by *Pseudomonas aeruginosa*
- Second-degree burn
- Cigarette burns from child abuse

Treatment

- Warm compresses
- Local wound care with gentle cleansing and debridement
- Topical and systemic antibiotics

Prognosis

- Heals with scarring
- Can rarely progress to cellulitis
- Infection can rarely be associated with post-streptococcal glomerulonephritis

References

Gucluer H, Ergun T, Demircay Z. Ecthyma gangrenosum. Int J Dermatol 1999; 38: 299–302

Mancini AJ. Bacterial skin infections in children: the common and the not so common. Pediatr Ann 2001; 29: 26–35

Stulberg DL, Penrod MA, Blatny RA. Common bacterial skin infections. Am Fam Physician 2002; 66: 119–24

Travers JB, Norris DA, Leung DY. The keratinocyte as a target for staphylococcal bacterial toxins. Symposium Proceedings. J Invest Dermatol 2001; 6: 225–30

Cellulitis

Major points

- Acute infection and inflammation of the deep dermis and subcutaneous fat
- Presents with warm, red, tender, edematous plaques with ill-defined borders (Figure 7.7)

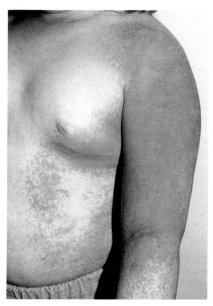

Figure 7.7 Cellulitis – caused by streptococcus with marked erythema

- Typically blue to purple dusky erythema if caused by *Haemophilus influenzae* (usually on the face)
- Most commonly seen on the face, neck or extremities (Figures 7.8 and 7.9)
- Predisposing factors: immunosuppression and diabetes mellitus
- Typically accompanied by regional lymphadenopathy, fever and constitutional symptoms

Pathogenesis

- Initiated by a break in the skin (e.g trauma or primary dermatosis) that serves as a portal of entry for the organism or preceded by upper respiratory infection, otitis media, sinusitis or tooth abscess
- Most common etiologic organisms: *Streptococcus pyogenes* or *Staphylococcus aureus*
- Preseptal or periorbital cellulitis (infection anterior to the orbital septum) is typically caused by *S. pyogenes* or *S. aureus*, but can also be caused by *Streptococcus pneumoniae*, especially in patients <5 years old
- Orbital cellulitis (infection behind the orbital septum) is most commonly caused by *S. aureus*, but can also be caused by *S. pyogenes*, *S. pneumoniae*, or *H. influenzae*

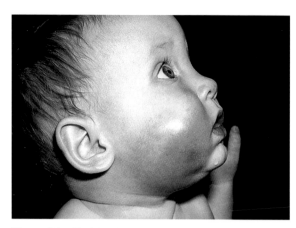

Figure 7.8 Facial cellulitis – caused by *Haemophilus influenzae* with a violaceous hue

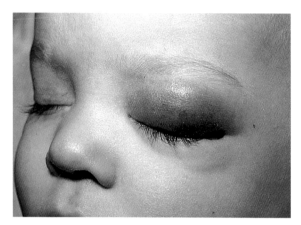

Figure 7.9 Orbital cellulitis with meningitis caused by *Haemophilus influenzae*

- Additional causative agents in neonates include group B streptococci and rarely *E. coli*
- Inoculation through animal bites: *Pasteurella multocida* from cats and dogs, *Eikenella corrodens* from humans

Diagnosis

- Clinical findings
- Typically accompanied by leukocytosis
- Gram stain and bacterial culture from lesional aspirate is positive in 25% of cases
- Histology reveals edema and intense neutrophilic inflammation in the dermis and fat; tissue Gram stain or bacterial culture is positive in the minority of cases
- Blood cultures may be positive if there is associated bacteremia
- Computed tomography may be indicated if there is ocular involvement
- Lumbar puncture is indicated if the patient is <1 year old or if there are signs of toxicity or sepsis

Differential diagnosis

- Allergic contact dermatitis
- Urticaria
- Drug eruption
- Cold panniculitis
- Insect bite
- Wells syndrome

Treatment

- Therapy is based on the age of the patient, location of the infection, and the immune status of the patient
- Systemic antibiotics are required
- Localized infection on the extremity can be treated with oral penicillinase-resistant antibiotic with outpatient follow-up in 24 hours to re-assess status of patient
- Patients <5 years old should also be covered for *S. pneumoniae*
- Intravenous antibiotics and hospitalization are warranted if refractory to oral antibiotics, or with facial involvement
- Orbital cellulitis is an emergency and requires hospitalization, intravenous antibiotic therapy and evaluation by an ophthalmologist and otolaryngologist

Prognosis

- Good prognosis if diagnosed and appropriately treated early
- Delay in diagnosis or treatment is associated with increased complications
- Complications: subcutaneous abscess (Figure 7.10), necrotizing fasciitis, lymphangitis, thrombophlebitis, bacteremia, osteomyelitis, septic arthritis and systemic involvement of the heart valves, eyes or central nervous system (CNS); post-streptococcal glomerulonephritis can also occur

References

Capdevila O, Grau I, Vadillo M, et al. Bacteremic pneumococcal cellulitis compared with bacteremic cellulitis caused by Staphylococcus aureus and Streptococcus pyogenes. Eur J Clin Microbiol Infect Dis 2003; 22: 337–41

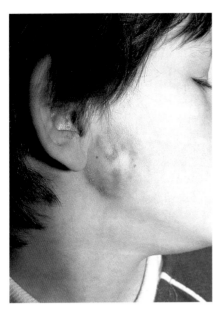

Figure 7.10 Abscess – caused by *Staphylococcus aureus*

Cohen PR, Kurzrock R. Community-acquired methicillin-resistant Staphylococcus aureus skin infection: an emerging clinical problem. J Am Acad Dermatol 2004; 50: 277–80

Darmstadt GL. Bacterial skin infections in adolescents. Adolesc Med 2001; 12: 243–68

Eady EA, Cove JH. Staphylococcal resistance revisited: community-acquired methicillin resistant Staphylococcus aureus—an emerging problem for the management of skin and soft tissue infections. Curr Opin Infect Dis 2003; 16: 103–24

Fisher RG, Benjamin DK. Facial cellulitis in childhood: a changing spectrum. South Med J 2002; 95: 672–4

Givner LB. Periorbital versus orbital cellulitis. Pediatr Infect Dis J 2002; 21: 1157–8

Erysipelas

Major points

- Acute, superficial cellulitis with infection and inflammation in the dermis and upper subcutaneous tissue involving the superficial dermal lymphatics
- Infection follows inoculation through breaks in the skin (e.g. trauma, fissures, primary dermatosis such as intertrigo, tinea pedis or ulceration)
- Predisposing factors include lymphatic/venous obstruction, diabetes mellitus and nephrotic syndrome

- Typically involves the face, scalp or leg; the lower extremity has replaced the face as the most common location of involvement
- Presents as a red, shiny, warm, indurated plaque with well-demarcated, advancing border (Figure 7.11)
- Can also be vesicular, bullous or petechial
- Fever and constitutional symptoms can precede the cutaneous eruption

Pathogenesis

- Bacteria enter the skin through some disruption of skin integrity leading to bacterial proliferation causing intense lymphatic inflammation
- Most commonly caused by infection with *Streptococcus pyogenes*
- Can also be due to infection with *S. aureus, S. pneumoniae* and group G, B, C, D streptococci

Diagnosis

- Clinical findings
- ASO and anti-DNAase B titers may be elevated
- Gram stain and bacterial culture of the portal of entry may identify the organism
- Histology reveals marked dermal and lymphatic edema with surrounding neutrophilic infiltrate

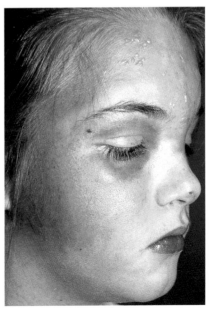

Figure 7.11 Erysipelas – quickly-spreading erythema with pain caused by streptococcus

- Latex particle agglutination for streptococcal antigens in skin biopsy specimens may be positive

Differential diagnosis

- Systemic lupus erythematosus
- Dermatomyositis
- Relapsing polychondritis
- Acute tuberculoid leprosy
- Contact dermatitis
- Urticaria

Treatment

- Systemic penicillin or cephalexin for at least 10 days; can use erythromycin or clarithromycin if penicillin allergic

Prognosis

- May resolve with postinflammatory hyperpigmentation
- Can rarely progress to bacteremia, thrombophlebitis, abscess formation, necrotizing fasciitis, gangrene or bony changes
- Post-streptococcal renal and cardiac involvement can occur
- Recurrence occurs in up to 20% of cases

References

Bisno AL, Stevens DL. Streptococcal infections of skin and soft tissues. N Engl J Med 1996; 334: 240–5

Bonnetblanc JM, Bedane C. Erysipelas: recognition and management. Am J Clin Dermatol 2003; 4: 157–63

Dahl PR, Perniciaro C, Holmkvist KA, et al. Fulminant group A streptococcal necrotizing fasciitis: clinical and pathologic findings in 7 patients. J Am Acad Dermatol 2002; 47: 489–92

Eriksson B, Jorup-Ronstrom C, Karkkonen K, et al. Erysipelas: clinical and bacteriologic spectrum and serological aspects. Clin Infect Dis 1996; 23: 1091–8

Hedrick J. Acute bacterial skin infections in pediatric medicine: current issues in presentation and treatment. Paediatr Drugs 2003; 5 (Suppl 1): 35–46

Perianal streptococcal dermatitis

Major points

- Superficial infection of the perianal skin
- Associated with concurrent pharyngeal infection in >50% of cases
- May be preceded by impetigo with secondary infection of the perianal skin
- Typically presents between 6 months and 10 years of age
- More common in males
- Presents acutely with well-demarcated, bright red, tender erythema surrounding the anus (Figure 7.12)
- Chronic infection leads to perianal fissures, crusting and psoriasiform plaques
- Associated with perianal itching and pain leading to painful defecation and fecal retention
- Rarely associated with constitutional symptoms
- Can precipitate guttate psoriasis in children

Pathogenesis

- Local infection in the dermis caused by *Streptococcus pyogenes*

Diagnosis

- Perianal swab with positive bacterial culture for *S. pyogenes* or latex agglutination are confirmatory
- Histology is not well-described and is rarely required

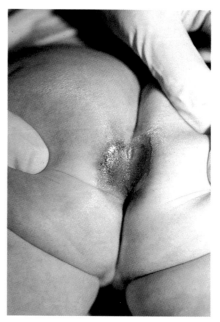

Figure 7.12   Perianal streptococcus with typical bright shiny erythema

Differential diagnosis

- Psoriasis
- Intertrigo
- Candidiasis
- Seborrheic dermatitis
- Pinworm infestation
- Inflammatory bowel disease
- Sexual abuse

Treatment

- Oral penicillin or cephalexin for 10 days
- Alternatives: oral erythromycin or clarithromycin in penicillin-allergic patients
- Oral clindamycin has been successful in recurrent cases
- Mupirocin ointment topically along with systemic antibiotics have also been utilized to treat recurrences

Prognosis

- Typically heals without sequelae
- Frequently recurrent
- Can lead to behavioral defecating difficulties if untreated

References

Anonymous. Kindergarten-based outbreak of perianal group A streptococcal infection. Arch Dis Child 2003; 88: 811

Barzilai A, Choen HA. Isolation of group A streptococci from children with perianal cellulitis and from their siblings. Pediatr Infect Dis J 1998; 17: 358–60

Mogielnicki NP, Schwartzman JD, Elliott JA. Perineal group A streptococcal disease in a pediatric practice. Pediatrics 2000; 106: 276–81

Petersen JP, Kaltoft MS, Misfeldt JC, et al. Community outbreak of perianal group A streptococcal infection in Denmark. Pediatr Infect Dis J 2003; 22: 105–9

Velez A, Moreno JC. Febrile perianal streptococcal dermatitis. Pediatr Dermatol 1999; 16: 23–4

Blistering distal dactylitis

Major points

- Superficial blistering infection of the skin
- Typically affects school-aged children
- Presents with tense, tender, dusky, erythematous-based vesicles over the anterior fat pad of the fingers and toes (Figure 7.13)

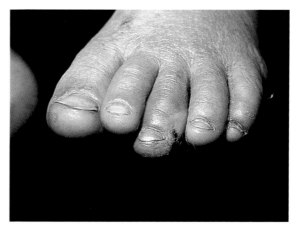

Figure 7.13   Blistering dactylitis caused by *Staphylococcus aureus*

- Can involve multiple digits
- May be associated with fever and constitutional symptoms
- Resolves with desquamation
- Can be associated with asymptomatic infection of the nasopharynx or conjunctiva

Pathogenesis

- Caused by a localized infection with group A streptococcus
- Can rarely be due to infection with group B streptococcus or *S. aureus*

Diagnosis

- Positive Gram stain and bacterial culture from blister fluid

Differential diagnosis

- Herpetic whitlow
- Friction blisters

Treatment

- Incision and drainage
- Systemic penicillinase-resistant antibiotics

Prognosis

- Resolves without sequelae
- Can be recurrent

References

Barnett BO, Frieden IJ. Streptococcal skin diseases in children. Semin Dermatol 1992; 11: 3–10

Ney AC, English JC, Greer KE. Coexistent infections on a child's distal phalanx: blistering dactylitis and herpetic whitlow. Cutis 2002; 69: 46–8

Woroszylski A, Duran C, Tamayo L, et al. Staphylococcal blistering dactylitis: report of two patients. Pediatr Dermatol 1996; 13: 292–3

Scarlet fever

Synonym: scarlatina

Major points

- Most common in children aged 2 to 10 years
- Uncommon in children <2 years old because of maternal anti-exotoxin antibodies
- Typically begins with fever and sore throat
- Exanthem follows after 1–2 days; typically starts on upper trunk and then generalizes with typical sandpaper texture and sparing of the palms and soles (Figures 7.14–7.16)
- Resolves with fine brawny desquamation
- Erythema is accentuated in the skin folds which can develop petechiae (Pastia's lines)
- Facial flushing with circumoral pallor is common
- Enanthem with petechiae of the palate and uvula (Forschheimer spots), or bright red mucous

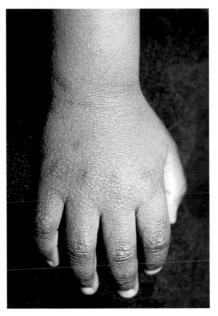

Figure 7.15 Scarlet fever – typical sandpaper rash on the hand

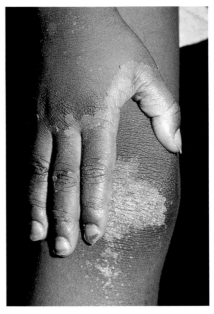

Figure 7.16 Scarlet fever – desquamation 1 week later, typically concentrated on hands, feet and knees

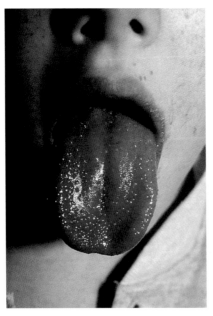

Figure 7.14 Scarlet fever – strawberry tongue with loss of papillae

membranes and a white-coated tongue with dilated papillae (white strawberry tongue) that sloughs producing a glistening red tongue with dilated papillae (red strawberry tongue)

- May have associated lymphadenopathy, fever and constitutional symptoms

Pathogenesis

- Initiated by infection of the pharynx, skin, soft tissue or surgical sites with *S. pyogenes* or group C or G streptococci
- Clinical manifestations are caused by streptococcal pyrogenic exotoxins A, B or C produced by the infectious organism

Diagnosis

- Clinical presentation
- Leukocytosis with increased number of bands and eosinophilia
- Rising antistreptolysin-O titer during the acute phase and declining titer with convalescence
- Rapid antigen detection may be positive, but can be falsely negative early in the disease course
- Positive Gram stain and bacterial culture of the throat or wound is confirmatory
- Histology: dilated dermal blood and lymphatic vessels especially around hair follicles along with perivascular mononuclear cell infiltration

Differential diagnosis

- Viral exanthem
- Exanthematous drug eruption
- Kawasaki disease
- Toxic shock syndrome
- Staphylococcal scalded skin syndrome
- Measles
- Rubella
- Mononucleosis

Treatment

- Penicillin is the treatment of choice
- Alternatives: erythromycin, clarithromycin, or azithromycin

Prognosis

- Typically good with early treatment
- Early complications can include otitis media, mastoiditis, pneumonia, bacteremia and osteomyelitis
- Rheumatic fever is a rare sequela; risk is reduced with early treatment
- Acute glomerulonephritis is a rare sequela and treatment of skin infection does not reduce its risk of development

- 80% of children develop lifelong antibodies to the exotoxins, eliminating the chance of recurrence

References

Bialecki C, Feder HM Jr, Grant-Kels JM. The six classic childhood exanthems: a review and update. J Am Acad Dermatol 1989; 21: 891–903

Espinosa de los Monteros LE, Bustos IM, Flores LV, Avila-Figueroa C. Outbreak of scarlet fever caused by an erythromycin-resistant Streptococcus pyogenes emm22 genotype strain in a day-care center. Pediatr Infect Dis J 2001; 20: 807–9

Shiseki M, Miwa K, Nemoto Y, et al. Comparison of pathogenic factors expressed by group A Streptococci isolated from patients with streptococcal toxic shock syndrome and scarlet fever. Microb Pathol 1999; 27: 243–52

Staphylococcal scalded skin syndrome

Synonym: Ritter disease

Major points

- Typically presents in children <5 years old
- Initially begins with fever, malaise, irritability, skin tenderness and erythema
- Rapidly progresses to diffuse erythroderma that is accentuated in the flexural areas with characteristic perioral erythema (Figures 7.17–7.21)

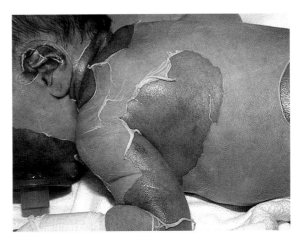

Figure 7.17   Staphylococcal scalded skin syndrome – in a neonate; mother had a positive vaginal culture for *Staphylococcus aureus*

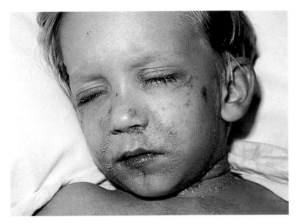

Figure 7.18 Staphylococcal scalded skin syndrome – typical painful erythema and crusting around the face

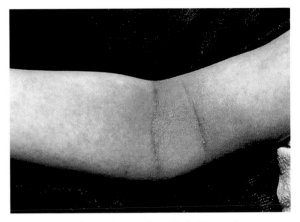

Figure 7.20 Staphylococcal scalded skin syndrome – painful erythema caused by exfoliative toxin

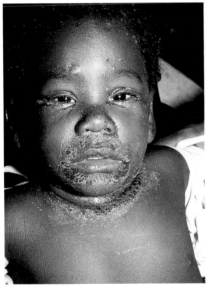

Figure 7.19 Staphylococcal scalded skin syndrome – typical crusting and scaling on the face

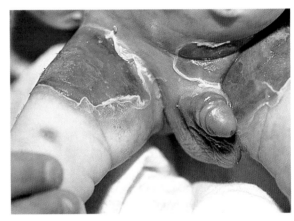

Figure 7.21 Staphylococcal scalded skin syndrome – localized to the diaper area

- Followed by diffuse exfoliation or bullous desquamation with perioral, perinasal and periocular crusting and radial fissuring and underlying shiny erythema

Pathogenesis

- Primary colonization or infection with *S. aureus* phage group II (types 3A, 3B, 3C, 55, 71) of the nasopharynx, conjunctivae, cutaneous wounds, umbilical cord stump or urinary tract

- Causative organisms produce epidermolytic toxins A and B that are hematogenously spread
- Exotoxins have serine protease activity causing cleavage of desmosomal desmoglein 1 leading to a granular layer split and generalized sloughing of the superficial epidermis

Diagnosis

- Culture of the primary source (e.g. nasopharynx, conjunctivae or umbilical cord)
- Gram stain and culture of the exfoliated skin is negative for organisms unless secondarily infected
- Tzanck smear may reveal acantholytic cells
- Histologic evaluation of the exfoliated skin in frozen sections reveals only stratum corneum

- Histology of skin reveals a subcorneal vesicle with the cleavage plane within the granular layer, a few acantholytic cells and limited inflammation

Differential diagnosis

- Scarlet fever
- Kawasaki disease
- Toxic shock syndrome
- Bullous impetigo
- Bullous mastocytosis
- Drug-induced toxic epidermal necrolysis

Treatment

- Gentle cleansing with antibacterial cleansers may prevent secondary infection
- Emollients, mupirocin, or topical silver sulfadiazine to denuded areas
- Oral penicillinase-resistant antibiotics in cases with limited cutaneous involvement
- Parenteral antibiotics are required if there is extensive cutaneous involvement or signs of systemic involvement

Prognosis

- Typically heals without scarring in 14 days
- May be scarring if secondarily infected
- Extensive desquamation can lead to fluid and electrolyte imbalance
- Can develop pneumonia, endocarditis, cellulitis or bacteremia
- Mortality is less than 4% from sepsis

References

Faden H. Neonatal staphylococcal skin infections. Pediatr Infect Dis J 2003; 22: 389

Ladhani S, Joannou CL. Difficulties in diagnosis and management of the staphylococcal scalded skin syndrome. Pediatr Infect Dis J 2000; 19: 819–21

Ladhani S, Joannou CL, Lochrie DP, et al. Clinical, microbial, and biochemical aspects of the exfoliative toxins causing staphylococcal scalded skin syndrome. Clin Microbiol Rev 1999; 12: 224–42

Patel GK, Finlay AY. Staphylococcal scalded skin syndrome: diagnosis and management. Am J Clin Dermatol 2003; 4: 165–75

Sarkar R, Sharma RC, Koranne RV, Sardana K. Erythroderma in children: a clinico-etiological study. J Dermatol 1999; 26: 507–11

Meningococcemia

Major points

- Severe, acute bacterial septicemia
- Most common in infants of 6–12 months of age; 50% of all cases are <5 years of age
- Increased susceptibility with asplenia or complement deficiency
- Begins with prodrome of fever, headache and upper respiratory symptoms, followed by meningeal irritation and neurologic symptoms
- Progression is variable but typically rapid
- Cutaneous findings: acrocyanosis of the ears, nose, lips, legs and genitalia (often the first cutaneous finding), petechiae, purpura, confluent ecchymoses with central necrosis that can progress to gangrene (Figure 7.22)
- Chronic meningococcemia is rare in children; has been associated with complement deficiencies or prior meningococcal disease

Pathogenesis

- Infection with *Neisseria meningitidis*; typically from nasopharyngeal carriage or inhalation of infected secretions with bacterial seeding of the blood and widespread dissemination
- Endotoxin-mediated procoagulation and thrombosis leads to infarction and necrosis in multiple organ systems with consumption of protein C, protein S and antithrombin III
- Serogroups A and C are associated with epidemics; serotype B is associated with sporadic cases and is most common in childhood cases

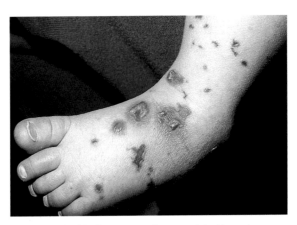

Figure 7.22 Meningococcemia – angulated irregular necrotic lesions

Diagnosis

- Clinical findings of an acutely ill child with fever, typical skin lesions and signs of sepsis
- Cultures of blood and cerebrospinal fluid (CSF) which reveal Gram-negative diplococci
- Latex agglutination of the CSF is the most rapid diagnostic test
- Gram stain of aspiration fluid or scraping from a petechial lesion occasionally reveals organisms
- Histology reveals thrombi in the dermal vessels with acute vasculitis and perivascular hemorrhagic necrosis; Gram-negative diplococci may be identified within or around vessels
- Cultures of skin are positive in up to 85% of cases; requires chocolate agar or Thayer–Martin medium with specific growth requirements

Differential diagnosis

- Gonococcemia
- Bacteremia with *Haemophilus influenzae* or *Streptococcus pneumoniae*
- Henoch–Schönlein purpura
- Leukocytoclastic vasculitis
- Endocarditis
- Rickettsial infections
- Rheumatic fever

Treatment

- Broad antibacterial coverage: ampicillin and cefotaxime or ceftriaxone with or without doxycycline until culture and sensitivity are available
- Supportive and intensive care
- Management of sepsis and other complications
- Polyvalent polysaccharide vaccines for serogroups A, C, Y and W-135 are available and recommended in those who are asplenic, those with complement deficiencies and those in closed communities (e.g. dormitories and the military); vaccination is 90% effective

Prognosis

- Fatal if not diagnosed and/or treated appropriately
- Morbidity and mortality increase with increasing purpuric lesions
- Fulminant, rapidly progressive disease is associated with >50% mortality
- 90% recovery rate if treated in the early stages of disease

- Complications occur in 11–19% of cases and include gangrene with skin necrosis, septic arthritis, myocarditis, pneumonia, renal failure, adrenal involvement (Waterhouse–Friderichsen syndrome), neurologic involvement and seizures

References

Darmstadt GL. Acute infectious purpura fulminans: pathogenesis and medical management. Pediatr Dermatol 1998; 15: 169–83

Domingo P, Muniz-Diaz E, Baraldes MA, et al. Associations between Fc gamma receptor IIA polymorphisms and the risk and prognosis of meningococcal disease. Am J Med 2002; 112: 19–25

Malley R, Huskins WC, Kuppermann N. Multivariable predictive models for adverse outcome of invasive meningococcal disease in children. J Pediatr 1996; 129: 702–10

Ploysangam T, Sheth AP. Chronic meningococcemia in childhood: case report and review of the literature. Pediatr Dermatol 1996; 13: 483–7

Powars D, Larsen R, Johnson J, et al. Epidemic meningococcemia and purpura fulminans with induced protein C deficiency. Clin Infect Dis 1993; 17: 254–61

Pitted keratolysis

Major points

- Bacterial infection of the stratum corneum of the weight-bearing plantar surfaces
- Rarely affects palmar surfaces
- Malodorous; occasionally painful but typically asymptomatic
- Presents with shallow, discrete pits or erythematous plaques with shallow ulcerations (Figure 7.23)
- Associated with humid climates, hyperhidrosis, extended immersion in water or walking barefoot in wet environments

Pathogenesis

- Multiple causative organisms have been identified and may exist synergistically: *Corynebacterium, Micrococcus, Dermatophilus, Actinomyces* or *Kytococcus*
- Extracellular enzymes classified as serine proteases are produced in cultures and have been shown to degrade human keratin

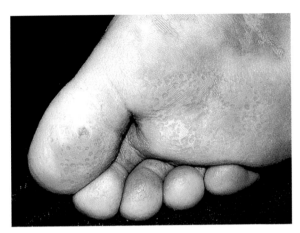

Figure 7.23   Pitted keratolysis with typical multiple shallow craters on the feet

Diagnosis

- Clinical appearance

Differential diagnosis

- Tinea pedis
- Plantar warts
- Dyshidrotic eczema

Treatment

- Topical antibiotics including erythromycin, clindamycin or mupirocin
- Castellani's paint
- Aluminum chloride
- Topical benzoyl peroxide
- Dakin solution (diluted bleach water 0.25%)

Prognosis

- Can be recurrent but responds rapidly to treatment

References

Longshaw CM, Wright JD, Farrell AM, Holland KT. Kytococcus sedentarius, the organism associated with pitted keratolysis, produces two keratin-degrading enzymes. J Appl Microbiol 2002; 93: 810–16

Shah AS, Kamino H, Prose NS. Painful, plaque-like pitted keratolysis occurring in childhood. Pediatr Dermatol 1992; 9: 251

Takama H, Tamada Y, Yano K, et al. Pitted keratolysis: clinical manifestations in 53 cases. Br J Dermatol 1997; 137: 282–5

Cat scratch disease

Synonym: cat scratch fever, benign lymphoreticulosis

Major points

- Benign, self-limited infection
- > 90% of patients have a history of exposure to a kitten
- Inoculation site characterized by a maculopapule, vesiculopapule or pustule, develops 3–10 days after exposure; most common on the upper extremity, head or neck
- Primary inoculation occurs in the eye in 7% of cases leading to conjunctivitis or ocular granuloma
- Regional lymphadenopathy is the hallmark of the disease and develops 3–50 days following the primary inoculation
- Other rare associated cutaneous findings: morbilliform eruption, petechiae, urticaria, erythema multiforme and erythema nodosum
- May be accompanied by constitutional symptoms: fever, malaise, headache, anorexia, sore throat and nausea
- Systemic involvement in 4% of patients, typically those who are immunocompromised: thrombocytopenic purpura, pneumonitis, hypercalcemia, endocarditis, CNS involvement, hepatitis and hepatosplenic abscesses

Pathogenesis

- Caused by the pleomorphic, Gram-negative bacillus *Bartonella henselae*
- Domestic cats, especially kittens <6 months of age, are the reservoir; fleas are implicated in the transmission between animals; rarely, dogs have been associated with infection
- Transmission to humans by cutaneous inoculation through a scratch, bite or lick of an infected animal

Diagnosis

- Clinical history and examination
- Serologic tests for *B. henselae*, but may be falsely positive
- Biopsy of the skin or lymph node reveals areas of necrobiosis in the dermis characterized by a central acellular zone surrounded by palisading histiocytes and a few giant cells with a surrounding zone of lymphoid cells
- Small bacilli seen with Warthin–Starry silver stain from the skin or lymph node

- Culture of skin or blood is difficult without specific growth requirements

Differential diagnosis

- Bacterial lymphadenitis
- Viral lymphadenopathy (e.g. HIV, Epstein–Barr virus, cytomegalovirus)
- Toxoplasmosis
- Histoplasmosis
- Atypical mycobacteria
- Sporotrichosis
- Sarcoidosis
- Lymphoreticular malignancy

Treatment

- Not required as skin lesions resolve spontaneously over 2–4 weeks and lymphadenopathy typically resolves in 4 months
- Multiple antibiotics have been used and are reportedly effective in speeding recovery if used early in the disease course: azithromycin, rifampin, gentamicin or trimethoprim/sulfamethoxazole
- Warm compresses
- Needle aspiration or incision and drainage of lymph nodes may relieve symptoms, but can lead to a chronic draining fistula
- Lymph node excision may be undertaken for persistent lymphadenopathy or to aid in diagnosis
- Disease in the reservoir animal is also self-limited and does not require specific treatment or disposal

Prognosis

- Patients with normal immune function have an excellent prognosis; disease resolves spontaneously over 1–3 months
- Associated with rare neurological sequelae
- Immunocompromised patients have a higher rate of systemic involvement and a more aggressive course (bacillary angiomatosis) which can lead to disseminated intravascular coagulation, shock and death

References

Chian CA, Arrese JE, Pierard GE. Skin manifestations of Bartonella infections. Int J Dermatol 2002; 41: 461–6

Metzkor-Cotter E, Kletter Y, Avidor B, et al. Long-term serological analysis and clinical follow-up of patients with cat scratch disease. Clin Infect Dis 2003; 37: 1149–54

Murakami K, Tsukahara M, Tsuneoka H, et al. Cat scratch disease: analysis of 130 seropositive cases. J Infect Chemother 2002; 8: 349–52

Somech R, Spirer Z. Uncommon presentation of some common pediatric diseases. Adv Pediatr 2003; 50: 269–304

Atypical mycobacterial diseases

Major points

- Nontuberculous acid-fast organisms that encompass a group of ~ 30 pathogens found in soil, animals, food, milk and water
- Genus *Mycobacterium* classified into four groups by Runyon:
  1. Group I
     a. Photochromogens
     b. Produces yellow pigment on Lowenstein–Jensen medium at 37°C with light exposure
     c. Includes *M. kansasii, M. marinum, M. simiae*
  2. Group II
     a. Scotochromogens
     b. Produces yellow-orange pigment with dark exposure
     c. Includes *M. scrofulaceum, M. szulgai, M. gordonae, M. xenopi*
  3. Group III
     a. Nonphotochromogens
     b. Does not produce pigment
     c. Includes *M. avium-intracellulare, M. haemophilum, M. ulcerans, M. malmoense*
  4. Group IV
     a. Rapid growers; growth within 3–5 days in culture
     b. Does not produce pigment
     c. Includes *M. fortuitum* and *M. chelonei*
- Low pathogenicity unless traumatic exposure or underlying immunocompromised state
- Most common cutaneous atypical mycobacterial infection is caused by *M. marinum* (formerly known as *M. balnei*) acquired from a swimming pool, aquarium or fish tank
- Cutaneous lesions: pink, red, purple or brown papules and nodules that can spread to adjacent surrounding skin and develop ulceration or crusting (Figures 7.24 and 7.25)

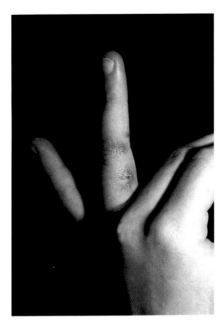

Figure 7.24 Atypical mycobacterial infection – fish tank granuloma caused by *Mycobacterium marinum*

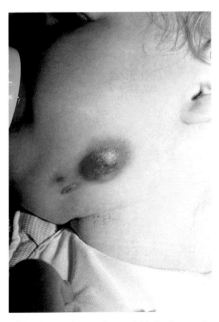

Figure 7.25 Atypical mycobacterial infection – abscess caused by *Mycobacterium intracellulare*

- Lesions are most commonly found on the extremities, especially the fingers, knees, elbows and feet, and appear ~3 weeks after exposure

Pathogenesis

- *M. marinum* is an aerobic acid-fast bacterium that inhabits warm water (open seas, natural pools, swimming pools or aquariums) and can affect fish, especially tropical fish, aquatic animals and humans
- Causative organism is inoculated into the skin either traumatically or through abrasions while working or playing in an affected environment

Diagnosis

- Consistent history and physical examination
- Intradermal testing with purified protein derivative (PPD) may be positive and can be supportive
- Tissue culture for *M. marinum* can be positive in up to 70% of cases with proper growth requirements
- Histologic features depend on the stage of development:
  1. <2–3 months: nonspecific mixed inflammation
  2. ~4 months: small epithelioid granulomas with a few multinucleated giant cells
  3. >6 months: typical tuberculoid granulomas which may have central necrosis with or without epidermal hyperkeratosis and papillomatosis
- Acid-fast organisms may be identified by Fite stain of skin biopsy specimens from early lesions

Differential diagnosis

- Bacterial abscess (e.g. *S. aureus*)
- Verruca vulgaris
- Cutaneous tuberculosis
- Sarcoidosis
- Foreign-body granuloma
- Sporotrichosis
- Blastomycosis
- Leishmaniasis

Treatment

- Multiple systemic antibiotics: tetracycline, minocycline, doxycycline, trimethoprim–sulfamethoxazole, clarithromycin and rifampin effective if given for at least 8 weeks
- Surgical excision can be used if unresponsive to antibiotics
- Proper cleaning of the reservoir (e.g. fish tank) should be undertaken if feasible

Prognosis

- Resolves with scarring

- Can resolve without treatment in 1–2 years but may persist for over a decade without treatment
- Can produce secondary draining sinuses, synovitis, bursitis, arthritis or osteomyelitis
- Rare cases of fatal disseminated disease

References

Ang P, Rattana-Apiromyakij N, Goh CL. Retrospective study of Mycobacterium marinum skin infections. Int J Dermatol 2000; 9: 343–7

Aubry A, Chosidow O, Caumes E, et al. Sixty-three cases of Mycobacterium marinum infection: clinical features, treatment, and antibiotic susceptibility of causative isolates. Arch Intern Med 2002; 162: 1746–52

Bartralot R, Pujol RM, Garcia-Patos V, et al. Cutaneous infections due to nontuberculous mycobacteria: histopathological review of 28 cases. Comparative study between lesions observed in immunosuppressed patients and normal hosts. J Cutan Pathol 2000; 27: 124–9

Pumberger W, Hallwirth U, Pawlowsky J, Pomberger G. Cervicofacial lymphadenitis due to atypical mycobacteria: a surgical disease. Pediatr Dermatol 2004; 21: 24–9

Speight EL, Williams HC. Fish tank granuloma in a 14-month-old girl. Pediatr Dermatol 1997; 14: 209–12

Tuberculosis

Major points

- Classification of cutaneous lesions is based on route of transmission and immunologic response
- Exogenous source
  1. Previously uninfected: primary inoculation tuberculosis or primary tuberculosis complex
     a. Typically occurs in a wound: abrasion, insect bite, ear piercing, circumcision site
     b. Lesion develops 2–4 weeks after inoculation
     c. Presents as a red-brown papule with 'apple jelly' translucence on diascopy that may ulcerate or crust
     d. Associated with regional lymphadenopathy or lymphangitis
  2. Previously infected: reinfection tuberculosis or tuberculosis verrucosa cutis
     a. Very rare in children
     b. Presents with large verrucous papule or plaque at the site of re-inoculation
     c. Due to strong immunity and hypersensitivity against *M. tuberculosis*

3. Bacillus Calmette–Guérin (BCG) vaccination
   a. Site of injection develops an enlarging papule which ulcerates and then heals spontaneously over 2–4 weeks
   b. May have associated lymphadenopathy
   c. Rarely develops a local abscess, scrofuloderma, generalized eruption or lupus vulgaris
4. Scrofuloderma
   a. Caused by direct extension of the organism to the skin overlying an infected lymph node or bone
   b. Lesions are most common over the cervical lymph nodes
   c. May ulcerate or form draining sinuses
   d. Heals with characteristic cord-like scar
5. Tuberculosis cutis orificialis
   a. Autoinoculation of the mucous membranes
   b. Occurs at the mouth, nose, anus, urinary meatus or genitalia from infected secretions or visceral involvement
   c. Presents as painful punched-out ulcers with undermined edges
   d. Indicates failing resistance to disease
- Hematogenous spread
  1. Lupus vulgaris
     a. Chronic, slowly progressive cutaneous form
     b. Associated with strong immunity to *M. tuberculosis*
     c. Presents with atrophic red-brown plaques on the head and neck in ~90% of cases
     d. Lesions can ulcerate and cause ectropion or eclabium
  2. Miliary or disseminated tuberculosis
     a. Presents with generalized macules, papules, pustules, nodules or purpura associated with fulminant pulmonary or meningeal involvement
     b. Systemically ill with poor prognosis
  3. Metastatic tuberculosis
     a. Occurs in patients with decreased immunity or malnutrition
     b. Presents with ulcerated nodules and sinuses
  4. Congenital tuberculosis
     a. Intrauterine infection through placental circulation
     b. Presents at 4–8 weeks of age with discrete crusted papules on the face, trunk and extremities

- Tuberculids – cutaneous reaction related to an immunologic response to the organism; associated with an underlying focus of distant infection with hematogenous spread
  1. Papulonecrotic tuberculid
     a. Most commonly seen in children
     b. Presents with successive crops of dusky-red papules with or without central necrosis on the extensor extremities which heal spontaneously with varioliform scars
     c. Typically have infected lymph nodes
  2. Lichen scrofulosorum
     a. Occurs in children and young adults
     b. Presents with clusters of lichenoid papules and discoid plaques on the trunk
     c. Resolves spontaneously and can recur
     d. Associated with infection of the bone or lymph nodes
  3. Erythema induratum (Bazin disease)
     a. Typically seen in girls and young women
     b. Presents with ulcerated nodules on the posterior calves with underlying panniculitis and vasculitis

Pathogenesis

- Caused by infection with *Mycobacterium tuberculosis*
- Can be spread by exogenous or endogenous routes

Diagnosis

- Positive tuberculin test with PPD
- Histology: variety of inflammatory reaction patterns including nonspecific acute inflammation, epithelial hyperplasia, non-necrotic granulomas and necrotic granulomas
- Fite stain of skin biopsy specimen may reveal acid-fast bacilli
- Culture of tissue
- Polymerase chain reaction for *M. tuberculosis* DNA in tissue

Differential diagnosis

- Cat scratch disease
- Atypical mycobacterial infection
- Syphilis
- Leprosy
- Sporotrichosis
- Tularemia
- Sarcoidosis
- Cutaneous lymphoma

Treatment

- Isoniazid (10–15 mg/kg per day) and rifampin (10–20 mg/kg per day) for 9 months
- Pyrazinamide, ethambutol or streptomycin is added for the initial 2 months of therapy if drug resistance is a consideration (Hispanic or Asian population), or if the duration of therapy is limited to 6 months

Prognosis

- Variable course and prognosis depending on classification and systemic involvement
- Cutaneous tuberculosis typically heals with scarring

References

Antaya RJ, Gardner ES, Bettencourt MS, et al. Cutaneous complications of BCG vaccination in infants with immune disorders: two cases and a review of the literature. Pediatr Dermatol 2001; 18: 205–9

Caksen H, Arslan S, Oner AF, et al. Multiple metastatic tuberculous abscesses in a severely malnourished infant. Pediatr Dermatol 2002; 19: 90–1

Jacinto SS, Lopez de Leon P, Mendoza C. Cutaneous tuberculosis and other skin diseases in hospitalized, treated pulmonary tuberculosis patients in the Philippines. Cutis 2003; 72: 373–6

Kivanc-Altunay I, Baysal Z, Ekmekci TR, Koslu A. Incidence of cutaneous tuberculosis in patients with organ tuberculosis. Int J Dermatol 2003; 42: 197–200

Tan H, Karakuzu A, Arik A. Scrofuloderma after BCG vaccination. Pediatr Dermatol 2002; 19: 323–5

Thami GP, Kaur S, Kanwar AJ, Mohan H. Lichen scrofulosorum: a rare manifestation of a common disease. Pediatr Dermatol 2002; 19: 122–6

Leprosy

Synonym: Hansen disease

Major points

- Chronic infection of the skin, nasal mucosa, nerves and eyes
- Clinical manifestations and disease course is dependent on the immune response of the host to *Mycobacterium leprae*
- Endemic in India, Southeast Asia, China, Central and East Africa, Central and South America, Louisiana, Hawaii and California

- Incubation period ~5 years
- Disease classification
  1. Tuberculoid leprosy
     a. <3 skin lesions which are anesthetic and anhidrotic
     b. Highest immune resistance and reactivity
     c. Organisms are not identified in tissues (paucibacillary)
     d. Nerve involvement
     e. Strong positive reaction to the lepromin skin test
  2. Borderline tuberculoid leprosy
     a. Few (3–10) skin lesions
     b. May have enlarged nerves with mild motor impairment
  3. Borderline borderline leprosy
     a. Indeterminate type
     b. Multiple asymmetric annular plaques
     c. Host resistance is unstable
     d. Organisms may be identified
  4. Borderline lepromatous leprosy
     a. Skin lesions are symmetrical and numerous
     b. Nerve involvement is not prominent
  5. Lepromatous leprosy
     a. Diffuse skin infiltration with characteristic leonine facies and loss of the eyebrows
     b. No host resistance or reactivity
     c. Organisms are numerous (multibacillary)
     d. No reaction to lepromin skin test
- Childhood disease typically presents within the tuberculoid or indeterminate spectrum with hypopigmented macules (Figure 7.26)
- Children can also present with nerve involvement alone causing thickened peripheral nerves with sensory loss (e.g. temperature is lost first, followed by light touch and pinprick)

Pathogenesis

- Infection caused by acid-fast bacillus *Mycobacterium leprae*
- Low infectivity
- Transmission is not fully known although droplet infection via an upper respiratory route is suspected
- Genetic predisposition may play a role in disease development
- Animal reservoirs: armadillos, monkeys and chimpanzees

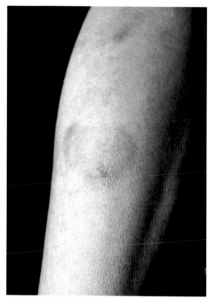

Figure 7.26   Leprosy – anesthetic plaque in a patient from Vietnam

Diagnosis

- Slit skin smears stained with Ziehl–Neelsen reveals organisms
- Organisms cannot be cultured *in vitro*
- Histology varies depending on disease state
  1. Tuberculoid leprosy: noncaseating granulomas of epithelioid cells, Langhans giant cells and lymphocytes throughout the dermis; granulomas may extend along nerves; acid-fast bacilli are identified by Fite stain in <50% of cases
  2. Lepromatous leprosy: collections and sheets of histiocytes with a few lymphocytes; foamy macrophages (Virchow cells); Grenz zone; organisms are numerous within macrophages

Differential diagnosis

- Pityriasis alba
- Tinea corporis
- Tinea versicolor
- Nummular eczema
- Granuloma annulare
- Vitiligo
- Sarcoidosis
- Syphilis
- Tuberculosis
- Lupus erythematosus

Treatment

- Dapsone (1 mg/kg per day) for 1 year in all types
- Rifampin (10 mg/kg per day) should be added for 6 months in cases of tuberculoid, borderline tuberculoid or indeterminate disease
- Clofazimine (1 mg/kg per day) should be added for 2 years in cases of borderline, borderline lepromatous and lepromatous disease
- Type I reaction (downgrading or reversal reaction that represents an enhanced cell-mediated response to *M. leprae*) and type II reactions (erythema nodosum leprosum due to circulating immune complexes with potential multisystem involvement) are treated with systemic corticosteroids

Prognosis

- Chronic disease with unpredictable course unless treated
- Reactional phenomenon can occur and leads to tissue damage, especially nerve injury with persistent neurologic sequelae
- 50% of patients will experience a reaction after starting antibiotic therapy

References

Boggild AK, Keystone JS, Kain KC. Leprosy: a primer for Canadian physicians. Can Med Assoc J 2004; 170: 71–8

Cosma CL, Sherman DR, Ramakrishnan L. The secret lives of the pathogenic mycobacteria. Ann Rev Microbiol 2003; 57: 641–76

Fakhouri R, Sotto MN, Manini MI, Margarido LC. Nodular leprosy of childhood and tuberculoid leprosy: a comparative, morphologic, immunopathologic and quantitative study of skin tissue reaction. Int J Lepr Other Mycobact Dis 2003; 71: 218–26

Jayalakshmi P, Tong M, Sing S, Ganesapillai T. Leprosy in children. Int J Lepr Other Mycobact Dis 1997; 65: 95–7

Ramos-e-Silva M, Rebello PF. Leprosy. Recognition and treatment. Am J Clin Dermatol 2001; 2: 203–11

Rook GA, Martinelli R, Brunet LR. Innate immune responses to mycobacteria and the downregulation of atopic responses. Curr Opin Allergy Clin Immunol 2003; 3: 337–42

Syphilis

Synonym: lues

Major points

- Incubation period: 9–90 days after initial exposure
- Often associated with other sexually transmitted diseases including HIV
- Congenital syphilis (See Chapter 2)
- Primary stage
  1. Initial lesion at the site of inoculation (chancre)
  2. Presents as a painless ulcer that heals over 1–6 weeks
  3. Typically found on the genitalia, but can also be seen on the lips, tongue, areola or hands (Figure 7.27)
- Secondary stage
  1. Begins 2–10 weeks after healing of the primary chancre
  2. Results from hematogenous spread
  3. Constitutional signs: generalized lymphadenopathy, hepatosplenomegaly
  4. Classic findings: diffuse papulosquamous eruption, specifically involving the palms and soles (Figures 7.28 and 7.29)
  5. Other skin findings: condyloma lata, (Figure 7.30) split papules, moth-eaten alopecia and mucous patches
- Subclinical, latent phase
  1. No signs or symptoms except for reactive serology
  2. May last 1–40 years

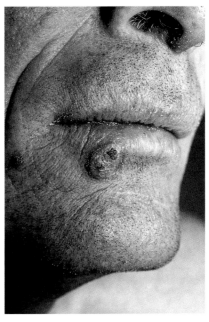

Figure 7.27 Syphilitic chancre in an adult

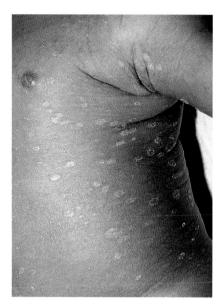

Figure 7.28   Secondary syphilis – age 6 weeks acquired congenitally

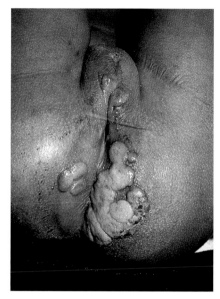

Figure 7.30   Secondary syphilis – condylomata lata (previously published in *Pediatric Dermatology* 1989; 6: 51–2, with permission)

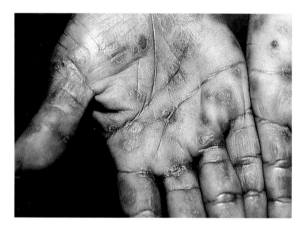

Figure 7.29   Secondary syphilis – typical copper-colored palmar lesions

- Tertiary or late stage
  1. Develops in one-third of untreated cases; rare in children
  2. Typically presents 3–5 years after the initial infection
  3. Presents with nodular lesion or gummas
  4. Can involve the bones, CNS and cardiovascular systems

Pathogenesis

- Caused by the spirochete *Treponema pallidum*

- Sexually transmitted disease with penetration of the organism through mucous membranes or abrasions in the stratum corneum
- Nonsexual transmission from an infected parent to a child is rare; sexual abuse should be assumed until proven otherwise

Diagnosis

- Nontreponemal antigen tests include the rapid plasma reagent (RPR) and Venereal Disease Research Laboratory (VDRL) test; typically positive within 5–6 weeks of infection; negative with therapy and in late syphilis
- Treponemal antigen tests are more sensitive and specific and include the microhemagglutination assay for *T. pallidum* (MHA-TP) or fluorescent treponemal antibody absorption (FTA-ABS) test; typically positive at 2–3 weeks after infection and remains positive for life
- Dark field examination and direct fluorescent antibody tests on lesional exudate or tissue
- Histology varies with stage of disease
  1. Primary syphilis: acanthosis, ulcer infiltrated by lymphocytes and plasma cells; Warthin–Starry silver stain may reveal the spirochete at the dermal–epidermal junction or around vessels

2. Secondary syphilis: epidermal psoriasiform hyperplasia, spongiosis, vacuolar alteration, papillary dermal edema, and a lymphohistiocytic perivascular and periadnexal infiltrate with variable number of plasma cells; spirochetes can be seen in one-third of cases with silver staining

3. Tertiary syphilis: granulomatous inflammation with central necrosis and peripheral infiltrate of lymphocytes, macrophages and plasma cells; spirochetes are typically not present

Differential diagnosis

- Primary: herpes simplex, chancroid, granuloma inguinale
- Secondary: pityriasis rosea, psoriasis, drug eruptions, lichen planus, sarcoidosis
- Tertiary: leprosy, tuberculosis, sarcoidosis

Treatment

- Parenteral penicillin G is the treatment of choice in all stages of syphilis, and is the only antibiotic with documented efficacy in pregnancy and in neurosyphilis
  1. Primary and secondary: benzathine penicillin G 50 000 units/kg intramuscularly up to 2.4 million units, in a single dose
  2. Latent: benzathine penicillin G 50 000 units/kg IM up to 2.4 million units with three doses at 1-week intervals
  3. Neurosyphilis: aqueous crystalline penicillin G 200 000–300 000 units/kg per day intravenously for 10 days
- Penicillin-allergic patients can be treated with:

1. Doxycycline 100 mg twice a day for 2–4 weeks depending on the duration of infection; associated with discoloration of teeth if <8 years old

2. Tetracycline 500 mg four times a day for 2–4 weeks depending on the duration of infection; associated with discoloration of teeth if <8 years old

3. Erythromycin 500 mg four times a day for 2 weeks

Prognosis

- Variable depending on the stage of disease
- Untreated, the disease is slowly progressive and fatal with CNS and cardiac involvement

References

Burstein GR. Workowski KA. Sexually transmitted diseases treatment guidelines. Curr Opin Pediatr 2003; 15: 391–7

Golden MR. Marra CM. Holmes KK. Update on syphilis: resurgence of an old problem. J Am Med Assoc 2003; 290: 1510–14

Hollier LM, Cox SM. Syphilis. Semin Perinatol 1998; 22: 323–31

Ozturk F, Gurses N, Sancak R, et al. Acquired secondary syphilis in a 6-year-old girl with no history of sexual abuse. Cutis 1998; 62: 150–1

Pandhi D, Kumar S, Reddy BS. Sexually transmitted diseases in children. J Dermatol 2003; 30: 314–20

Rubins S, Janniger CK, Schwartz RA. Congenital and acquired early childhood syphilis. Cutis 1995; 56: 132–6

Vural M, Ilikkan B, Polat E, et al. A premature newborn with vesiculobullous skin lesions. Eur J Pediatr 2003; 162: 197–9

8

VIRAL AND RICKETTSIAL DISEASES

GENERAL

- Exanthems
  1. Morbilliform (measles-like)
  2. Petechial
  3. Scarlatiniform (scarlet-fever like)
  4. Vesiculobullous
  5. Papulonodular
  6. Asymmetric periflexural exanthem
- Enanthems (oral lesions)
  1. Nonspecific
  2. Specific
- Epidermal growths
  1. Verrucous
  2. Papular

Measles (Rubeola)

Major points

- Classic measles: prodrome of fever, malaise and upper respiratory symptoms followed by high fever, cough, coryza (rhinitis), conjunctivitis
- Incubation period 9–14 days
- Cough 'barking', sounds like croup
- Coryza (runny nose)
- Conjunctivitis with photophobia
- Lymphadenopathy, especially cervical
- Koplik spots (enanthem): 1-mm white spots ('grains of sand') on intensely erythematous background, usually on buccal mucosa (Figure 8.1)
- Characteristic rash begins on face as blotchy erythema, progresses downward to involve trunk and extremities with multiple discrete very

erythematous macules and papules which can become petechial (Figure 8.2)
- Complications (more common in young children, or those malnourished or chronically ill):
  1. Bacterial otitis media
  2. Bacterial pneumonia
  3. Encephalitis
  4. Myocarditis/pericarditis
  5. Thrombocytopenia
  6. Hepatitis
  7. Acute glomerulonephritis
- Atypical measles
  1. Usually in patients who have had killed measles vaccine, or failed vaccination

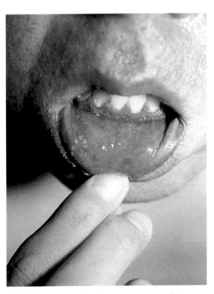

Figure 8.1 Rubeola – Koplik spots: tiny white papules on oral mucosa

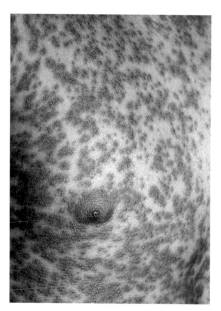

Figure 8.2   Rubeola – intense morbilliform eruption

2. Symptoms: high fever, abdominal pain, pneumonitis, acral petechiae, vesicles, vesiculopustular eruption, vasculitis

Pathogenesis

- Measles virus replicates in nasopharynx before disseminating
- Lymphoid hyperplasia occurs with wide distribution of virus-infected cells
- Rash is result of viremia with lodging of antigen and virus in the capillaries, followed by cell-mediated response
- Koplik spots contain viral nucleocapsids
- Lifelong immunity follows natural measles infection

Diagnosis

- Characteristic rash and symptoms
- Positive serologic test for measles IgM antibody
- Viral isolation from nasopharyngeal secretions, blood or urine
- Rise in measles IgG antibody, acute and convalescent sera at first encounter and after 2–4 weeks
- Viral antigen detected by immunofluorescence in cell smears from nasal aspirates early in illness

Differential diagnosis

- Rocky Mountain spotted fever

- Drug eruptions
- Vasculitis

Treatment

- Isolation of patient; highly contagious
- Symptomatic treatment
- Antibiotics for secondary infection
- Immune globulin 0.25 ml/kg of body weight, intramuscularly; immunocompromised children 0.5 ml/kg (maximum 15 ml) given within 6 days attenuates the infection in exposed persons
- Immunization with live attenuated vaccine reduces the incidence of measles in contacts
- Vitamin A supplementation 200 000 IU orally for age >1 year; 100 000 IU for 6 months to 1 year. Repeat next day and 4 weeks later if there is ophthalmologic evidence of vitamin deficiency

Prognosis

- Lifelong immunity follows natural measles infection or immunization
- High morbidity and mortality rate in malnourished or immunosuppressed patients

References

Bialecki C, Feder HM, Grant-Kels JM. The six classic childhood exanthems: a review and update. J Am Acad Dermatol 1989; 21: 891–903

Butler JC, Havens PL, Sowell AL, et al. Measles severity and serum retinal (vitamin A) concentration among children in the United States. Pediatrics 1993; 91: 1176–81

Frieden IJ, Resnick SD. Childhood exanthems. Old and new. Pediatr Clin North Am 1991; 38: 859–87

Rall GF. Measles virus 1998–2002: progress and controversy. Annu Rev Microbiol 2003; 57: 343–67

Report of the Committee on Infectious Diseases. Red Book, 26th edn. American Academy of Pediatrics: Elk Grove Village, IL, 2003: 419–29

Somech R, Spirer Z. Uncommon presentation of some common pediatric diseases. Adv Pediatr 2003; 50: 269–304

Venczel L, Rota J, Dietz V, et al. The Measles Laboratory Network in the region of the Americas. J Infect Dis 2003; 187 (Suppl 1): S140–5

Rubella

Major points

- Incubation period ~18 days (14–21 days)

- Prodrome may be mild or negligible, lasts 1–5 days, with fever up to 39°C, headache, malaise, sore throat, conjunctivitis
- 50% of infections are asymptomatic
- Rash may be absent in 40% of cases
- Enanthem (Forschheimer sign) present in 20%; consists of red macules or petechiae on soft palate
- Lymph node enlargement begins in prodrome in suboccipital, postauricular and cervical glands
- Rash appears on face and spreads downwards to trunk and limbs, made up of pink macules, which become confluent; clears quickly in 3–4 days
- Complications few in childhood
- Complications in adults and older children: monoarticular arthritis, which lasts ~1 month; rarely, purpura or encephalitis
- Rubella in pregnancy
  1. Fetal damage in 90% of cases in first 11 weeks of pregnancy (rubella embryopathy)
  2. Between 12 and 16 weeks' gestation, risk of deafness is 25%
  3. Major defects: deafness, mental retardation, heart damage, eye damage (cataracts, glaucoma), microcephaly, growth retardation
- Neonatal period
  1. Thrombocytopenic purpura which clears spontaneously in several weeks
  2. Jaundice (rubella hepatitis)
  3. Bone lesions
  4. Recurrent exanthem which may recur during first 5 years
  5. 'Blueberry muffin' appearance with blue/purple macules, papules in a generalized pattern due to extramedullary hematopoiesis
- Infectivity
  1. Patients infective for 2 days before rash and 7 days after rash begins
  2. In congenital rubella, virus can be shed up to 5–6 years
- Epidemics occur in spring, mainly in older children and adults

Pathogenesis

- Rubella virus member of Rubivirus genus, RNA virus, Togaviridae
- Virus spreads through direct or droplet contact from nasopharyngeal secretions
- Rash may be result of viral dissemination to skin
- Mechanism of embryopathy unknown

Diagnosis

- Morphology of rash with enlarged lymph nodes suggestive of diagnosis
- Serology with four-fold increase in antibody titers in acute and convalescent serum
- Specific IgM antibody in previous infection
- Viral isolation from peripheral blood leukocytes, stool or urine for months to years after birth in patients with rubella embryopathy or from nasal mucosa in acute disease

Differential diagnosis

- Acute viral disease in children or adults (Table 8.1) or drug eruptions
- Congenital infections (toxoplasmosis, syphilis, cytomegalovirus (CMV), herpes simplex), neonatal lupus erythematosus, Wiskott–Aldrich syndrome, hereditary platelet disorders

Treatment

- Symptomatic treatment for acute disease
- Nonsteroidal anti-inflammatory agents for arthritis
- Prophylaxis
  1. Active immunization with live attenuated rubella virus. Administration in pregnancy is contraindicated. Arthralgia is common

Table 8.1   Viral morbilliform eruptions
Characteristic disease pattern
Measles
Rubella
Roseola
Erythema infectiosum
Infectious mononucleosis
Pityriasis rosea
Hand, foot and mouth disease
Nonspecific morbilliform eruptions
Hepatitis A, B, C, D, E
Mumps
Echovirus
Coxsackievirus
Respiratory syncytial virus
Cytomegalovirus
Adenoviruses
Dengue fever
Ehrilichiosis
Colorado tick fever
HIV

2. Immune serum globulin given 0.5 ml/kg intramuscularly

Prognosis

- Good in acute disease
- Poor in rubella embryopathy. Multidisciplinary approach and birth defects clinic is advisable

References

Bale JF Jr. Congenital infections. Neurol Clin 2002; 20: 1039–60, vii

Bialecki C, Feder HM, Grant-Kels JM. The six classic childhood exanthems: a review and update. J Am Acad Dermatol 1989; 21: 891–903

Hartley AH, Rasmussen JE. Infectious exanthems. Pediatr Rev 1988; 9: 321–9

Report of the Committee on Infectious Diseases. Red Book, 26th edn. American Academy of Pediatrics: Elk Grove Village, IL, 2003: 536–41

Spika JS, Wassilak S, Pebody R, et al. Measles and rubella in the World Health Organization European region: diversity creates challenges. J Inf Dis 2003; 187 (Suppl 1): S191–7

Vander Straten MR, Tyring SK. Rubella. Dermatol Clin 2002; 20: 225–31

Roseola (exanthem subitum, sixth disease)

Major points

- Incubation period ~9 days
- Occurs mainly in infants under 2 years of age
- Abrupt high fever (39.5–40°C) for 2–5 days, with child looking otherwise well
- When the temperature falls, rash breaks out
- Rash consists of pink, morbilliform maculopapules and fades within 1–2 days
- Rash starts on neck and trunk, and later spreads to extremities and face
- Occasionally febrile seizures occur. Encephalitis rare
- Subclinical infection common
- Other features:
  1. Mild edema of eyelids
  2. Cervical lymphadenopathy
  3. Cough
  4. Otitis media
  5. Hematuria

Pathogenesis

- Caused by human herpesvirus-6 (HHV-6), member of the family Herpesviridae; a large, double-stranded DNA virus
- HHV-6 preferentially attacks circulating lymphocytes
- After initial infection, virus persists and can be detected in saliva

Diagnosis

- Clinical picture usually specific with lack of symptoms during febrile stage, and eruption begins as fever subsides
- HHV-6 can be identified by culture of peripheral blood lymphocytes
- Serodiagnosis with rise in antibody production
- Skin lesions can demonstrate virus

Differential diagnosis

See Table 8.1: drug eruptions

Treatment

- Symptomatic treatment of fever with antipyretics and tepid sponge baths
- Follow-up at 2 days is recommended to confirm the diagnosis or rule out other causes of morbilliform rash and fever
- Isolation of the hospitalized patient is not necessary

Prognosis

- Benign in infants
- Most older children and adults are immune, but may have a mild mononucleosis-like illness with fever, rash, cervical lymphadenopathy and possibly hepatitis for up to 3 months
- HHV-6 has been isolated from peripheral B cells in HIV patients, and may become reactivated in immunosuppressed patients with fever, hepatitis, bone marrow suppression and pneumonia
- By age 4 years, almost all individuals are seropositive

References

Bialecki C, Feder HM, Grant-Kels JM. The six classic childhood exanthems: a review and update. J Am Acad Dermatol 1989; 21: 891–903

Blauvelt A. Skin diseases associated with human herpesvirus 6, 7, and 8 infection. Symposium Proceedings. J Invest Dermatol 2001; 6: 197–202

De Araujo T, Berman B, Weinstein A. Human herpesviruses 6 and 7. Dermatol Clin 2002; 20: 301–6

Dockrell DH. Human herpesvirus 6: molecular biology and clinical features. J Med Microbiol 2003; 52: 5–18

Report of the Committee on Infectious Diseases. Red Book, 26th edn. American Academy of Pediatrics: Elk Grove Village, IL, 2003: 357–9

Erythema infectiosum (fifth disease)

Major points

- Common in school-aged children
- Classical presentation: intense confluent redness of both cheeks ('slapped cheeks') with circumoral pallor (Figure 8.3)
- Later symmetric, lacy, reticulated, macular, erythematous eruption on arms, legs, chest, abdomen or buttocks (Figure 8.4)
- Eruption lasts 3–5 days, but can have exacerbations up to 4 months, especially after exercise, fever, or sun-exposure
- Mild systemic symptoms and fever seen in 15–30%
- Occasionally, other eruptions may occur: morbilliform, vesicular, purpuric (particularly in a 'gloves and socks' distribution)
- Symmetric arthritis of hands, wrists and knees may occur which resolves in 1–2 months; more common in adults
- Red cell aplasia and transient aplastic crisis may occur in patients with chronic hemolytic anemias (e.g. sickle cell disease) lasting 7–10 days; may be persistent
- Chronic infection may result in systemic necrotizing vasculitis
- In pregnant women, fetal death may occur, caused by aplastic crisis in the fetus with resultant hydrops fetalis
- Risk of fetal death is <10% in first half of pregnancy, and nonsignificant in second half
- Conjunctivitis may occur
- Probaby not contagious once skin eruption occurs except in patients with aplastic crisis who can be contagious for at least 1 week after onset of rash

Pathogenesis

- Caused by parvovirus B19, a small DNA virus, which can be identified in skin lesions by electron microscopy

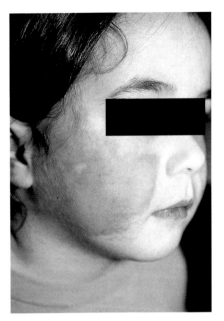

Figure 8.3   Erythema infectiosum (fifth disease) – 'slapped cheeks'

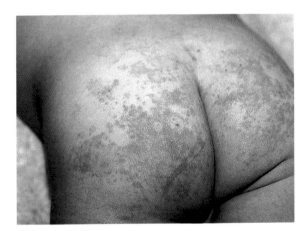

Figure 8.4   Erythema infectiosum – typical reticulated erythema

- Virus replicates in erythroid bone marrow cells causing transient aplastic crises in children with chronic hemolytic anemias
- Spread by respiratory secretions and blood
- Patients with aplastic crises are highly contagious before onset of clinical symptoms until a week or longer afterwards
- Incubation period usually 4–14 days but can be up to 20 days

Diagnosis

- Cutaneous pattern characteristic
- Serum specific parvovirus B19-IgM antibody within 30 days of onset of illness is diagnostic. Serum IgG antibody indicates previous infection and immunity
- Best method for detecting chronic infection is demonstrating virus by nucleic acid hybridization assay or polymerase chain reaction (PCR) assay
- Viral B19 antigens can be detected by radioimmunoassay or enzyme assay

Differential diagnosis

- Sunburn
- Drug eruptions (morbilliform)
- Collagen vascular diseases (reticulated pattern)
- See Table 8.1

Treatment

- Supportive care
- Isolation from patients at risk for complications (pregnant women, chronic hemolytic anemia patients)
- Contact isolation for hospitalized children with aplastic crises or immunosuppressed patients
- Intravenous immunoglobulin may be effective in immunosuppressed children
- Good hand washing techniques

Prognosis

- Excellent in normal children
- Children with arthritis, pregnant women, immunosuppressed patients and those with chronic hemolytic anemias should be followed until complications have subsided

References

Frieden IJ, Resnick SD. Childhood exanthems. Old and new. Pediatr Clin North Am 1991; 38: 859–87

Heegaard ED, Brown KE. Human parvovirus B19. Clin Microbiol Rev 2002; 15: 485–505

Katta R. Parvovirus B19: a review. Dermatol Clin 2002; 20: 333–42

Qari M, Qadri SMH. Parvovirus B19 infection. Postgrad Med 1996; 100: 239–52

Report of the Committee on Infectious Diseases. Red Book, 26th edn. American Academy of Pediatrics: Elk Grove Village, IL, 2003: 459–61

Silver MM, Hellmann J, Zielenska M, et al. Anemia, blueberry muffin rash and hepatomegaly in a newborn infant. J Pediatr 1996; 12: 579–86

Young NS, Brown KE, Parvovirus B19. N Engl J Med 2004; 350: 586–97

Gianotti–Crosti syndrome

Synonym: papular acrodermatitis of childhood, papulovesicular acrolated syndrome

Major points

- Characterized by numerous skin-colored or pink flat topped lichenoid symmetrical papules, 5–10 mm in size (Figures 8.5 and 8.6)
- Lesions begin individually and then often coalesce
- Distribution mainly on the arms, legs and face, and sparing trunk
- Associated findings:
  1. Low-grade fever and mild upper respiratory symptoms
  2. Lymphadenopathy
  3. Diarrhea
  4. Cough
  5. Hepatosplenomegaly
  6. Enanthem
- Age usually 8 months to 4 years
- Duration of rash 2–8 weeks

Pathogenesis

- Various viral causes: Epstein–Barr virus (EBV), echovirus, coxsackie B virus, hepatitis A, B, or C, CMV, respiratory syncytial virus, parainfluenza virus, parvovirus B19, rubella virus, poliovirus, adenovirus, rotavirus, HHV-6, and immunizations with diphtheria, pertussis or influenza vaccines

Diagnosis

- Characteristic clinical picture
- Biopsy usually not necessary
- Histology: spongiosis, exocytosis of lymphocytes, edema of the papillary dermis and a perivascular lymphocytic infiltrate

Differential diagnosis

- Molluscum contagiosum
- Viral exanthem (nonspecific)
- Scarlet fever
- Kawasaki syndrome

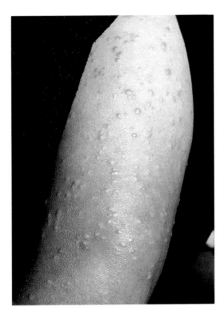

Figure 8.5 Gianotti–Crosti syndrome – lichenoid monomorphic papules on extremities

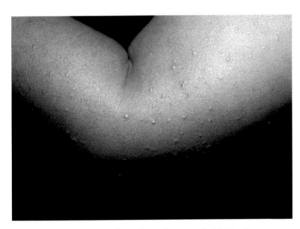

Figure 8.6 Gianotti–Crosti syndrome – individual lichenoid papules

- Measles
- Rubella

Treatment
- Usually no treatment is needed
- If rash is symptomatic, topical corticosteroids may be helpful

Prognosis
- Rash resolves within 2–8 weeks

References

Caputo R, Gelmetti C, Ermacora E, et al. Gianotti–Crosti syndrome: a retrospective analysis of 308 cases. J Am Acad Dermatol 1992; 26: 207–10

Chuh AA. Diagnostic criteria for Gianotti–Crosti syndrome: a prospective case–control study for validity assessment. Cutis 2001; 68: 207–13

Hoffmann B, Schuppe H-C, Adams O, et al. Gianotti–Crosti syndrome associated with Epstein–Barr virus infection. Pediatr Dermatol 1997; 14: 273–7

Nelson JS, Stone MS. Update on selected viral exanthems. Curr Opin Pediatr 2000; 12: 359–64

Report of the Committee on Infectious Diseases. Red Book, 26th edn. American Academy of Pediatrics: Elk Grove Village, IL, 2003: 419–29

Unilateral laterothoracic exanthem

Synonym: Asymmetric periflexural exanthem

Major points
- Female/male ratio >1
- Average age ~2 years, and most cases under 4 years
- More common in White children
- More common in spring
- Morbilliform, erythematous eczematous papules (occasionally with a pallid halo) on unilateral trunk (Figure 8.7)
- Begins as a discrete patch with small lichenoid papules, then extends into axilla over 3 weeks, becoming inflamed
- Lesions become confluent, then gradually clear, leaving some postinflammatory hyperpigmentation
- Similar lesions may appear on other side and involve extremities
- Pruritus uncommon
- Lesions last up to 6 weeks, with rare recurrences
- Usually no systemic symptoms

Pathogenesis
- Viral cause suggested by clinical symptoms, but no clear agent has been identified

Diagnosis
- Clinical appearance
- Histology: superficial perivascular dermatitis with some foci of lichenoid dermatitis

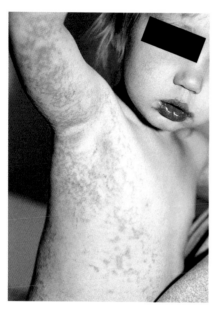

Figure 8.7   Unilateral laterothoracic exanthem – beginning on the lateral trunk

Differential diagnosis

- Atopic dermatitis
- Molluscum contagiosum
- Contact dermatitis
- Drug eruption

Treatment

- Topical steroids and antihistamines may be helpful if pruritus is present

Prognosis

- Self-limited
- May leave postinflammatory hyperpigmentation

References

Gutzmer R, Herbst RA, Kiehl P, et al. Unilateral laterothoracic exanthem (asymmetrical periflexural exanthem of childhood): report of an adult patient. J Am Acad Dermatol 1997; 37: 484–5

McCuaig CC, Russo P, Powell J, et al. Unilateral laterothoracic exanthem. J Am Acad Dermatol 1996; 34: 979–84

Resnick SD. New aspects of exanthematous diseases of childhood. Dermatol Clin 1997; 15: 257–66

Taieb A, Megraud F, Legrain V, et al. Asymmetric periflexural exanthem of childhood. J Am Acad Dermatol 1993; 29: 391–3

Echovirus

Major points

- Morbilliform eruption, occasionally with petechiae
- Found worldwide and ubiquitous
- Incubation period 3–5 days
- Spread by fecal–oral route
- Despite enteric replication, gastrointestinal symptoms uncommon
- Severe symptoms can occur rarely: encephalitis, polio-like paralysis, neonatal hepatic necrosis
- Attack rates highest in infants and toddlers
- Occurs usually in summer in epidemics, particularly in crowded living conditions
- Echovirus 16 ('Boston exanthem') seen in epidemic form and may mimic roseola with morbilliform rash and sometimes vesicles appearing after 2–3 days of fever
  1. Adenopathy common
  2. Aseptic menigitis occasional
- Echovirus 9 usually shows a morbilliform eruption with acral petechiae which lasts 2–7 days
  1. Can be epidemic, usually in summer and fall in temperate climates. No seasonal pattern in tropics
  2. Primarily in preschool children
  3. Fever, sore throat, abdominal pain and vomiting
- Echoviruses 2, 4, 6, 11, 25, 30 show similar signs and symptoms
  1. Aseptic meningitis common

Pathogenesis

- Echoviruses (33 types), small RNA viruses in picornavirus group

Diagnosis

- Culture of echovirus from stool and throat washings, cerebrospinal fluid, or blood; biopsy if indicated
- Serum for acute and convalescent titers of antibodies (at 4 weeks) can be drawn and tested if tissue culture results are positive (enteroviruses can persist in the lower gastrointestinal tract for 8–12 weeks and may not be causative)

Differential diagnosis

- Coxsackie viruses
- Roseola (human herpesvirus-6)

- Atypical measles
- Rocky Mountain spotted fever
- Meningococcemia
- Streptococcal infection
- Epstein–Barr virus (EBV) infection
- Hepatitis
- Rubella
- Dengue fever
- Typhus

Treatment

- Symptomatic treatment
- Very contagious
- Follow-up visits usually not necessary
- Intravenous immunoglobulin with a high antibody titer to the infecting virus may be beneficial in immunocompromised patients or life-threatening neonatal infection

Prognosis

- Excellent unless complications cause permanent damage

References

Frieden IJ, Resnick SD. Childhood exanthems. Old and new. Pediatr Clin North Am 1991; 38: 859–87

Kim KS, Hufnagel G, Chapman NM, Tracy S. The group B coxsackieviruses and myocarditis. Rev Med Virol 2001; 11: 355–68

Report of the Committee on Infectious Diseases. Red Book, 26th edn. American Academy of Pediatrics: Elk Grove Village, IL, 2003: 269–70

Infectious mononucleosis

Major points

- Can occur in all ages, with peak found in adolescents and young adults
- Onset is usually insidious
- Spectrum of disease is extremely variable, ranging from asymptomatic to fatal
- Presenting symptoms
  1. Fatigue
  2. Fever
  3. Generalized lymphadenopathy
  4. Sore throat with exudative pharyngitis
  5. Headache
  6. Splenomegaly
  7. Jaundice
  8. Hepatomegaly
  9. Arthritis
  10. Rash (~15%): pink, fleeting morbilliform eruption lasting 1–5 days
- Treatment with ampicillin or penicillin for sore throat results in morbilliform rash in up to 80%: bright red papules or urticarial plaques; may persist for 7–10 days
- Palmar erythema may be prominent
- Neurologic symptoms: spatial and visual distortion, encephalitis, meningitis, neuritis, or Guillain–Barré syndrome
- Acute phase lasts 2–3 weeks; begins with fever and sore throat
- Extreme fatigue may persist for 3 months
- Rare complications: splenic rupture, thrombocytopenia, agranulocytosis, hemolytic anemia, orchitis and myocarditis
- Incubation period is 4–8 weeks in adolescents, shorter in prepubertal children
- Transmission by close personal contact (oral, fecal) or blood transfusion
- Asymptomatic carriage is common

Pathogenesis

- Caused by several different viruses:
  1. Epstein–Barr virus (herpesvirus-4)
     a. More common in adolescents and is the cause in 85%
     b. EBV replicates in B-lymphocytes, which in normal patients are inhibited by natural killer and T-cell responses
     c. In patients with cellular immune deficiencies, fatal dissemination or B-cell lymphoma can occur
  2. More common in infants and young children:
     a. Cytomegalovirus (herpesvirus-5)
     b. Human herpesvirus 6, 7
     c. Rubella
     d. Human parvovirus B19

Diagnosis

- EBV antibody tests
  1. Nonspecific serologic tests for heterophile antibody, Paul–Bunnell test and slide agglutination
  2. Viral capsid antigen (VCA)-IgG antibody found in high titers early in infection

3. IgM anti-VCA antibody and early antigen (EA) antibody; useful in identifying recent infections
4. Serum antibodies against EBV nuclear antigen (EBNA) demonstrate past or recent infection
5. PCR or culture of saliva or peripheral blood mononuclear cells for EBV

- Patients who are negative for EBV should be tested for CMV and other causes

Differential diagnosis

- Streptococcal pharyngitis
- Parvovirus B19 infection
- Idiopathic thrombocytopenic purpura
- Systemic lupus erythematosus
- Malignancies

Treatment

- In mild cases, no treatment is necessary
- In severe cases with complications, prednisone 2–3 mg/kg per day for 3 days
- Ampicillin or penicillin should be avoided
- Avoid contact sports where abdominal injury may cause splenic rupture
- Weekly visits to assess the course of disease and complications
- In severe disease, hospitalization may be necessary
- Isolation not necessary

Prognosis

- Excellent unless there are complications

References

Ikediobi NI, Tyring SK. Cutaneous manifestations of Epstein–Barr virus infection. Dermatol Clin 2002; 20: 283–9

Ohga S, Nomura A, Takada H, Hara T. Immunological aspects of Epstein–Barr virus infection. Crit Rev Oncol Hematol 2002; 44: 203–15

Report of the Committee on Infectious Diseases. Red Book, 26th edn. American Academy of Pediatrics: Elk Grove Village, IL, 2003: 271–3

Yachie A, Kanegane H, Kasahara Y. Epstein–Barr virus-associated T-/natural killer cell lymphoproliferative diseases. Semin Hematol 2003; 40: 124–32

Hepatitis

Major points

- Although viral hepatitis is not usually associated with an exanthem, it can cause a morbilliform, urticarial, lichenoid or scarlatiniform eruption
- Hepatitis A and hepatitis E
  1. Incubation period is 15–50 days, average 25–30 days
  2. Symptoms: abrupt fever, jaundice, anorexia, nausea, malaise and occasionally upper respiratory symptoms
  3. Subclinical cases are more common, especially in younger children
  4. Sometimes have a preceding morbilliform eruption with following jaundice and development of icterus and hepatic tenderness
  5. Pruritus may occur
- Hepatitis B, hepatitis C, hepatitis D
  1. Spectrum of symptoms from asymptomatic seroconversion to clinical hepatitis with jaundice
  2. Anicteric infection is most common in young children
  3. Chronic infection can lead to cirrhosis, chronic active hepatitis or hepatocellular carcinoma
  4. Symptoms:
     a. Morbilliform, urticarial and serum-sickness-like eruptions are the most common skin manifestations
     b. Joint swelling
     c. Fixed urticaria, lichen planus
     d. Lasts 7–10 days, and resolves with the onset of hepatic symptoms
     e. Leukocytoclastic vasculitis or periarteritis nodosa
- Papular acrodermatitis of childhood (See Gianotti–Crosti syndrome)

Pathogenesis

- Hepatitis A virus (HAV), single-stranded RNA viruses replicate in liver
  1. Viral shedding into bowel during infectious stage, usually 1–3 weeks
  2. Viremia may occur and produce rash
  3. Hepatitis A and E are primarily waterborne, transmitted by human fecal contamination of food, causing local outbreaks
- Hepatitis B virus (HBV), double-stranded DNA virus, replicates by reverse transcription
  1. Reproduces as complete virus particles and capsids which circulate in the blood

2. Incubation period is 45–160 days, average 120 days
3. Transmitted by blood or body fluids such as wound exudates, semen, saliva
4. Chronic carrier is primary reservoir
5. HBV can survive 1 week on dry objects
6. Groups at high risk: intravenous drug users, multiple heterosexual partners, homosexual men, hemodialysis patients
- Hepatitis C virus, single-stranded RNA virus in a separate genus in Flaviviridae family
- Hepatitis delta virus, unique single-stranded RNA virus which needs a co-infection with hepatitis B in order to enter hepatocytes and can result in fulminant or chronic hepatitis
- Hepatitis E, single-stranded RNA virus, similar to calicivirus, acquired by fecal–oral route; incubation period ~40 days

Diagnosis

- Serum aminotransferase elevated
- Serologic tests for IgM antihepatitis antibodies by enzyme-linked immunosorbent assay (ELISA) or radioimmunoassay diagnostic
- Hepatitis A
  1. Presence of IgM anti-HAV antibodies usually indicates recent infection, disappearing within 6 months
  2. IgG anti-HAV antibodies develop after IgM anti-HAV antibodies, and indicate past infection
- Hepatitis B
  1. Acute active infection
     a. Hepatitis B surface antigen positive (HBsAg+)
     b. Hepatitis B core antigen positive (HBcAg+)
     c. Hepatitis B e antigen positive (HBeAg+)
     d. IgM anti-hepatitis B core antibody positive (Anti-HBcAb+)
  2. Chronic infection
     a. HBsAg+
     b. IgG anti-hepatitis B surface antibody negative (Anti-HBsAb–)
     c. IgG anti-hepatitis B core antibody positive (Anti-HBcAb+)
  3. Immunized: IgG anti-hepatitis B surface antibody positive (Anti-HBsAb+)
  4. Prior infection: Anti-HBsAb+, HBsAg–
- Hepatitis C: Anti-HCV+

Differential diagnosis

- Viral exanthems, particularly rubella, parvovirus B19
- Urticaria
- Leukocytoclastic vasculitis of other etiologies
- Contact dermatitis
- Atopic dermatitis
- Lichen planus

Treatment

- Bed rest, supportive measures
- Exposed individuals should receive human immune serum globulin 0.02 ml/kg, as soon as possible after exposure
- In HBV, hepatitis B immunoglobulin (HBIG), 0.06 ml/kg within 24 hours of exposure, and hepatitis B vaccine within 7 days of exposure. Repeat vaccination should be given 1 and 6 months later
- For perinatal exposure to HBV, 0.5 ml of HBIG within 12 hours of birth, and initial dose of vaccine at 7 days, 1 month and 6 months
- Education and good hygiene measures, as HAV may survive on objects in the environment for weeks
- Report to local public health officials
- Hepatitis B immunoprophylaxis is recommended
- Hepatitis C (chronic): interferon-α

Prognosis

- Course is usually benign, but can progress to liver failure

References

Fontana RJ, Everson GT, Tuteja S, et al. Controversies in the management of hepatitis C patients with advanced fibrosis and cirrhosis. Clin Gastroenterol Hepatol 2004; 2: 183–97

Ganem D, Prince AM. Hepatitis B virus infection – natural history and clinical consequences. N Engl J Med 2004; 350: 1118–29

Report of the Committee on Infectious Diseases. Red Book, 26th edn. American Academy of Pediatrics: Elk Grove Village, IL, 2003: 309–43

Roberts EA. Neonatal hepatitis syndrome. Semin Neonatol 2003; 8: 357–74

Shearer CM, Jackson JM, Callen JP. Symmetric polyarthritis with livedo reticularis: a newly recognized manifestation of hepatitis C virus infection. J Am Acad Dermatol 1997; 37: 659–61

Herpes simplex

Major points

- Lesions are typically grouped vesicles on erythematous base
  1. Although characteristically around the mouth or genital region, can be found anywhere
  2. On mucous membranes, blister roof easily becomes eroded
  3. Regional lymphadenopathy often prominent
  4. Generally heals within 8 days
  5. Herpes simplex virus (HSV) is ubiquitous and transmitted from direct contact with infected oral secretions or lesions
  6. Incubation period: 2 days to 2 weeks
- Manifestations in children and infants >1 month of age (Figure 8.8)
  1. Gingivostomatitis is commonly first manifestation of primary HSV infection, with fever, irritability, foul breath and inability to take liquids orally
     a. Usually asymptomatic or diagnosed as a nonspecific 'viral' enanthem
     b. Lasts 7–14 days
     c. May need hospitalization if oral intake is poor
  2. Eczema herpeticum (Kaposi varicelliform eruption): diffuse infection concentrated in areas of dermatitis or other skin disorders (e.g. burns, Darier disease) with characteristic grouped vesicles on erythematous bases and punched out erosions (Figure 8.19)
     a. High fever, lassitude, hundreds of vesicles
     b. May be primary infection with HSV
     c. Can be recurrent
  3. Immunocompromised patients: severe local lesions may occur with central necrosis; visceral involvement may occur
- Neonatal herpes infection (<4 weeks of age)
  1. 75–80% caused by HSV-2; the rest by HSV-1
  2. Characteristics of different presentations:
     a. Generalized systemic infection with multiorgan involvement and encephalitis
     b. Localized CNS disease
     c. Disease localized to skin, eyes, or mucous membranes (Figure 8.10)
     d. Intrauterine infection, usually in first trimester, which causes malformations and small-for-gestational-age infants

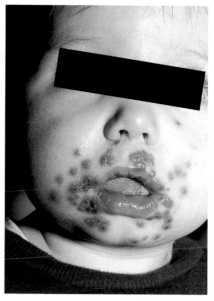

Figure 8.8   Herpes simplex – primary infection

  3. Presents at birth to 6 weeks of age, with disseminated disease occurring in first 2 weeks of life
  4. Typical skin lesions present in 80%
  5. Asymptomatic cases probably do not occur
  6. Often severe with high mortality and morbidity, even with antiviral therapy
  7. Recurrent skin lesions common in surviving infants
  8. Incidence: 1 in 3000–20 000 live births
  9. Infants frequently born prematurely

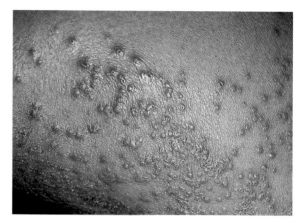

Figure 8.9   Eczema herpeticum – generalized herpes simplex infection in a teenager with atopic dermatitis

10. Transmitted during birth through an infected birth canal, or by ascending infection. (In USA, 0.01–0.39% of women shed HSV at birth)
11. Postnatal transmission from infected parent can occur if lesions on mouth, hands, or nipples
12. Transmission from nursery workers rarely occurs
13. Risk of HSV infection in infant born vaginally to mother with first herpetic infection is 33–50%; with recurrent HSV is 3–5%

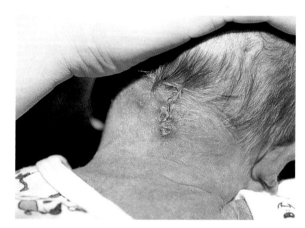

Figure 8.10   Herpes simplex – in an 8-day-old neonate

- Genital herpes infection
  1. Usually caused by HSV-2; occasionally HSV-1
  2. Vesicles or shallow ulcerations, usually painful, in perineal area or on genitalia
  3. Transmitted from direct contact with infected secretions through sexual activity
  4. Genital herpes in prepubertal children should be investigated for sexual abuse
- Eye infections
  1. May be primary or recurrent
  2. Cause superficial conjunctivitis
  3. May involve deeper layers of cornea or chorioretinitis
  4. Potentially leading to scarring and loss of vision
- Herpetic whitlow
  1. Typically involves fingertips
  2. More common in thumbsuckers with inoculation from oral lesions (Figure 8.11)

- Herpes gladiatorum
  1. Occurs in wrestlers from direct skin-to-skin inoculation
- Recurrent erythema multiforme minor can occur with reactivation of herpes virus
- Herpes encephalitis: associated with fever, convulsions, irritability, alterations of consciousness, or focal neurological changes

Pathogenesis

- Herpes simplex: large, enveloped DNA virus with two major types which have genomic and antigenic differences
  1. Type 1 (HSV-1) causes lesions above waist, but can be found anywhere
  2. Type 2 (HSV-2) usually involves genitalia
- Epidermotropic; produces infection within keratinocytes
- Persists in nerve ganglia in latent form and can become reactivated following various factors: fever, ultraviolet light, trauma, menses
- Transmitted during primary and recurrent infections, either symptomatic or asymptomatic
- With recurrent lesions, first 24 hours has highest concentration of virus with development of vesicles
- Active infection occurs despite high titers of specific antibody; antibody cannot interact with active virus, which is transferred from cell to cell

Diagnosis

- Cell culture with special transport media will grow virus readily
  1. Open and swab skin vesicles

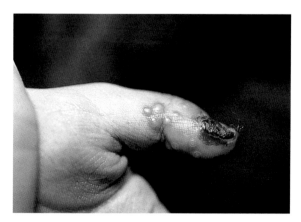

Figure 8.11   Herpes simplex – herpetic whitlow in a thumb sucker

2. In neonates, take cultures from skin, nasopharynx, eyes, urine, blood, stool and CSF and maternal lesions, cervix or vulva
- Direct fluorescent antibody staining or immunoassay detection of vesicle scraping
- Polymerase chain reaction (PCR)
- Tzanck preparation: multinucleated keratinocytes and eosinophilic intranuclear inclusions; smear material from base of blister on slide and stain with Wright stain

Differential diagnosis

- Cutaneous lesions
  1. Cellulitis
  2. Pyoderma
  3. Impetigo
- Gingivostomatitis
  1. Aphthous stomatitis
  2. Erythema multiforme
  3. Herpangina caused by enteroviruses, particularly coxsackie A virus
- Herpes keratitis
  1. Adenovirus (usually bilateral)
- Genital herpes simplex
  1. Gonorrhea
  2. Syphilis
- Neonatal herpes simplex
  1. TORCH complex (toxoplasmosis, other (syphilis, viruses), rubella, CMV, herpes simplex)
  2. Staphylococcal infection
  3. Candida infection

Treatment

- Acyclovir indicated for primary infections, and occasionally for recurrences (see Chapter 21)
- Topical agents (as adjunct): acyclovir 5% ointment, docosamol 10% cream (Denavir) in conjunction with parenteral antiviral therapy) 1–2% trifluridine, 1% iododeoxyuridine, 3% vidarabine
- Topical steroids are contraindicated unless used in conjunction with antiviral therapy
- Refer to an ophthalmologist if eye involvement
- Isolation of patients in hospital
- HSV in wrestlers or rugby players
  1. Inspection of skin of players during athletic competition
  2. Exclusion from competition until lesions are healed or deemed noninfectious by viral cultures
  3. Wash mats with freshly prepared 1/64 household bleach solution (one-quarter of a cup diluted to 1 gallon of water) between matches

Prognosis

- Generally heals in ~8 days
- Neonates and those who are immunocompromised have guarded prognosis
- All lesions are potentially recurrent

References

Amir J, Harel L, Smetana Z, Varsano I. The natural history of primary herpes simplex type 1 gingivostomatitis in children. Pediatr Dermatol 1999; 16: 259–63

Arvin AM, Prober CG. Herpes simplex virus type 2 – a persistent problem. N Engl J Med 1997; 337: 1158–9

Donovan B. Sexually transmissible infections other than HIV. Lancet 2004; 363: 545–56

Drago F, Rebora A. The new herpesviruses. Arch Dermatol 1999; 135: 71–5

Kimberlin DW. Neonatal herpes simplex infection. Clin Microbiol Rev 2004; 17: 1–13

Kimberlin DW, Lin C-Y, Jacobs RF, et al. Natural history of neonatal herpes simplex virus infections in the acyclovir era. Pediatrics 2001; 108: 223–9

Report of the Committee on Infectious Diseases. Red Book, 26th edn. American Academy of Pediatrics: Elk Grove Village, IL, 2003: 344–53

Waggoner-Fountain LA, Grossman LB. Herpes simplex virus. Pediatr Rev 2004; 25: 86–93

Wollenberg A, Zoch C, Wetzel S, et al. Predisposing factors and clinical features of eczema herpeticum: a retrospective analysis of 100 cases. J Am Acad Dermatol 2003; 49: 198–205

Varicella

Synonym: chickenpox

Major points

- Clinical characteristics
  1. Abrupt onset of generalized pruritic, scattered vesicular rash with mild fever and mild systemic symptoms (Figures 8.12–8.14)

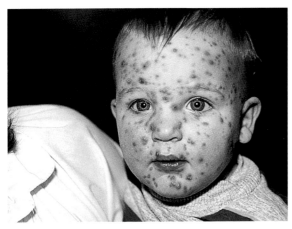

Figure 8.12   Varicella – typical multiple lesions in different stages of development

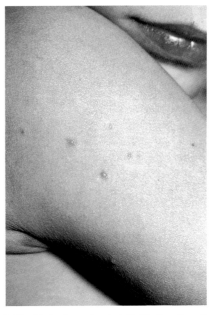

Figure 8.13   Varicella – classic initial lesion described as a 'dew drop on a rose petal'

2. Initial lesions resemble 'dew drops on a rose petal'
3. Crops of lesions in different stages of development; break out for 2–5 days
4. Individual lesions go from papules to vesicles to crusts within 24–48 hours
5. When shed, crusts leave shallow erosions
6. Lesions may be concentrated in areas of skin injury or sun exposure
7. Oral cavity lesions frequent, as are other mucous membrane lesions
8. Total duration 7–10 days
- Epidemiology
  1. Incubation period 10–21 days (average 14–16 days)
  2. Highly contagious
  3. Most contagious for 1–2 days before and shortly after onset of rash, but lasts until vesicles have crusted
  4. Person-to-person transmission by direct contact with infected patients (varicella or zoster) or air-borne spread from respiratory secretions
  5. Children who acquire their infection at home (secondary family cases) may have more severe disease than index case
  6. Late winter and early spring more common
  7. Most common in children <10 years
  8. Immunity is usually life-long
- Complications
  1. Bacterial superinfection with *Staphylococcus aureus* or *Streptococcus*
  2. Thrombocytopenia

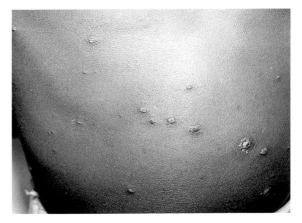

Figure 8.14   Varicella – typical multiple lesions on the trunk

3. Pneumonia
4. Arthritis
5. Hepatitis
6. Encephalitis or meningitis
7. Glomerulonephritis
8. More severe in adolescents and adults
9. Reye syndrome
10. Acute cerebellar ataxia
11. Immunocompromised children can have progressive varicella with continued eruption of

lesions and high fever from 2 weeks to several months

12. Children receiving corticosteroids or chronic salicylate therapy may have more severe disease or complications
13. Fetal infection (first or early second trimester) can result in varicella embryopathy (congenital varicella syndrome) with limb atrophy and scarring; attack rate 1.2% (higher between 13 and 20 weeks' gestation)
14. Fetuses exposed to varicella-zoster virus can develop unapparent varicella and then zoster early in life
15. Severe neonatal varicella results when infant's mother develops varicella from 5 days before to 2 days after delivery; mortality rate 30%

Pathogenesis

- Caused by varicella-zoster virus (human herpes virus-3)
- Herpes viruses are epidermotropic and produce infection within the keratinocytes with epidermal cell death

Diagnosis

- Clinical diagnosis
- Viral culture is usually positive in the first 3–4 days of eruption
- Immunofluorescent staining with monoclonal antibodies of vesicular scrapings; PCR
- Tzanck smear demonstrates multinucleated epithelial cells containing intranuclear inclusions
- Acute and convalescent-phase sera for anti-varicella-zoster virus antibody
- Serologic tests: enzyme immunoassay (EIA), latex agglutination (LA), indirect fluorescent antibody (IFA) and fluorescent antibody-to-membrane antigen (FAMA) assays
- Histology: balloon degeneration within keratinocytes, multinucleated giant epithelial cell and nuclear inclusions

Differential diagnosis

- Insect bite reactions
- Molluscum contagiosum
- Pityriasis lichenoides et varioliformis acuta
- Rickettsialpox
- Dermatitis herpetiformis
- Herpes simplex (disseminated)
- Orf

- Coxsackie infections
- Echoviruses 4, 9, 11, 17, 25
- Variola
- Vaccinia (cowpox)

Treatment

- Healthy children usually do not require treatment
- Symptomatic treatment: wet dressings, soothing baths, oral antipruritics
- Acyclovir (see Chapter 21)
- Varicella-zoster immune globulin (VZIG) within 72 hours of exposure can modify the course, but is not helpful once the disease is established. (Consult Red Book)
- Hospitalized patients should be isolated
- Contact with elderly, neonates and immunocompromised children should be avoided
- School children with uncomplicated cases may return to school on the 6th day after the onset of the rash or when there are no new lesions, and existing lesions have crusted over; children with zoster based on similar criteria may return to school when lesions have crusted
- Varicella vaccine is a cell-free live-attenuated preparation
  1. Single dose recommended for patients between 12 months and 12 years with a 97% seroconversion rate
  2. Persons >13 years should have second dose 4–8 weeks after initial vaccination
- Secondary bacterial infection should be treated with antibiotics

Prognosis

- Excellent in a healthy child
- Immunosuppressed children have higher rate of complications
- Virus persists in latent form after initial infection
- Reactivation causes herpes zoster ('shingles')

References

Arvin AM. Varicella vaccine – the first six years. N Engl J Med 2001; 344: 1007–9

English R. Varicella. Pediatr Rev 2003; 24: 372–9

Hall S, Maupin T, Seward J, et al. Second varicella infections: are they more common than previously thought? Pediatrics 2002; 109: 1068–73

LaRussa P. The success of varicella vaccine. Pediatr Ann 2002; 31: 710–15

LaRussa P, Steinberg SP, Shapiro E, et al. Viral strain identification in varicella vaccines with disseminated rashes. Pediatr Infect Dis 2000; 19: 1037–9

MMWR. Varicella-related deaths among adults – United States, 1997. Morbid Mortal Weekly Rep 1997; 46: 409

Report of the Committee on Infectious Diseases. Red Book, 26th edn. American Academy of Pediatrics: Elk Grove Village, IL, 2003: 672–86

Vazquez M, LaRussa PS, Gerxon AA, et al. The effectiveness of the varicella vaccine in clinical practice. N Engl J Med 2001; 344: 955–60

Herpes zoster

Major points

- Patients have previously had varicella infection or vaccine
- Clinical characteristics:
  1. Lesions begin as erythematous macules, then become grouped vesicles on erythematous base in dermatomal distribution (may be one to three sensory dermatomes) (Figure 8.15)
  2. Most common dermatomes involved are on the trunk and buttocks
  3. Mild febrile illness lasts 7–10 days
  4. Pruritus may be severe
  5. Pain can occur and is localized to the area involved
  6. Generalized lesions may be seen in immunocompromised patients, with lesions appearing outside the dermatomes, with visceral complications

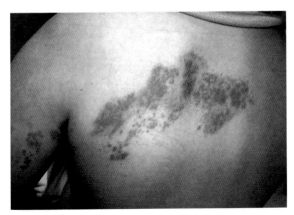

Figure 8.15 Herpes zoster – typical dermatomal distribution of vesicles

- Complications
  1. Scarring (Figure 8.16)
  2. Motor paralysis
  3. Keratitis
  4. Ramsay-Hunt syndrome: involvement of geniculate ganglion with pain in the ear, vesicles on pinnae and facial palsy
  5. Postherpetic neuralgia (rare in children)

Pathogenesis

- Caused by a recrudescence of a latent infection with varicella zoster virus (human herpes virus-3)

Diagnosis

- Clinical diagnosis
- See Varicella above, for testing

Differential diagnosis

- Herpes simplex infection
- Impetigo
- Pain can mimic internal disease: encephalitis, appendicitis

Treatment

- Acyclovir either oral or intravenously (see Chapter 21)
- Topical antibiotic ointments (e.g. mupirocin, bacitracin)
- Oral antipruritics: hydroxyzine 10–25 mg every 6 hours, diphenhydramine 10–25 mg every 6 hours
- Prednisone 1–2 mg/kg per day to prevent postherpetic neuralgia and to decrease inflammation

Prognosis

- Excellent in immunocompetent host
- May be prolonged in immunocompromised host
- May cause scarring

References

Brown TJ, McCrary M, Tyring SK. Antiviral agents: nonantiviral drugs. J Am Acad Dermatol 2002; 47: 581–99

English R. Varicella. Pediatr Rev 2003; 24: 372–9

Johnson RW. Herpes zoster in the immunocompetent patient: management of post-herpetic neuralgia. Herpes 2003; 10: 38–45

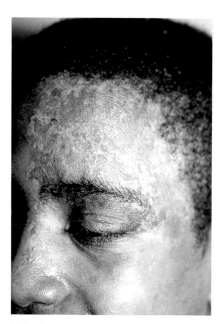

Figure 8.16   Post-herpes zoster scarring

Kakourou T, Theodoridou M, Mostrous G, et al. Herpes zoster in children. J Am Acad Dermatol 1998; 39: 207–10

Liang MG, Heidelberg KA, Jacobson RM, McEvoy MT. Herpes zoster after varicella immunization. J Am Acad Dermatol 1998; 38: 761–3

McCrary ML, Severson J, Tyring SK. Varicella zoster virus. J Am Acad Dermatol 1999; 41: 1–14

Thomas SL, Hall AJ. What does epidemiology tell us about risk factors for herpes zoster? Lancet Infect Dis 2004; 4: 26–33

Hand, foot and mouth disease

Major points

- Abrupt onset of scattered papules/vesicles, oval or linear in shape, in an acral distribution
- Individual (not grouped) lesions are seen on palms, fingertips, soles and mouth; occasionally, more numerous lesions may involve extremities (Figures 8.17 and 8.18)
- Lesions usually number <100
- Fever may be mild or nonexistent
- Oral lesions are discrete, shallow, oval erosions
- There is diarrhea, particularly in young children
- Epidemics occur in summer and early fall in temperate climates
- Incubation period: 3–5 days

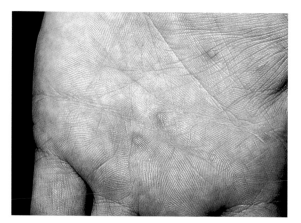

Figure 8.17   Hand, foot and mouth disease caused by coxsackie virus

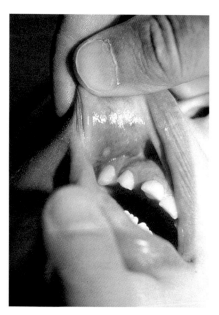

Figure 8.18   Hand, foot and mouth disease – oral lesion with erythematous halo

- Fecal–oral acquisition; virus may be excreted in feces for up to 12 weeks
- Contagious from 2 days before onset of rash to 2 days after
- Enteroviruses may survive on fomites
- Clinical attack rates highest in young children

Pathogenesis

- Caused by several coxsackie virus groups: A16, A2, A5, A10 and A71

Diagnosis

- Virus isolation from throat, stool and rectal swabs, and occasionally blood
- Antibodies from sera (onset of illness and 4 weeks after) showing rise in titer

Differential diagnosis

See Table 8.1
- Acropustulosis of infancy
- Insect bites
- Urticaria

Treatment

- None usually necessary
- Treat dehydration if it occurs in infants
- IVIG containing high antibody titer may be helpful for immunocompromised patients
- Good handwashing, personal hygiene, especially after diaper changes

Prognosis

- Excellent

References

Chang LY, King CC, Hsu KH, et al. Risk factors of enterovirus 71 infection and associated hand, foot, and mouth disease/herpangina in children during an epidemic in Taiwan. Pediatrics 2002; 109: 88

Chang LY, Lin TY, Huang YC, et al. Comparison of enterovirus-71 and coxsackievirus A16 clinical illnesses during the Taiwan enterovirus epidemic, 1998. Pediatr Infect Dis J 1999; 18: 1092–6

Frieden IJ, Resnick SD. Childhood exanthems. Old and new. Pediatr Clin North Am 1991; 38: 859–87

Messner J, Miller JJ, James WD, Honig PJ. Accentuated viral exanthems in areas of inflammation. J Am Acad Dermatol 1999; 40: 345–6

Report of the Committee on Infectious Diseases. Red Book, 26th edn. American Academy of Pediatrics: Elk Grove Village, IL, 2003: 269–70

Thomas I, Janniger CK. Hand, foot and mouth disease. Cutis 1993; 52: 265–6

Verrucae

Major points

- Human papillomaviruses (HPV) cause benign epithelial tumors (warts) of skin and mucous membranes
- Cutaneous warts are common in school-aged children
- Transmitted from person to person by direct contact. Enters areas of minor trauma to skin
- Severe or widespread infections occur in patients with compromised cellular immunity (e.g. transplantation, HIV infection) or atopic patients
- Anogenital warts are primarily transmitted by sexual contact, but may be acquired at delivery from an infected mother
- Evidence of genital HPV infection has been detected in up to 38% of sexually active adolescent females
- Incubation period: unknown; estimated 3 months to several years
- Common warts (caused by HPV 2, 4): dome-shaped papules with finger-like projections giving a rough appearance or texture of cauliflower (Figures 8.19 and 8.20)
  1. Usually asymptomatic and multiple
  2. Commonly occur on hands and around nails but can be anywhere, including lips and mouth
  3. Thrombosed capillaries give appearance of tiny dark dots
- Flat warts (caused by HPV 3, 10) common on face and extremities; usually small, multiple, flat topped papules (Figure 8.21)
- Plantar warts (caused by HPV 1, 4 and others) on weight-bearing areas; can be painful, hyperkeratotic; multiple lesions grouped together ('mosaic' appearance) (Figure 8.22)
- Anogenital or venereal warts (caused by HPV 6, 11, 16, 18) can range from asymptomatic papules to condylomata acuminata (cauliflower-like growths ranging from a few millimeters to several centimeters) (Figure 8.23)
  1. In males, found on shaft of the penis, meatus, scrotum and perineal areas
  2. In females, located on labia, vagina, cervix or perianal areas
  3. Perianal warts can cause itching, burning, local pain or bleeding
- Laryngeal papillomas found in children <3 years of age
  1. Manifest as hoarse crying or respiratory obstruction
  2. Acquired via aspiration of infected secretions from mother during passage through infected birth canal

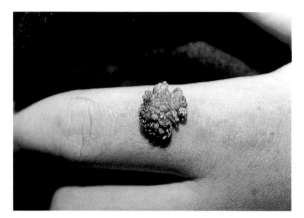

Figure 8.19   Verruca vulgaris

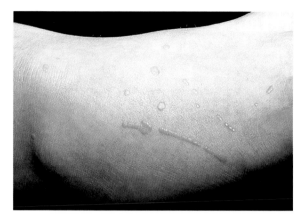

Figure 8.21   Plantar verrucae demonstrating the Koebner phenomenon

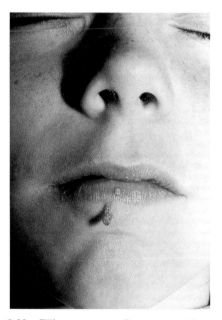

Figure 8.20   Filiform verrucae often occur on the face

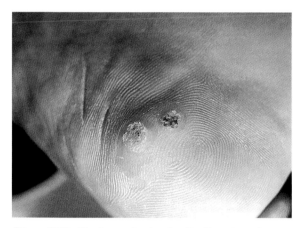

Figure 8.22   Plantar warts showing the thrombosed capillaries

- Epidermodysplasia verruciformis: inherited deficiency of cell-mediated immunity to particular HPV types
  1. Presents in childhood as flat warts
  2. Malignant transformation occurs in adults in one-third of cases, particularly in sun-exposed areas

Pathogenesis

- Caused by papillomavirus, Papovaviridae family, DNA viruses

- >80 types have been identified, but most warts are caused by a few types
- Papillomaviruses are common in mammals and are species-specific
- HPV is located in epidermal cell nucleus and induces keratinocyte proliferation with relatively normal differentiation

Diagnosis

- Clinical diagnosis
- Histology: vacuolated epidermal cells with hypergranulosis and eosinophilic inclusions
- PCR detection of certain viral types

Differential diagnosis

- Common warts: molluscum contagiosum, cysts
- Plantar warts: calluses

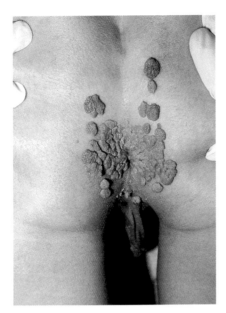

Figure 8.23 Condyloma acuminata in a sexually abused child caused by human papillomavirus

- Anogenital warts: syphilis (condyloma lata); molluscum contagiosum
- Flat warts: lichen planus, lichen nitidus, seborrheic keratosis, epidermal nevus

Treatment

- Nongenital warts often resolve spontaneously in <2 years
  1. Destruction: liquid nitrogen (–195°C), salicylic acid paints (17%), CO_2 laser, pulsed dye laser, electrodesiccation, tape occlusion
  2. Tretinoin (0.025% or 0.05% cream) (off label) may be helpful for flat warts
- Anogenital warts
  1. Podophyllum resin 25%
  2. Podofilox
  3. Destructive methods such as liquid nitrogen, trichloroacetic acid, CO_2 laser, or surgical excision
  4. Imiquimod 5% approved for >12 years
  5. Recurrences common
  6. Cervical HPV infections can be associated with epithelial dysplasia, and in certain types of HPV (16, 18, 31) may predispose the patient to cervical cancer
  7. In children who are not sexually active, suspicion of child abuse should be raised and

reported to appropriate authorities; inspect genitalia for signs of abuse
  8. If history of unusual behavior, withdrawal, sleep disturbances, phobias, enuresis or encopresis, consider child abuse

Prognosis

- Although most warts spontaneously regress, some persist for years
- Multiple treatments are often needed

References

Brown TJ, McCrary M, Tyring SK. Antiviral agents: nonantiviral drugs. J Am Acad Dermatol 2002; 47: 581–99

Focht DR, Spicer C, Fairchok MP. The efficacy of duct tape vs. cryotherapy in the treatment of verruca vulgaris (the common wart). Arch Pediatr Adolesc Med 2002; 156: 971–4

Grussendorf-Conen E-I, Jacobs S. Efficacy of imiquimod 5% cream in the treatment of recalcitrant warts in children. Pediatr Dermatol 2002; 19: 263–6

Handley J, Hands E, Armstrong K, et al. Common association of HPV 2 with anogenital warts in prepubertal children. Pediatr Dermatol 1997; 14: 339–43

Hengge UR, Cusini M. Topical immunomodulators for the treatment of external genital warts, cutaneous warts and molluscum contagiosum. Br J Dermatol 2003; 149: 15–19

Kopera D. Verrucae vulgaris: flashlamp-pumped pulsed dye laser treatment in 134 patients. Int J Dermatol 2003; 42: 905–8

Majewski S, Pniewski T, Malejczyk M, Jablonska S. Imiquimod is highly effective for extensive, hyperproliferative condyloma in children. Pediatr Dermatol 2003; 20: 440–2

Torrelo A. What's new in the treatment of viral warts in children? Pediatr Dermatol 2002; 19: 191–9

Molluscum contagiosum

Major points

- Several (usually 2–20) skin-colored or pearly 1–6 mm discrete papules with central umbilication (Figures 8.24 and 8.25)
- Eczematous dermatitis often surrounds larger lesions
- Common locations: face, axilla and groin; can be anywhere
- May be sexually transmitted, mainly in teens and adults. In children, groin lesions common and

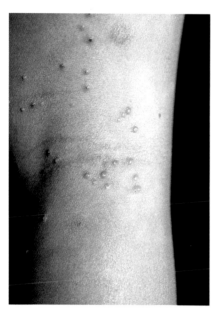

Figure 8.24   Molluscum contagiosum – skin-colored papules, some with central umbilication

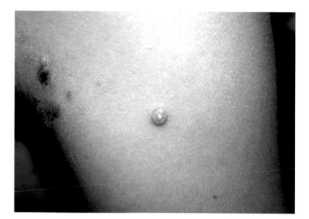

Figure 8.25   Molluscum contagiosum – large lesion with several smaller ones nearby

should not be considered a sexually transmitted disease unless there are other stigmata of sexual abuse
- Patients with atopic dermatitis often have hundreds of lesions
- Infection occurs after contact with infected person, contaminated object, or swimming pool
- Incubation period 2–7 weeks but may be longer, up to 6 months
- Infectious as long as lesions are present
- Lesions may spontaneously suppurate, crust and resolve, being mistaken for secondary infection
- Conjunctivitis or keratitis may complicate lesions on eyelids
- Patients with HIV may have larger and more numerous lesions, suggesting that cell-mediated immunity helps eliminate the virus

Pathogenesis

- Caused by a poxvirus (Poxviridae) which induces epidermal cell proliferation

Diagnosis

- Clinical diagnosis
- Extrusion of keratinous material from a papule and inspecting it microscopically with Wright stain or

potassium hydroxide will show characteristic pear-shaped 'molluscum bodies'
- Histology: pear-shaped eosinophilc 'molluscum bodies' in the keratinocytes; bodies contain cytoplasmic masses of virus material
- Virus can be seen with electron microscopy

Differential diagnosis

- Warts
- Closed comedones
- Epidermal cysts
- Milia
- Folliculitis
- Pyogenic granuloma
- Keratoacanthoma

Treatment

- Lesions self-limiting and benign
- Can leave small pox-like scars, and can become very inflamed before resolving
- Mechanical removal of each papule can be performed with a dermal curette with prior application of anesthetic cream
- Other treatments:
  1. Liquid nitrogen
  2. Opening the lesions and squeezing out the contents
  3. Cantharidin
  4. Tretinoin or salicylic acid preparations may cause irritation and are somewhat unpredictable for treatment
  5. Imiquimod 5% cream (off label)

6. Cidofovir (off label)
- Recurrences common
- Treat every 2–4 weeks until cleared
- Molluscum is contagious; therefore, bathing or swimming together and sharing towels should be avoided

Prognosis

- Most cases are self-limited within 6–9 months; however, some persist for years

References

Bayerl C, Feller G, Goerdt S. Experience in treating molluscum contagiosum in children with imiquimod 5% cream. Br J Dermatol 2003; 149 (Suppl 66): 25–8

Hengge UR, Cusini M. Topical immunomodulators for the treatment of external genital warts, cutaneous warts and molluscum contagiosum. Br J Dermatol 2003; 149 (Suppl 66): 15–19

Hengge UR, Esser S, Schultewolter T, et al. Self-administered topical 5% imiquimod for the treatment of common warts and molluscum contagiosum. Br J Dermatol 2000; 143: 1026–31

Majewski L, Jablonska S. Human papillomavirus-associated tumors of the skin and mucosa. J Am Acad Dermatol 1997; 36: 659–85

Meadows KP, Tyring SK, Pavia AT, Rallis TM. Resolution of recalcitrant molluscum contagiosum virus lesions in human immunodeficiency virus-infected patients treated with cidofovir. Arch Dermatol 1997; 133: 987–90

Myskowski PL. Molluscum contagiosum. New insights, new directions. Arch Dermatol 1997; 133: 1039–60

Silverberg N. Pediatric molluscum contagiosum: optimal treatment strategies. Paediatr Drugs 2003; 5: 505–12

Orf

Synonym: ecthyma contagiosum

Major points

- Widespread in sheep and goats, affecting mainly young lambs that contract it from one another or persistent virus in pastures
- Incubation period: 5–6 days
- Begins as small, firm, red tender papule, enlarging to form a hemorrhagic pustule or bulla, which becomes crusted or umbilicated in the center (Figure 8.26)
- Usually 2–5 cm, solitary or few in number
- Common on fingers and hands

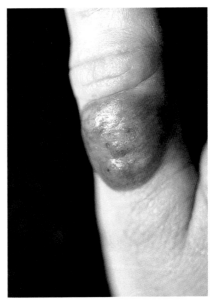

Figure 8.26   Orf – bullous, erythematous nodule on finger

Pathogenesis

- Caused by poxviridae inoculated from sheep or goats

Diagnosis

- Clinical diagnosis with appropriate history
- Histology: inter- and intracellular edema, vacuolization and ballooning degeneration of the epidermis

Differential diagnosis

- Pyoderma
- Brown recluse spider bite

Treatment

- Secondary infection should be treated
- Removal of the bulk of lesion by biopsy may hasten healing

Prognosis

- Spontaneous recovery in 6 weeks

References

Haig DM, McInnes C, Deane D, et al. The immune and inflammatory response to orf virus. Comp Immunol Microbiol Infect Dis 1997; 20: 197–204

Weedon D. Skin Pathology. Churchill Livingstone: Edinburgh, 1997: 586–7

Human immunodeficiency virus

Major points

- Acquired immunodeficiency syndrome (AIDS): severe end of the clinical spectrum of HIV infections
- AIDS in children accounts for 2% of reported cases in the USA; most acquired from mothers
- Clinical manifestations (See Table 8.2)
  1. Generalized lymphadenopathy
  2. Hepatomegaly
  3. Splenomegaly
  4. Failure to thrive
  5. Candidiasis (oral or esophageal)
  6. Recurrent diarrhea
  7. Parotitis
  8. Cardiomyopathy
  9. Hepatitis
  10. Nephropathy
  11. CNS disease
  12. Developmental delay
  13. Seborrheic dermatitis (persistent)
  14. Pneumonia with *Pneumocystis carinii* (PCP); lymphoid interstitial pneumonia
  15. Recurrent bacterial infections with *Staphylococcus aureus* (Figure 8.27)
  16. Dermatophyte infections, widespread
  17. Scabies; severe, crusted
  18. Eosinophilic folliculitis
  19. Drug eruptions (especially with trimethoprim–sulfamethoxazole)
  20. Opportunistic infections (see Table 8.2)

Table 8.2   Revised case definition of AIDS-defining conditions for adults and adolescents ≥ 13 years of age

Candidiasis of bronchi, trachea, or lungs
Candidiasis, esophageal
Cervical cancer, invasive
Coccidioidomycosis, disseminated or extrapulmonary
Cryptococcosis, extrapulmonary
Cryptosporidiosis, chronic intestinal
Cytomegalovirus disease (other than liver, spleen or lymph nodes)
Cytomegalovirus retinitis
Encephalopathy, HIV related
Herpes simplex: chronic ulcer >1 month's duration, or bronchitis, pneumonitis, or esophagitis
Histoplasmosis, disseminated or extrapulmonary
Isosporiasis, chronic intestinal
Kaposi sarcoma
Lymphoma, Burkitt
Lymphoma, immunoblastic
Lymphoma, primary or brain
Mycobacterium avium complex or *M. kansasii*, disseminated or extrapulmonary
Mycobacterium tuberculosis
Mycobacterium, other species disseminated
Pneumocystis carinii pneumonia
Pneumonia, recurrent
Progressive multifocal leukoencephalopathy
Salmonella septicemia, recurrent
Toxoplasmosis of brain
Wasting syndrome due to HIV
CD4+ T-lymphocyte count < 200 cells/µl or CD4+ percentage < 15%

Modified from Centers for Disease Control and Prevention. 1993 revised classification system for HIV infection and expanded case surveillance definition for AIDS among adolescents and adults. MMWR 1992; 41 (No. RR-17):1–19 and Red Book 2003: 360–82

  21. Malignancies (uncommon in pediatric HIV) (see Table 8.2)
- Epidemiology
  1. Humans are reservoir
  2. HIV has been isolated from blood, CSF, pleural fluid, human milk, semen, cervical secretions, saliva, urine and tears
  3. Transmission:
     a. Sexual contact
     b. Percutaneous or mucous membrane exposure to contaminated blood or body fluids

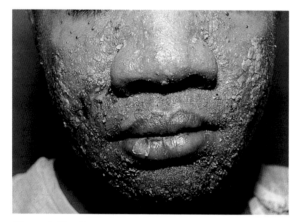

Figure 8.27 Human immunodeficiency virus infection with secondary *Staphylococcus aureus*

c. Mother-to-infant before or around the time of birth
   d. Breastfeeding
   e. Transfusion of blood or blood products
- Incubation period:
  1. HIV-infected neonates are usually asymptomatic in the first months of life
  2. Median onset of symptoms is 3 years of age if acquired perinatally (may be >5 years)

Pathogenesis

- Caused by human immunodeficiency virus type 1 (HIV-1), a RNA cytopathic human retrovirus; HIV-2 is more common in West Africa
- HIV is tropic for T-helper lymphocytes (CD4+) and other cells such as monocytes, macrophages and CNS cells
- Retroviruses integrate into cell genome and replicate
- Virus persists for life in infected individuals
- Increasing loss of cell-mediated immunity with lymphopenia, decrease in T-helper lymphocytes (CD4+), and decrease in normal CD4+/CD8+ cell ratio
- Response of T lymphocytes to mitogens is lost; patients become anergic
- Loss of humoral immune function with elevated IgG and IgA
- Panhypogammaglobulinemia
- Viral load of circulating virus may be high (300 000 RNA copies/ml) or low (40 000 RNA copies/ml)

Diagnosis

- For patients >18 months, serum antibody tests using enzyme immunoassays (EIA) are used for screening. Repeat testing should be performed, and confirmed with Western blot immunofluorescent antibody test
- Some patients with hypogammaglobulinemia or advanced disease may not have HIV antibodies
- Polymerase chain reaction (PCR) and HIV cultures are performed in reference laboratories
- Modified p24 antigen assay is less sensitive than PCR or culture but may be present early in infection
- For infants born to HIV-seropositive women, diagnosis may be difficult, as neonates are usually seropositive at birth, whether infected or not

1. HIV culture or PCR are preferred
2. May need to be repeated at 4–6 months of age

Differential diagnosis

- Immunodeficiency states (e.g. severe combined immunodeficiency)
- Malnutrition
- Child abuse
- Infections, viral and bacterial
- Nutritional deficiencies

Treatment

- Physicians should consult an HIV specialist if possible
- Treatment with antiretroviral agents for HIV-infected mothers during pregnancy can reduce the risk of vertical transmission
- Antiretroviral therapy
- Antibiotics or antifungal agents as appropriate for infections
- Newly diagnosed patients with HIV infection must be reported to public health department

Prognosis

- Opportunistic infections, progressive neurological disease and severe wasting are associated with poor prognosis
- Viral load and CD4+ count are good predictors of prognosis

References

Fauci AS. The AIDS epidemic. N Engl J Med 1999; 341: 1046–50

Hachem ME, Bernardi S, Pianosi G, et al. Mucocutaneous manifestations in children with HIV infection and AIDS. Pediatr Dermatol 1998; 15: 429–34

Harris PS, Saag MS. Dermatologic manifestations of human immunodeficiency virus infection. Curr Prob Dermatol 1997; 9: 209–62

Mocroft A, Youle M, Phillips AN, et al. The incidence of AIDS-defining illnesses in 4883 patients with human immunodeficiency virus infection. Arch Intern Med 1998; 158: 491–7

Report of the Committee on Infectious Diseases. Red Book, 26th edn. American Academy of Pediatrics: Elk Grove Village, IL, 2003: 360–82

Rico JM, Myers SA, Sanchez MR. Guidelines of care for dermatologic conditions in patients infected with HIV. J Am Acad Dermatol 1997; 37: 450–72

Wananukul S, Deekajorndech T, Panchareon C, Thisyakorn U. Mucocutaneous findings in pediatric AIDS related to degree of immunosuppression. Pediatr Dermatol 2003; 20: 289–94

Ward HA, Russo GG, Shrum J. Cutaneous manifestations of antiretroviral therapy. J Am Acad Dermatol 2002; 46: 284–93

Rocky mountain spotted fever

Major points

- Clinical characteristics:
  1. Fever, headache, myalgias, nausea, vomiting, anorexia
  2. Rash begins on wrists and ankles as an erythematous macular eruption which later becomes petechial and spreads to the trunk (Figure 8.28)
     a. Palms and soles are often involved
     b. Rarely, no rash is present; more common in infants
  2. Thrombocytopenia
  3. Anemia
  4. Leukocytopenia
  5. Duration of illness ~3 weeks
  6. Involvement of various organ systems: CNS, cardiac, pulmonary, gastrointestinal tract, renal and other organs
  7. Disseminated intravascular coagulation in severe cases
  8. Shock leading to death

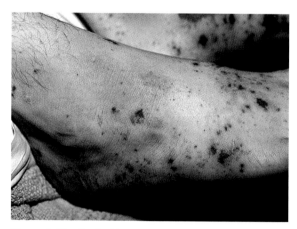

Figure 8.28 Rocky Mountain spotted fever with vasculitis and purpura

- Epidemiology
  1. Incubation period: 2–14 days (usually 1 week)
  2. Transmitted to humans by the bite of ticks, which are reservoirs and vectors of *Rickettsia rickettsii*
  3. Ticks: *Dermacentor variabilis* (dog tick), *Dermacentor andersoni* (wood tick) in upper Rocky Mountain states, and *Amblyomma americanum* (Lone Star tick) in south central USA
  4. Organism is transmitted transovarially and between stages in ticks
  5. Increased risk: persons exposed to ticks frequently (e.g. pet owners, outdoorsmen)
  6. More common in children <15 years of age
  7. Most common in April through October
  8. Widespread in USA, with most cases reported in southeastern and south central states; also reported in Canada, Mexico, Central and South America

Pathogenesis

- Caused by *Rickettsia rickettsii*, an obligate intracellular pathogen and member of the spotted fever group of rickettsiae

Diagnosis

- Culture of organism not recommended because of danger of transmission
- Skin biopsy of rash with immunofluorescent staining for *R. rickettsii* is specific but not readily available
- Four-fold increase in one of multiple rickettsial group-specific tests; or decrease in antibody titer between acute and convalescent sera by indirect immunofluorescence antibody (IFA), complement fixation (CF), latex agglutination (LA), indirect hemagglutination (IHA), or microagglutination tests
  1. Antibodies can be detected by IFA 7–10 days after illness starts
  2. IFA and IHA are the most sensitive and specific tests
  3. CF and microagglutination are highly specific but lack sensitivity
  4. Weil–Felix serologic test (Proteus Ox-19 and Ox-2 agglutinins) is nonspecific and not sensitive
  5. PCR test from blood and skin specimens is available in reference laboratories but positivity depends upon number of organisms

Differential diagnosis

- Drug eruptions
- Petechiae
- Vasculitis
- Ehrlichiosis
- Toxic shock syndrome
- Disseminated intravascular coagulation
- Measles
- Parvovirus B19 ('gloves and socks' syndrome)

Treatment

- Doxycycline 2–4 mg/kg per day in one to two doses given orally or intravenously (adult dose 1–2 g/day) is drug of choice for all ages. Tetracycline staining of teeth is dose related and doxycycline is less likely to stain developing teeth than other tetracyclines. Since ehrlichiosis and Rocky Mountain Spotted Fever overlap clinically, tetracyclines are effective against both infections, whereas chloramphenicol is not
- Chloramphenicol 50–100 mg/kg per day given intravenously or orally in four doses (adult dose 2–4 g/day)
- Treatment is given until the patient has been afebrile for 2–3 days (usually 7–10 days)
- Preventative measures: protective clothing, tick/insect repellents to skin and clothes
- Thorough inspection of the skin after being outdoors and removal of ticks

Prognosis

- Early treatment is needed for a good outcome
- Mortality highest in males, in persons >30 years, in non-Whites, and in persons with no known tick-bite history
- Delay in disease recognition increases risk of death or neurological sequelae

References

Case Records of the Massachsetts General Hospital (Case 32-1997). N Engl J Med 1997; 337: 1149–56

Jacobs RF. Human monocytic ehrlichiosis: similar to Rocky Mountain spotted fever but different. Pediatr Ann 2002; 31: 180–4

Masters EJ, Olson GS, Weiner SJ, Paddock CD. Rocky Mountain spotted fever: a clinician's dilemma. Arch Int Med 2003; 163: 769–74

McGinley-Smith DE, Tsao SS. Dermatoses from ticks. J Am Acad Dermatol 2003; 49: 363–92

Report of the Committee on Infectious Diseases. Red Book, 26th edn. American Academy of Pediatrics: Elk Grove Village, IL, 2003: 532–4

Sexton DJ, Kaye KS. Rocky mountain spotted fever. Med Clin North Am 2002; 86: 351–60, vii-viii

Lyme disease

Synonym: erythema chronicum migrans

Major points

- Clinical manifestation divided into three stages:
  1. Early localized
     a. Erythema migrans at site of tick bite (Figure 8.29)

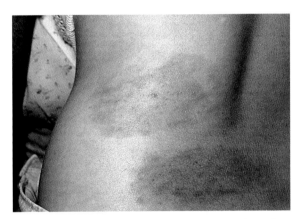

Figure 8.29 Lyme disease – typical annular patches of erythema chronicum migrans

    b. Begins as a red macule or papule, expanding during days to weeks to form a large annular erythematous lesion >5 cm (average 15 cm) with central clearing

    c. Rash can vary greatly and may be vesicular or necrotic in the center

    d. Fever, malaise, headache, mild neck stiffness and arthralgia

  2. Early disseminated

    a. Multiple lesions of erythema migrans which are similar to but usually smaller than the primary lesion

    b. Lesions usually occur 3–5 weeks after the tick bite

    c. Common manifestations: palsies of cranial nerves (especially 7th cranial nerve),

meningitis, conjunctivitis, arthralgias,
myalgias, headache and fatigue
   d. Rare manifestation: carditis
3. Late disease
   a. Occurs several months to several years after
the tick bite
   b. Recurrent arthritis (pauciarticular, affecting
large joints, particularly knees)
   c. Chronic arthritis is uncommon in children
treated in early stages with antibiotics
   d. CNS: encephalopathy, neuropathy
- Epidemiology
1. Usually occurs April through October
2. Incubation period 3–31 days (average 7–14
days)
3. Occurs in three distinct geographic regions in
the USA (although it has been reported in 48
states): northeast (Massachusetts to Maryland),
upper midwest (Minnesota, Wisconsin), west
coast (northern California)
4. Reported in Canada, Europe, former Soviet
Union, China, Japan
5. Tick vectors
   a. *Ixodes scapularis* (previously called *Ixodes
dammini*) in east and midwest
   b. *Ixodes pacificus* in west

Pathogenesis

- Caused by spirochete *Borrelia burdorferi*, acquired
by tick bite

Diagnosis

- Clinical diagnosis
- Borrelia cultures require special media and are not
readily available
- Serological testing:
1. IgM specific antibody titers peak 3–6 weeks
after onset of disease
2. IgG antibody titers rise slowly and peak weeks
to months later
3. Titers persist for years and should not be used
to assess treatment
4. Localized erythema migrans, because it occurs
1–2 weeks after tick bite, usually does not
show rising titers. Some patients treated early
never develop elevated titers
- Enzyme immunosorbent assay (EIA): may give
false-positive results; should be confirmed with
immunoblot

- Immunofluoresence assay (IFA): may give false-
positive results; should be confirmed with
immunoblot
- Western immunoblot test: should be used to
corroborate positive or equivocal EIA or IFA results
1. Both IgM and IgG should be assessed if early
in disease
2. IgM not recommended if illness >1 month's
duration
3. Comparing acute- and convalescent-phase sera
may be needed in some cases
- PCR is specific but limited in availability
- Widespread practice of ordering serologic tests for
nonspecific symptoms should be discouraged, as
positive tests are frequently false-positives

Differential diagnosis

- Granuloma annulare
- Gyrate erythema
- Tinea corporis
- Urticaria
- Drug eruption

Treatment

- Early treatment usually prevents development of
later stages
- Clinical response is slow, and symptoms may
persist for weeks
- Jarisch–Herxheimer reaction with fever, chills and
malaise can occur transiently when therapy is
started; nonsteroidal anti-inflammatory agents may
be helpful
- Early localized disease:
1. Doxycycline 100 mg twice a day, orally for
14–21 days for children >8 years and
nonpregnant women
2. Amoxicillin 25–50 mg/kg per day, divided into
three doses (maximum 2 g per day) for 14–21
days
- Multiple erythema migrans:
1. Same oral regimen as early disease for 21 days
- Isolated facial palsy:
1. Same oral regimen as early disease but for
21–28 days
2. Treatment has no effect on palsy, but prevents
further complications
- Arthritis:
1. Same oral regimen as for early disease but for
28 days

- Persistent or recurrent arthritis:
  1. Ceftriaxone 75–100 mg/kg, intravenously or intramuscularly, once a day (maximum 2 g/day) for 14–21 days; or
  2. Penicillin 300 000 U/kg per day intravenously, given in divided doses every 4 hours (maximum, 20 million U/day) for 14–21 days
- Carditis/meningitis or encephalitis:
  1. Ceftriaxone 75–100 mg/kg intravenously or intramuscularly, once a day (maximum 2 g/day) for 14–21 days; or
  2. Penicillin 300 000 U/kg per day, intravenously, given in divided doses every 4 hours (maximum, 20 million U/day) for 14–21 days
- Control measures:
  1. Avoid tick-infested areas
  2. Cover skin with clothing as much as possible
  3. Permethrin can be sprayed on clothing to prevent tick attachment
  4. Repellents containing diethyltoluamide (DEET) can be applied sparingly to skin; can be neurotoxic in high doses
  5. Bathe with soap and water after outdoor exposure
  6. Inspect the skin and remove ticks daily
  7. Prophylactic antimicrobial treatment after tick bite is not usually recommended routinely, especially if the tick attachment is <24–48 hours
  8. Analysis of ticks to determine infectivity is not recommended

Prognosis

- Excellent for early disease
- Guarded for disseminated or late disease

References

American Academy of Pediatrics. Committee on Infectious Diseases. Prevention of Lyme disease. Pediatrics 2000; 105: 142–7

Bachman DT, Srivastava G. Emergency department presentations of Lyme disease in children. Pediatr Emerg Care 1998; 14: 356–61

Eppes SC. Diagnosis, treatment, and prevention of Lyme disease in children. Paediatr Drugs 2003; 5: 363–72

Hengge UR, Tannapfel A, Tyring SK, et al. Lyme borreliosis. Lancet Infect Dis 2003; 3: 489–500

Huppertz HI. Lyme disease in children. Curr Opin Rheumatol 2001; 13: 434–40

McGinley-Smith DE, Tsao SS. Dermatoses from ticks. J Am Acad Dermatol 2003; 49: 363–92

Report of the Committee on Infectious Diseases. Red Book, 26th edn. American Academy of Pediatrics: Elk Grove Village, IL, 2003: 407–11

Singh-Behl D, La Rosa SP, Tomecki KJ. Tick-borne infections. Dermatol Clin 2003; 21: 237–44

Stanek G, Strle F. Lyme borreliosis. Lancet 2003; 362: 1639–47

9

FUNGAL DISEASES

SUPERFICIAL FUNGAL INFECTIONS

Candida

Major points

- Oral candidiasis (thrush)
  1. Affects ~5% of healthy infants
  2. Clinical presentation: white, raised patches on buccal mucosa, tongue and palate; may be described as having a 'cheesy' appearance or as 'pseudomembranous' patches; scraping reveals a raw, red base (Figure 9.1)
  3. May be acquired from passage through the birth canal in a healthy newborn

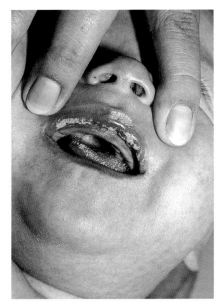

Figure 9.1 Candida – thrush on the lips and tongue

  4. Infants or older children with persistent oral thrush should be evaluated for predisposing factors (e.g. immunodeficiency, HIV)
- Diaper candidiasis
  1. Clinical presentation: brightly erythematous ('beefy red') confluent patches with a sharply demarcated serpiginous border and satellite pustules; small rings of scale, edema, oozing
- Candidal paronychia
  1. Seen in children who suck their fingers, in people who are exposed to excessive moisture, or in diabetics
  2. Clinical presentation: chronic inflammation of the skin surrounding the nails; periungual erythema, edema and separation of the nail fold from the nail plate
- Congenital candidiasis/neonatal candidiasis (see Chapter 2)
- Chronic mucocutaneous candidiasis (CMC)
  1. Recurrent or severe infections of the skin, mucous membranes and nails with *Candida*, most frequently *C. albicans*
  2. Persistent infection, sometimes granulomatous, and resistant to therapy
  3. Rare disorder
  4. Majority of cases begin in the first 3 years of life
  5. Male/female ratio = 1
  6. Absence of visceral or disseminated sepsis
  7. Often associated with genetic, immunologic or endocrine dysfunction
  8. Most common immune defect is a specific inability to respond to antigens of *C. albicans*
- Systemic candidiasis
  1. Candidal infection in the blood, urine or cerebrospinal fluid (CSF)

2. Affects 2–4% of very-low-birth-weight infants
3. Associated with long-term hospitalization, invasive instrumentation, immunosuppression
4. Cutaneous findings: erythematous macules, papules and plaques
- Other manifestations of candida infection: folliculitis, candidal intertrigo, vaginitis and vulvovaginitis, esophagitis and laryngitis, intravenous line sepsis, candiduria
- Risk factors for invasive infection:
    1. High risk: HIV, extreme prematurity, neutropenia, diabetes, chemotherapy, corticosteroid therapy
    2. Increased risk: neutrophil defects (chronic granulomatous disease or myeloperoxidase deficiency), intravenous hyperalimentation, broad-spectrum antimicrobial therapy

Pathogenesis

- Causative pathogen is a yeast-like fungus of the genus *Candida*
- Most common is *Candida albicans* (50–60%), which is part of the normal flora of the gastrointestinal tract and mucocutaneous areas of humans; it is not part of the normal skin flora
- The yeast phase is the dominant form; the pseudohyphal (mycelial) phase is the invasive form; the chlamydospore is the resting state
- Mechanism of invasion is unclear
- Host defense factors against invasion include: intact stratum corneum, humoral immunity
- Person-to-person transmission rarely occurs
- Patients with immunodeficiency (e.g. HIV/AIDS, prematurity, organ transplantation, chemotherapy) are at risk for invasive/recurrent disease
- Other risk factors: endocrine dysfunction, malnutrition, prematurity, use of antibiotics

Diagnosis

- Characteristic clinical findings
- KOH preparation shows pseudohyphae and budding yeast
- Culture is helpful but may be misleading; *Candida* can be cultured from non-infected skin
- Diagnosis of invasive candidiasis requires isolation of the organism from typically sterile body fluid or tissue (e.g. blood, CSF, bone marrow, biopsy)
- For early-onset, recurrent or recalcitrant candidal infections, suspect CMC and evaluate

for underlying endocrine and autoimmune disorders

Differential diagnosis

- Oral candidiasis
    1. Lichen planus
    2. Food in the mouth
    3. Leukoplakia
    4. Squamous cell carcinoma
- Diaper candidiasis
    1. Irritant contact dermatitis
    2. Psoriasis
    3. Allergic contact dermatitis
- Candidal paronychia
    1. Bacterial infection
    2. Herpetic whitlow

Treatment

- Oral candidiasis
    1. Oral nystatin suspension 100 000 U/ml four times a day PO, 'swish and swallow'
    2. Clotrimazole troches
    3. Elimination of predisposing factors (e.g. antibiotics)
    4. In the immunocompromised: oral fluconazole or itraconazole
- Skin infections
    1. Topical nystatin is effective and inexpensive
    2. Other topical antifungals: miconazole, clotrimazole, naftifine, ketoconazole, econazole, ciclopirox
- Vulvovaginal candidiasis
    1. Topical azoles are more effective than nystatin
    2. Clotrimazole, miconazole, ketoconazole, others
- Diaper candidiasis
    1. Topical nystatin or antifungal creams
    2. Oral nystatin may be of benefit, especially if there is thrush
    3. Protective barrier (e.g. zinc oxide-containing ointments) after dermatitis has resolved
    4. Elimination of predisposing factors, frequent diaper change, use of superabsorbent disposable diapers
- Chronic mucocutaneous candidiasis
    1. Usually refractory to traditional topical antifungal therapies and imidazole preparations
    2. Systemic antifungal agents: oral fluconazole, oral itraconazole and low-dose IV amphotericin B (0.3 mg/kg per day, maximum 1.5 mg/kg per day) have been used successfully

3. Immune enhancers
4. Maintenance on antifungal therapy may be necessary

- Systemic candidiasis
  1. Early treatment is critical, based on clinical suspicion, as culture may take days
  2. IV amphotericin B: drug of choice for disseminated disease
  3. Alternative treatment: fluconazole IV or PO
  4. Duration based on clinical response, presence or absence of neutropenia
  5. Flucytosine may be used as adjuvant in cases with CNS involvement; can act synergistically with amphotericin B

Prognosis

- Based on the severity of disease and underlying predisposing factors
- Disseminated or invasive candidiasis can be rapidly fatal
- Chronic mucocutaneous candidiasis has a high frequency of relapse; severe infections with other organisms may occur and result in serious morbidity or death

References

Friedlander SF, Rueda M, Chen BK, Caceres-Rios HW. Fungal, protozoan, and helminthic infections. In: Pediatric Dermatology, 3rd edn. Schachner LA, RC Hansen, eds. CV Mosby: St Louis, 2003: 1093–129

Garcia Hidalgo L. Dermatological complications of obesity. Am J Clin Dermatol 2002; 3: 497–506

Kaufman D. Strategies for prevention of neonatal invasive candidiasis. Semin Perinatol 2003; 27: 414–24

Mengesha YM, Bennett ML. Pustular skin disorders: diagnosis and treatment. Am J Clin Dermatol 2002; 3: 389–400

Report of the Committee on Infectious Diseases. Red Book, 26th edn. American Academy of Pediatrics: Elk Grove Village, IL, 2003: 229–32

Rowen JL. Mucocutaneous candidiasis. Semin Perinatol 2003; 27: 406–13

Tinea corporis

Synonym: ringworm

Major points

- Dermatophyte infection of body surfaces, not otherwise designated to a specific body site
- More prevalent in warm or moist climates
- Clinical presentation: red, scaly papules coalescing into annular plaques; may see erythema, vesicles, pustules, bulla, crusting; often unilateral; may be pruritic (Figures 9.2–9.4)
- Tinea incognito – alteration in appearance when topical corticosteriod is applied (source of diagnostic confusion)
- Tinea gladiatorum – tinea corporis affecting wrestlers; lesions usually on neck and upper arms where there is physical contact

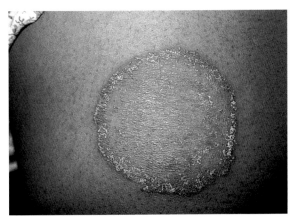

Figure 9.2 Tinea corporis – annular erythematous scaly plaque, acquired from a cat

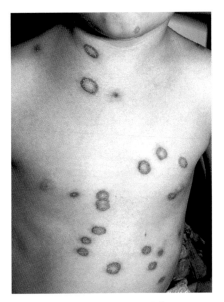

Figure 9.3 Tinea corporis – multiple inflammatory, annular lesions

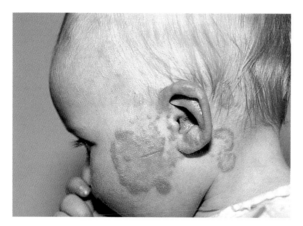

Figure 9.4   Tinea corporis – acquired from a kitten

- Tinea profunda – unusual clinical presentation of a boggy mass resembling a kerion
- Majocchi granuloma – perifollicular or follicular granulomatous inflammatory response to dermatophyte, often associated with topical steroid usage (Figure 9.5)
- Hypersensitivity eruption (dermatophytic or id reaction) – pruritic, fine papulovesicular eruption on trunk, hands, or face caused by a hypersensitivity reaction to fungal infection

Pathogenesis

- Most common causes: *Trichophyton tonsurans, T. rubrum* and *T. mentagrophytes, Microsporum canis* and *Epidermophyton floccosum*
- Transmission by direct contact with infected humans, animals, or fomites

Diagnosis

- KOH preparation – scraping should be performed from scale with demonstration of hyphae in epidermal cells
- Culture on dermatophyte test medium (DTM) or Sabouraud dextrose agar

Differential diagnosis

- Nummular eczema
- Granuloma annulare
- Candidiasis
- Erythema annulare centrifugum
- Psoriasis
- Pityriasis rosea
- Subacute cutaneous or discoid lupus erythematosus

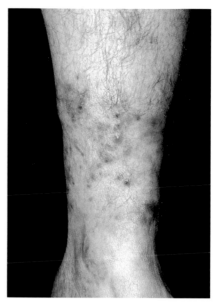

Figure 9.5   Majocchi granuloma from tinea pedis treated with topical steroids

Treatment

- Topical treatment usually sufficient in limited disease:
  1. Miconazole, clotrimazole, terbinafine, tolnaftate, naftifine, or ciclopirox, ketoconazole, econazole, oxiconazole, butenafine, or sulconazole until 1–2 weeks after clearance
  2. Minimum duration of therapy recommended is 4 weeks
  3. Treat until there is no scaling
- Oral antifungals for poor response or in extensive disease
  1. Griseofulvin 20 mg/kg per day PO for 4 weeks given 1–2 times a day
  2. Oral itraconazole, fluconazole and terbinafine (off label)
- Use of combination antifungal/corticosteroid (e.g. Lotrisone) can be associated with persistent/recurrent infection

Prognosis

- Cases resolve with treatment

References

Adams BB. Tinea corporis gladiatorum: a cross-sectional study. J Am Acad Dermatol 2000; 43: 1039–41

Alston SJ, Cohen BA, Braun M. Persistent and recurrent tinea corporis in children treated with combination antifungal/corticosteroid agents. Pediatrics 2003; 111: 201–3

Greenberg HL, Shwayder TA, Bieszk N, Fivenson DP. Clotrimazole/betamethasone diproprionate: a review of costs and complications in the treatment of common cutaneous fungal infections. Pediatr Dermatol 2002; 19: 78–81

Gupta AK, Chaudhry M, Elewski B. Tinea corporis, tinea cruris, tinea nigra, and piedra. Dermatol Clin 2003; 21: 395–400

Report of the Committee on Infectious Diseases. Red Book, 26th edn. American Academy of Pediatrics: Elk Grove Village, IL, 2003: 619–20

Tinea pedis

Synonym: athlete's foot fungus

Major points

- Prevalence in industrialized countries approaches 10%; men have a 20% risk of developing tinea pedis; increases in incidence with age (probably due to increased exposure)
- Uncommon in young children; common in adolescents and adults
- Clinical presentation: scaly, pruritic, erythematous eruption on the plantar and dorsal surfaces of the feet with maceration, peeling, and fissuring in the lateral toe web spaces (especially in the 3rd and 4th interdigital spaces); may see vesicles (Figures 9.6 and 9.7)
- Toenails can be affected and dystrophic
- Commonly occurs in association with tinea cruris
- Often a family history is positive (usually an affected parent)
- Hypersensitivity reaction to the fungus (dermatophytid or id reaction) may be present on the hands and feet with pruritic vesicles and papules

Pathogenesis

- Causative organisms: *Trichophyton rubrum* (60%), *Trichophyton mentagrophytes* (25%), *Epidermophyton floccosum* (10%) and mixed (5%)
- Transmission is by person-to-person contact; often source of exposure in children is a parent
- Fungi also found in damp areas – swimming pools, locker rooms

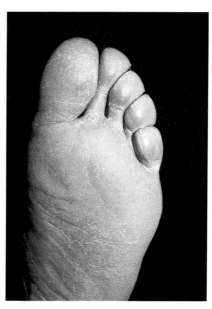

Figure 9.6   Tinea pedis – typical scaling on bottom of foot

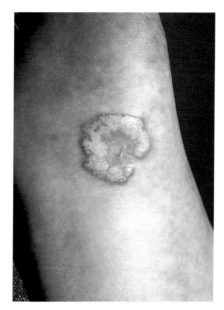

Figure 9.7   Tinea pedis – bullous, annular lesion with a positive KOH preparation

Diagnosis

- Characteristic clinical manifestations
- KOH preparation – scraping reveals branching hyphae
- Fungal culture to confirm on DTM or Sabouraud media

Differential diagnosis

- Dyshidrotic eczema
- Contact dermatitis
- Atopic dermatitis
- Juvenile plantar dermatosis ('sweaty-sock syndrome')
- Psoriasis
- Pitted keratolysis

Treatment

- Topical antifungal therapy
  1. Miconazole, haloprogin, clotrimazole, ciclopirox, terbinafine, butenafine, tolnaftate, ketoconazole, econazole, naftifine, oxiconazole, or sulconazole
  2. Duration of treatment ~2–3 weeks
- Oral antifungals for severe, chronic, or recalcitrant tinea pedis
  1. Oral griseofulvin for 6–8 weeks
  2. Oral itraconazole or terbinafine (not US Food and Drug Administration (FDA)-approved for this indication)
- Superimposed bacterial infections treated with antibacterial agents (topical or systemic); soak feet in dilute bleach water (Dakin solution 0.25%) once daily for 15 minutes
- Prevention of recurrences:
  1. Foot hygiene: keep feet cool and dry; drying between toes; absorbent socks; air shoes between wearings
  2. Topical antifungal powder (e.g. ZeaSORB AF®)

Prognosis

- Rarely, may be complicated by bacterial superinfection including lymphangitis, lymphadenitis and cellulitis

References

Gupta AK, Chow M, Daniel CR, Aly R. Treatments of tinea pedis. Dermatol Clin 2003; 21: 431–62

McBride A, Cohen BA. Tinea pedis in children. Am J Dis Child 1992; 146: 844–7

Report of the Committee on Infectious Diseases. Red Book, 26th edn. American Academy of Pediatrics: Elk Grove Village, IL, 2003: 621–3

Sweeney SM, Wiss K, Mallory SB. Inflammatory tinea pedis/manum masquerading as bacterial cellulitis. Arch Pediatr Adolesc Med 2002; 156: 1149–52

Weinstein A, Berman B. Topical treatment of common superficial tinea infections. Am Fam Physician 2002; 65: 2095–102

Zaias N, Rebell G. Clinical and mycological status of the Trichophyton mentagrophytes (interdigitale) syndrome of chronic dermatophytosis of the skin and nails. Int J Dermatol 2003; 42: 779–88

Tinea capitis

Syndrome: Scalp ringworm

Major points

- Most common in preschool or school-age children (ages 3–9 years)
- Incidence is highest in Black children
- Most common cause is *Trichophyton tonsurans* in North America (>90%)
- Clinical presentation is an incomplete alopecia especially prominent on the crown and occipital regions, with scaling
- Other clinical presentations:
  1. Asymptomatic scaling
  2. Widespread scaling with minimal hair loss (seborrheic dermatitis-like pattern) (Figures 9.8–9.10)
  3. Black-dot tinea – discrete areas of hair loss with stubs of broken hairs resembling dots
  4. Kerion – painful, inflamed, crusted mass with purulent discharge; often with associated fever and regional lymphadenopathy (Figure 9.11)
  5. Favus – inflammation and scarring characterized by yellow cup-shaped crusts (scutula), around a hair; rare in the USA
- Classified as ectothrix (spores on the surface of the hairs) which fluoresces with Wood's lamp or endothrix (spores inside the hair shaft) which does not fluoresce
- Hypersensitivity reaction (dermatophytic or id reaction); pruritic, fine, papulovesicular eruption on trunk, hands, or face may occur (Figure 9.12)

Pathogenesis

- Caused by dermatophytic fungi; common etiologic agents are *T. tonsurans* (anthropophilic) and *Microsporum canis* (zoophilic)
- Transmission is person-to-person or fomites such as combs, clothing, bedding, toys and furniture

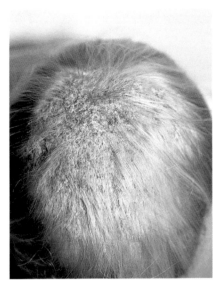

Figure 9.8 Tinea capitis – scaly patch of hair loss with *Microsporum canis*

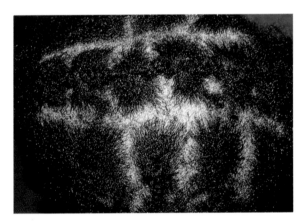

Figure 9.9 Tinea capitis – typical diffuse scaling mistaken for dandruff

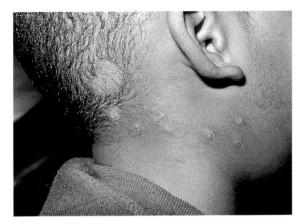

Figure 9.10 Tinea capitis – scaling typical of *Trichophyton tonsurans* with additional tinea corporis

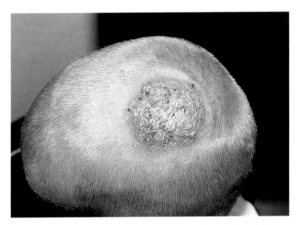

Figure 9.11 Kerion – marked inflammation and crusting in the scalp

- Asymptomatic individuals, especially family members, act as reservoirs for infection (~25% of family members affected)

Diagnosis

- Clinical examination
- KOH preparation: observe spores within broken-off hairs, rarely hyphae
- Culture – collect specimen by rubbing a sterile cotton swab over the scalp and inoculating in fungal media or DTM
- Skin biopsy may be necessary to confirm diagnosis in unusual cases, especially Majocchi granuloma

- Histology: neutrophils in the upper stratum corneum; stain for fungi with periodic acid-Schiff (PAS) or methenamine silver stain

Differential diagnosis

- Alopecia areata
- Trichotillomania
- Staphylococcal infection
- Traction alopecia
- Seborrheic dermatitis
- Psoriasis

Treatment

- Topical antifungals not fully effective
- Oral griseofulvin:

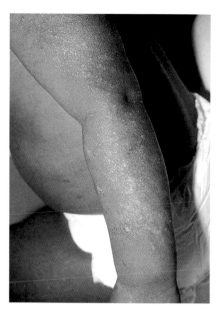

Figure 9.12   Hypersensitivity reaction to tinea capitis

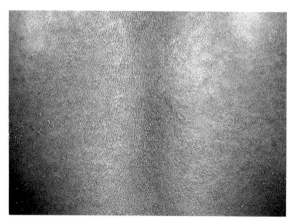

Figure 9.13   Tinea versicolor with hyperpigmented scaly plaques

1. Microsize griseofulvin 20 mg/kg per day (maximum 1 g/24 hours)
2. Ultramicrosize griseofulvin 10 mg/kg per day (maximum 750 mg/24 hours)
3. Take BID with fatty foods to increase absorption
4. Minimal duration of treatment is 4–6 weeks; continue for 2 weeks past clinical resolution
- Adjuvant treatment to decrease fungal shedding and curb spread of infection:
  1. Selenium sulfide 2.5% shampoo 2–3 times a week
  2. Ketoconazole 1–2% shampoo 2–3 times a week
- Newer oral antifungal therapies shown to be safe and effective: (see doses in Chapter 21) terbinafine, itraconazole, fluconazole
- Obtain follow-up cultures until negative result is obtained
- Evaluate household contacts and treat if necessary
- For severe inflammatory kerion: prednisone 1 mg/kg per day in addition to antifungal therapy, can hasten reduction of scaling and pruritus
- Secondary bacterial infection in a kerion should be treated with appropriate antibiotic therapy for *Staphylococcus* coverage

Prognosis

- Usually resolves without permanent alopecia
- With severe inflammatory disease, scarring and permanent hair loss may occur, but tends to be rare and spotty

References

Abdel-Hamid IA, Agha SA, Moustafa YM, El-Labban AM. Pityriasis amiantacea: a clinical and etiopathologic study of 85 patients. Int J Dermatol 2003; 42: 260–4

Chen BK, Friedlander SF. Tinea capitis update: a continuing conflict with an old adversary. Curr Opin Pediatr 2001; 13: 331–5

Gupta AK, Adam P, Dlova N, et al. Therapeutic options for the treatment of tinea capitis caused by Trichophyton species: griseofulvin versus the new oral antifungal agents, terbinafine, itraconazole, and fluconazole. Pediatr Dermatol 2001; 18: 533–8

Gupta AK, Cooper EA, Ginter G. Efficacy and safety of itraconazole use in children. Dermatol Clin 2003; 21: 521–35

Gupta AK, Cooper EA, Lynde CW. The efficacy and safety of terbinafine in children. Dermatol Clin 2003; 21: 511–20

Report of the Committee on Infectious Diseases. Red Book, 26th edn. American Academy of Pediatrics: Elk Grove Village, IL, 2003: 617–18

Onychomycosis

Synonym: tinea unguium

Major points

- Less common in children than adults; rare in children <6 years old

- Prevalence of onychomycosis in children is 0.3–0.44%
- Mycotic nail infection accounts for roughly 30% of nail diseases seen in childhood
- Most commonly affects the toenails
- Most common type in children is distal and lateral subungual onychomycosis
- Higher prevalence in children with Down syndrome or HIV infection
- Usually associated with tinea pedis

Pathogenesis

- Most common causative agent is *Trichophyton rubrum*, followed by *Candida* sp. and *T. interdigitale*
- Transmission usually from a family member

Diagnosis

- KOH preparation – scrape underneath the nail plate or take fine clippings or filings through the entire thickness of the nail with visualization of hyphae
- Histology of nail clipping with PAS staining can demonstrate fungal elements
- For severe disease, must exclude immunodeficiency, HIV, endocrinopathies

Differential diagnosis

- Psoriasis
- Lichen planus
- Alopecia areata
- Twenty-nail dystrophy

Treatment

- Mild cases may respond to topical therapy:
  1. Terbinafine or ketoconazole creams
  2. Ciclopirox 8% lacquer (Penlac)
- Oral antifungals needed for moderate to severe disease: griseofulvin, itraconazole, terbinafine, fluconazole
- Adjuvant surgical debridement or excision of affected nail may be of benefit for severely affected nails
- Foot hygiene to reduce recurrence: keep feet cool, clean and dry; absorbent socks; antifungal foot powders; well-fitting shoes; avoid barefoot contact with areas with a high density of fungal spores, such as bathroom floors, gymnasiums and locker rooms

Prognosis

- May be recurrent

References

Arrese JE, Pierard GE. Treatment failures and relapses in onychomycosis: a stubborn clinical problem. Dermatology 2003; 207: 255–60

Faergemann J, Baran R. Epidemiology, clinical presentation and diagnosis of onychomycosis. Br J Dermatol 2003; 149 (Suppl 65): 1–4

Ghannoum MA, Hajjeh RA, Scher R, et al. A large-scale North American study of fungal isolates from nails: the frequency of onychomycosis, fungal distribution and antifungal susceptibility patterns. J Am Acad Dermatol 2000; 43: 641–8

Gupta AK, Chang P, Del Rosso JQ, et al. Onychomycosis in children: prevalence and management. Pediatr Dermatol 1998; 15: 464–71

Gupta AK, Skinner AR. Onychomycosis in children: a brief overview with treatment strategies. Pediatr Dermatol 2004; 21: 74–9

Gupta AD, Skinner AR. Onychomycosis in children: a brief overview with treatment strategies. Pediatr Dermatol 2004; 21: 74–9

Scher RK, Baran R. Onychomycosis in clinical practice: factors contributing to recurrence. Br J Dermatol 2003; 149 (Suppl 65): 5–9

Tinea versicolor

Synonyms: pityriasis versicolor

Major points

- Worldwide distribution
- Superficial chronic fungal infection
- Common in temperate regions: prevalence of ~1% during warmer parts of the year
- More common in tropical and subtropical regions: incidence of up to 40% in tropics
- Majority of cases occur during adolescence
- 5–7% of cases occur in children <13 years
- Male/female ratio = 1
- Family history is often positive
- Clinical presentation:
  1. Discrete or confluent hypopigmented or hyperpigmented (fawn-colored or brown) oval macules and patches with slight, fine scale (Figures 9.13 and 9.14)

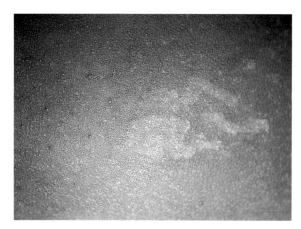

Figure 9.14   Tinea versicolor with typical furfuraceous scale

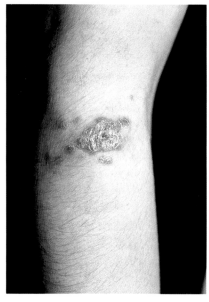

Figure 9.15   Sporotrichosis – grouped erythematous papules and nodules

2. Distribution over back, upper chest and shoulders, neck and proximal extremities
3. The face is commonly affected in children (rarely in adults)
4. Lesions fail to tan normally and are more prominent in summer months
- Other related conditions:
  1. *Pityrosporum* folliculitis
  2. Obstructive dacryocystitis – from colonization of the lacrimal sac

3. Confluent and reticulate papillomatosis – may represent a host response to *P. orbiculare*
4. Systemic infection in patients receiving intralipid therapy: neonates with cardiovascular disease, or immunosuppressed

Pathogenesis

- Causative agent is *Pityrosporum orbiculare* (*Malassezia furfur*)
- Lipophilic yeast, part of the normal flora of the skin
- Not contagious
- *P. orbiculare* changes from the round, budding blastospore form to the hyphal form under predisposing conditions:
  1. Exogenous factors: heat, humidity or moisture, or occlusive clothing
  2. Endogenous factors: adrenalectomy, diabetes, pregnancy, malnutrition, systemic corticosteroids, immunosuppression, hyperhidrosis, seborrheic dermatitis

Diagnosis

- Characteristic skin findings
- Wood's lamp may aid in diagnosis of subclinical patches
- KOH preparation – 'spaghetti and meatballs' appearance of budding yeast cells and hyphae
- Culture/biopsy usually unnecessary

Differential diagnosis

- Vitiligo
- Pityriasis alba
- Postinflammatory hypopigmentation
- Psoriasis
- Seborrheic dermatitis
- Erythrasma
- Dermatophytosis

Treatment

- Topical therapy
  1. Selenium sulfide 2.5% applied once a day for 7 days for 10 minutes, and washed off; then on the first and third day of the month for 6 months
  2. Propylene glycol 50% in water applied once or twice a day
  3. Topical azoles: ketoconazole, miconazole, oxiconazole once or twice a day

4. Topical terbinafine 1% cream
- Systemic therapy: ketoconazole 400 mg in a single dose, repeated 1 week later; exercise to induce sweating increases skin concentration and increases effectiveness of systemic therapy

Prognosis

- Repigmentation may take months or years
- Recurrence rates high, 60–80%, with topical therapy

References

Gupta AK, Batra R, Bluhm R, Faergemann J. Pityriasis versicolor. Dermatol Clin 2003; 21: 413–29

Report of the Committee on Infectious Diseases. Red Book, 26th edn. American Academy of Pediatrics: Elk Grove Village, IL, 2003: 623–4

Terragni, L, Lassagni A, Oriani A, Gelmetti C. Pityriasis versicolor in the pediatric age. Pediatr Dermatol 1991; 8: 9–12

Vander Straten MR, Hossain MA, Ghannoum MA. Cutaneous infections dermatophytosis, onychomycosis, and tinea versicolor. Infect Dis Clin North Am 2003; 17: 87–112

DEEP FUNGAL INFECTIONS

Sporotrichosis

Major points

- Worldwide distribution
- Clinical presentation: subacute or chronic cutaneous and subcutaneous infection
  1. Lymphocutaneous sporotrichosis – commonly on upper or lower extremities or face; incubation period 1–3 weeks; begins with small, firm, subcutaneous, violaceous nodules with regional lymphadenopathy; over the next 2 weeks, secondary nodules and streaking appear following the course of lymphatics; often ulcerates; facial localization common in children (Figure 9.15)
  2. Fixed cutaneous sporotrichosis – erythematous papules, nodules, or verrucous plaques (may ulcerate) with scale or crust surrounded by violaceous halo; does not extend past point of inoculation
  3. Children more commonly have solitary lesions

- Severe disease manifestations: disseminated visceral, osteoarticular meningeal, and pulmonary sporotrichosis
- Usually affects normal hosts; disease more severe in immunosuppressed people

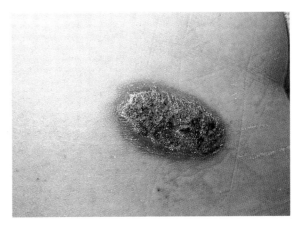

Figure 9.16 Blastomycosis – isolated verrucous plaque on the leg

- Risk factors for severe disease: strong association with HIV infection, diabetes, chronic obstructive pulmonary disease (COPD)
- Pulmonary and disseminated sporotrichosis is rare in children

Pathogenesis

- Causative agent is *Sporothrix schenckii*, a dimorphic fungus which exists as a mold in nature and as yeast *in vivo* at a temperature of 37°C
- The organism grows in sphagnum moss, thorny plants (especially roses), decaying vegetation, soil and hay
- Infection occurs with exposure to environmental foci at the site of minor trauma; specific activities associated with disease include rose gardening, topiary production, Christmas tree farming, hay baling, masonry; inoculation may occur after motor vehicle or other accidents or animal (especially cat) bites/scratches
- Pulmonary sporotrichosis – transmitted by inhalation of spores
- T-cell-mediated immunity is important in host defense; disease more severe in patients with AIDS

Diagnosis

- Culture scrapings or exudates from site of infection on Sabouraud dextrose agar at room temperature; read at 4–7 days; conversion to yeast form demonstrated on brain–heart infusion agar at 37°C
- Skin biopsy for culture/examination with special stains (e.g. PAS) demonstrates organisms
- No definitive serologic test available

Differential diagnosis

- Bacterial infection
- Pyoderma
- Spider or insect bite
- Non-tuberculous mycobacteria infection
- Nocardiosis
- Deep fungal infections: blastomycosis, paracoccidiomycosis, chromoblastomycosis
- Tularemia
- Leishmaniasis

Treatment

- Itraconazole 100 mg/day PO for 3–6 months
- Saturated solution of potassium iodide (SSKI)
  1. For a 50–70 kg person: 5 drops (50 mg/drop) three times daily, increasing 1 drop per dose per day to a maximum of 30–35 drops TID for 4–6 weeks after resolution of the lesion (do not increase if there is severe nausea)
  2. For infants and smaller children: 1 drop TID, increasing to a maximum of 10 drops TID for 4–6 weeks until resolution of lesions
- Local heat therapy applied ~1 hour/day for many months (baths at ~45°C, hot compress, hand-held heater); watch for burns
  1. Basis for treatment is that growth of some strains is inhibited by temperature of >35°C, killed at a temperature of 39°C
- Amphotericin B – for pulmonary, disseminated and meningeal disease, and in children with immunodeficiency

Prognosis

- May lead to scarring or hyperpigmentation

References

Burch JM, Morelli JG, Weston WL. Unsuspected sporotrichosis in childhood. Pediatr Infect Dis J 2001; 20: 442–5

De Araujo T, Marques AC, Kerdel F. Sporotrichosis. Int J Dermatol 2001; 40: 737–42

Koga T, Matsuda T, Matsumoto T, Furue M. Therapeutic approaches to subcutaneous mycoses. Am J Clin Dermatol 2003; 4: 537–43

Queiroz-Telles F, McGinnis MR, Salkin I, Graybill JR. Subcutaneous mycoses. Infect Dis Clin North Am 2003; 17: 59–85, viii

Report of the Committee on Infectious Diseases. Red Book, 26th edn. American Academy of Pediatrics: Elk Grove Village, IL, 2003: 558–9

Blastomycosis

Synonyms: North American blastomycosis, Gilchrist disease

Major points

- Endemic in midwest and south central USA, the Great Lakes region, upstate New York, Eastern Canada, Manitoba
- Cases have been reported in Africa, and rarely in Central and South America, Europe, India and the Middle East
- Rare in children
- Clinical findings: acute, primary pulmonary infection (often subclinical) occurs after a 30–45-day incubation period; this may resolve or progress to chronic pulmonary infection or dissemination with extrapulmonary manifestations, such as cutaneous findings (secondary cutaneous blastomycosis)
- Skin is involved in 40–80% of cases where there is extrapulmonary disease
- Cutaneous lesions are verrucous or ulcerative with heaped-up borders; usually slowly enlarging; erythema nodosum has been reported; may see subcutaneous nodules (Figure 9.16)
- Other organs involved include: bones and joints, genitourinary system, CNS (mass lesion or meningitis)
- Primary cutaneous blastomycosis – relatively rare, inoculation occurs after trauma (e.g. dog bite, open wounds); lymphangitis and regional lymphadenopathy often accompany the skin lesion; no evidence of systemic infection; the organism can be recovered from the skin lesion
- Immunosuppression is a risk factor for disease, and also for more aggressive disease with higher mortality
- Intrauterine or congenital infections occur rarely

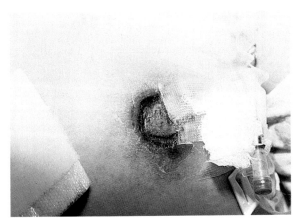

Figure 9.17 Mucormycosis – acquired from infected tape

Pathogenesis

- Causative agent is *Blastomyces dermatitidis*, a dimorphic fungus, growing in a mycelial form at room temperature and in a yeast form at 37°C; reproduces with characteristic broad-based budding
- The organism is found in warm, damp soil
- Transmission to humans is most often via lungs; aerosolized conidia are inhaled and transform to the yeast form at body temperature
- Person-to-person transmission does not occur
- Cellular immunity and adequate neutrophil and humoral responses are among the factors necessary for host defense

Diagnosis

- Clinical findings
- Histology: thick-walled, broad-based budding yeasts
- Specimen collection:
  1. Sputum: organisms can be seen on KOH preparation or by special stains
  2. Wet preparation or special stains of exudates from cutaneous lesions, synovial fluid, or soft tissue abscesses usually reveal organisms
  3. CSF is usually negative
- Culture needed for definitive diagnosis
- Serologic assays not sensitive or specific

Differential diagnosis

- Pyoderma gangrenosum
- Squamous cell carcinoma

- Other cutaneous infections: sporotrichosis, nocardiosis, atypical mycobacteria, tularemia, leishmaniasis

Treatment

- Amphotericin B IV has greatest proven treatment success (cure rates up to 97%)
- Itraconazole 4–10 mg/kg per day has been used to treat non-life-threatening blastomycosis in children; treatment course is many months

Prognosis

- May result in chronic pulmonary disease
- In immunosuppressed patients, serious disease is frequent with complications of CNS disease, acute respiratory distress syndrome, fungemia and high mortality rates

References

Bradsher RW, Chapman SW, Pappas PG. Blastomycosis. Infect Dis Clin North Am 2003; 17: 21–40

Lemos LB, Baliga M, Guo M. Blastomycosis: the great pretender can also be an opportunist. Initial clinical diagnosis and underlying diseases in 123 patients. Ann Diagn Pathol 2002; 6: 194–203

Pappas PG, Dismukes WE. Blastomycosis, Gilchrist's disease revisited. Curr Clin Top Infect Dis 2002; 22: 61–77

Report of the Committee on Infectious Diseases. Red Book, 26th edn. American Academy of Pediatrics: Elk Grove Village, IL, 2003: 219–20

Zampogna JC, Hoy MJ, Ramos-Caro FA. Primary cutaneous North American blastomycosis in an immunosuppressed child. Pediatr Dermatol 2003; 20: 128–30

Mucormycosis

Major points

- Acute, rapidly progressive, fatal disease occurring in immunosuppressed patients caused by opportunistic fungi
- Cutaneous mucormycosis:
  1. Superficial: gradual onset with slow progression, associated with the use of contaminated adhesive tape; no vascular or deep tissue involvement (Figure 9.17)
  2. Gangrenous: progresses rapidly with painful ulcers and eschars; vascular invasion with

hematogenous spread common; poor prognosis; usually occurs in the setting of skin trauma (e.g. IM injection, open fracture, insect bites, motor vehicle accidents) in patients with an underlying predisposing condition
   a. Premature infants: associated with contaminated adhesive tape use or wooden tongue depressors for limb splinting; very grave prognosis in this setting
   b. Older children with underlying myeloproliferative disease
- Other clinical presentations:
   1. Rhinocerebral: most common, affects diabetics with underlying ketoacidosis
   2. Pulmonary: more common in patients with hematologic malignancies
   3. Gastrointestinal: usually seen only with severe malnutrition; high (98%) mortality rate
   4. Disseminated: more common in patients with hematologic malignancies
- Infection affects patients with neutropenia, diabetes, generalized immunosuppression (hematologic malignancy, bone marrow or solid organ transplantation, HIV/AIDS), deferoxamine therapy, trauma, burns
- Rarely occurs in immunocompetent individuals

Pathogenesis

- Caused by fungi in the family Mucoraceae; opportunistic 'bread molds'
- Most common pathogen is *Rhizopus oryzae*
- Organism is present in decaying fruits and vegetables, seeds, soil and animal excreta
- Infection occurs after skin/soft tissue trauma, ingestion of spores (gastrointestinal form), use of contaminated tape in a patient with underlying predisposing factors
- Angiotrophic nature of the fungus results in vascular invasion and destruction leading to skin necrosis and ulceration
- Infection occurs in patients with impaired neutrophil or mononuclear cell phagocytic function

Diagnosis

- Early diagnosis is critical
- Tissue biopsy usually needed for diagnosis – direct microscopic examination with hematoxylin and

eosin (H&E), PAS staining or Gomori's methenamine silver
- Organism grows on routine bacterial and fungal culture media

Differential diagnosis

- Aspergillosis
- Ecthyma gangrenosum (pseudomonas infection)

Treatment

- Extensive surgical debridement of necrotic tissue required (due to poor penetration of antifungal agents)
- Amphotericin B, IV
- Correction of underlying disease

Prognosis

- High mortality rates; especially with infection in infants
- Older children have somewhat better prognosis
- Prognosis is best for the cutaneous form of the disease
- Mortality rates:
   1. Cutaneous 16%
   2. Rhinocerebral 67%
   3. Pulmonary 83%
   4. Disseminated and gastrointestinal disease ~100%
- Early detection, extensive surgical debridement, and systemic amphotericin B necessary for survival

References

Boyd AS, Wiser B, Sams HH, King LE Jr. Gangrenous cutaneous mucormycosis in a child with a solid organ transplant: a case report and review of the literature. Pediatr Dermatol 2003; 20: 411–15

Leitner C, Hoffmann J, Zerfowski M, Reinert S. Mucormycosis: necrotizing soft tissue lesion of the face. J Oral Maxillofacial Surg 2003; 61: 1354–8

Prabhu RM, Patel R. Mucormycosis and entomophthoromycosis: a review of the clinical manifestations, diagnosis and treatment. Clin Microbiol Infect 2004; 10: 31–47

10

INFESTATIONS AND ENVIRONMENTAL HAZARDS

Scabies

Major points

- Papules on wrists, fingerwebs, periaxillary skin, genitalia and abdomen
- In infants, lesions more generalized: feet, scalp and face
- Multiple excoriations, erythematous papules, honey-colored crusts, some pustules and secondary impetigo
- Pruritus, often increased in evening/night
- Erythematous nodules (nodular scabies) more common on trunk and axillae, particularly in infants (Figure 10.1)
- Debilitated or immunosuppressed individuals who are unable to scratch may be severely affected
- Burrows (linear superficial lesions) are diagnostic; usually seen on wrists, interdigital webs, or feet of infants (Figures 10.2 and 10.3)

- Symptoms may vary: asymptomatic carriers, or few scattered itchy papules, or hundreds of lesions, or thick crusts which have hundreds of mites (crusted scabies)
- High index of suspicion in pruritic patients
- Family members are often itchy, although degree of itching may vary

Pathogenesis

- Caused by eight-legged human mite, *Sarcoptes scabiei*, <0.4 mm in length
- Female mite remains within stratum corneum where she lays eggs and can move 0.5–5 mm/day; female mite lives 30–40 days; burrows up to 5 mm/day; lays 2–3 eggs/day; eggs take 10–14 days to mature
- Human contact or contagious clothing or bed sheets (fomites) necessary for transmission

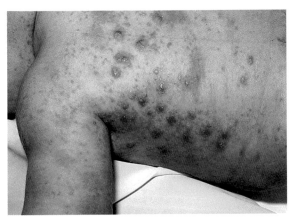

Figure 10.1 Nodular scabies – usually more prominent in the axillary areas

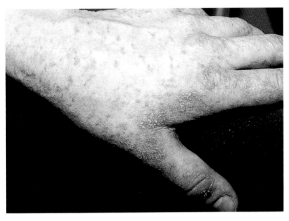

Figure 10.2 Scabies – typical pruritic papules on the hands and finger webs

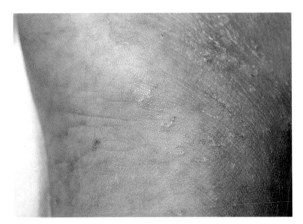

Figure 10.3 Scabies – burrow showing linear tunnel with tiny, dark dot at end which is the mite

- Newly infested individuals may not itch for 3–6 weeks and may be a source of infestation

Diagnosis

- Confirmed by scraping an unscratched burrow, demonstrating a mite, egg, feces (scybala) microscopically (Figure 10.4)

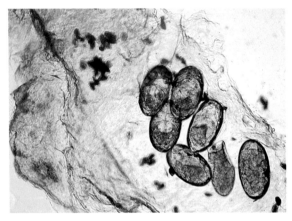

Figure 10.4 Scabies – typical eggs and feces seen microscopically

- Technique of scraping:
  1. Scrape several lesions, preferably unscratched burrows with a no. 15 blade
  2. Place scales on glass slide, cover with immersion oil or KOH and coverslip
  3. Microscope objective on low power: 4× or 10×
- Adult female mite has a round body, eight legs, length ~0.3 mm; male is half that size

Differential diagnosis

- Atopic dermatitis
- Lichen planus
- Dermatitis herpetiformis
- Papular urticaria (insect bites)
- Impetigo
- Folliculitis
- Contact dermatitis
- Histiocytosis

Treatment

- Permethrin cream 5% (see Table 10.1)
  1. Dispense 60 g per patient; no refills
  2. Apply thin layer of cream from neck down to toes
  3. Be sure to include finger webs, armpits, groin
  4. Leave cream on for 8–12 hours (overnight)
  5. Take a hot shower or bath in the morning
  6. Wash clothes used in previous 3 days through the hot cycle of the washer
  7. Reapply cream (same technique) 1 week later
  8. Do not apply cream more than twice
- Gamma benzene hexachloride lotion or cream 1% (lindane, Kwell®, Gamene®)
  1. Dispense 60 g per patient; no refills
  2. A bath is not recommended before applying the lotion

Table 10.1   Instruction sheet for scabies treatment

Permethrin cream 5%

A bath is not necessary before applying the cream. If you take a bath, wait half an hour before applying the cream. Apply a thin layer from the neck down to the toes. Be sure not to forget finger webs, fingernails, armpits and groin. Leave cream on for 8–12 hours (overnight). After this, take a hot shower or bath to remove the cream. At the time of the shower, wash clothing and bed linen used in the previous 3 days in the hot cycle of the washer. Reapplication is necessary 1 week later (left on 8–12 hours – same routine). Be sure to keep your return appointment with your doctor.

Do not apply this cream more than is recommended by your doctor

3. Apply a thin layer of cream or lotion from the neck down to the toes. Be sure to include finger webs, armpits and groin
4. Leave cream on for 8–12 hours (overnight)
5. In the morning, take a hot shower or bath
6. At time of shower, wash clothing and bed linen used in previous 3 days in hot cycle of washer
7. Reapply cream or lotion (same technique) 1 week later (left on for 8–12 hours) with same routine
8. Lindane should not be used by pregnant women, women who are breast feeding, or very young infants
9. Do not apply this lotion more than is recommended

- Precipitated sulfur ointment 6–10% (for infants, small children, and pregnant patients)
  1. Apply thin layer of ointment from neck down to toes
  2. Be sure to apply between fingers, toes, in armpits and groin
  3. For babies who have lesions on their heads, apply ointment directly to these areas
  4. Leave ointment on for 24 hours
  5. After this time, the patient may bathe
  6. Reapply ointment in the same manner. Leave on for 24 hours
  7. Again reapply ointment; three times each for 24 hours (total 72 hours)
  8. After 72 hours, wash clothing and bed linen used in previous 3 days in hot cycle of washer and dryer
  9. Sulfur ointment is messy and odiforous, and may stain clothing
- Ivermectin (oral) 150–400 μg/kg for teens and adults (off label)
  1. Single dose orally is 95% effective; repeat at 2 weeks if necessary
  2. Administered as 6-mg scored tablets (range 9–18 mg depending upon weight)
- Other points:
  1. Follow-up in 2–3 weeks to prevent patient from continually treating themselves for itching.
  2. Patients may need hydrocortisone 1–2.5% cream or ointment to calm residual itching
  3. Be sure to treat all family members and others with close personal contact
  4. People do not get human scabies from animals

References

Avila-Romay A, Alvarez-Franco M, Ruiz-Maldonado R. Therapeutic efficacy, secondary effects, and patient acceptability of 10% sulfur in either pork fat or cold cream for the treatment of scabies. Pediatr Dermatol 1991; 8: 64–6

Hoke AW, Maibach HI. Scabies management: a current perspective. Cutis 1999; 64: 2–16

Huynh TH, Norman RA. Scabies and pediculosis. Dermatol Clin 2004; 22: 7–11

Kim K-J, Rosh K-H, Choi J-H, et al. Scabies incognito presenting as urticaria pigmentosa in an infant. Pediatr Dermatol 2002; 19: 409–11

Meinking TL, Taplin D, Hermida JL, et al. The treatment of scabies with ivermectin. N Engl J Med 1995; 333: 26–30

Paller AS. Scabies in infants and small children. Semin Dermatol 1993; 12: 3–8

Pruksachatkunakorn C, Damrongsak M, Sinthupuan S. Sulfur for scabies outbreaks in orphanages. Pediatr Dermatol 2002; 19: 448–53

Usha V, Gopalakrishnan Nair TV. A comparative study of oral ivermectin and topical permethrin cream in the treatment of scabies. J Am Acad Dermatol 2000; 42: 236–40

Pediculoses (louse infestations)

Major points

- Body louse infestations present with excoriated papules and pustules on trunk and perineum
- *Pediculosis capitis* usually presents with pruritic papules at nape of neck (Figure 10.5)
- Nits and lice can be detected in scalp or clothing, especially seams of clothing
- Nits are white ovoid bodies, tightly adherent to hair shafts
- Head lice are infrequent in Black patients
- Pubic lice ('crabs') occasionally with blue-black crusted macules (maculae ceruleae)
- Pubic lice can also be seen in eyelashes or the scalp of young children

Pathogenesis

- Caused by *Pediculus humanus* (human body louse) with subspecies *capitis* (head lice) or *humanus* (body lice) and *Pthirus pubis* (crab lice)
- Lice are six-legged insects, 1–4 mm long; they attach to skin or hair and ingest blood

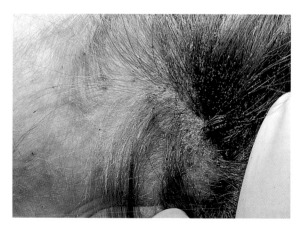

Figure 10.5   Pediculosis (lice) – pruritic papules and nits at the nape of the neck

- The female louse produces new offspring every 2 weeks, attaching to hair and depositing eggs along the hair shaft
- Crowded living conditions are ideal for spreading infestation through direct contact
- Fomites (e.g. hairbrushes, hats, scarves, coats, clothes)
- Body lice carry typhus in some endemic areas

Diagnosis

- Observation of nits or lice by visual inspection or microscopically (Figure 10.6)

Differential diagnosis

- Scabies
- Insect bites (mosquitoes, fleas)

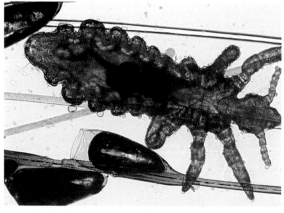

Figure 10.6   Pediculosis (lice) – louse with nits microscopically (courtesy of Dr Anne Lind)

- Dermatitis herpetiformis
- Factitial excoriations
- Pseudonits (retained external hair root sheath)

Treatment

- *Pediculosis Capitis* (Head lice)
  1. Permethrin 1% (Nix®) one application of cream rinse, left on for 10 minutes after shampoo, then rinsed out
  2. Pyrethrins with piperonyl butoxide (RID®, A-200 Pyrinate Shampoo®) two applications (5–7 days apart) applied undiluted to the scalp, left on 10 minutes, then rinsed out
  3. Lindane 1% shampoo (by prescription) 10-minute application then rinsed out; repeat in 1 week
  4. Malathion 0.5% (Ovide®) excellent ovicidal, but odiferous. Apply to hair, let dry for 8–12 hours, then shampoo out. Repeat in 1 week. Caution: flammable
  5. Ivermectin 200–250 μg/kg in a single oral dose (off label)
  6. Other hints
     a. Apply cream rinse and comb hair to remove nits
     b. Chemicals used to 'dissolve' nits (of questionable value): vinegar, glacial acetic acid, Step 2® (formic acid); use with combing
     c. Metal nit combs – helpful if hair is thick
     d. Nit picking – if hair is thin (may want to cut individual hairs)
     e. R & C Spray® – for use on clothing, furniture which cannot be washed or dry cleaned; do not use on people
     f. Pseudonits – flakes of skin on hair shafts which may resemble nits; to differentiate, observe microscopically
- *Pediculosis corporis* (Body lice)
  1. Proper hygiene, clean clothes, clean housing conditions
  2. Lindane lotion 1% (left on 8 hours, then washed off)
- *Pediculosis pubis* (crab lice)
  1. Lindane 1% shampoo
     a. 5-minute application, then wash out
     b. Repeat in 1 week
     c. Nits should be removed

2. Synergized pyrethrins (OTC)-(RID®, R & C Shampoo®, A-200®)
   a. Apply undiluted, leave on 10 minutes, then wash off
   b. Second application in 1 week
3. Treat sexual contacts or other appropriate contacts
4. Eyelash involvement
   a. Use petrolatum 3–5 times a day for 8 days
   b. Remove nits
   c. Do not use lindane or pyrethrins on the eyelids

References

Burgess IF. Human lice and their control. Annu Rev Entomol 2004; 49: 457–81

Drugs for head lice. Medical Letter 1997; 39 (Issue 992): 6–7

Frankowski B, Weiner LB. Head lice. Pediatrics 2002; 110: 638–43

Huynh TH, Norman RA. Scabies and pediculosis. Dermatol Clin 2004; 22: 7–11

Ko CJ, Elston DM. Pediculosis. J Am Acad Dermatol 2004; 50: 1–12

Meinking TL, Serrano L, Hard B, et al. Comparative *in vitro* pediculicidal efficacy of treatments in a resistant head lice population in the United States. Arch Dermatol 2002; 138: 220–4

Williams LK, Reichert A, MacKenzie WR, et al. Lice, nits and school policy. Pediatrics 2001; 107: 1011–15

Papular urticaria (insect bite reactions)

Major points

- Clinical points
  1. Erythematous pruritic papules (Figure 10.7)
  2. May be grouped in clusters; where the insect bit several times, it looks like 'breakfast, lunch and dinner'
  3. Occasional vesicles or bullae, especially in young children
  4. May be anywhere on the body, but typically on exposed skin
  5. Children aged 18 months to 10 years typically affected
  6. Recurrent crops common
  7. One child in the family may be the only person bitten

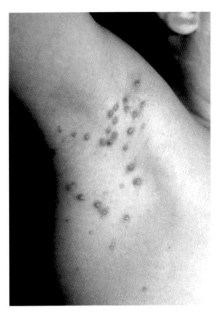

Figure 10.7   Papular urticaria (insect bite reactions) – multiple, erythematous, pruritic papules

  8. Common in spring or summer
  9. Some immunosuppressed children or those with HIV infections can have severe exaggerated reactions
  10. Harvest mites (chiggers)
   a. *Trombiculidae splendens*
   b. Bright red mites
   c. Tends to occur in intertriginous areas and around waistband
   d. Larval form takes blood meal then drops off

Pathogenesis

- Lesions caused by delayed hypersensitivity reaction to insect bite
- Fleas (dog or cat), mosquitoes, bedbugs, lice, scabies or mites (fowl, grain, grass) can be implicated in most cases

Diagnosis

- Clinical recognition
- May need biopsy confirmation in rare or unusual cases
- Histology: wedge-shaped perivascular lymphoid infiltrate with eosinophils, endothelial prominence and spongiosis or focal epidermal necrosis

Differential diagnosis

- Viral exanthems (varicella and others)
- Scabies
- Atopic dermatits
- Pityriasis lichenoides et varioliformis acuta

Treatment

- Avoid offending insects
- Veterinarian should inspect household pets for fleas or mites
- Insecticides used in house can kill fleas in carpet or furniture
- Protective clothing with long sleeves and long trousers
- Insect repellents containing DEET 10% or less may be applied to clothing or skin (Caution: can be neurotoxic)
- Pruritic lesions can be individually treated with a topical steroid (low strength to medium) 2–3 times a day
- Oral antihistamines (diphenhydramine, hydroxyzine) may help reduce itching

Prognosis

- Excellent, once offending agent is removed

References

Asada H, Miyagawa S, Sumikawa Y, et al. CD4+ T-lymphocyte-induced Epstein–Barr virus reactivation in a patient with severe hypersensitivity to mosquito bites and Epstein–Barr virus-infected NK cell lymphocytosis. Arch Dermatol 2003; 139: 1601–7

Demain JG. Papular urticaria and things that bite in the night. Curr Allergy Asthma Rep 2003; 3: 291–303

Diven DB, Newton RC, Ramsey KM. Heightened cutaneous reactions to mosquito bites in patients with acquired immunodeficiency syndrome receiving zidovudine. Arch Intern Med 1988; 148: 2296

Goddard J. Physician's Guide to Arthropods of Medical Importance, Boca Raton, FL: 4th edn. CRC Press, 2003

Moffitt JE. Allergic reactions to insect stings and bites. South Med J 2003; 96: 1073–9

Tokura Y, Ishihara S, Tagawa S, et al. Hypersensitivity to mosquito bites as the primary clinical manifestation of a juvenile type of Epstein–Barr virus-associated natural killer cell leukemia/lymphoma. J Am Acad Dermatol 2001; 45: 569–78

Hymenoptera stings

Major points

- Bee, wasp, or hornet stings followed by local reaction:
  1. Immediate pain and burning followed by intense, local, erythematous reaction with swelling, pruritus and an urticarial plaque (Figure 10.9)
  2. Honeybee leaves stinger in skin which can be gently removed by scraping with a fingernail or blade to prevent further envenomation
  3. Other Hymenoptera (e.g. yellow jackets) may sting repeatedly
- Systemic reactions (1–3% of population):
  1. Angioedema or generalized urticaria within 10 minutes
  2. Laryngeal edema and/or bronchospasm
  3. Rare anaphylaxis, shock and death

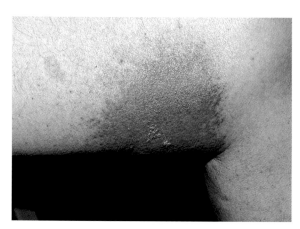

Figure 10.8   Hymenoptera sting – marked erythema and pruritus 2 days after a sting

- Fire ant bites (*Solenopsis*) – intense local inflammatory response followed by superficial pustules; bites/stings are usually multiple

Pathogenesis

- Hymenoptera order of insects includes bees, wasps, hornets and ants
- Venom contains phospholipase A2 which liberates acute inflammatory mediators
- Other active agents: hyaluronidase, histamine, acid phosphatase, norepinephrine and others

Diagnosis

- Clinical diagnosis and history

Differential diagnosis

- Urticaria
- Snake bite
- Lacerations
- Animal bite

Treatment

- Apply ice or cold compresses
- Systemic reactions may require subcutaneous epinephrine (adrenaline), steroids, antihistamines and treatment of shock if necessary
- In highly sensitive patients, consider desensitization
- Potent or ultrapotent topical steroid for persistent reactions
- Avoidance and pest control

Prognosis

- Excellent for local reactions.
- Guarded in sensitive patients with severe systemic symptoms

References

Cohen PR. Imported fire ant stings: clinical manifestations and treatment. Pediatr Dermatol 1992; 9: 44–8

Ditto AM. Hymenoptera sensitivity: diagnosis and treatment. Allergy Asthma Proc 2002; 23: 381–4

Golden DB. Stinging insect allergy. Am Fam Physician 2003; 67: 2541–6

Caterpillar dermatitis (lepidopterism)

Major points

- Lepidoptera (order) consists of butterflies and moths
- Incidental contact with insect larvae, especially hairs or spines of caterpillars
- Presents with widespread red macules and urticarial wheals
- Chronic cutaneous lesions: lichen simplex chronicus, post-inflammatory hyperpigmentation
- Other symptoms: inflammation of skin, eyes, respiratory system with dermatitis, conjunctivitis, keratitis, rhinitis, wheezing

- Rare systemic findings: tachycardia, arrhythmia, chest pain, dyspnea, peripheral neuropathy, convulsions, shock
- Treatment of symptoms: antihistamines, antipruritic lotions, mid-potency topical corticosteroids
- Stripping skin with adhesive tape will help remove remaining hairs
- Symptoms last hours to 10 days

References

Gardner TL, Elston DM. Painful papulovesicles produced by the puss caterpillar. Cutis 1997; 60: 125–6

Kuspis DA, Rawlins JE, Krenzelok EP. Human exposures to stinging caterpillar: Lophocampa caryae exposures. Am J Emerg Med 2001; 19: 396–8

Maier H, Spiegel W, Kinaciyan T, et al. The oak processionary caterpillar as the cause of an epidemic airborne disease: survey and analysis. Br J Dermatol 2003; 149: 990–7

Severs GA, Elston DM. What's eating you? Megalopyge opercularis. Cutis 2003; 71: 445–8

Spider bites

Major points

- Two spiders in USA which cause most problems: black widow spider (*Lactrodectus mactans*) and brown recluse spider (*Loxosceles reclusa*)
- Initial bites may be either painful (black widow spider) or nonpainful until several hours later (brown recluse spider)
- Hemorrhagic painful blister or skin necrosis follows, which may extend for several days until size reaches its maximum (Figure 10.9)
- Common on exposed skin (e.g. ankles or hands)
- Systemic reactions: vomiting, headache, chills, malaise, thrombocytopenia, hemolysis and hemoglobinuria; probably related to amount of venom injected

Pathogensis

- Spiders with powerful jaws which penetrate skin, inject venom and produce a reaction
- *Loxosceles reclusa* found in midwestern USA (particularly Arkansas, Tennessee, Texas and Missouri); mainly in attics, cellars and abandoned buildings

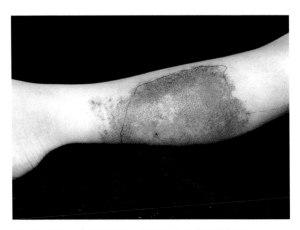

Figure 10.9   Spider bite – necrosis and pain from *Loxosceles reclusa*

1. Size 8–10 mm, brown, with thin legs, and has a distinct violin shape on its dorsal thorax
- *Lactrodactus mactans*
  1. Causes acute pain and edema at site of bite; systemic symptoms caused by neurotoxin α-lactrotoxin
  2. Often found in old outhouses and bite exposed buttocks

Diagnosis

- Identify spider if possible
- Central necrosis and pain may be prominent

Differential diagnosis

- Vascular infarction
- Vasculitis
- Bacteremia
- Ecthyma gangrenosum
- Streptococcal gangrene
- Herpes zoster
- Cutaneous diphtheria
- Anthrax

Treatment

- Ice packs directly to site will reduce spread of venom in tissues
- Elevation of area and bed rest advised until necrosis has stopped, usually several days
- Surgical excision not recommended and may spread toxin
- Dapsone may be helpful early
- 25% of bites become infected with *Staphylococcus aureus* – use antibiotics to cover

- Close follow-up until lesion stabilized
- Corticosteroids for systemic symptoms (e.g. hemolysis or thrombocytopenia); best given IV and patient observed for other symptoms for ~3 days
- Recognition of spider and its habitat is important in avoiding these bites. In endemic areas, shake out clothes before getting dressed and shake bed clothes before retiring
- Antivenin if available if reation severe

References

Elston DM. What's eating you? Loxosceles reclusa (brown recluse spider). Cutis 2002; 69: 91–2, 94–5

Isbister GK, Graudins A, White J, Warrell D. Antivenom treatment in arachnidism. J Toxicol Clin Toxicol 2003; 41: 291–300

Orion E, Matz H, Ruocco V, Wolf R. Parasitic skin infestations II, scabies, pediculosis, spider bites: unapproved treatments. Clin Dermatol 2002; 20: 618–25

Sams HH, Dunnick CA, Smith ML, King LE. Necrotic arachnidism. J Am Acad Dermatol 2001; 44: 561–73

Sams HH, Hearth SB, Long LL, et al. Nineteen documented cases of Loxosceles reclusa envenomation. J Am Acad Dermatol 2001; 44: 603–8

Wendell RP. Brown recluse spiders: a review to help guide physicians in nonendemic areas. South Med J 2003; 96: 486–90

Williams ST, Khare VK, Johnston GA. Severe intravascular hemolysis associated with brown recluse spider envenomation. Am J Clin Pathol 1995; 104: 463–7

Tick bites

Major points

- Usually painless, and often noticed when engorged tick is found (Figure 10.10)
- Local urticaria, pruritus, or erythema can occur several days after the bite (Figure 10.11)
- Common locations: scalp, axilla and groin
- Persistent pruritic papule may occur from retained tick mouthparts forming a granulomatous reaction
- *Borrelia burgdorferi*, which causes Lyme disease, can be carried by ticks. Observation of an expanding ring of erythema (erythema chronicum migrans) at the site of tick attachment is seen within 3 weeks after the bite (See Chapter 8)

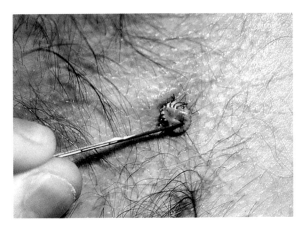

Figure 10.10   Tick embedded in skin, thought to be a 'changing mole'

- Rare reaction: tick paralysis with fever, nausea, abdominal cramping, headache and ascending symmetric paralysis similar to Guillain–Barré syndrome

Pathogenesis

- Major species
  1. *Dermacentor variabilis* (American dog tick); carrier of Rocky Mountain spotted fever
  2. *Amblyomma americanum* (Lone Star tick) in Southern USA; carrier of Rocky Mountain spotted fever and Ehrlichia
  3. *Ixodes dammini* (deer tick) in Eastern USA; carrier of *Borrelia burgdorferi* (Lyme disease)
  4. *Ixodes ricinus* in Europe; carrier of *Borrelia* (erythema chronicum migrans)

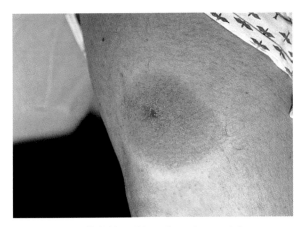

Figure 10.11   Tick bite with erythematous patch

- Ticks occur in wooded areas primarily in warmer months; also occur from handling dogs or clothing
- Larval and nymphal stages attach their heads into skin for blood meal, and become engorged
- Ticks cut skin surface with sharp chelicerae, introducing the proboscis, and secreting saliva into wound. Saliva contains an anticoagulant, an anesthetic and a cement substance, as well as possible *Borrelia*. As tick engorges, *Borrelia* proliferate in the tick gut and enters patient's blood after 24–48 hours

Diagnosis

- Careful clinical inspection and history
- Nymphal stages are small and may be overlooked (size 1–2 mm, 'seed ticks')

Differential diagnosis

- Nevocellular nevus
- Skin tag
- Pyogenic granuloma

Treatment

- Remove tick:
  1. Grasp the body of tick as close to the mouthparts as possible
  2. Apply slow, gentle, firm, outward pressure until the tick releases its mouthparts
  3. Not recommended: burning tick with a match, applying noxious substances to skin, squeezing, twisting or jerking the tick
- Cleanse skin with alcohol and apply topical antibiotic ointment
- Dispose of the tick by putting it in a jar of alcohol for a few minutes, then flush down the toilet
- Keep the tick for examination later; may be helpful in endemic Lyme disease areas
- Prevention is important
  1. Avoid tick-infested areas, especially tall grass and dense brush
  2. Wear long sleeves, and long trousers tucked into boots
  3. Wear insect repellents containing DEET
  4. Inspect children and dogs after exposure

References

Eppes SC. Diagnosis, treatment, and prevention of Lyme disease in children. Paediatr Drugs 2003; 5: 363–72

McGinley-Smith DE, Tsao SS. Dermatoses from ticks. J Am Acad Dermatol 2003; 49: 363–92

Meinking T, Taplin D. Infestations. In Pediatric Dermatology, 3rd edn. Schachner L, Hansen R. eds. Mosby: New York, 2003: 1141–80

Spach DH, Liles WC, Campbell GL, et al. Tick-borne diseases in the United States. N Engl J Med 1993; 329: 936–47

Stanek G, Strle F. Lyme borreliosis. Lancet 2003; 362: 1639–47

Wilson ME. Prevention of tick-borne diseases. Med Clin North Am 2002; 86 :219–38

Cutaneous larva migrans

Synonym: creeping eruption

Major points

- Within a few hours, there is pruritic dermatitis at the site of exposure
- Serpiginous, linear, erythematous, slightly raised, pruritic tracts 2–3 mm wide with bizarre patterns (Figure 10.12)
- Vesicles, pain or edema in area
- Feet most frequently affected
- Peripheral eosinophilia (can be up to 35% of cells)

Pathogenesis

- Caused by *Ancylostoma braziliensis* or *A. caninum*, the dog and cat hookworm (most common in southeastern North America)
  1. History of playing along southeastern or central shoreline of USA or in sandbox where cat or dog excreta may have been deposited
  2. Larvae hatch and penetrate bare skin where they migrate and die within 4–6 weeks
  3. Larvae can migrate 1–2 cm/day
- Other organisms less commonly causing larva migrans: *Bunostmum phlebotomum* (cattle hookworm), *A. duodenale*, and *Necator americanus*

Diagnosis

- Characteristic history and inspection: linear, serpiginous, pruritic lesions

Differential diagnosis

- Annular erythema
- Erythema chronicum migrans
- Tinea corporis

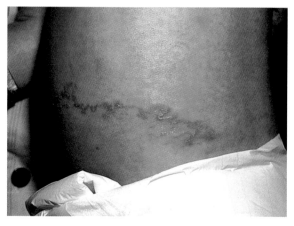

Figure 10.12   Cutaneous larva migrans – typical erythematous, serpiginous, linear streak

- Tinea pedis
- Nummular eczema
- Visceral larva migrans

Treatment

- For *A. braziliensis*, topical thiabendazole 15% cream applied 3–4 times/day for 5–7 days; apply cream beyond erythematous lesions
- Freeze advancing burrow with liquid nitrogen
- Return visit 4–5 days after starting treatment to determine therapeutic response
- Ivermectin 12 mg PO, single dose 0.2 mg/kg (off label)
- High potency topical steroids for itching

Prognosis

- Lesions are self-limited because humans are 'dead-end' hosts
- Duration is variable, usually lasting 4–6 weeks

References

Albanese G, Venturi C, Galviati G. Treatment of larva migrans cutanea (creeping eruption): a comparison between albendazole and traditional therapy. Int J Dermatol 2001; 40: 67–71

Brenner MA, Patel MB. Cutaneous larva migrans: the creeping eruption. Cutis 2003; 72: 111–15

Caumes E, Datry A, Paris L, et al. Efficacy of ivermectin in the therapy of cutaneous larva migrans. Arch Dermatol 1992; 128: 994–5

Caumes E. Treatment of cutaneous larva migrans. Clin Infect Dis 2000; 30: 811–14

Davies HD, Sakuls P, Keystone JS. Creeping eruption. Arch Dermatol 1993; 129: 588–91

Elgart ML. Creeping eruption. Arch Dermatol 1998; 134: 619–20

Van den Enden E, Stevens A, Van Gompel A. Treatment of cutaneous larva migrans. N Engl J Med 1998; 339: 1246–7

Animal bites

Major points

- Dog and cat bites (pets) are most common
- Victim usually a child who is teasing or playing with the animal
- Location usually the hand
- Human bites and monkey bites are often infected with aerobic or anaerobic mouth organisms
- Wild animals such as skunks, bats, foxes, coyotes, raccoons, other carnivores and some monkeys should be considered rabid until proven otherwise

Pathogenesis

- Most common organism causing secondary infection is *Pasteurella multocida*

Diagnosis

- History of a bite and clinical appearance

Differential diagnosis

- Other bites or stings

Treatment

- Culture wound for bacteria, then wash and leave open if possible (except face)
- Antibiotics should be given: amoxicillin–clavulanic acid, cefuroxime or clindamycin and a fluoroquinolone
- Tetanus immunization if needed
- Rabies immunization considered if needed

Prognosis

- Excellent unless lesions are large or multiple
- Scarring is possible
- Secondary infection

References

Gandhi RR, Liebman MA, Stafford BL, et al. Dog bite injuries in children: a preliminary survey. Am Surg 1999; 65: 863–4

Jones N, Khoosal M. Infected dog and cat bites. N Engl J Med 1999; 340: 1841–2

Overall KL, Love M. Dog bites to humans – demography, epidemiology, injury, and risk. J Am Vet Med Assoc 2001; 218: 1923–34

Presutti RJ. Prevention and treatment of dog bites. Am Fam Physician. 2001; 63: 1567–72

Weiss HB, Friedman DI, Coben JH. Incidence of dog bite injuries treated in emergency departments. J Am Med Assoc 1998; 279: 51–3

Snake bites

Major points

- Snakes
  1. Family Viperidae
     a. Crotalinae (pit vipers). North America: rattlesnake, cottonmouth, copperhead
     b. Viperinae (true vipers). Africa, Europe, other continents: vipers, adders
  2. Elapidae
     a. Tropical and warm temperate zones: coral snakes, cobras, mambas
  3. Hydrophidae
     a. Hydrophinae. Indopacific region: sea snakes
- 7000 bites recorded annually in USA, 2000 by venomous snakes
- Degree of toxicity depends upon potency of the venom, amount injected, size of person bitten, and size of snake
- Pain occurs immediately after bite followed by edema, numbness, ecchymosis and painful lymphadenopathy within 30 minutes
- Typical victims are males, aged 17–27 years
- Most bites are on extremities, between April and September
- Skin will have distinct fang punctures
- Immediate pain occurs, followed by edema, numbness, ecchymosis and painful lymphadenopathy within 30 minutes (Figure 10.13)
- Systemic symptoms (must be differentiated from terror): nausea, vomiting, sweating, fever, slurred speech, bleeding

Pathogenesis

- Pit-viper venom increases permeability of capillary membranes, causing edema, hypotension, hemolysis and other symptoms

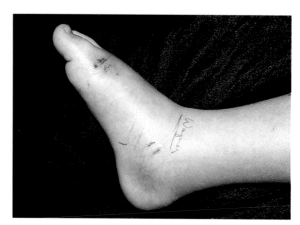

Figure 10.13   Snake bite from copperhead showing marked swelling, necrosis and pain

- Venoms are mixtures of potent proteolytic enzymes and low molecular-weight peptides with toxic effects

Diagnosis

- Clinical diagnosis with history

Differential diagnosis

- Other venomous animal or insect bites

Treatment

- Call regional Poison Control Center (National hotline: 800-222-1222)
  1. Identify species
  2. Aggressive supportive care, laboratory evaluation, and observation for at least 8–12 hours
  3. Antivenom if available and indicated
  4. Polyvalent pit viper antivenin should be used for severe snake bites (except the coral snake) as soon as possible
- Clean and cover the wound; baseline circumferential measurements of necrosis
- Limb should be immobilized in a functional position
- Tetanus toxoid
- Antibiotic coverage, if indicated
- Hospitalization with careful observation for dropping blood count and hemolysis
- Surgical debridement may need to be performed 3–10 days after the bite

Prognosis

- Severity depends upon size and species of snake, amount and degree of toxicity of venom, location,

first-aid treatments provided, timing of definitive treatment and state of health of the victim
- Common necrosis of skin with scar formation
- Rarely fatal

References

Dart RC, McNally J. Efficacy, safety, and use of snake antivenoms in the United States. Ann Emerg Med 2001; 37: 181–8

Gold BS, Dart RC, Barish RA. Bites of venomous snakes. N Engl J Med 2002; 347: 347–56

Hall EL. Role of surgical intervention in the management of crotaline snake envenomation. Ann Emerg Med 2001; 37: 175–80

Juckett G, Hancox JG. Venomous snakebites in the United States: management review and update. Am Fam Physician 2002; 65: 1367–74

Lalloo DG, Theakston RD. Snake antivenoms. J Toxicol Clin Toxicol 2003; 41: 277–90; 317–27

Rosen PB, Leiva JI, Ross CP. Delayed antivenom treatment for a patient after envenomation by Crotalus atrox. Ann Emerg Med 2000; 35: 86–8

Cercarial dermatitis (swimmer's itch)

Major points

- Clinical characteristics
  1. Begins with urticarial lesions (usually 10–30 but can be >200) and prickling sensation starting half an hour after exposure to infected water (Figure 10.14)
  2. Within 24 hours, pruritic erythematous papules occur in exposed areas not covered by a swimsuit
  3. Headache, fever and superinfection occasionally seen
- Occurs in freshwater lakes of upper Great Lakes region of North America and throughout the world

Pathogenesis

- Caused by *Schistosoma cercariae* (larval form of schistosomes)
- Humans are accidental hosts in life cycle of schistosomes
- Primary hosts (waterfowl, birds, mice, deer, etc.) deposit eggs in excreta in water
- Eggs hatch forming miracidia which infect snails, where they transform into cercariae

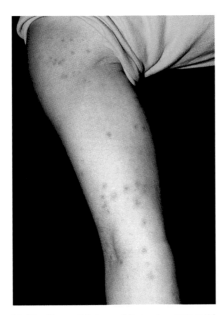

Figure 10.14   Cercarial dermatitis (swimmer's itch)

- In host, cercariae attach to skin and penetrate into dermis and blood vessels, passing to the gastrointestinal tract; eggs are discharged into feces, completing the life cycle
- In humans, ceracariae do not penetrate the blood vessels, but die in the superficial papillary dermis
- Cercarial proteins stimulate delayed-type hypersensitivity response manifest as an erythematous rash and itching

Diagnosis

- Typical distribution after history of swimming in fresh water

Differential diagnosis

- Seabather's eruption
- Insect bites
- Impetigo
- Varicella
- Insect bites
- Contact dermatitis
- Scabies
- Jellyfish stings

Treatment

- Topical steroid creams (low or mid-strength), drying lotions, oatmeal baths and oral antihistamines may help pruritus

- Severe eruption can be treated with oral prednisone 1 mg/kg per day for 5 days
- Treat secondary infection if present
- Not contagious
- Prevention is difficult. Barrier clothing or application of petrolatum prior to swimming may be of some benefit

Prognosis

- Lesions are self-limited

References

Folster-Holst R, Disko R, Rowert J, et al. Cercarial dermatitis contracted via contact with an aquarium: case report and review. Br J Dermatol 2001; 145: 638–40

Gonzales E. Schistosomiasis, cercarial dermatitis, and marine dermatitis. Dermatol Clin 1989; 7: 291–300

Sangueza OP, Lu D, Sangueza M, Pereira CP. Protozoa and worms. In Dermatology. Bolognia JL, Jorizzo JL, Rapini R, eds. Mosby: London, 2003: 1295–320

Seabather's eruption

Synonym: marine dermatitis

Major points

- Clinical characteristics
  1. Erythematous macules, papules or wheals that itch or burn
  2. May progress to vesiculopapules and heal with crusts in 7–10 days
  3. Occurs under covered areas (e.g. swimsuit, bathing cap, wet suit areas), beginning shortly after bathing in seawater
  4. Symptoms usually noticed after exiting water
  5. Systemic symptoms (e.g. fatigue, malaise, fever, lymphadenopathy)

Pathogenesis

- Caused by stinging larvae of sea anemones, Portuguese man-of-war, or thimble jellyfish; type determined by geographical location

Diagnosis

- Clinical lesions in typical bathing suit distribution after salt water swimming

Differential diagnosis

- Atopic dermatitis
- Jellyfish stings

- Swimmer's itch
- Insect bites
- Contact dermatitis
- Caterpillar dermatitis
- Varicella
- Viral eruptions
- Urticaria

Treatment

- Wash and dry skin immediately after bathing
- Symptomatic relief with topical steroids, antipruritic lotions, or oral antihistamines
- Oral prednisone 1 mg/kg per day if symptoms are severe
- Avoid occluding clothes, such as T-shirts, wet suits

Prognosis

- Self-limited eruption; resolves in 2 weeks

References

Adams BB. Dermatologic disorders of the athlete. Sports Med 2002; 32: 309–21

Freudenthal AR, Joseph PR. Seabather's eruption. N Engl J Med 1993; 329: 542–4

Segura Puertas L, Burnett JW, Heimer de la Cotera E. The medusa stage of the coronate scyphomedusa Linuche unguiculata ('thimble jellyfish') can cause seabather's eruption. Dermatology 1999; 198: 171–2

Tomchik RS, Russell MT, Szmant AM, Black NA. Clinical perspectives on seabather's eruption, also known as 'sea lice'. J Am Med Assoc 1993; 269: 1669–72

Wong DE, Meinking TL, Rosen LB, et al. Seabather's eruption. J Am Acad Dermatol 1994; 30: 399–406

11

HYPERSENSITIVITY DISORDERS/ UNCLASSIFIED DISORDERS

Urticaria

Major points

- 15–20% of children will have at least one episode by adolescence
- Classified as acute if it lasts for <6 weeks, chronic if >6 weeks
- Usually acute (not chronic) in children
- Etiologic factor can often be identified in children
- Frequent association with atopy
- Presents with circumscribed, slightly elevated, erythematous, edematous plaques that persist for minutes to hours; typical wheal and flare; usually pruritic; often presents at points of pressure (e.g. belt-line, palms, soles); individual lesions rarely last for more than 24–48 hours, but new lesions often arise as older ones clear (Figures 11.1 and 11.2)
- Food-related urticaria often has associated itching and swelling of the lips, mucous membranes,

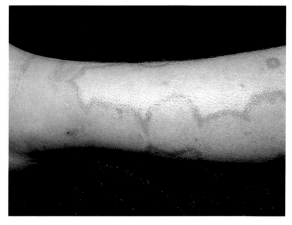

Figure 11.2 Urticaria – annular plaques which have become confluent. These lesions were gone the next day

palate and tongue with gastrointestinal (GI) symptoms (e.g. diarrhea)
- Papular urticaria occurs on the lower extremities of children as a result of insect bites
- Dermatographism – sharply demarcated wheal and erythematous flare occurring within seconds of stroking the skin
- Giant urticaria – large lesions of 6–10 cm in diameter
- Anaphylaxis – life-threatening medical emergency characterized by the sudden onset of urticaria, angioedema, dyspnea and hypotension
- Angioedema – deep edema of the subcutaneous tissue manifesting as diffuse swelling; often affects the hands, feet, eyelids and lips
  1. Mild angioedema accompanies ordinary urticaria in 10% of infants and children

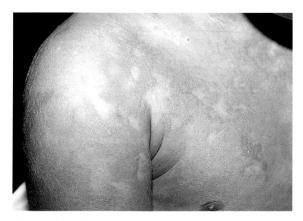

Figure 11.1 Urticaria – generalized pruritic wheals

2. Occurs more severely in:
   a. Anaphylaxis
   b. Serum sickness
   c. Hereditary angioedema – autosomal dominant deficiency in C1 esterase inhibitor

Pathogenesis

- Results from dilatation of capillaries, arterioles and venules with increased permeability
- Mediators: histamine released from circulating mast cells and basophils, anaphylotoxins, kinins, arachadonic acid metabolites, acetylcholine (cholinergic urticaria)
- Mechanism/etiologic factors:
  1. Immunologic factors: type I IgE-mediated hypersensitivity reaction; type II hypersensitivity reaction; type III hypersensitivity reaction (serum sickness); activation of alternate complement pathway
  2. Nonimmunologic factors: cholinergic effects, direct effect of physical agents, drugs
  3. Modulating factors: alcohol, heat, fever, exercise and emotional stress, endocrine factors
  4. Genetic factors: may play a role in chronic urticaria
  5. Infections: association with streptococcal pharyngitis, otitis media, sinusitis, upper respiratory infection, mononucleosis, hepatitis, coxsackie infections, mycoplasma infections, parasitic infections, fungal infections
  6. Drugs:
     a. Allergic reaction: penicillins, others
     b. Histamine liberators (even in normal individuals): codeine, morphine, cocaine, meperidine, quinine, thiamine, pilocarpine, polymyxin, dextran, D-tubocurarine
  7. Foods/additives: cow's milk allergy (infants), eggs, nuts, shellfish and other sea foods, chocolate, strawberries, grains
  8. Insect bites and stings: fleas, bed bugs, mites, bees, fire ants
  9. Acute contact urticaria: nettles, cat scratch, animal saliva, sea lice, moth or butterfly scales
  10. Physical agents or pressure
  11. Localized heat or cold
  12. Sun exposure (solar urticaria)
  13. Exposure to water (aquagenic urticaria)

Diagnosis

- Complete history and physical examination looking for infection, drug history, travel, environmental history, pet exposure, food history
- Test for dermatographism
- Other tests as indicated: ice cube test (cold urticaria), exercise test or methacholine test (cholinergic urticaria), pressure test (pressure urticaria), tepid towel test (aquagenic urticaria)
- Laboratory studies as indicated: streptococcal throat culture, complete blood count (CBC), streptozyme, erythrocyte sedimentation rate (ESR), urinalysis, complement levels, transaminases (AST and ALT), mycoplasma titers, sinus films, chest X-ray, urine culture, stool for ova and parasites, C1 esterase inhibitor level (if angioedema is present)

Differential diagnosis

- Erythema multiforme
- Systemic lupus erythematosus
- Dermatomyositis
- Porphyria
- Dermatitis herpetiformis
- Bullous pemphigoid
- Vasculitis
- Guttate psoriasis
- Pityriasis rosea

Treatment

- H1-type oral antihistamines
  1. Over-the-counter oral medications such as chlorpheniramine and diphenhydramine (Benadryl) are often adequate
  2. Prescription medications: hydroxyzine (Atarax®) or azatadine
  3. Continue treatment for at least 1 week after resolution of hives
- Identification and removal of etiologic agent if possible (e.g. food, drug) or treat infection
- Reassurance
- For anaphylaxis: epinephrine and airway/cardiovascular support; wear Medical Alert bracelet

Prognosis

- Acute urticaria – excellent prognosis in the absence of serious disease

- 20–30% of cases of acute urticaria will evolve into chronic or recurrent disease
- Chronic urticaria – prognosis for early resolution better than in adults
  1. Urticaria only: average duration 6 months
  2. Angioedema only: average duration 1 year
  3. Urticaria with angioedema: average duration 5 years
  4. Cholinergic urticaria: average duration 7 years
  5. Dermatographism: average duration 2 years

References

Beattie PE, Dawe RS, Ibbotson SH, Ferguson J. Characteristics and prognosis of idiopathic solar urticaria. Arch Dermatol 2003;139:1149-54

Greaves MW. Chronic idiopathic urticaria. Cur Opin Allergy Clin Immunol 2003; 3: 363–8

Kozel MMA, Bossuyt PMM, Mekkes JR, Bos JD. Laboratory tests and identified diagnoses in patients with physical and chronic urticaria and angioedema: a systematic review. J Am Acad Dermatol 2003; 48: 409–16

Mortureux P, Leaute-Labreze C, Legrain-Lifermann V, et al. Acute urticaria in infancy and early childhood. Arch Dermatol 1998; 134: 319–23

Muller BA. Urticaria and angioedema: a practical approach. Am Fam Physician 2004; 69: 1123–8

Poon M, Reid C. Do steroids help children with acute urticaria? Arch Dis Child 2004; 89: 85–6

Sackesen C, Sekerel BE, Orhan F, et al. The etiology of different forms of urticaria in childhood. Pediatr Dermatol 2004; 21: 102–108

Zembowicz A, Mastalerz L, Setkowicz M, et al. Safety of cyclooxygenase 2 inhibitors and increased leukotriene synthesis in chronic idiopathic urticaria with sensitivity to nonsteroidal anti-inflammatory drugs. Arch Dermatol 2003; 139: 1577–82

Erythema multiforme

Synonym: erythema multiforme minor

Major points

- Acute, self-limited cutaneous disease
- Herpes simplex virus (HSV 1 or 2) is the major precipitating factor
- Most common in young adults, rare in younger children
- Clinical features:

1. Rare prodrome, mild if present, with low-grade fever, cough, decreased appetite
2. Fixed red papules which develop into target/iris lesions
3. Target or iris lesions – regular circular macule or plaque that enlarges centrifugally, forming three zones of color change, and may coalesce with other lesions; central zone appears as dusky erythematous macule with bulla and/or crust (indicating epidermal damage) surrounded by lighter area and a purplish red external ring (Figure 11.3)
4. Vesicles and bullae
5. Symmetrically distributed in acral distribution on extensor surfaces of extremities and face
6. Mucous membrane involvement can be mild or absent, or may have painful oral erosions
7. Predilection for sun-exposed skin
8. May exhibit Koebner phenomenon
9. Frequently recurrent
10. May or may not have a history of preceding HSV 1 or HSV 2 infection (~50%)
11. Itching and/or burning sensation may occur

Pathogenesis

- Presumed to be a delayed hypersensitivity reaction with cytotoxic attack on keratinocytes bearing foreign (e.g. viral) antigens
- HSV has been the most prevalent precipitating factor identified in erythema multiforme minor; can be detected by polymerase chain reaction (PCR) of skin

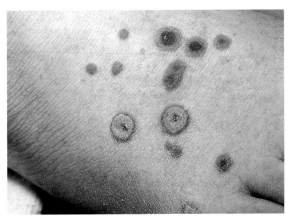

Figure 11.3 Erythema multiforme – target lesions with bullous component

- Other etiologic factors: drugs, *Histoplasma* infection and orf
- Histology: interface dermatitis with exocytosis, apoptotic keratinocytes and a perivascular mononuclear cell infiltrate

Diagnosis

- Characteristic clinical findings
- Skin biopsy if diagnosis is in doubt
- No laboratory studies usually necessary

Differential diagnosis

- Giant urticaria
- Drug reaction
- Polymorphous light eruption
- Bullous pemphigoid
- Vasculitis
- Systemic lupus erythematosus

Treatment

- Symptomatic treatment:
  1. Oral antihistamines for itching/burning
  2. Oral antacids for oral ulcers, for soothing effect
- Topical antibiotics to prevent secondary infection
- Preventative treatment: prophylactic oral acyclovir can prevent recurrences, use for 6–12 months
- Intermittent acyclovir ineffective unless used early during outbreak
- Systemic steroids if given early for recurrences

Prognosis

- Lesions fade over 1–3 weeks without specific treatment
- Usually lesions heal without sequelae, but may have mild scarring or hypopigmentation
- HSV-associated erythema multiforme commonly recurs
- Patients on immunosuppressive drugs tend to have more frequent and longer recurrences

References

Ayangco L, Rogers RS. Oral manifestations of erythema multiforme. Dermatol Clin 2003; 21: 195–205

Weston WL. Erythema multiforme and Stevens–Johnson syndrome. In Dermatology. Bolognia JL, Jorizzo JL, Rapini RP, et al., eds. Mosby: London, 2003: 313–21

Weston WL, Brice SL, Jester JD, et al. Herpes simplex virus in childhood erythema multiforme. Pediatrics 1992; 89: 32–4

Weston WL, Morelli JG. Herpes simplex virus-associated erythema multiforme in prepubertal children. Arch Pediatr Adolesc Med 1997; 151: 1014–16

Stevens–Johnson syndrome/toxic epidermal necrolysis

Major points

- Stevens–Johnson syndrome (SJS) and toxic epidermal necrolysis (TEN) are on a spectrum and have considerable overlap (see Chapter 13)
- Severe cutaneous reaction in which the individual appears acutely ill
- Rare in infants and children compared to teens and adults
- Combined incidence of SJS and TEN is approximately 1.5–2 cases per million per year in the general population
- Stevens–Johnson syndrome (erythema multiforme major):
  1. Drugs are the major precipitating factor
  2. *Mycoplasma pneumoniae* infection associated in children and teens
  3. Clinical features:
     a. 1–14 day prodrome of high fever, sore throat, malaise
     b. Rapid onset of cutaneous blistering with epidermal detachment beginning with target lesions (Figures 11.4–11.6)

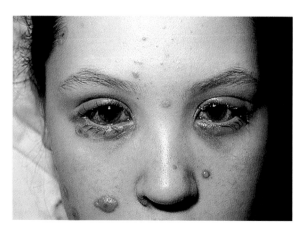

Figure 11.4   Stevens–Johnson syndrome – marked eye involvement

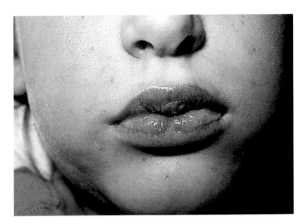

Figure 11.5 Stevens–Johnson syndrome – early erythema and tenderness of the lips

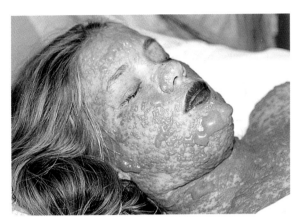

Figure 11.7 Toxic epidermal necrolysis – diffuse blistering over 90% of the skin surface

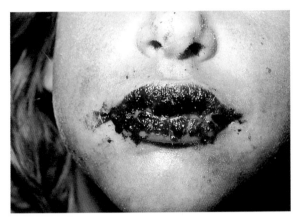

Figure 11.6 Stevens–Johnson syndrome – same patient as Figure 11.5 5 days later showing intense erythema and bleeding on the lips

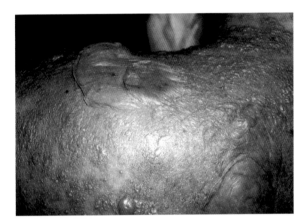

Figure 11.8 Toxic epidermal necrolysis – positive Nikolsky sign

  c. Involvement of two or more mucosal sites
  d. Fever, lymphadenopathy, toxic symptoms
  e. Total body surface area of epidermal detachment ≤10% classified as SJS; 10–30% classified as SJS–TEN overlap; >30% as TEN
- Toxic epidermal necrolysis:
 1. Drugs are the cause in >95% of cases
 2. Clinical features:
  a. 1–3 day prodrome of fever, stinging eyes, cutaneous tenderness
  b. Rapid onset of blistering with epidermal detachment (Figures 11.7 and 11.8)
  c. Positive Nikolsky sign
  d. Total body surface area of epidermal detachment >30%

Pathogenesis

- Same factors precipitate SJS and TEN:
 1. Drugs:
  a. Antibiotics: penicillin, doxycycline, tetracycline
  b. Anticonvulsants: carbamazapine, phenytoin, phenobarbital, lamotrigine, valproic acid
  c. Sulfonamides
  d. Nonsteroidal anti-inflammatory drugs (NSAIDs): ibuprofen, naproxen
 2. Specific cause identified in only 50% of cases
- Immune-mediated: drug activates CD95 (fas) ligand which binds to an apoptotic receptor located on the keratinocyte cell surface
- Histology:

1. Extensive epidermal damage with keratinocyte necrosis, basal cell layer vacuolation and blister formation at the dermal–epidermal junction
2. Dermal edema
3. Perivascular infiltrates

Diagnosis

- Characteristic clinical findings and course
- Skin biopsy

Differential diagnosis

- Staphylococcal scalded skin syndrome
- Kawasaki disease
- Toxic shock syndrome
- Serum sickness-like drug eruption

Treatment

- Severe cases best treated in an intensive care unit, preferably a burn unit
- Supportive measures:
  1. Removal of offending drug and any cross-reacting drug
  2. Fluid and electrolyte balance
  3. Nutritional support
  4. Prevention of complications (e.g. cultures and antibiotics for infection only when indicated)
  5. Physical therapy to prevent contractures
- Management of skin wounds:
  1. Topical antibiotic therapy e.g. 1% silver sulfadiazine (Silvadene®) twice daily (unless sensitive to sulfa)
  2. Debridement is indicated for extensive disease but may not be necessary for localized disease
  3. Hydrotherapy in a tank, bathtub, or shower to aid debridement
  4. Pre-medication with pain medicines
  5. Consider biological dressings
- Systemic treatments:
  1. Intravenous immunoglobulin (IVIG) 0.5–2 g/kg administered over 3 days
  2. Corticosteroids are controversial
     a. If used, should be early and high dose short duration (<5 days)
     b. Some evidence suggests IV pulsed methylprednisolone is preferable
     c. May cause increased septic complications

Prognosis

- High morbidity and mortality rates

- Mortality ~30% in SJS and 25–70% in TEN
- Poor prognostic factors in TEN: neutropenia, large percentage of body surface skin loss
- Disease has a protracted course lasting from 15 days to months
- Recovery is long and may require home physical therapy, tutoring and psychological support
- Sequelae: scarring, contractures, ocular sequelae (eyelid immobility, corneal scarring, blindness), esophageal and anal strictures, vaginal stenosis, urethral meatal stenosis, hair and nail loss
- Recurrences rare; most caused by re-exposure to same offending medication

References

Bachot N, Roujeau JC. Differential diagnosis of severe cutaneous drug eruptions. Am J Clin Dermatol 2003; 4: 561–72

Bachot N, Roujeau JC. Intravenous immunoglobulins in the treatment of severe drug eruptions. Curr Opin Allergy Clin Immunol 2003; 3: 269–74

Bannasch H, Kontny U, Kruger M, et al. A semisynthetic bilaminar skin substitute used to treat pediatric full-body toxic epidermal necrolysis. Arch Dermatol 2004; 140: 160–2

Hebert AA, Bogle MA. Intravenous immunoglobulin prophylaxis for recurrent Stevens–Johnson syndrome. J Am Acad Dermatol 2004; 50: 286–8

Martinez AE, Atherton DJ. High-dose systemic corticosteroids can arrest recurrences of severe mucocutaneous erythema multiforme. Pediatr Dermatol 2000; 17: 87–90

Metry DW, Jung P, Levy ML. Use of intravenous immunoglobulin in children with Stevens–Johnson syndrome and toxic epidermal necrolysis: seven cases and review of the literature. Pediatrics 2003; 112: 1430–6

Prendiville J. Stevens–Johnson syndrome and toxic epidermal necrolysis. Adv Dermatol 2002; 18: 151–73

Ringheanu M, Laude TA. Toxic epidermal necrolysis in children–an update. Clin Pediatr 2000; 39: 687–94

Erythema nodosum

Major points

- Uncommon skin disorder
- Prevalence of 2.4 per 10 000 in adults; rarer in children
- Sex ratio in children before puberty is roughly equal (in contrast to the female predominance in adults)

- Often associated with infection:
  1. Beta-hemolytic streptococcus (especially pharyngitis)
  2. Other causes: *Yersinia, Mycoplasma pneumoniae,* tuberculosis
- Less commonly associated chronic diseases: inflammatory bowel disease, Hodgkin disease, sarcoidosis
- Clinical presentation:
  1. Tender, erythematous or bruise-like nodules or plaques with irregular and indistinct borders (Figure 11.9)
  2. No ulceration or suppuration
  3. Usually located bilaterally on the anterior and lateral legs
  4. Other body sites: upper limbs, trunk, face, plantar surfaces in children
  5. Upper respiratory symptoms/fever/arthralgias related to etiologic agent (i.e. infection)
  6. Clinical course is <6 weeks
  7. Resolves without scarring

Pathogenesis

- Autoimmune or hypersensitivity disease
- Etiologic factors: infections, chronic diseases, idiopathic
- Histology: septal panniculitis

Diagnosis

- Characteristic clinical findings usually sufficient for diagnosis
- Skin biopsy in atypical, protracted cases

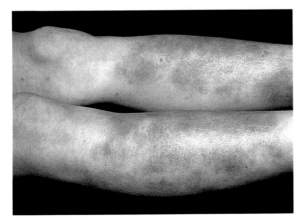

Figure 11.9 Erythema nodosum – tender plaques on the anterior shins caused by streptococcal disease

- Laboratory studies: CBC, ESR, liver enzymes, throat swab, stool culture, CXR, anti-streptolysin titer, *Yersinia* serologic test

Differential diagnosis

- Nodular vasculitis (Bazin disease) from tuberculosis
- Henoch–Schönlein purpura
- Eosinophilic cellulitis
- Infectious cellulitis
- Other panniculitides
- Child abuse
- Trauma

Treatment

- Bed rest and restriction of physical activities for ~2 weeks
- Analgesic medications or nonsteroidal anti-inflammatory drugs (NSAIDs)
- Treatment of underlying condition

Prognosis

- Course is benign and self-limited
- Lesions last ~10–14 days and resolve without scarring
- Recurrences are rare

References

Boh EE, al-Smadi RM. Cutaneous manifestations of gastrointestinal diseases. Dermatol Clin 2002; 20: 533–46

Crawford GH, Kim S, James WD. Skin signs of systemic disease: an update. Adv Dermatol 2002; 18: 1–27

Hern AE, Shwayder TA. Unilateral plantar erythema nodosum. J Am Acad Dermatol 1992; 26: 259–60

Kakourou T, Drosatou P, Psychou F, et al. Erythema nodosum in children: a prospective study. J Am Acad Dermatol 2001; 44: 17–21

Labbe L, Perel Y, Maleville J, Taieb A. Erythema nodosum in children: a study of 27 patients. Pediatr Dermatol 1996; 13: 447–50

Ter Poorten MC, Thiers BH. Panniculitis. Dermatol Clin 2002; 20: 421–33, vi

Annular erythemas

Major points

- Heterogeneous group of disorders characterized by annular erythematous eruption

- Transient:
  1. Erythema gyratum atrophicans transiens neonatale
     a. Presents in newborns
     b. Patchy, generalized erythema that resolves into atrophic hypopigmented patches
  2. Annular erythema of infancy
     a. Onset in infancy, usually ages 3–11 months
     b. Erythematous plaques that enlarge centrifugally to form rings and arcs; lesions appear and vanish over 36–48 hours (Figure 11.10)

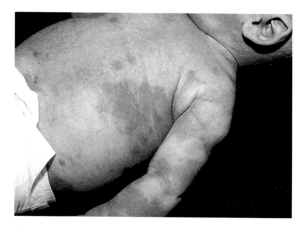

Figure 11.10   Annular erythema of infancy – this rash resolved in 2 weeks without treatment

  3. Annular erythema in infants born to mothers with autoimmune disease (e.g. neonatal lupus erythematosus)
- Chronic:
  1. Erythema annulare centrifugum (EAC)
     a. Rare in children but has been reported in neonates
     b. Dusky red, erythematous papules and plaques that expand in a centrifugal pattern, usually on trunk and proximal extremities, fine scale at advancing edge
     c. May accompany an underlying infection or neoplasm
  2. Familial annular erythema
     a. Presents shortly after birth
     b. Erythematous papules that enlarge centrifugally to form rings; may have vesiculated borders or inner collarette of scale
     c. Family history of disorder

  3. Erythema chronicum migrans (ECM)
     a. Manifestation of Lyme disease caused by infection with *Borrelia burgdorferi* (see Chapter 8)
     b. Enlarging erythematous ring develops at the site of a tick bite, up to a diameter of 20–30 cm
- Nonspecific annular erythemas

Pathogenesis

- Inflammatory hypersensitivity disorder of unknown etiology

Diagnosis

- Characteristic clinical findings
- Skin biopsy
- Histology consistent with diagnosis: superficial and deep lymphohistiocytic infiltrate in a perivascular distribution with presence of eosinophils and sometimes neutrophils

Differential diagnosis

- Erythema multiforme
- Annular urticaria
- Tinea corporis
- Seborrheic dermatitis

Treatment

- Tends to resolve without treatment in the absence of underlying disease
- Antihistamines, antibiotics, corticosteroids (systemic and local), antifungals (oral and topical) have been reported to have no effect on disease course
- ECM and accompanying Lyme disease should be treated with antibiotics (see Chapter 8); skin lesion resolves with treatment

Prognosis

- Complete resolution without treatment has been reported to occur after a course of partial remissions and exacerbations over a period of months to years
- Course can be chronic

References

Anzai H, Kikuchi A, Kinoshita A, Nishikawa T. Recurrent annular erythema in juvenile chronic myelogenous leukaemia. Br J Dermatol 1998; 138: 1058–60

Bottoni U, Innocenzi D, Bonaccorsi P, et al. Erythema annulare centrifugum: report of a case with neonatal onset. J Eur Acad Dermatol Venereol 2002; 16: 500–3

Cox NH, McQueen A, Evans TJ, Morley WN. An annular erythema of infancy. Arch Dermatol 1987; 123: 510–13

Stachowitz S, Abeck D, Schmidt T, Ring J. Persistent annular erythema of infancy associated with intestinal Candida colonization. Clin Exp Dermatol 2000; 25: 404–5

Toonstra J, de Wit FE. 'Persistent' annular erythema of infancy. Arch Dermatol 1984; 120: 1069–72

Watanabe T, Tsuchida T, Ito Y, et al. Annular erythema associated with lupus erythematosus/Sjogren's syndrome. J Am Acad Dermatol 1997; 36: 214–18

Weyers W, Diaz-Cascajo C, Weyers I. Erythema annulare centrifugum: results of a clinicopathologic study of 73 patients. Am J Dermatopathol 2003; 25: 451–62

Granuloma annulare

Major points

- Benign, self-limited dermatosis
- Subcutaneous indurated dermal papules/plaques in an annular configuration
- Several different types:
  1. Localized form – most common, usually seen on the dorsa of the hands and feet and lower extremities, but may be seen anywhere (Figure 11.11)
  2. Subcutaneous form – deep dermal or subcutaneous nodules with no overlying epidermal change, commonly on the pretibial area of children aged 2–5 years (Figure 11.12)
  3. Perforating form (generalized perforating granuloma annulare) – rare, grouped papules, some of which have a central area where damaged collagen ulcerates through the epidermis
  4. Generalized form – hundreds of small papules forming ringed lesions that coalesce into reticulate patterns or linear bands
- Association with insulin-dependent diabetes mellitus in adults, not children

Pathogenesis

- Etiology unknown
- Proposed to be an immune-mediated response to an unknown antigenic stimulus with degeneration of collagen in the dermis, reactive inflammation and fibrosis
- Histology: palisading granuloma with necrobiotic collagen, fibrin and mucin deposits; in perforating

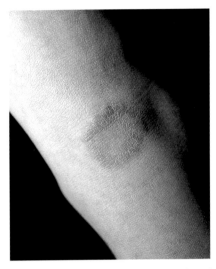

Figure 11.11 Granuloma annulare – typical ring of papules

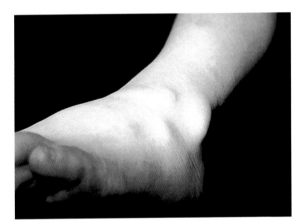

Figure 11.12 Granuloma annulare – deep subcutaneous nodules

granuloma annulare the granulomas perforate the epidermis, extruding necrobiotic material

Diagnosis

- Characteristic clinical findings
- Skin biopsy if atypical
- No specific laboratory abnormalities associated

Differential diagnosis

- Tinea corporis
- Sarcoidosis
- Rheumatoid nodules
- Necrobiosis lipoidica

Treatment

- Reassurance of benign condition
- Mid-range topical corticosteroid with or without occlusion
- Intralesional steroids for persistent lesions

Prognosis

- Lesions persist for several years then resolve spontaneously
- Mainly a cosmetic problem

References

Choi JC, Bae JY, Cho S, et al. Generalized perforating granuloma annulare in an infant. Pediatr Dermatol 2003; 20: 131–3

Grogg KL, Nascimento AG. Subcutaneous granuloma annulare in childhood: clinicopathologic features in 34 cases. Pediatrics 2001; 107: 42

Kuwahara, RT, Naylor MF, Skinner RB. Treatment of granuloma annulare with topical 5% imiquimod cream. Pediatr Dermatol 2003; 20: 90

Rheumatoid nodules

Major points

- Subcutaneous nodules similar to the ones seen in rheumatoid arthritis in adults with no other clinical signs or laboratory evidence of systemic disease
- Seen in otherwise healthy children most commonly at 2–10 years of age
- Clinical presentation:
  1. Subcutaneous nodules
  2. Often multiple
  3. Distribution usually on the limbs, over the occiput, prepatellar and malleolar regions, pretibial areas, heels, fingers, elbows and proximal ulnar regions
  4. Occasional reports of associated arthralgias
- Not thought to be a precursor for juvenile rheumatoid arthritis (JRA); however, there have been rare reported cases of development of JRA
- May be the same entity as subcutaneous granuloma annulare (pseudorheumatoid nodules)

Pathogenesis

- Etiology unknown
- Thought to be an immunologic mechanism; IgG and IgM have been found in nodules

- Reported following trauma or acute tonsillitis
- Histology:
  1. Similar to that of subcutaneous granuloma annulare
  2. Central necrotic zone surrounded by palisading histiocytes and mononuclear inflammatory cells

Diagnosis

- Clinical presentation
- Absence of clinical or laboratory evidence of JRA

Differential diagnosis

- Granuloma annulare
- Rheumatoid nodules associated with JRA
- Calcinosis cutis
- Osteoma cutis

Treatment

- No specific treatment usually needed
- Intralesional steroids

Prognosis

- Nodules may regress and disappear over time
- Generally, does not progress to JRA

References

Cawkwell GD. Benign rheumatoid nodules. Arch Pediatr Adolesc Med 1994; 148: 1219–20

Nalbant S, Corominas H, Hsu B, et al. Ultrasonography for assessment of subcutaneous nodules. J Rheumatol 2003; 30: 1191–5

Yamamoto T, Matsunaga T, Nishioka K. Rheumatoid neutrophilic dermatitis, rheumatoid papules, and rheumatoid nodules in a patient with seronegative rheumatoid arthritis. J Am Acad Dermatol 2003; 48: 634–5

Yavuz H, Ozel A, Yilmaz O, et al. Benign rheumatoid nodules. Am J Dis Child 1993; 147: 1011–12

Necrobiosis lipoidica diabeticorum

Major points

- Skin lesions strongly associated with diabetes mellitus (DM) type I but has been reported with type II DM
- Prevalence of 0.06% in children with diabetes and may precede onset of DM
- Female/male ratio >1

- Average age of onset: 15 years
- Clinical presentation:
  1. Painless papules which enlarge to form a central, waxy, atrophic, depressed area with an elevated violaceous peripheral ring (Figure 11.13)
  2. Central color is reddish-brown to orange-yellow
  3. Telangiectasias may be seen within plaques
  4. Usually over the bilateral anterior tibias
  5. Often multiple plaques
  6. May rarely be seen on the upper extremities or trunk
  7. Tend to ulcerate

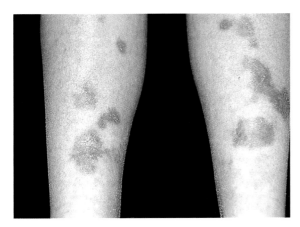

Figure 11.13   Necrobiosis lipoidica diabeticorum – erythematous, shiny plaques on shins with central atrophy

Pathogenesis

- Etiology unknown
- Microangiopathy or other vascular etiology, lipid disorder, and immunologic mechanisms have been proposed
- Histology: diffuse palisading and interstitial granulomatous inflammation

Diagnosis

- Characteristic clinical findings
- Skin biopsy
- Evaluation for diabetes

Differential diagnosis

- Granuloma annulare
- Sarcoidosis

- Panniculitis
- Morphea

Treatment

- Treat underlying diabetes to achieve good glycemic control
- Corticosteroids:
  1. Potent topical corticosteroids – for early lesions
  2. Intralesional corticosteroids – injected into the active border of established lesions
- Oral pentoxifylline (Trental®)

Prognosis

- Ulcerated lesions heal slowly and may ulcerate again
- May indicate a greater risk for diabetic retinopathy and nephropathy

References

de Silva DM, Schofield OM, Walker JD. The prevalence of necrobiosis lipoidica diabeticorum in children with type 1 diabetes. Br J Dermatol 1999; 141: 593–4

Pestoni C, Ferreirós MM, de la Torre C, Toribio J. Two girls with necrobiosis lipoidica and type I diabetes mellitus with transfollicular elimination in one girl. Pediatr Dermatol 2003; 20: 211–14

Retting KR. Necrobiosis lipoidica diabeticorum. Clin Pediatr 2000; 39: 439–40

Szabo RM, Harris GD, Burke WA. Necrobiosis lipoidica in a 9-year-old girl with new-onset type II diabetes mellitus. Pediatr Dermatol 2001; 18: 316–19

Kawasaki disease

Major points

- Characterized by high fever, lymphadenopathy and mucocutaneous lesions
- Most serious complications are coronary artery abnormalities:
  1. Aneurysms, diffuse ectasia, vasculitis
  2. Develop in 20–25% of cases of untreated Kawasaki disease
  3. Giant aneurysm carries the worst prognosis – risk of developing coronary thrombosis, stenosis or myocardial infarction
  4. Smaller aneurysms tend to resolve; giant aneurysms do not

- Most common cause of acquired heart disease among children in the USA
- Occurs predominantly in children <5 years age
- Hospitalization rate for US children aged <5 years is ~17 per 100 000 (approximates the disease incidence)
- Increased risk in younger children, males (ratio of 1.5 : 1), and individuals of Asian descent
- Increased rates in winter and spring months, with higher socioeconomic status, and in certain geographic regions of the USA (higher in the Northeast and West)
- Clinical course can be divided into three phases:
  1. Acute febrile phase (7–14 days):
     a. Fever
     b. Conjunctival injection
     c. Mouth and lip changes – dryness, redness, fissuring, crust, 'strawberry tongue'
     d. Swelling and erythema of hands and feet
     e. Rash – polymorphous exanthem on the body and/or extremities, especially in diaper area (Figures 11.14 and 11.15)
     f. Cervical lymphadenopathy
  2. Subacute phase (from the end of fever for ~25 days)
     a. Desquamation of fingers and toes (Figure 11.16)

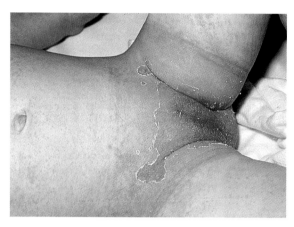

Figure 11.15   Kawasaki disease – perineal rash with peeling

     b. Arthritis and arthralgias
     c. Thrombocytosis
  3. Convalescent phase (6–8 weeks)
     a. Clinical symptoms resolve
     b. Continues until ESR becomes normal

Pathogenesis

- Etiology unknown
- Immunoregulatory abnormalities – response to a bacterial (or viral) protein toxin acting as a superantigen has been proposed
- Presumed etiology is infectious – viral (e.g. Epstein–Barr virus and retrovirus), *Streptococcus viridans*, staphylococci, *Propionibacterium* species and parvovirus

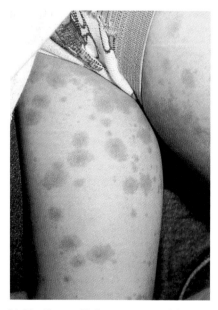

Figure 11.14   Kawasaki disease – targetoid, erythematous macules

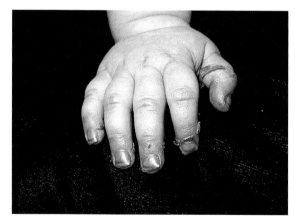

Figure 11.16   Kawasaki disease – desquamation of the fingertips

Diagnosis

- Based on history and physical examination
- Jones criteria:
    1. High fever for ≥5 days without other explanation
    2. Four of the following five criteria:
        a. Conjunctival injection
        b. Oropharyngeal changes: injected or fissured lips, hyperemia of pharynx, strawberry tongue
        c. Extremity changes: erythema of palms or soles, hand or foot edema, periungual desquamation
        d. Polymorphous rash (especially on trunk)
        e. Acute nonsuppurative cervical lymphadenopathy
- Cases of 'atypical' or 'incomplete' Kawasaki disease:
    1. Fewer than four of the five criteria
    2. Coronary complications
    3. More common in infants <6 months age
- Electrocardiogram and echocardiogram – to look for cardiovascular manifestations
- Common laboratory abnormalities: leukocytosis, thrombocytosis, elevated ESR and C-reactive protein, sterile pyuria

Differential diagnosis

- Viral exanthem
- Scarlet fever
- Staphylococcal scalded skin syndrome
- Stevens–Johnson syndrome
- Drug reactions
- Toxic shock syndrome

Treatment

- Combined intravenous immunoglobulin (IVIG) and aspirin therapy
    1. IVIG – 2 g/kg as a single dose before day 10 of fever can reduce risk of coronary artery disease from ~20% to <5%
    2. Aspirin – 30–100 mg/kg per day in four divided doses until defervescence, and then reduced to 3–5 mg/kg per day as a single daily dose
- Ongoing fever or other signs of inflammation 24–72 hours or longer after treatment may warrant additional doses of IVIG

- Treatment of cardiac complications – thrombolytics, surgical revascularization, cardiac transplantation
- Use of corticosteroids is controversial

Prognosis

- 85% of children treated in the first 10 days after onset will have prompt defervesence and resolution of signs of inflammation
- Prognosis is favorable for those children who do not develop coronary artery abnormalities
- In children with coronary artery aneurysms:
    1. 50% regress within 2 years
    2. For giant aneurysms (>8 mm), risk for stenosis, complete obstruction, or myocardial infarction
- Myocardial infarction is the major cause of mortality – most commonly occurs after years in patients with giant aneurysms

References

Genizi J, Miron D, Spiegel R, et al. Kawasaki disease in very young infants: high prevalence of atypical presentation and coronary arteritis. Clin Pediatr 2003; 42: 263–7

Holman RC, Curns AT, Belay ED, et al. Kawasaki syndrome hospitalizations in the United States, 1997 and 2000. Pediatrics 2003; 112: 495–501

Meissner HC, Leung DYM. Kawasaki syndrome: where are the answers? Pediatrics 2003; 112: 672–5

Proft T, Fraser JD. Bacterial superantigens. Clin Exp Immunol 2003; 133: 299–306

Taubert KA, Shulman ST. Kawasaki disease. Am Fam Physician 1999; 59: 3093–102, 3107–8

Pyoderma gangrenosum

Major points

- Clinical features:
    1. Begins as a small pustule, erythematous nodule, or bulla that spreads concentrically from the center to develop necrotic ulceration with a mucopurulent base, violaceous undermined border, and peripheral erythema (Figure 11.17)
    2. Clinical variants: ulcerative, pustular, bullous, or vegetative
    3. History given of preceding minor trauma or irritation is common

4. May progress to become atrophic paper-like skin or cribriform scars
5. Single or multiple lesions
6. Most frequent on anterior legs; may occur on face, trunk, or buttocks

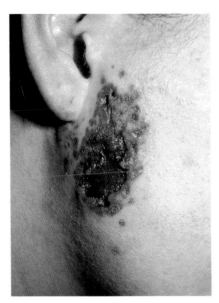

Figure 11.17   Pyoderma gangrenosum – deep scarring and painful erythema

7. Exquisitely painful
8. Pathergy may be reported
- Often occurs in association with systemic disorders:
  1. Inflammatory bowel disease
  2. Arthritis
  3. Hematologic disease: leukemia, monoclonal gammopathy, polycythemia vera, lymphoma
  4. Immunodeficiency disorders: hypogammaglobulinemia, IgA deficiency, impaired leukocyte deficiency, HIV
  5. Most common in children: inflammatory bowel disease and arthritis
- Idiopathic (no associated disease identified) in 20–30% of cases

Pathogenesis

- Cause is unknown
- Proposed to be an exaggerated inflammatory response caused by an underlying immunologic abnormality

1. Frequent association with systemic diseases with presumed autoimmune etiology or immunologic defects
2. Associated immune abnormalities have been reported, including: immunoglobulin levels, cell-mediated immunity and neutrophil function
- Pathergy has been reported in ~20% of cases
- Histology: necrosis and ulceration of the epidermis and dermis, acute inflammatory cell infiltrate and the margin of the lesion, chronic inflammatory cell infiltrate at the base

Diagnosis

- Skin biopsy – to exclude deep fungal infection and vasculitis
- Look for underlying conditions
- Common laboratory abnormalities: elevated ESR, mild anemia, various immune defects (e.g. abnormal immunoglobulins)

Differential diagnosis

- Deep fungal infection
- Vasculitis
- Sweet syndrome
- Spider bite

Treatment

- Treat underlying disorder
- Systemic treatment
  1. Oral or pulsed IV corticosteroids
  2. Dapsone (oral)
- Adjuvant topical antibiotic therapy
- Topical or intralesional corticosteroids at edge of active lesion
- Dressings – oxygen-permeable or semi-permeable
- Other options if above treatments fail: cyclophosphamide, azathioprine, methotrexate, mercaptopurine, melphalan, minocycline, tetracycline, clofazimine, cyclosporine A, thalidomide
- Surgical debridement can extend the lesion; not recommended

Prognosis

- Atrophy or scarring common
- Successful treatment of underlying disorder may result in clearing
- Chronic relapsing disease may occur and may be difficult to manage

References

Crowson AN, Mihm MC Jr, Magro C. Pyoderma gangrenosum: a review. J Cutan Pathol 2003; 30: 97–107

Dourmishev AL, Miteva I, Schwartz RA. Pyoderma gangrenosum in childhood. Cutis 1996; 58: 257–62

Gettler S, Rothe M, Grin C, Grant-Kels J. Optimal treatment of pyoderma gangrenosum. Am J Clin Dermatol 2003; 4: 597–608

Mekkes JR, Loots MA, Van Der Wal AC, Bos JD. Causes, investigation and treatment of leg ulceration. Br J Dermatol 2003; 148: 388–401

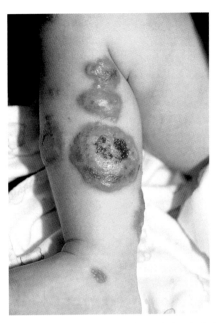

Figure 11.18   Sweet syndrome – large, indurated plaques

Sweet syndrome

Synonym: acute febrile neutrophilic dermatosis

Major points

- Cardinal features: fever, neutrophilic leukocytosis in the peripheral blood; tender, red plaques on limbs, face and neck; dense dermal infiltrate of neutrophils on histology
- Can occur at all ages
  1. Peak onset in middle age
  2. Pediatric cases account for 5% of all total reported cases
  3. Can occur in infants as young as 7 weeks
- Cutaneous manifestations:
  1. Abrupt onset of lesions that enlarge and coalesce over days to weeks
  2. Bright red to purple, painful, tender, sharply demarcated plaques (Figure 11.18)
  3. May have scaling, crusting, hemorrhagic bullae, or ulceration
  4. May be warm to touch
  5. Lesions range in size from 4 mm to >12 cm
  6. Lesions are usually multiple
  7. Solitary lesions usually have a predilection for the face
  8. Distribution is asymmetric; over the upper extremities, neck, face more than trunk, lower extremities
  9. Pathergy has been reported
- Extracutaneous manifestations:
  1. Fever
  2. Neutrophilic leukocytosis
  3. Serum sickness-like symptoms: myalgias, malaise, nausea, headache
  4. Meningeal symptoms
  5. Gastrointestinal distress
  6. Musculoskeletal symptoms: arthralgias, arthritis
  7. Renal involvement (11–72%): proteinuria, hematuria, acute renal failure, glomerulonephritis
  8. Ocular findings: iritis, episcleritis, conjunctivitis
  9. Lung involvement
  10. Hepatic involvement
- Associated with many conditions (Table 11.1):
  1. Antecedent infection (especially upper respiratory infection)
  2. Autoimmune/inflammatory diseases
  3. Malignancy (in 20% of cases) – primarily hematologic malignancies
  4. Drugs and vaccinations (especially granulocyte colony-stimulating factor; G-CSF)

Pathogenesis

- Likely to be a reactive process resulting from immunologic hypersensitivity to a variety of agents (e.g. infection, neoplasm, drug, autoimmune processes)
- Interleukin-1 has been implicated as a mediator for both cutaneous and systemic inflammation
- Association with G-CSF treatment supports neutrophil activation as a mechanism

Table 11.1   Conditions associated with Sweet syndrome

Inflammatory/autoimmune
Ulcerative colitis
Crohn disease
Bowel bypass syndrome
Systemic lupus erythematosus
Rheumatoid arthritis
Sjögren syndrome
Behçet syndrome
Pyoderma gangrenosum
Subacute thyroiditis
Cirrhosis

Infections
Staphylococcus
Streptococcus
Yersinia
Salmonella
Tuberculosis
Histoplasmosis
Meningitis
Hepatitis
HIV

Malignancy
Acute myelogenous leukemia
Chronic myelogenous leukemia
Acute lymphocytic leukemia
Chronic lymphocytic leukemia
Lymphoma
Myelodysplastic syndromes
Breast cancer
Prostate cancer
Ovarian cancer
Endometrial cancer
Vaginal cancer
Testicular cancer
Rectal cancer

Other
Drugs (most commonly granulocyte colony-
    stimulating factor)
Immunizations
Pregnancy
Photoinduction
Renal stones

Adapted from Fitzgerald RL, McBurney IE, Nesbitt LT. Sweet's syndrome. Int J Dermatol 1996; 35: 9–15

- Histology:
    1. Dense, dermal infiltrate of mature neutrophils
    2. Epidermis is usually normal, but may have reactive changes
    3. Classic definition of Sweet syndrome requires the absence of vasculitis; however, vasculitis (vessel damage) may be seen especially in lesions present for a long duration – thought to be a result of toxic metabolites released by activated neutrophils

Diagnosis

- Diagnostic criteria (two major and one minor criteria needed for diagnosis):
    1. Major criteria:
        a. Abrupt onset of tender or painful erythematous plaques or nodules
        b. Predominantly neutrophilic infiltration in the dermis
    2. Minor criteria:
        a. Preceded by respiratory infection, GI infection, vaccination or associated with: inflammatory disease, hematoproliferative disorder, solid malignant tumor, or pregnancy
        b. Malaise and fever (>38°C)
        c. Laboratory values at onset: ESR >20 mm, C-reactive protein, segmented neutrophils >70% in peripheral blood smear, leukocytosis (three out of four values necessary)
        d. Excellent response to systemic corticosteroid or potassium iodide treatment
- Rule out infectious causes, including HIV
- Underlying condition (e.g. malignancy) should be investigated
- Laboratory findings are nonspecific: ESR, C-reactive protein, CBC, renal function tests
- Skin biopsy usually necessary

Differential diagnosis

- Drug reaction
- Cellulitis
- Herpes simplex infection
- Pyoderma gangrenosum
- Secondary syphilis
- Erythema multiforme
- Vasculitis
- Leukemia cutis

Treatment

- Systemic glucocorticoids:
  1. Oral steroids 0.5–1.5 mg/kg per day for 10 days followed by a slow taper
  2. Lesions usually clear in several days with treatment
- Other drugs: potassium iodide, dapsone, cyclosporine, colchicine, clofazimine, indomethacin, methotrexate, isotretinoin, pulse steroids with chlorambucil

Prognosis

- Most cases respond well to oral steroids with rapid clearing of lesions
- Healing may result in hyperpigmentation, milia, or scarring
- Untreated lesions usually resolve in 6–8 weeks, but may take months
- Recurrences are common
- Prognosis depends upon severity of underlying systemic condition

References

Callen JP. Neutrophilic dermatoses. Dermatol Clin 2002; 20: 409–19

Crawford GH, Kim S, James WD. Skin signs of systemic disease: an update. Adv Dermatol 2002; 18: 1–27

Fitzgerald RL, McBurney IE, Nesbitt LT. Sweet's syndrome. Int J Dermatol 1996; 35: 9–15

Kourtis AP. Sweet syndrome in infants. Clin Pediatr 2002; 41: 175–7

Malone JC, Slone SP, Wills-Frank LA, et al. Vascular inflammation (vasculitis) in Sweet syndrome. Arch Dermatol 2002; 138: 345–9

Von den Driesch P. Sweet's syndrome (acute neutrophilic dermatosis). J Am Acad Dermatol 1994; 3: 535–56

Sarcoidosis

Major points

- Systemic granulomatous disorder characterized by the presence of noncaseating granulomas
- Rare in pediatric age group; more common in adolescents and young adults
- Male/female ratio = 1
- Two distinct forms of juvenile sarcoidosis:
  1. Early-onset:
     a. Presents in ages 1–5 years
     b. Triad of arthritis/rash/uveitis with typical pulmonary disease often absent
     c. Predominantly Whites
     d. Often confused with JRA
     e. Less favorable prognosis – progressive and debilitating course
  2. Older children:
     a. Presents in adolescence
     b. Similar to adult disease with lung/lymph node/eye involvement
     c. Predominantly Blacks
- Clinical manifestations are protean; multiple organ systems can be involved
- Most common clinical features:
  1. Lung involvement:
     a. Most common organ involved
     b. Accounts for majority of morbidity and mortality
     c. Dry cough and dyspnea
     d. Bilateral hilar lymphadenopathy with or without parenchymal involvement
     e. Abnormal chest X-ray and pulmonary function tests
  2. Cutaneous manifestations:
     a. Red to yellowish-brown papules, plaques, or nodules; erythema nodosum; hypo- or hyperpigmentation (Figure 11.19)
     b. Most frequent on the face, but may occur on trunk, extremities, buttocks
     c. Lupus pernio (sarcoidosis of the nose) – rare in children
  3. Eye involvement:
     a. Common, serious and progressive
     b. Granulomatous uveitis
     c. Conjunctival granulomatous nodules
     d. Complications: optic neuritis, band keratopathy, cataracts, glaucoma, retinal vasculitis
  4. Lymphadenopathy
  5. Other organ systems involved: CNS, kidneys, liver, spleen, heart and blood vessels, musculoskeletal system

Pathogenesis

- Etiology unknown
- Postulated to represent an altered immune response to unknown agent(s) resulting in granuloma formation

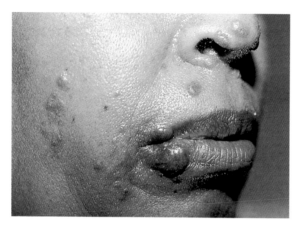

Figure 11.19   Sarcoidosis – typical firm papules on the face in an adult

- Genetic predisposition
- Histology: discrete, compact, noncaseating, epithelioid cell granulomas

Diagnosis

- Biopsy: demonstration of noncaseating granulomas in one or more organs
    a. Fungal and other infections should be ruled out using special stains
    b. Least invasive biopsy site should be chosen based on clinical presentation (e.g. skin, palpable lymph nodes)
- Characteristic clinical findings
- Radiographic imaging:
    1. Chest X-ray: bilateral hilar lymphadenopathy
    2. CT or MRI for involvement in the orbit, CNS, muscle/bone
- Ophthalmologic evaluation
- Laboratory studies are nonspecific: calcium levels and serum angiotensin converting enzyme may be elevated

Differential diagnosis

- Systemic juvenile rheumatoid arthritis
- Lymphoma
- Tuberculosis
- Other diffuse interstitial pulmonary diseases
- Infections with granulomatous reactions

Treatment

- Asymptomatic patients and mild disease; watchful waiting without treatment may be appropriate; may spontaneously resolve

- Patients with multisystem disease:
    1. Oral corticosteroid treatment for serious lung, ocular, neurological, cardiac disease
    2. Methotrexate if refractory to steroid treatment or as a steroid-sparing agent
    3. Other agents used: cyclosporine, azathioprine, cyclophosphamide

Prognosis

- Majority of older children recover with minimal or no therapy with improved pulmonary status (similar to adults)
- Poor prognosis associated with severe involvement at presentation, multiorgan involvement, early-onset form of disease

References

Cimaz R, Ansell BM. Sarcoidosis in the pediatric age. Clin Exp Reumatol 2002; 20: 231–7

Fetil E, Ozkan S, Ilknur T, et al. Sarcoidosis in a preschooler with only skin and joint involvement. Pediatr Dermatol 2003; 20: 416–18

Lindsley CB, Petty RE. Overview and report on international registry of sarcoid arthritis in childhood. Curr Rheumatol Rep 2000; 2: 343–8

Mana J, Marcoval J, Graells J, et al. Cutaneous involvement in sarcoidosis: relationship to systemic disease. Arch Dermatol 1997; 133: 882–8

Ramanan AV, Denning DW, Baildam EM. Cutaneous childhood sarcoidosis – a rare disease refractory to treatment. Rheumatology 2003; 42: 1570–1

Shetty AK, Gedalia A. Sarcoidosis: a pediatric perspective. Clin Pediatr 1998; 37: 707–17

Shetty AK, Gedalia A. Sarcoidosis in children. Curr Probl Pediatr 2000; 30: 153–76

NUTRITIONAL DISORDERS

Anorexia and bulimia nervosa-associated skin disorders

- Xerosis
- Acral changes: coldness, cyanosis, periungual erythema
- Hypertrichosis
- Telogen effluvium
- Brittle hair and nails

- Carotenemia
- Oral changes: cheilitis and perleche, aphthae, gum erosions, dental caries
- Russell sign: calluses on the dorsum of hands from repetitive forced vomiting

Kwashiorkor

- Protein intake deficiency with normal caloric intake
- Causes:
  1. All maize diet (e.g. in impoverished areas)
  2. Chronically ill children
  3. Restricted diet (e.g. food fads, food aversion)
- Cutaneous findings:
  1. Generalized hyperpigmentation
  2. Black patches of thickened epidermis over pressure point which desquamate ('peeling paint' appearance) (Figure 11.20)
  3. Dry, hypopigmented hair
  4. Desquamation around eyes, mouth
  5. Erosions in mouth, intertriginous areas with fissuring
- Extracutaneous findings: massive edema/anasarca, extreme irritability, apathy

Marasmus

- Total calorie starvation
- Cutaneous findings:
  1. Thin, dry, lax skin
  2. Hair is thin, falls out readily
  3. Occasionally seen: fine scaling, desquamation, hyperpigmentation
- Extracutaneous findings:
  1. Loss of subcutaneous fat and muscle
  2. Individual remains alert

Vitamin deficiencies

- Vitamin A (retinol) deficiency
  1. Cutaneous findings: scaliness, atrophy of sebaceous and sweat glands, follicular hyperkeratosis (phrynoderma), dull scalp hair
  2. Extracutaneous findings: poor night vision, conjunctival xerosis, Bitot spots in the eyes, impaired bone growth, cranial nerve lesions
  3. Causative drugs/factors: fat malabsorption, liver disease

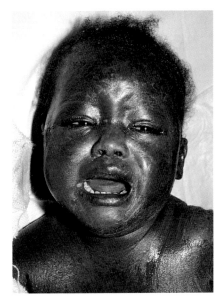

Figure 11.20   Kwashiorkor – protein malnutrition in a child who was thought to be allergic to milk, so milk was eliminated from her diet

- Vitamin B$_1$ (thiamine) deficiency – beriberi
  1. Wet (cardiac) beriberi: myocarditis with high-output congestive heart failure, edema
  2. Dry (neurologic) beriberi: peripheral neuropathy with wrist/foot drop, motor and digestive disturbances
  3. Wernicke–Korsakoff syndrome: encephalopathy with psychosis, ataxia, memory loss, confabulation, confusion
  4. Orogenital dermatitis
  5. Causative factors: rice-dependent diets, chronic alcoholism
- Vitamin B$_2$ (riboflavin) deficiency
  1. Cutaneous findings: oculo-orogenital syndrome, angular cheilitis, black tongue, glossitis, seborrheic dermatitis/dyssebacia, scrotal dermatitis
  2. Extracutaneous findings: anemia, mental retardation
  3. Causative drugs/factors: borate poison, neonatal phototherapy for hyperbilirubinemia, protein deficiency, hypothyroidism
- Vitamin B$_3$ (niacin) deficiency – pellagra
  1. Classic triad (3 Ds): diarrhea, dermatitis, dementia
  2. Cutaneous findings: dermatitis on sun-exposed skin, Casal necklace – photosensitive eruption

around the neck, angular stomatitis, glossitis, oral and perirectal sores

3. Causative drugs/factors: gastrointestinal (malabsorptive) disease, drugs, plain corn diet, alcoholism

- Vitamin B_6 (pyridoxine) deficiency
  1. Cutaneous findings: periorificial dermatitis, pellagra-like rash, seborrhea, conjunctivitis, stomatitis, glossitis
  2. Extracutaneous findings: anorexia, GI symptoms, anemia, lymphopenia, confusion
  3. Causative factors: drugs, uremia, cirrhosis

- Vitamin B_{12} (cobalamin) deficiency
  1. Cutaneous findings: hyperpigmentation of flexural areas, palms, soles, nails, oral cavity, glossitis, poliosis
  2. Extracutaneous findings: megaloblastic anemia, paresthesias, ataxia, hypotonia in infants, mental status changes
  3. Causative drugs/factors:
     a. In infants – born to strict vegan mother or mothers with pernicious anemia, malnutrition due to low socioeconomic status
     b. Others: decreased gastric synthesis of intrinsic factor (pernicious anemia), tropical sprue, strict vegetarianism, ileal destruction or bypass, chronic alcoholism

- Vitamin C (ascorbic acid) deficiency – scurvy
  1. Cutaneous findings: follicular hyperkeratosis, perifollicular petechiae, 'corkscrew' hairs, poor wound healing, koilonychias, gingival hemorrhage, sclerodermatous changes
  2. Extracutaneous findings: weakness, fatigue, depression

- Vitamin D deficiency – rickets
  1. No cutaneous alterations seen with deficiency
  2. Extracutaneous findings: rickets, muscle weakness
  3. Causative drugs/factors: excessive lack of sunlight, malabsorption, liver disease, vitamin D resistance, renal disease

- Biotin deficiency
  1. Cutaneous findings: acrodermatitis enteropathica, intertriginous and periorificial dermatitis, conjunctivitis, glossitis, cheilitis, xerosis, alopecia
  2. Extracutaneous findings: neuropsychiatric symptoms

3. Causative drugs/factors: raw egg-white ingestion (avidin impedes absorption of biotin), anticonvulsant drugs, total parenteral nutrition, chronic GI disease, short bowel

- Vitamin K deficiency
  1. Deficiency results in impairment of the coagulation cascade; vitamin K is required for synthesis of factors II, VII, IX, X and proteins C and S
  2. Cutaneous findings: purpura, ecchymoses, hemorrhage
  3. Extracutaneous findings: GI, nasal, subgaleal, intracranial hemorrhage
  4. Causative drugs/factors: neonates (inadequate intake and decreased production), warfarin, antibiotics, liver disease, fat malabsorption

- Folic acid deficiency
  1. Similar to vitamin B_{12} deficiency
  2. Cutaneous findings: hyperpigmentation of tongue and genitals, glossitis, angular cheilitis
  3. Extracutaneous findings: megaloblastic anemia
  4. Causative drugs/factors: phenytoin, barbiturates, methotrexate, celiac disease, goat's milk diet, pregnancy

References

Avci Z, Turul T, Aysun S, Unal I. Involuntary movements and magnetic resonance imaging findings in infantile cobalamine (Vit B 12) deficiency. Pediatrics 2003; 112: 684–6

Barthelemy H, Chouvet B, Cambazard F. Skin and mucosal manifestations in vitamin deficiency. J Am Acad Dermatol 1986; 15: 1263–74

Grob JJ, Collet-Villette AM, Aillaud MF, et al. Spontaneous adult scurvy in a developed country: new insight in an ancient disease. Arch Dermatol 1990; 126: 249–51

Glorio R, Allevato M, De Pablo A, et al. Prevalence of cutaneous manifestations in 200 patients with eating disorders. Int J Dermatol 2000; 39: 348–53

Hegyi J, Schwartz RA, Hegyi V. Pellagra: dermatitis dementia, and diarrhea. Int J Dermatol 2004; 43: 1–5

Lucky AW, Powell J. Cutaneous manifestations of endocrine, metabolic, and nutritional disorders. In Pediatric Dermatology, 3rd edn. Schachner LA, Hansen RC, eds. Mosby: New York, 2003: 937–8

Lutter CK, Rivera JA. Nutritional status of infants and young children and characteristics of their diets. J Nutr 2003; 133: 2941S–9S

Miller SJ. Nutritional deficiency and the skin. J Am Acad Dermatol 1989; 21: 1–30

Schulze UME, Pettke-Rank CV, Kreienkamp M, et al. Dermatologic findings in anorexia and bulimia nervosa of childhood and adolescence. Pediatr Dermatol 1999; 16: 90–4

Sigman GS. Eating disorders in children and adolescents. Pediatr Clin North Am 2003; 50: 1139–77

Acrodermatitis enteropathica

Synonym: zinc deficiency

Major points

- Classic presentation: dermatitis, diarrhea, alopecia, extreme irritability
- Types:
  1. Genetic (autosomal recessive)
  2. Nutritional, found sporadically in premature and full-term infants
  3. Endemically in the Middle East (growth failure and delayed pubertal maturation); caused by concurrent ingestion of high amounts of a zinc-binding ligand, phytate
  4. Iatrogenic zinc deficiency associated with total parenteral nutrition
- Genetic form: usually occurs 1–2 weeks after weaning from breast feeding, and rarely during breast feeding; in bottle-fed infants it occurs 4–10 weeks of age
- Dermatitis: periorificial (around mouth, eyes, genital area) and acral areas: erythematous, vesiculobullous or psoriasiform eruption with exudation and crusting (Figure 11.21)
- Secondary superinfection with *Candida* and staphylococci common
- Nail changes: pustular paronychia with subsequent nail dystrophy
- Hair fine and sparse, leading to total alopecia
- Photophobia, blepharitis, conjunctivitis, cheilitis
- Other: failure to thrive, apathy, ataxia, immune abnormalities, poor wound healing

Pathogenesis

- Zinc is essential for normal function of all cells
- May be caused by defect in intestinal absorption of zinc or from deficient intake, malabsorption (as in cystic fibrosis) (Figures 11.22 and 11.23) and other chronic illnesses
- In the genetic form, caused by mutation in the intestinal zinc-specific transporter SLC39A4 on chromosome 8q24.3

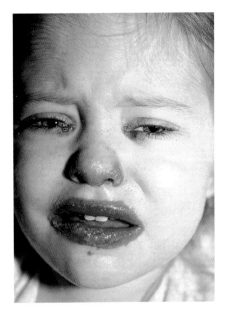

Figure 11.21   Acrodermatitis enteropathica – erythematous, eroded, periorificial plaques

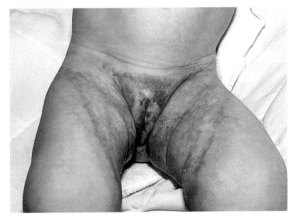

Figure 11.22   Cystic fibrosis presenting with edema and acrodermatitis enteropathica lesions

Diagnosis

- Low plasma zinc levels are pathognomonic (blood must be collected in special acid-washed or plastic tubes)
- Low serum alkaline phosphatase (a zinc-dependent metalloenzyme)

Differential diagnosis

- Seborrheic dermatitis
- Psoriasis

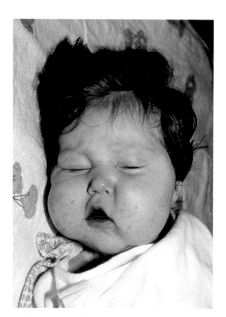

Figure 11.23   Cystic fibrosis – edema is obvious in the cheeks

- Candidal infection
- Fatty acid deficiency
- Biotin deficiency

Treatment

- Rapid and dramatic improvement with supplementation
- Zinc is in nuts, whole grains, green leafy vegetables, shellfish
- Daily requirement is 1–3 mg/kg per day, or 10–20 mg for adults

Prognosis

- Excellent response when treated
- Can be fatal without supplementation

References

Brar BK, Pall A, Gupta RR. Acrodermatitis enteropathica-like rash in an exclusively breast fed infant with zinc deficiency. J Dermatol 2003; 30: 259–60

Kim BE, Wang F, Dufner-Beattie J, et al. Zn2+-stimulated endocytosis of the mZIP4 zinc transporter regulates its location at the plasma membrane. J Bio Chem 2004; 279: 4523–30

Michalczyk A, Varigos G, Catto-Smith A, et al. Analysis of zinc transporter, hZnT4 (Slc30A4), gene expression in a mammary gland disorder leading to reduced zinc secretion into milk. Hum Genet 2003; 113: 202–10

Muniz AE, Bartle S, Foster R. Edema, anemia, hypoproteinemia, and acrodermatitis enteropathica: an uncommon initial presentation of cystic fibrosis. Pediatr Emerg Care 2004; 20: 112–4

Nakano A, Nakano H, Nomura K, et al. Novel SLC39A4 mutations in acrodermatitis enteropathica. J Invest Dermatol 2003; 120: 963–6

Perafan-Riveros C, Franca LF, Alves AC, Sanches JA Jr. Acrodermatitis enteropathica: case report and review of the literature. Pediatr Dermatol 2002; 19: 426–31

Quirk CM, Seykora J, Wingate BJ, Cotsarelis G. Acrodermatitis enteropathica associated with anorexia nervosa. J Am Med Assoc 2002; 288: 2655—6

Wang K, Zhou B, Kuo YM, et al. A novel member of a zinc transporter family is defective in acrodermatitis enteropathica. Am J Hum Genet 2002; 71: 66–73

12

PHOTODERMATOSES AND PHYSICAL INJURY AND ABUSE

PHOTODERMATOSES

General

- Sun exposure in childhood is normal; excessive sun exposure may result in sunburn (toxic response) or, in some cases, abnormal reactions (e.g. lupus)
- Tanning is a sign of ultraviolet (UV) injury, and should not be considered 'healthy'
- Long-term consequences of chronic sun damage: skin cancer and photoaging

Phototoxicity/sunburn

Major points

- Sunburn depends upon a number of factors:
  1. Length of exposure
  2. Skin phototype (Table 12.1)
  3. Direction of sun's rays (summer > winter)
  4. Time of day (10.00 to 15.00 are strongest rays)
  5. Geographical location (nearer equator)
  6. Altitude (higher > lower)
  7. Age (infants > young children > adults)
- Erythema and tenderness begin 30 minutes to 4 hours after sun exposure; peaks at 24 hours; may last for 72 hours (Figures 12.1 and 12.2)
- Most prominent on areas which receive direct light (e.g. nose, cheeks, shoulders) with less reaction in shielded areas (e.g. under nose and chin, and on upper eyelids)
- With intense exposure: blistering, edema and later desquamation
  1. Sleep often disturbed
  2. Tenderness of skin
  3. Reduced sweating

Table 12.1	Skin phototypes	
Skin type	Reactivity to sun	Examples
I	Always burns; never tans	Light skin, blond or red hair, blue or brown eyes, and freckles (e.g. Celts)
II	Always burns; tans minimally or lightly	Light skin; red, blond, or brown hair; blue, hazel or brown eyes (e.g. Northern Europeans)
III	Sometimes burns; tans gradually and uniformly	Brown hair, blue or brown eyes (e.g. Southern Europeans)
IV	Burns minimally or never; always tans	Dark brown hair, dark eyes, light brown skin (e.g. Latinos, Asians)
V	Moderately pigmented skin; never burns, always tans well	Medium brown skin, dark brown hair (e.g. Middle Easterners, Latinos)
VI	Deeply pigmented; never burns, always tans well	Dark skin, dark hair (e.g. Black Africans)

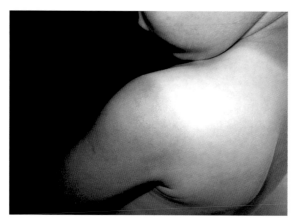

Figure 12.1   Phototoxicity – from excessive sun exposure

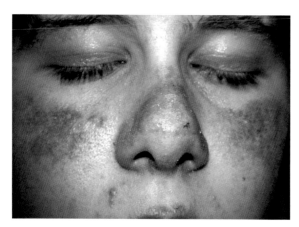

Figure 12.2   Phototoxicity from doxycycline

4. In severe burns, collapse from heat stroke, fever, headache and fatigue
- Ultraviolet light
  1. UV light consists of UVA, UVB, UVC
  2. UVB does not generate a perception of warmth unless skin is already burned (i.e. a person does not realize the damage until it is too late)
  3. On cloudy days, visible light and infrared rays (both cause a sensation of warmth) are filtered out; however, 80% of UVB can get through
  4. Much of lifetime sun exposure occurs before 18 years

Pathogenesis

- Acute ultraviolet injury is caused by radiation damage

1. First change is vasodilatation, probably caused by prostaglandins as mediators
2. Metabolic changes occur within epidermal cells, which demonstrate clumping of tonofilaments and abnormalities of cytoplasm and nucleus which produce dyskeratotic 'sunburn cells', recognizable by light microscopy. These cells lose their epidermal cell attachments, and produce intraepidermal blisters
3. By 48 hours, damage throughout epidermis
4. By 72 hours, regeneration begins
5. At 96 hours, great increase in number of melanocytes that have arborized their dendrites, beginning the tanning process
- Tanning response occurs in two distinct phases:
  1. Immediate response caused by photo-oxidation of melanin chromoproteins
  2. Delayed tanning develops with increased melanosome formation and increased transfer of melanosomes to keratinocytes; starts at 2 days and peaks at 19 days
  3. Melanin absorbs UVB and also acts as a 'sponge' by mopping up free radicals which damage the epidermis
- UV radiation effects are cumulative
  1. Long-term effects: fine, deep wrinkling, actinic keratoses, skin cancer (especially basal cell carcinoma and squamous cell carcinoma), laxity, mottled pigmentation and telangiectasias
  2. Malignant melanoma: more common in patients with a history of several severe sunburns

Diagnosis

- Clinical symptoms and history
- Histology: epidermal spongiosis, 'sunburn cells' (dyskeratotic damaged epidermal cells), dermal vasodilatation, edema, neutrophils, monocytes, reduced number of Langerhans cells
- Photosensitizing agents can induce a reaction with short exposure (5–30 minutes) (Table 12.2)

Differential diagnosis

- Porphyria
- Lupus erythematosus
- Viral eruptions (e.g. fifth disease)
- Xeroderma pigmentosum

Table 12.2 Exogenous photosensitizers	
	Examples
Drugs	Antibiotics (sulfonamides, tetracyclines, griseofulvin), phenothiazines, diuretics (furosemide, thiazides), quinine, isoniazid, tranquilizers, antidepressants, anti-inflammatory agents (naproxen), antiarrhythmics, antihypertensives
Plants	Furocoumarins
Dyes	Methylene blue, toluidine blue, xanthenes, fluorescein, eosin, erythrosine, acridine
Polycyclic hydrocarbons	Pitch, coal tars, anthracene, acridine, fluoranthrene
Perfumes/ cosmetics	Bergamot oil, musk ambrette, 6-methylcoumarin, halogenated salicylanilides
Sunscreens	PABA, benzophenones, cinnamates
Tatoos	Cadmium sulfide

Treatment

- Prevention
  1. Good sun protection habits should be stressed at an early age
  2. Infants <6 months should not have much direct sun exposure, but should be protected with clothing and umbrellas; more likely to develop heat stroke because of decreased ability to sweat
  3. Sun-protective clothing (e.g. Solumbra)
  4. Shade (e.g. umbrellas)
  5. Sunscreens (see Chapter 21) with the regular use of SPF 15 sunscreen during first 18 years of life, the lifetime incidence of nonmelanoma skin cancers can be reduced 78%
- Acute sunburn
  1. Cool wet compresses
  2. Aspirin, non-steroidal agents and indomethacin inhibit prostaglandin synthesis, and may modify sunburn if given within 24–48 hours of exposure, but will not repair damage already done to epidermal cells
  3. Steroids either topically or orally are not beneficial

4. Topical anesthetics (e.g. benzocaine) can be sensitizing and only bring temporary relief. Not recommended
5. Efficacies of topical aloe vera, jojoba oil and vitamin E have not been well studied

Prognosis

- Self-limited
- Chronic sun exposure has long-term effects

References

Cokkinides VE, Weinstock MA, O'Connell MC, Thun MJ. Use of indoor tanning sunlamps by US youth, ages 11–18 years, and by their parent or guardian caregivers: prevalence and correlates. Pediatrics 2002; 109: 1124–30

Drake LA, Dinehart SM, Farmer ER, et al.Guidelines of care for photoaging/photodamage. J Am Acad Dermatol 1996; 35: 462–4

Driscoll MS, Wagner RF Jr. Clinical management of the acute sunburn reaction. Cutis 2000; 66: 53–8

Garssen J, van Loveren H. Effects of ultraviolet exposure on the immune system. Crit Rev Immunol 2001; 21: 359–97

Geller AC, Colditz G, Oliveria S, et al. Use of sunscreen, sunburning rates, and tanning bed use among more than 10 000 US children and adolescents. Pediatrics 2002; 109: 1009–14

Kim HJ. Photoprotection in adolescents. Adolesc Med State Art Rev 2001; 12: 181–93

Photoallergic dermatitis

Major points

- Chemicals can produce abnormal reactions when light energy is absorbed, causing either phototoxic or photoallergic reactions
- Photosensitizing agents may be either endogenous or exogenous
  1. Endogenous photosensitivity (e.g. porphyria); primary action spectrum is in the UVA range, 400–410 nm
  2. Exogenous photosensitizers produce phototoxic reactions which clinically resemble exaggerated sunburn (see Table 12.2)
  3. Topical photosensitizers (e.g. furocoumarins, lime oil, oil of cedar, vanilla oils, oil of lavender and sandalwood oil) cause photosensitivity reactions beginning 24 hours after exposure (see Phytophotodermatitis)

- Ranges from mild erythema or eczematous patches to severe blistering; may present with only postinflammatory hyperpigmentation
- Most photosensitization caused by UVA (320–400 nm)

References

Crouch RB, Foley PA, Baker CS. Analysis of patients with suspected photosensitivity referred for investigation to an Australian photodermatology clinic. J Am Acad Dermatol 2003; 48: 714–20

Darvay A, White IR, Rycroft RJ, et al. Photoallergic contact dermatitis is uncommon. Br J Dermatol 2001; 145: 597–601

Moore DE. Drug-induced cutaneous photosensitivity: incidence, mechanism, prevention and management. Drug Safety 2002; 25: 345–72

Morison WL. Clinical practice. Photosensitivity. N Engl J Med 2004; 350: 1111–17

Phytophotodermatitis

Major points

- Caused by exposure to furocoumarins (psoralens) from plants
- Clinical picture:
  1. Redness, blisters and post-inflammatory hyperpigmentation, which often occur in bizarre shapes or linear streaks (Figure 12.3)
  2. Can present with hyperpigmented streaks without history of erythema or blistering

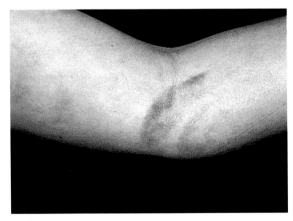

Figure 12.3 Phytophotodermatitis caused by lime juice and sun exposure

3. Limes, certain perfumes, celery and certain grasses have higher content of furocoumarins
4. History of exposure is helpful

Differential diagnosis

- Allergic contact dermatitis
- Postinflammatory hyperpigmentation
- Incontinentia pigmenti
- Lentiginous nevus

Treatment

- Avoid photosensitizing chemicals
- Apply moderate potency topical corticosteroid 2–3 times daily for 2–3 weeks
- Over-the-counter bleaching creams with hydroquinone may be helpful for postinflammatory hyperpigmentation, although usually not needed

Prognosis

- Excellent; lesions fade slowly

References

Bowers AG. Phytophotodermatitis. Am J Contact Dermatitis 1999; 10: 89–93

Coffman K, Boyce WT, Hansen RC. Phytophotodermatitis simulating child abuse. Am J Dis Child 1985; 139: 239–40

Goskowicz MO, Friedlander SF, Eichenfield LF. Endemic 'Lime' disease: phytophotodermatitis in San Diego County. Pediatrics 1994; 93: 828–30

Solis RR, Dotson DA, Trizna Z. Phytophotodermatitis: a sometimes difficult diagnosis. Arch Fam Med 2000; 9: 1195–6

Polymorphous light eruption

Major points

- Broad term for a group of sun-sensitive disorders which have distinct clinical patterns
- Four major types:
  1. Papular polymorphous light eruption (PMLE)
     a. Most common type, manifests as a papular, itchy dermatitis beginning in spring and tending to improve throughout summer (Figure 12.4)
     b. Sudden onset of pruritic, discrete, erythematous papules and plaques

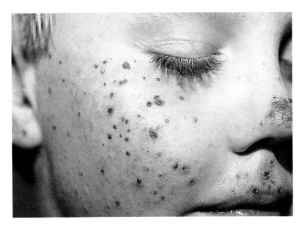

Figure 12.4   Polymorphous light eruption – vesicles on the face

c. Begins within hours to days of sun exposure
d. Lasts 1–7 days
e. Not scarring
f. Not all areas of sun exposure affected
g. Female/male ratio >1
h. Some improvement or resolution with time
2. Actinic prurigo (Hutchinson summer prurigo)
   a. Most commonly seen in school-aged children
   b. More common in Native Americans
   c. Dermatitis starts in the early spring with acute itchy facial and forearm dermatitis with edematous papules and vesicles
   d. With time, crusting, thickening and lichenification
   e. Eruption clears, only to recur the next spring; however, some children have the eruption all year
   f. Chronic cheilitis, especially of the lower lip
   g. Autosomal dominant in some families
3. Juvenile spring eruption (hydroa aestivale)
   a. Primarily seen in northern European boys, aged 5–12 years
   b. Discrete papules of 2–3 mm or vesicles on ears and cheeks lasting about a week (Figure 12.5)
   c. Tends to recur each spring
   d. Some patients develop more typical papular PMLE

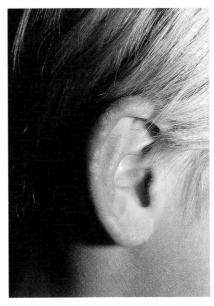

Figure 12.5   Juvenile spring eruption – limited to the ears

4. Hydroa vacciniforme
   a. Discrete, deep-seated vesicles on ears, nose and face which lead to hemorrhage and scarring
   b. Lesions last up to 4 weeks
   c. Occasional keratitis and uveitis
   d. Begins before age 10 years
   e. Male/female ratio >1
   f. Rare

Pathogenesis

- Considered to be caused by delayed-type hypersensitivity response to a UV radiation-induced antigen
- One-quarter of affected individuals sensitive to UVB alone, one-quarter to UVB and UVA together, and one-half to UVA only
- Probably genetic, with incomplete expression and penetrance

Diagnosis

- Suspect diagnosis on clinical basis. Biopsy or phototesting may be needed
- Histology shows:
  1. Superficial and deep lymphocytic infiltrate
  2. Papillary dermal edema and hemorrhage
  3. Variable epidermal changes

4. Spongiotic dermatitis resembling eczema
5. Late lesions demonstrate chronic infiltration of lymphocytes and spongiosis

Differential diagnosis

- Atopic dermatitis
- Contact dermatitis
- Systemic lupus erythematosus
- Erythropoietic protoporphyria
- Sunburn/phototoxicity
- Photoallergic reactions
- Tinea corporis
- Drug-induced photosensitivity
- Solar urticaria

Treatment

- Sun avoidance
- Restriction of daily activities outdoors between 10.00 and 16.00 (peak UV times)
- Clothing: wide-brimmed hat, long-sleeved shirt and sunscreens
- Topical corticosteroids in an ointment vehicle 2–3 times a day
- Wet dressings for acute weeping lesions
- Treatment of secondary bacterial infection if present
- β-carotene (Solatene) 60–180 mg/day for an adult
- For severe cases, oral psoralen plus UVA (PUVA) under controlled conditions may help induce hardening
- Frequent follow-up visits if dermatitis is not under control; less frequent as child improves
- Hydroxychloroquine (Plaquenil®) 100–200 mg BID (adult dose) for severe cases

Prognosis

- Variable; some patients may improve with time or with chronic sun exposure; however, many patients continue to have symptoms

References

Boonstra HE, van Weelden H, Toonstra J, van Vloten WA. Polymorphous light eruption: a clinical, photobiologic, and follow-up study of 110 patients. J Am Acad Dermatol 2000; 42: 199–207

Fusaro RM, Johnson JA. Hereditary polymorphic light eruption of American Indians: occurrence in non-Indians with polymorphic light eruption. J Am Acad Dermatol 1996; 34: 612–17

Hann SK, Im S, Park Y-K, Lee S. Hydroa vacciniforme with unusually severe scar formation: diagnosis by repetitive UVA phototesting. J Am Acad Dermatol 1991; 25: 401–3

Hasan T, Ranki A, Jansen CT, Karvonen J. Disease associations in polymorphous light eruption. Arch Dermatol 1998; 134: 1081–5

Leenutaphong V. Hydroa vacciniforme: an unusual clinical manifestation. J Am Acad Dermatol 1991; 25: 892–5

Patel DC, Bellaney GJ, Seed PT, et al. Efficacy of short-course oral prednisolone in polymorphic light eruption: a randomized controlled trial. Br J Dermatol 2000; 143: 828–31

Rhodes LE. Polymorphic light eruption reassessed. Arch Dermatol 2004; 140: 351–2

van de Pas CB, Hawk JL, Young AR, Walker SL. An optimal method for experimental provocation of polymorphic light eruption. Arch Dermatol 2004; 140: 286–92

Van Praag MCG, Boom BW, Vermeer BJ. Diagnosis and treatment of polymorphous light eruption. Int J Dermatol 1994; 33: 233–8

Solar urticaria

Major points

- Pruritic wheals occur within minutes of sun exposure and last <24 hours
- Locations on sun-exposed areas
- Onset usually >10 years of age
- Tolerance (i.e. 'hardening') can occur after repeated exposure
- Onset usually between 10 and 50 years of age
- Slight female predominance

Pathogenesis

- Allergic response to photo-induced allergen
- Mast cells play a major role
- Types of solar urticaria based on action spectra: usually visible light, but UVA and UVB or combinations may be responsible

Diagnosis

- Clinical characteristics
- Histology: similar to urticaria with dermal edema, perivascular neutrophilic and eosinophilic infiltrates

Differential diagnosis

- Urticaria
- Polymorphous light eruption

- Porphyria
- Drug reactions

Treatment

- Sun avoidance with clothing and sunscreens
- Nonsedating antihistamines
- Systemic steroids (short course for 5–10 days) initially may be helpful
- PUVA may induce tolerance

Prognosis

- May be chronic and intermittent

References

Beattie PE, Dawe RS, Ibbotson SH, Ferguson J. Characteristics and prognosis of idiopathic solar urticaria: a cohort of 87 cases. Arch Dermatol 2003; 139: 1149–54

Grabbe J. Pathomechanisms in physical urticaria. Symposium Proceedings. J Invest Dermatol 2001; 6: 135–6

Roelandts R. Diagnosis and treatment of solar urticaria. Dermatol Ther 2003; 16: 52–6

GENODERMATOSES WITH SUN SENSITIVITY

Porphyria

Major points

- Group of disorders of porphyrin metabolism which can have sun sensitivity as a primary feature (Table 12.3)
- Erythropoietic protoporphyria (EPP)
  1. Most common type in children
  2. Usually presents in preschool child with burning, itching or stinging of skin after short exposure to sun, even through window glass
  3. Younger children may be irritable but may not have typical skin lesions
  4. Intense sun exposure may result in severe facial edema, urticaria, vesiculation and crusting
  5. Chronic changes: thickened skin-colored papules on the dorsal hands, and pitted scarring on nose and face (Figures 12.6 and 12.7)
  6. Perioral linear papules may result from previous vesicular damage

Pathogenesis

- Caused by enzyme defects in heme biosynthesis which lead to blockade of porphyrin

pathway and accumulation of porphyrins and precursors
- Porphyrin molecules absorb visible light and generate molecular level excited states leading to free radical formation with subsequent cell membrane damage and cell death

Diagnosis

- Histology: thickening of superficial blood vessels and a perivascular deposit of periodic acid-Schiff (PAS)-positive material which, on direct immunofluorescence, contains IgG
- Blood, urine and stool porphyrin levels have characteristic patterns

Differential diagnosis

- Phototoxicity
- Photoallergic reactions
- Polymorphous light eruption
- Solar urticaria
- Contact dermatitis

Treatment

- Sun avoidance with clothing and sunscreens blocking UVA (physical sunscreens with titanium dioxide are best)
- β-carotene (Solatene) 60–180 mg/day may be helpful
- Because of potential chronic liver changes, liver function tests should be followed every 6–12 months
- Genetic counseling advised. Family members should be screened and liver functions followed
- Low-dose hydroxychloroquine

Prognosis

- Chronic, life-long sun sensitivity, skin damage and possible liver disease

References

Ahmed I. Childhood porphyrias. Mayo Clin Proc 2002; 77: 825–36

Bruce AJ, Ahmed I. Childhood-onset porphyria cutanea tarda: successful therapy with low-dose hydroxychloroquine (Plaquenil). J Am Acad Dermatol 1998; 38: 810–14

Cummins R, Wagner-Weiner L, Paller A. Pseudoporphyria induced by celecoxib in a patient with juvenile rheumatoid arthritis. J Rheumatol 2000; 27: 2938–40

De Silva B, Banney L, Uttley W, et al. Pseudoporphyria and nonsteroidal antiinflammatory agents in children with juvenile idiopathic arthritis. Pediatr Dermatol 2000; 17: 480–3

Table 12.3   Porphyrias

Type	Characteristics	Gene	Laboratory investigations
Erythropoietic porphyria (EP)	Begins in infancy Marked photosensitivity with pain Vesicles, bullae Hypertrichosis Mutilating scars Hemolytic anemia Splenomegaly Erythrodontia	Uroporphyrinogen III synthetase (UROS) Gene locus: 10q25.2-q26.3 Autosomal recessive	Urine: elevated URO I, COPRO I Urine: fluorescent Stool: elevated COPRO I Blood: fluorescent RBCs
Erythropoietic protoporphyria (EPP)	Onset in first decade Mild to severe photosensitivity Burning, stinging after sun exposure Edematous plaques with erythema, purpura Waxy or depressed scars on nose, dorsal hands Liver: cholelithiasis, hepatic failure	Ferrochelatase (FECH) Gene locus: 18q21.3 Autosomal dominant	Blood: elevated FEP Blood: elevated RBC & plasma PROTO Blood: fluorescent RBCs Urine: normal porphyrins Stool: elevated PROTO
Acute intermittent porphyria (AIP)	Onset 2nd to 4th decade No photosensitivity Recurrent attacks of abdominal pain, weakness, neuropathy, behavioral changes Attacks precipitated by drugs, events	PBG deaminase Gene locus: 11q23.3 Autosomal dominant	Urine: elevated ALA, PBG during attacks Stool: ALA, PBG during attacks Blood: plasma neg, RBC neg
Porphyria cutanea tarda (PCT)	Onset in 3rd to 4th decade Moderate photosensitivity Bullae, fragility, scars, milia, hyperpigmentation, facial hypertrichosis Precipitated by alcohol, estrogens, iron, hydrocarbons Liver iron overload	Uroporphyrinogen decarboxylase (UROD) Gene locus: 1p34 Autosomal dominant or sporadic	Urine: URO I>III, ISOCOPRO Stool: ISOCOPRO>PROTO Plasma + RBC neg
Variegate porphyria (VP)	Onset 2nd to 3rd decade Photosensitivity similar to PCT Acute attacks simlar to AIP Common in South Africa	Protoporphyrinogen oxidase Gene locus: 1q22, 6p21.3 Autosomal dominant	Urine: ALA and PBG elevated during attacks Urine: elevated URO & COPRO between attacks Stool: PROTO>COPRO both elevated during and between attacks
Hereditary coproporphyria (HCP)	Onset any age Skin lesions resemble PCT but milder Attacks like AIP but milder	Coproporphyrinogen oxidase Gene locus: 3q12 Autosomal dominant	Stool: COPRO III elevated during and between attacks Urine: COPRO III elevated during and between attacks Elevated ALA, PBG only during attacks

ALA, delta-aminolevulinic acid; PBG, porphobilinogen; URO, uroporphyrin; COPRO, coproporphyrin; PROTO, protoporphyrin; ISOCOPRO, isocoproporphyrin; RBCs, red blood cells; FEP, free erytrocyte protoporphyria

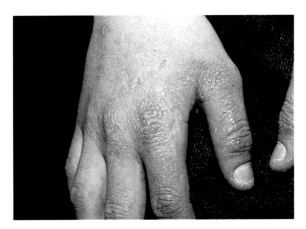

Figure 12.6 Erythropoietic protoporphyria – scars on hands

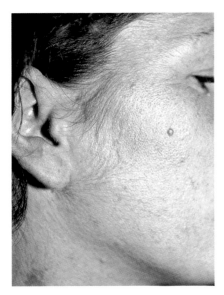

Figure 12.7 Porphyria cutanea tarda – hypertrichosis on the face

Fritsch C, Bolsen K, Ruzicka T, Goerz G. Congenital erythropoietic porphyria. J Am Acad Dermatol 1997; 36: 594–610

Gross U, Hoffmann GF, Doss MO. Erythropoietic and hepatic porphyrias. J Inherit Metab Dis 2000; 23: 641–61

Huang J-L, Zaider E, Roth P, et al. Congenital erythropoietic porphyria: clinical, biochemical, and enzymatic profile of a severely affected infant. J Am Acad Dermatol 1996; 34: 924–7

LaDuca JR, Bouman PH, Gaspari AA. Nonsteroidal antiinflammatory drug-induced pseudoporphyria: a case series. J Cutan Med Surg 2002; 6: 320–6

Paller AS, Eramo LR, Farrell EE, et al. Purpuric phototherapy-induced eruption in transfused neonates: relation to transient porphyrinemia. Pediatrics 1997; 100: 360–4

Pandhi D, Suman M, Khurana N, Reddy BSN. Congenital erythropoietic porphyria complicated by squamous cell carcinoma. Pediatr Dermatol 2003; 20: 498–501

Poh-Fitzpatrick MB, Wang X, Anderson KE, et al. Erythropoietic protoporphyria: altered phenotype after bone marrow transplantation for myelogenous leukemia in a patient heteroallelic for ferrochelatase gene mutations. J Am Acad Dermatol 2002; 46: 861–6

Xeroderma pigmentosum

Major points

- Presents in infancy with extreme sun sensitivity
- By 18 months of age, early sunburn reactions and freckling are evident after minimal sun exposure (Figure 12.8)
- Sunburn reactions persist for weeks
- Telangiectasias and atrophy of skin
- Actinic keratoses develop as red, scaly persistent macules and papules on sun-exposed areas
- In darker skinned patients, findings may be more subtle
- By 6–8 years, multiple basal cell carcinomas, squamous cell carcinomas and malignant melanoma are common
- Ocular findings, particularly photophobia and decreased vision, occur in ~20%
- Mild to severe mental retardation, especially evident in De Sanctis–Cacchione syndrome

Pathogenesis

- Defective repair of ultraviolet radiation damage to pyrimidine dimers in DNA in many cell types (e.g. epidermal cells, fibroblasts, lymphocytes, corneal cells, liver cells)
- Group A: most severe form; exhibits skin and central nervous system disorders (severe or mild) (DeSanctis–Cacchione syndrome); gene locus/gene: 9q22.3/ XPA
- Group B: gene locus/gene: 2q21/ ERCC3, XPB
- Group C: usually have only skin disorders; most common in USA, Europe, Egypt; gene locus/gene: 3p25/ XPC

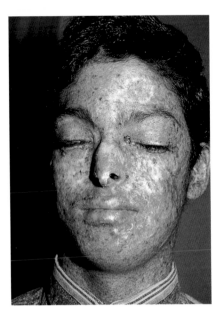

Figure 12.8   Xeroderma pigmentosum – multiple lentigines and scarring from previous skin cancer removal

- Group D: skin cancer, CNS disorders; may have Cockayne syndrome or trichothiodystrophy; gene locus/gene: 19q13.2-q13.3/ ERCC2, EM9
- Group E: few skin cancers, excision repair 40–50% of normal, gene locus: 11p12-p11
- Group F: mild skin symptoms, excision repair 10–20% of normal; gene locus: 16p13.3-p13.13; gene: ERCC4
- Group G: mental retardation, neurological abnormalities, photosensitivity, excision repair <5% of normal; gene locus: 13q33, gene: ERCC5

Diagnosis

- Sub-typing can be done in certain laboratories by studying the DNA repair mechanisms after UV light exposure in the clinical setting of XP

Differential diagnosis

- Multiple lentigines syndrome (LEOPARD syndrome)
- Erythropoietic protoporphyria
- Basal cell nevus syndrome

Treatment

- Treatment is symptomatic, with removal of skin cancers
- Early biopsy of suspicious lesions

- Prevention with complete sun avoidance: sun protective clothing, sunscreens, and night time habits of outdoor activities
- Should ideally be followed at a center which is familiar with this condition and treatment of skin cancers
- Frequent visits are important to evaluate incipient tumors

Prognosis

- Prognosis is poor. Morbidity from chronic skin cancers requiring surgery. Early death from metastatic skin cancer or melanoma. Some types have a better prognosis

References

Bootsma D, Hoeijmakers JHJ. The genetic basis of xeroderma pigmentosum. Ann Genet 1991; 34: 143–50

Cleaver JE, Thompson LH, Richardson AS, States JC. A summary of mutations in the UV-sensitive disorders: xeroderma pigmentosum, Cockayne syndrome, and trichothiodystrophy. Hum Mutat 1999; 14: 9–22

Kraemer KH, Lee MM, Scotto J. Xeroderma pigmentosum. Cutaneous, ocular, and neurologic abnormalities in 830 published cases. Arch Dermatol 1987; 123: 241–50

Stary A, Sarasin A. The genetics of the hereditary xeroderma pigmentosum syndrome. Biochimie 2002; 84: 49–60

Tsao H. Genetics of nonmelanoma skin cancer. Arch Dermatol 2001; 137: 1486–92

Cockayne syndrome

Major points

- Premature aging
- Microcephaly
- Photosensitivity – scaly erythema, begins at 1 year of age
- Short stature
- Mental retardation (progressive)
- Disproportionately large hands, feet, ears
- Atrophy of subcutaneous facial fat with sunken eyes
- Ocular defects
- Flexion contractures
- Short life span
- Autosomal recessive
- Gene locus/gene:
  1. Type 1: chromosome 5/ERCC8, CKN1
  2. Type 2: chromosome 10q11/ERCC6, CKN2

References

Berneburg M, Lehmann AR. Xeroderma pigmentosum and related disorders: defects in DNA repair and transcription. Adv Genet 2001; 43: 71–102

Licht CL, Stevnsner T, Bohr VA. Cockayne syndrome group B cellular and biochemical functions. Am J Hum Genet 2003; 73: 1217–39

Bloom syndrome

Major points

- Short stature (prenatal onset)
- Telangiectatic facial erythema (butterfly distribution)
- Photosensitivity (not true poikiloderma)
- Hypogonadism
- High incidence of malignancy, especially leukemias, lymphomas, gastrointestinal tract cancer
- Increased susceptibility to infections
- Autosomal recessive
- Male/female ratio >1
- Gene locus: 15q26.1
- Gene: BLM, RECQ3 helicase; protein product is member of DNA helicase

References

Chisholm CA, Bray MJ, Karns LB. Successful pregnancy in a woman with Bloom syndrome. Am J Med Genet 2001; 102: 136–8

Duker NJ. Chromosome breakage syndromes and cancer. Am J Med Genet 2002; 115: 125–9

Duker NJ. Chromosome breakage syndromes and cancer. Am J Med Genet 2002; 115: 125–9

Franchitto A, Pichierri P. Protecting genomic integrity during DNA replication: correlation between Werner's and Bloom's syndrome gene products and the MRE11 complex. Hum Mol Genet 2002; 11: 2447–53

Siegel DH, Howard R. Molecular advances in genetic skin diseases. Curr Opin Pediatr 2002; 14: 419–25

Rothmund–Thomson syndrome

Synonym: poikiloderma congenitale

Major points

- Generalized poikiloderma, begins in infancy and progresses until age 3–5 years; lesions begin as red edematous plaques sometimes accompanied by blistering
- Photosensitivity
- Ocular abnormalities
- Hyperkeratoses of palms, soles, hands, wrists, ankles and elsewhere (squamous cell carcinoma may develop)
- Scalp hair sparse and fine, may progress to partial or total alopecia
- Short stature (<4 feet) (<1.2 m)
- Autosomal recessive (female/male ratio >1)
- Gene locus: 8q24.3
- Gene: RECQL4 (DNA helicase)

References

Collins P, Barnes L, McCabe M. Poikiloderma congenitale: case report and review of the literature. Pediatr Dermatol 1991; 8: 58–60

Duker NJ. Chromosome breakage syndromes and cancer. Am J Med Genet 2002; 115: 125–9

Furuichi Y. Premature aging and predisposition to cancers caused by mutations in RecQ family helicases. Ann NY Acad Sci 2001; 928: 121–31

Hickson ID. RecQ helicases: caretakers of the genome. Nature Rev Cancer 2003; 3: 169–78

Kitao S, Shimamoto A, Goto M, et al. Mutations in RECQL4 cause a subset of cases of Rothmund–Thomson syndrome. Nature Genet 1999; 22: 82–4

Vennos EM, Collins M, James WD. Rothmund–Thomson syndrome: review of the world literature. J Am Acad Dermatol 1992; 27: 750–62

Pellagra – vitamin B₃ (niacin) deficiency

Major points

- Four D's: Diarrhea, Dementia, Dermatitis (on sun-exposed areas, angular stomatitis, glossitis, oral and perirectal sores), Death
- Causative drugs/factors: isoniazid, sulfonamides, anticonvulsants, antidepressants, plain corn diet (niacin not bioavailable), gastrointestinal disease (malabsorption), carcinoid syndrome, Hartnup disease

References

Karthikeyan K, Thappa DM. Pellagra and skin. Int J Dermatol 2002; 41: 476–81

Tyler I, Wiseman MC, Crawford RI, Birmingham CL. Cutaneous manifestations of eating disorders. J Cutan Med Surg 2002; 6: 345–53

COLD INJURIES

Pernio

Synonym: chilblains

Major points

- Abnormal inflammatory response to cold, damp, nonfreezing conditions
- May be associated with cryogloblulins
- Clinical:
  1. Single or multiple erythematous to violaceous macules, papules or nodules; rare blistering (Figure 12.9)
  2. Distribution: symmetrical on distal toes and fingers; less often on heels, nose and ears
- Pathogenesis unknown but thought to be of vascular origin
- Histology: nonspecific with papillary dermal edema, superficial and deep perivascular infiltrate comprising of lymphocytes

Treatment

- Warming the affected area
- Takes 1–2 weeks to recover

Differential diagnosis

- Systemic lupus erythematosus
- Leukemia
- Trauma
- Cryoglobulinemia

References

Goette DK. Chilblains (perniosis). J Am Acad Dermatol 1990; 23: 257–62

Klapman MH, Johnston WH. Localized recurrent postoperative pernio associated with leukocytoclastic vasculitis. J Am Acad Dermatol 1991; 24: 811–13

Weston WL, Morelli JG. Childhood pernio and cryoproteins. Pediatr Dermatol 2000; 17: 97–9

White KP, Rother MJ, Milanese A, Grant-Kels JM. Perniosis in association with anorexia nervosa. Pediatr Dermatol 1994; 11: 1–5

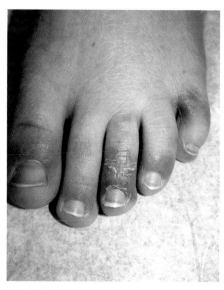

Figure 12.9 Pernio – erythematous painful nodules after cold exposure

Frostbite

Major points

- Erythema, edema, numbness initially followed by hyperemia and pain with re-warming
- Locations: usually nose, ears, fingertips, toes
- Ranges from first-degree frostbite to fourth-degree frostbite with full thickness loss of skin, muscle, tendon and bone

Pathogenesis

- Occurs when skin temperature drops below −2°C
- Combination of tissue freezing and vasoconstriction with damage due to inflammatory mediators

Diagnosis

- Clinical diagnosis: easily recognizable
- Histology: superficial dermal edema, subepidermal bullae, hemorrhage, necrosis

Treatment

- Rapid re-warming with water bath ~40°C

References

Biem J, Koehncke N, Classen D, Dosman J. Out of the cold: management of hypothermia and frostbite. Can Med Assoc J 2003; 168: 305–11

Huh J, Wright R, Gregory N. Localized facial telangiectasias following frostbite injury. Cutis 1996; 57: 97–8

Murphy JV, Banwell PE, Roberts AH, McGrouther DA. Frostbite: pathogenesis and treatment. J Trauma-Injury Infect Crit Care 2000; 48: 171–8

Nissen ER, Melchert PJ, Lewis EJ. A case of bullous frostbite following recreational snowmobiling. Cutis 1999; 63: 21–2

CHILD ABUSE

General

- Dr C. Henry Kempe in 1962 described 'battered child syndrome'
- Child abuse encompasses: physical abuse, neglect, sexual exploitation
- Physical abuse is the nonaccidental injury of a child
- Statistics: >2 million children abused in USA per year; 55% neglect, 27% physical, 16% sexual, 8% emotional
- Many teens run away from home
- 1200–1300 fatalities per year; 50% are <1 year old

Major points

- Victim usually 1–5 years of age, considered the 'vulnerable child'; often preverbal or handicapped
- No predilection for sex, race, social class, or income
- Morbidity is both physical and mental, with 25–30% permanent
- Tends to be self-propagating (i.e. one generation to the next)
- Mortality overall 3–4%, caused by head trauma, or abdominal organ rupture
- Classification of abuse:
  1. Definite abuse: definite act causing harm to child
     a. Seen by eyewitness
     b. Physical examination
     c. Skeletal survey
  2. Probable abuse: most information indicates an act of commission but was not beyond reasonable doubt; unlikely to be the result of an accident
  3. Household violence: not directed at a child
  4. Neglect: complete lack of parental supervision; inadequate food, shelter, clothing
  5. Medical neglect: inadequate medical care
  6. Accident: unpreventable by reasonable parental supervision
  7. Accident resulting from neglect: could have been prevented by reasonable parental supervision (e.g. more than one accidental poisoning)
- Cutaneous manifestations:
  1. Incidence 80–100% of child abuse cases
  2. Unusual findings should make one suspect abuse
     a. Lacerations in a child less than 1 year of age to the face or genitals
     b. Forced ingestions
  3. Common manifestations
     a. Bruises (blunt trauma)
        i   Child <1 year, especially facial bruises
        ii Unusual location (upper lip with torn frenulum, or back of buttocks)
        iii Multiple bruises
        iv Pinch marks on penis or ears
        v   Age of bruise is determined by color. Fresh–3 days: reddish blue, purple, black; 7–10 days: greenish yellow; >8 days: yellow brown; 2–4 weeks: resolution
        vi Linear bruising from rod or stick
        vii Loop marks such as small ropes, cords, belts (Figure 12.10)
        viii Normal (not abuse) bruises are common and found on shins, knees, elbows
     b. Imprints
        i   Buckles
        ii Slap imprints of fingers
        iii Human bites cause crushing injuries, not puncture wounds
     c. Binding or gagging around the ankles, wrists, or mouth means perpetuators are mentally disturbed
     d. Traumatic alopecia – hair pulled or yanked
     e. Thermal burns (Figure 12.11)
        i   4–8% of childhood burn patients have been abused
        ii 28% of tap water burn victims have been abused
        iii Hot water dunking
        iv Cigarette burns
        v   Microwave injuries (baby placed into the microwave oven causes injury to the

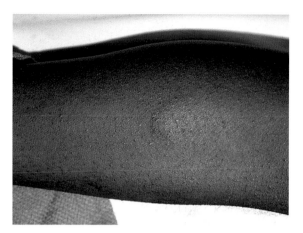

Figure 12.10   Child abuse – loop marks caused by a belt

skin and deeper structures, not the subcutaneous fat)

   vi Branding with a hot object (e.g. curling iron)

   vii Hot water vaporizer: holding the child's face too close which results in burn injuries

   viii Stun gun

  f. Child abuse until proven otherwise:

   i Circumferential burns in child <3 years

   ii Punched out, circular burns implying cigarette burns

   iii Forced immersion causing a doughnut pattern on the buttocks

   iv Gravity pattern of pouring hot fluids, particularly in areas the child could not cause

   v Uniform patterns

  g. Accidental burn prevention: recommend turning the water heater down to 120°F (49°C)

- Physical signs of neglect
  1. Emaciation
  2. Severe diaper dermatitis
  3. Dirty, unkempt
  4. Inappropriate dermatitis for the age (e.g. fire ant bites in a baby)
- Sexual abuse
  1. 90% are female children
  2. Natural father, stepfather or mother's boyfriend is usually the perpetrator
  3. Evidence of assaultive abuse (acute)
     a. Vaginal tears

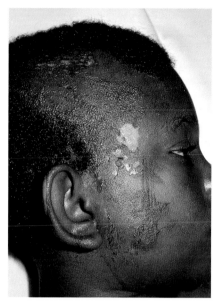

Figure 12.11   Child abuse – facial burn

    b. Anal tears

    c. Hematomas, bruises, petechiae

  4. Evidence of assaultive abuse (previous)

    a. Hymenal distortions

    b. Scarring

  5. Evidence of nonassaultive abuse

    a. Genital herpes simplex

    b. Condyloma accuminata

    c. Any sexually transmitted disease

    d. HIV; mean age of acquiring is 9 years; 64% in females

  6. Examination

    a. Hymenal orifice size with lateral and posterior traction should be <4 mm

    b. Cultures for *Neisseria gonorrhoeae*, *Trichomonas*, *Chylamydia*, herpes simplex, *Gardnerella vaginosis*

    c. Serological tests for syphilis, HIV

- Symptoms which may occur after sexual abuse:
  1. Depression
  2. Dysuria
  3. Encopresis
  4. Excessive masturbation
  5. Hematochezia
  6. Nightmares
  7. Promiscuous behavior
  8. School failure
  9. Sexually inappropriate behavior

10. Sleep disturbances
11. Suicide gestures
12. Substance abuse
13. Urinary tract infection
14. Vaginal bleeding or discharge
- Symptoms of noncutaneous child abuse:
  1. Head injury
  2. Shaking injuries
  3. Abdominal injury (kicking, slamming against an object)

Pathogenesis

- Nonaccidental injury to a child

Diagnosis

- Maintain a high index of suspicion
- Suspect child abuse in the following circumstances:
  1. Physical features
  2. Unusual behavior
  3. Family characteristics
  4. Actions of parents
- Clues which aid in diagnosis
  1. Injury inconsistent with history
  2. Changing history
  3. Delay in seeking medical attention
  4. Evidence of neglect
  5. Injury blamed on someone else
  6. Evidence of doctor shopping
  7. Extremely passive or fearful child
  8. High-risk family situation
     a. History of abuse to parent, sibling or patient
     b. Disorganized family relationships
     c. Parental history of drug or alcohol abuse or psychosis
     d. Child perceived as 'special'. Parent thinks the child 'deserves what he gets'
     e. No family support systems

Differential diagnosis

(See Table 12.4)

Treatment

- Evaluation and acute management (Table 12.5)
- Criteria for suspecting child abuse (Tables 12.6–12.8)
- Physicians are mandated to report child abuse or sexual abuse in all 50 states in the USA
  1. Report to child protective services

2. Anticipate hostility and explain your role as a child's advocate
3. Good photographs are imperative to document injuries
- Treat sexually transmitted diseases
- Refer for psychological counseling, social services
- Testify in court if necessary
- Provide support and follow-up care for the patient and family

Prognosis

- Poor prognosis unless intervention occurs
- Can be self-perpetuating in subsequent generations

References

American Academy of Pediatrics, and American Academy of Pediatric Dentistry. Oral and dental aspects of child abuse and neglect. Pediatrics 1999; 104: 348

Bar-on ME, Zanga JR. Child abuse: a model for the use of structured clinical forms. Pediatrics 1996: 98: 429–33

Carroll ST, Riffenburgh RH, Roberts TA, Myhre EB. Tattoos and body piercings as indicators of adolescent risk-taking behaviors. Pediatrics 2002; 109: 1021–7

Cohen JA, Mannarino AP, Zhitova AC, Capone ME. Treating child abuse-related posttraumatic stress and comorbid substance abuse in adolescents. Child Abuse Neglect 2003; 27: 1345–65

Dubowitz H, Black M, Harringon D. The diagnosis of child sexual abuse. Am J Dis Child 1992; 146: 688–93

Duhaime A-C, Christian CW, Rorke LB, Zimmerman RA. Nonaccidental head injury in infants – the 'shaken-baby syndrome'. N Engl J Med 1998; 338: 1822–9

Gutman LT, Herman-Giddens ME, Phelps WC. Transmission of human genital papillomavirus disease: comparison data from adults and children. Pediatrics 1993; 91: 31–8

Kivlahan C, Druse R, Furnell D. Sexual assault examinations in children. Am J Dis Child 1992; 146: 1365–70

Ledbetter EO. An ethical approach to intervention/prevention of child maltreatment. Adv Pediatr 2003; 50: 215–29

Raimer BG, Raimer SS, Hebeler JR. Cutaneous signs of child abuse. J Am Acad Dermatol 1981; 5: 203–12

Schachner LA, Hankin D. Assessing child abuse in the dermatologist's office. Adv Dermatol 1988; 3: 61–74

Stiffman MN, Schnitzer PG, Adam P, et al. Household composition and risk of fatal child maltreatment. Pediatrics 2002; 109: 615–21

Wissow LS. Child abuse and neglect. Review. N Engl J Med 1995; 332: 1425–31

Table 12.4   Differential diagnosis of child abuse

Clinical findings	Differential diagnosis	Differential tests
Bruising	Trauma	Skin biopsy
	Hemophilia	Partial thromoplastin time
	Von Willebrand disease	Bleeding time
	Henoch–Schönlein purpura	Rule out sepsis, and other causes of vasculitis
	Purpura fulminans	Rule out sepsis with cultures
	Ehlers–Danlos syndrome	Hyperextensibility of joints
Local erythema or bullae	Thermal burn	History
	Staphylococcal impetigo	Culture, Gram stain
	Bacterial cellulitis	Culture, Gram stain
	Pyoderma gangrenosum	Culture, Gram stain, biopsy
	Photosensitivity/phototoxicity	History of sensitizing agent (oral or topical)
	Frostbite	Clinical history and characteristics
	Herpes simplex or zoster	Tzanck smear, viral culture
	Epidermolysis bullosa	Skin biopsy, family history
	Contact dermatitis, allergic or irritant	Clinical characteristics, patch testing
	Lichen sclerosis	Clinical characteristics, skin biopsy
	Vulvar pemphigoid	Skin biopsy, direct immunofluorescence

DERMATITIS ARTEFACTA

Synonym: factitial dermatitis

Major points

- Created by self-induced lesions of the skin
- Motive is usually subconscious
- Female/male ratio >1
- Single or multiple skin lesions range from vesicles to purpura, often with bizarre or unnatural appearance and angulated borders (Figures 12.12 and 12.13)
- Patient usually denies doing it
- Munchausen syndrome by proxy
  1. Caused by parent inflicting injury on the child
  2. Readily seeks medical advice, multiple doctors
  3. Parent never leaves the bedside
  4. Perplexing problem to physicians
  5. Unexplained fever, cellulitis, seizures
  6. Injuries caused by caustic solutions, fingernails or implements
  7. Blood in the urine, vomit, sputum

Pathogenesis

- Psychocutaneous disorder where patients cause cutaneous lesions as a means to satisfy a psychological need of which they are not always consciously aware

Table 12.5   Evaluation and management of the abused child

Detailed history (medical and social)
Physical examination
Examine entire cutaneous surface (oral, rectal, genital mucosa, retina, tympanic membranes)
Laboratory data (complete blood count, serology, appropriate cultures)
Treatment of acute injuries or infections
Radiographs (skeletal survey)
Documentation in case records with photographs, diagrams, videos, as indicated
Report to a local child protective service agency by telephone followed by a detailed written report
Protection of the child from further injury

Diagnosis

- Lesions can mimic any dermatosis
- Difficult to make a diagnosis; other primary skin disorders must be ruled out
- Histology: early signs of injury without inflammatory response; material injected; can vary

Table 12.6 Checklist criteria for suspecting child abuse

Physical findings:
Fresh bruises; unusual locations or shapes
Old scars; unusual locations or shapes
Past or current burns; unusual shapes
Signs of rectal, genital injury

Medical experience, abuse or neglect suggested by:
Current medical problems
Prior medical problems
Prior emergency visits – ingestions or trauma
Prior hospitalizations
Current or past venereal disease or pregnancy
Poor compliance
Incomplete immunizations
Poor physical or developmental growth

Behavioral abnormalities with evidence of:
Withdrawal
Overcompliance
Compliant posturing
Phobias
Sleep problems
Recent onset of enuresis or encopresis
Sexualized play
Excessive interest in genitalia
Inappropriate or excessive masturbation

Psychosocial conditions with evidence of:
Disturbed parent–child interaction
Violent interaction between parents
Violent interaction between siblings
Violent interaction with friends and relatives
Parents abused as children
Parents victims of sexual abuse
Extra stresses on the family: marital discord,
  unemployment, alcoholism, substance abuse,
  recent death or illness in the family

Inappropriate custodial care of the child:
Inappropriate responsibilities for a child

Family isolation:
Lack of supportive relatives, friends or neighbors

Previous referrals for abuse or neglect

Adapted from Schachner L, Hankin DE. Assessing child abuse in childhood condyloma accuminatum. J Am Acad Dermatol 1985; 12: 157–60

Table 12.7 Findings specific for sexual abuse

Presence of semen, sperm, or acid phosphatase
Pregnancy
Fresh genital or anal injuries (lacerations, hematomas, ecchymoses, petechiae) in the absence of an adequate accidental explanation
Positive test or culture for syphilis or gonorrhea (not perinatally acquired)
HIV infection (if not acquired perinatally or through intravenous route)
Markedly enlarged hymenal opening for age with associated findings of hymen disruption, including absent hymen, hymenal remnants, or scars in the absence of an adequate accidental or surgical explanation

Table 12.8 Findings suggestive of sexual abuse

Genital or anal *Trichomonas*, *Chlamydia*, condyloma accuminatum, herpes simplex type 2, if not perinatally acquired
Disruptions of hymen tissue, including posterior or lateral angular, absence, and scars
Anal scars outside the midline
Anal skin tags outside the midline
Anal dilatation >15–20 mm without stool in the ampulla
Irregularity of the anal orifice after complete dilatation
Marked dilatation of the hymenal opening, persisting in different examination positions

widely depending upon how lesions were produced

Treatment

- Symptomatic initially
- Psychology referral
- Oral antidepressants

Prognosis

- Best for children in whom the lesions represent a response to transient stress
- In chronic cases, severity can wax and wane

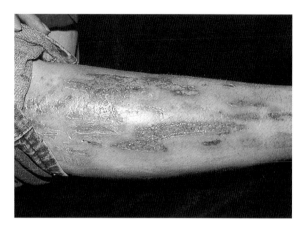

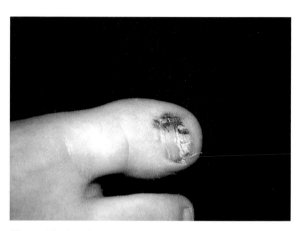

Figure 12.12 Factitial lesions – linear lesions without any signs of dermatitis (published in An Illustrated Dictionary of Dermatologic Syndromes by SB Mallory and S Leal-Khouri)

Figure 12.13 Habitual picking the great toenail

References

Driscoll MS, Rother MJ, Grant-Kels JM, Hale MS. Delusional parasitosis: a dermatologic, psychiatric, and pharmacologic approach. J Am Acad Dermatol 1993; 29: 1023–33

Hettler J. Munchausen syndrome by proxy. Pediatric Emerg Care 2002; 18: 371–6

Joe EK, Li VW, Magro CM, et al. Diagnostic clues to dermatitis artefacta. Cutis 1999; 63: 209–14

Koblenzer CS. Dermatitis artefacta. Clinical features and approaches to treatment. Am J Clin Dermatol 2000; 1: 47–55

Mallory SB, Leal-Khouri S. An illustrated Dictionary of Dermatologic Syndromes. Carnforth, UK: Parthenon Publishing, 1994

Puig L, Perez M, Llaurado A, et al. Factitial dermatosis of the breast: a possible dermatolgic manifestation of Munchausen's syndrome. Cutis 1989; 44: 292–4

13

DRUG ERUPTIONS

GENERAL

- Drug reactions occur in 1–3% of all hospitalized patients
- Reactions can occur through allergic, metabolic or toxic mechanisms
- Patients with allergy to one medicine are at risk of developing other drug allergies
- Disease states may cause eruptions or act as cofactors (e.g. Epstein–Barr virus (EBV) and ampicillin, or HIV and trimethoprim–sulfamethoxazole)
- Predisposing factors
  1. Personal or family history of skin disease
  2. Environmental exposure to other etiologic agents (e.g. sunlight)
- Some drugs have a very low incidence of drug eruption (Table 13.1)

TYPES OF REACTION

Morbilliform (maculopapular type) eruption

- Most common type of reaction causing ~40% of all reactions
- Symmetric erythematous blanchable macules and papules which coalesce into patches and plaques; can become pustular (Figures 13.1 and 13.2)
- Lesions tend to begin on extremities or in areas of pressure or trauma
- Variable involvement of mucous membranes, palms and soles

Table 13.1   Drugs with a low incidence of cutaneous reactions
Acetaminophen
Acyclovir
Aspirin
Aminophylline
Atropine
Chloral hydrate
Chlorpromazine
Cimetidine
Codeine
Desloratadine (Clarinex)
Digoxin
Diphenhydramine
Estrogens
Ferrous sulfate
Fexofenadine (Allegra)
Folic acid
Heparin
Hydroxyzine
Lidocaine hydrochloride
Magnesium sulfate
Methyldopa
Milk of magnesia
Morphine
Multivitamins
Nitroglycerin
Oral contraceptives
Potassium chloride
Prednisone/prednisolone
Promethazine hydrochloride
Propranolol
Regular insulin
Spironolactone
Tetracycline
Warfarin sodium

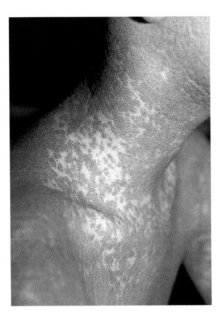

Figure 13.1   Morbilliform drug eruption from penicillin

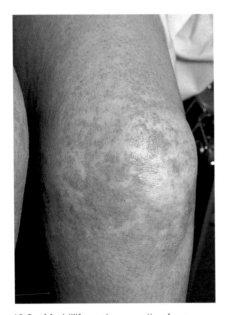

Figure 13.2   Morbilliform drug eruption from trimethoprim–sulfamethoxazole

- Usual time period between ingestion and drug eruption is 1–2 weeks
- Rash usually lasts 1–2 weeks
- Low-grade fever common
- Rash may not recur with rechallenge
- Main causes: Table 13.2

Table 13.2   Common causes of drug reactions
Amoxicillin
Amphotericin B
Ampicillin
Barbiturates
Blood products
Captopril
Carbamazepine
Cephalosporins
Chlorothiazide
Diazepam
Erythromycin
Furosemide
Gentamicin sulfate
Hydralazine
Hydrochlorothiazide
Isoniazid
Mercurial diuretics
Naproxen
Opiates
Penicillin
Phenytoin
Radiologic dyes
Thiazides
Trimethoprim–sulfamethoxazole

1. Ampicillin (patients with infectious mononucleosis have an incidence of >50%)
2. Trimethoprim–sulfamethoxazole (incidence >60% in HIV patients)
3. Penicillin derivatives
4. Antiepileptic drugs

Urticaria

- Red wheals occur which are very pruritic, ranging in size from pinpoint to >20 cm and last <24 hours (Figure 13.3)
- Immediate reactions: reactions occur within minutes to hours
- Accelerated reactions: reactions occur 12–36 hours after exposure
- Angioedema (deep dermal swelling) may involve mucous membranes
- Anaphylaxis can occur with subsequent administration of the offending drug
- Caused by the degranulation of mast cells with release of histamine and other mediators
- Most common offending drugs causing urticaria:
  1. Penicillins

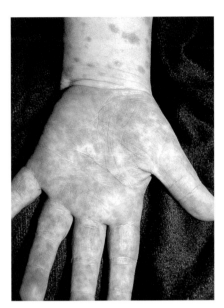

Figure 13.3 Urticarial drug eruption involving palms and soles

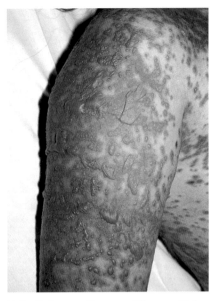

Figure 13.4 Bullous erythema multiforme which progressed into toxic epidermal necrolysis

2. Cephalosporins
3. Sulfonamides
4. Blood products
5. Radiographic dyes
6. Opiates
7. Curare
8. Aspirin
9. Nonsteroidal anti-inflammatory agents
10. Benzoates (in foods)
11. Food dyes (FD&C yellow dye no. 5)

Erythema multiforme

See Chapter 11
- Hypersensitivity caused by a drug, infection (e.g. herpes simplex or mycoplasma) or other cause
- Target-shaped lesions with urticaria or bullae (Figure 13.4)
- Onset is sudden and often associated with malaise and sore throat
- Stevens–Johnson syndrome – severe cutaneous lesions with mucous membrane involvement
- Most common drugs involved:
  1. Sulfonamides
  2. Phenytoin
  3. Barbiturates
  4. Penicillins
  5. Cephalosporins

Toxic epidermal necrolysis

See Table 13.3
- Most serious cutaneous drug reaction
- Skin turns red, and the epidermis peels in large sheets, leaving a moist very tender base (Figure 13.5)
- Usually caused by a drug
- Examples:
  1. Phenytoin
  2. Sulfonamides
  3. Nonsteroidal anti-inflammatory agents

Drug-induced hypersensitivity

See Table 13.4
- Multisystemic idiosyncratic drug reaction
- Fever, rash, lymphadenopathy, hepatitis, eosinophilia, leukocytosis
- Female/male ratio = 1
- Begins 7–60 days (mean 17 days) after starting suspected drug
- Rash (Figures 13.6 and 13.7)
  1. Begins as morbilliform on face, upper trunk
  2. Can progress to erythroderma or chronic exfoliative dermatitis
  3. Can have vesicles, bullae, petechiae, purpura, edema

Table 13.3   Findings associated with serious cutaneous drug eruptions

Cutaneous
Marked erythema
Edema, particularly facial
Cutaneous pain
Palpable purpura
Skin necrosis
Bullae
Positive Nikolsky sign
Mucous membrane involvement
Urticaria

Other findings
Fever >40°C
Arthralgias/arthritis
Pulmonary symptoms (shortness of breath, wheezing)
Hypotension

Laboratory abnormalities
Abnormal liver function tests
Elevated eosinophil count
Atypical lymphocytosis

Drugs implicated
Allopurinol
Amoxicillin
Ampicillin
Carbamazepine
Lamotrigine
Phenobarbital
Phenylbutazone
Phenytoin
Piroxicam
Sulfadiazine
Sulfadoxime
Sulfamethoxazole–trimethoprim
Sulfasalazine
Valproic acid

Adapted from: Stern RS, Wintroub BU. Cutaneous reactions to drugs. In Fitzpatrick's Dermatology in General Medicine, 5th edn. Freedberg IM, Eisen AZ, Wolff K, et al. McGraw Hill: New York, 1999: 1633–42

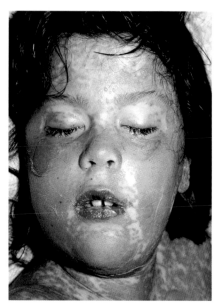

Figure 13.5   Toxic epidermal necrolysis – with sheets of denuded epidermis

   3. Renal (15%)
   4. Pulmonary (14%)
   5. Spleen
   6. Myositis
   7. Pancreatitis
* Can be associated with recent viral or bacterial infection (e.g. EBV, hepatitis B, parvovirus, *Streptococcus*, *Mycoplasma*)
* Treatment
   1. Oral prednisone 0.5–2.0 mg/kg per day
   2. Topical steroids
   3. Supportive care
   4. May need hospitalization
* Pathogenesis
   1. Possible defect in epoxide hydrolase enzymatic pathway which normally degrades toxic arene oxide metabolites formed during oxidation of antiepileptics; arene oxide metabolites may be directly cytotoxic or act as haptens, leading to hypersensitivity reaction
   2. Sulfonamides – possible defect in glutathione transferase-mediated enzymatic breakdown

Serum sickness

* Type III immune complex disease caused by deposition of circulating immune complexes in

   4. Mucous membrane findings subtle (erythema, petechiae)
* Systemic involvement
   1. Liver (61%)
   2. Hematologic (48%) – eosinophilia, leukocytosis, reactive lymphocytosis, leukopenia, anemia

Table 13.4   Drugs associated with hypersensitivity syndrome
Aromatic anticonvulsants Carbamazepine Phenobarbital Phenytoin Primidone **Nonaromatic anticonvulsants** Lamotrigine Valproic acid Ethosuxidimide **Sulfa drugs** Dapsone Sulfasalazine Sulfonamides Sulfamethoxazole **Others** Allopurinol Diltiazem Minocycline Terbinafine

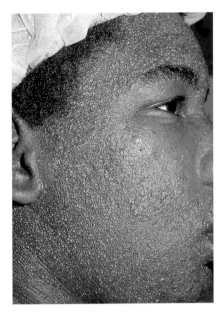

Figure 13.6   Drug-induced hypersensitivity from phenytoin

blood vessels and other tissues, activating the complement cascade
- Characterized by urticaria, morbilliform eruption, vasculitis, fever, arthralgia, lymphadenopathy, gastrointestinal disturbance, renal disease

Serum sickness-like reaction

- Characterized by rash (urticarial, maculopapular, erythema multiforme-like angioedema), fever, arthralgias, lymphadenopathy, eosinophilia (Figure 13.8)
- No circulating immune complexes, vasculitis or renal disease
- Usually starts 1–3 weeks after administration of offending drug
- Common drugs: cefaclor, amoxicillin, ampicillin, β-blockers, cefprozil, cephalexin, doxycycline, minocycline, penicillin, sulfonamide

Erythema nodosum

- Red, tender subcutaneous nodules, usually located on the anterior lower legs
- May be caused by drugs, infection, inflammatory bowel disease or other causes

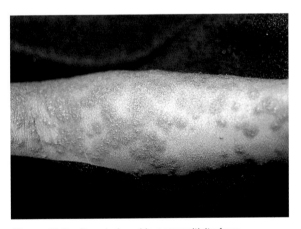

Figure 13.7   Drug-induced hypersensitivity from phenytoin with erythematous plaques

- Common drugs:
    1. Oral contraceptives
    2. Sulfonamides
    3. Sulfonylureas

Photosensitivity eruptions

See Table 13.5
- Action spectrum is long-wave ultraviolet light (UVA)

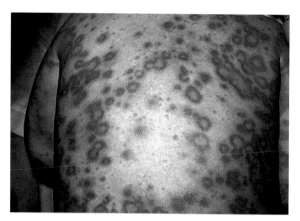

Figure 13.8 Serum sickness-like eruption from a cephalosporin

- Phototoxic reactions are characterized by an exaggerated sunburn reaction
  1. Does not involve immunologic mechanisms
  2. Severity is dose-related
  3. Phototoxic agents generally have a resonating chemical structure capable of absorbing photons of ultraviolet light and moving to an excited state, thus producing damage to cells
  4. Examples: psoralen, tetracyclines
- Photoallergic responses involve primarily type IV reactions
  1. Not dose-related
  2. Occurs in a sensitized individual
  3. Examples: chlorpromazine, sulfanilamide, thiazides, sulfonylureas
- Topical photosensitizers
  1. Drug applied to the skin and exposed to light causing an eczematous eruption
  2. Examples: para-amino benzoic acid (PABA), phenothiazines, coal tar, oil of bergamot, psoralens

Lichenoid drug eruption

- Purple-red, flat-topped, pruritic papules, similar to lichen planus
- Often photo-distributed
- Examples: gold, antimalarials, phenothiazines, captopril, β-blockers and thiazide diuretics

Fixed drug eruption

- Well-demarcated, red to brown plaque with dusky center

Table 13.5   Drugs and chemicals that cause photosensitivity reactions

Antidepressants	
Amitriptyline	Desipramine
Doxepin	Imipramine
Nortriptyline	
Antihistamines	
Cyproheptadine	Diphenhydramine
Antimetabolic drugs	
Actinomycin	Methotrexate
Doxorubicin	Vinblastine
5-fluorouracil	Hydroxyurea
Antimicrobials	
Ciprofloxacin	Doxycycline
Enoxacin	Griseofulvin
Minocycline	Nalidixic acid
Sulfasalazine	Tetracycline
Sulfamethoxazole–trimethoprim	
Antiparasitic drugs	
Chloroquine	Quinine
Diuretics	
Acetazolamide	Chlorothiazide
Furosemide	Hydrochlorothiazide
Nonsteroidal anti-inflammatory drugs	
Ketoprofen	Naproxen
Piroxicam	Sulindac
Psychiatric drugs	
Chlorpromazine	Haloperidol
Tricylic antidepressants	
Other agents	
Acetretin	Amiodarone
Captopril	Carbamazepine
Gold salts	Isotretinoin
Oral contraceptives	Promethazine
Psoralen	Quinidine

- Lesions appear at the same sites after each administration of the medication
- May become vesicular or bullous periodically with introduction of the offending medicine; chronically becomes a hyperpigmented patch (Figure 13.9)
- Location is usually hands, feet, face and genitalia, but can occur anywhere, including mucosal surfaces

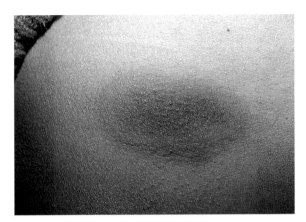

Figure 13.9 Fixed drug eruption – with typical dark center and erythematous halo

- Lesions are solitary or multiple
- Common offenders:
  1. Trimethoprim–sulfamethoxazole
  2. Ampicillin
  3. Amoxicillin
  4. Erythromycin
  5. Phenolphthalein
  6. Tetracycline
  7. Barbiturates
  8. Ibuprofen

Lupus-like reactions

- Difficult to tell the difference between lupus and drug-induced lupus reaction
- Erythema in the butterfly malar distribution and V of the neck
- Usually: antinuclear antibody-positive, antihistone antibody-positive, antidouble-stranded DNA antibody-negative
- Renal involvement less common in drug-induced lupus
- Examples: minocycline, procainamide, hydralazine (in patients who are slow acetylators), isoniazid, phenytoin, penicillamine

Pigmentary changes

- Mechanisms: drugs stimulate melanocytic activity or deposit drug in tissues (Figure 13.10)
- Examples:
  1. Heavy metals (gold, silver, mercury)
  2. Phenothiazines

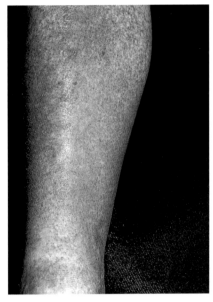

Figure 13.10 Gray pigmentation of the skin – caused by minocycline

  3. Antimalarials
  4. Cytotoxic agents (bleomycin)
  5. Hydantoin
  6. Tetracyclines

Vasculitis

- Palpable purpura with concentration on the lower extremities
- May involve other organs (e.g. liver, kidney, brain and joints)
- Examples: penicillin, phenytoin, thiazides

Acneiform eruptions

- Follicular papules and pustules in an acne distribution, often sudden in onset
- Causes: corticosteroids, oral contraceptives, halogens, hydantoin, lithium

Alopecia

- Anagen arrest caused by cytotoxic agents
- Telogen effluvium caused by anticoagulants, oral contraceptives and β-blockers
- Androgenetic alopecia caused by oral contraceptives

SPECIFIC DRUGS CAUSING REACTIONS

Penicillin

- Reactions range from 16 to 52 per 1000 recipients or 5–10% of the population
- Increased use of penicillin increases the risk of developing allergy
- Route of administration: parenterally administered drugs cause more reactions than those administered orally
- Certain diseases (e.g. infection with EBV, HIV, cytomegalovirus (CMV), etc.) may cause an increased risk of reaction
- Manifestations:
    1. Maculopapular and/or papulosquamous reactions most common (associated with IgM antibodies)
    2. Urticarial reactions – risk of developing anaphylaxis on subsequent exposure
- Penicillin can cause any of the four types of immunologic reactions
- Testing available to diagnose allergy to certain components of penicillin

Cephalosporins

- Erythema which progresses to 'purple urticaria' (not true erythema multiforme), with cutaneous swelling (especially feet), migratory pruritic lesions
- No adenopathy
- Serum-sickness-like picture
- Hypersensitivity occurs in ~3% of patients

Corticosteroids

- Occurs from oral, parenteral, or topical application of corticosteroids
- Manifestations:
    1. Acneiform eruptions
    2. Striae (Figure 13.11)
    3. 'Moon facies' caused by fat deposition in the cheeks
    4. 'Buffalo hump' caused by fat deposition on the upper back
    5. Telangiectasias
    6. Atrophy
    7. Masking of other dermatoses (e.g. tinea, scabies)

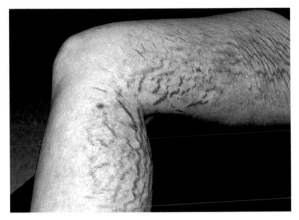

Figure 13.11   Striae caused by corticosteroids

Antiepileptic drugs

- Characteristic syndrome of maculopapular rash, fever, facial edema, lymphadenopathy, leukocytosis, hepatitis, nephritis, pneumonitis (see Drug-induced hypersensitivity)
- Most patients develop this syndrome within 2 months of starting the drug
- Cross-sensitivity with phenytoin, carbamazepine and phenobarbital
- Lamotrigine, which is structurally dissimilar, can also cause this reaction

Tetracyclines

- Phototoxic reactions
- Onycholysis
- Fixed drug eruptions
- Staining of teeth
- Hyperpigmentation
- Serum sickness-like reactions
- Drug-induced lupus (e.g. minocycline)
- Urticaria
- Morbilliform eruptions

Gold

- Reactions occur in about one-third to one-half of patients
- Clinical manifestations:
    1. Lichenoid reactions
    2. Papulosquamous reactions (resembling pityriasis rosea)
    3. Exfoliative dermatitis

4. Morbilliform eruptions
5. Erythema nodosum
- Chrysiasis can occur after prolonged use, resulting from deposition of gold salts in the skin, causing blue pigmentation of the skin and ocular conjunctiva

Antimetabolites (chemotherapy)

- Anagen effluvium (alopecia) caused by the sudden weakening of hair and subsequent breakage
- Stomatitis caused by toxic effect on mucosal cells which have a high mitotic rate
- Acneiform eruptions (e.g. actinomycin-D)
- Onychodystrophy (e.g. bleomycin, hydroxyurea, 5-fluorouracil)
- Chemical cellulitis/phlebitis/ulceration from intravenous extravasation

Lithium

- Aggravation of acne and psoriasis

Iodides and bromides

- Acneiform eruptions
- Granulomatous fungating lesions (halogenodermas)

Antimalarials

- Increased pigmentation (black or yellow) of skin and mucous membranes
- Lichenoid eruptions
- Erythema annulare centrifugum

Sulfonamides and thiazides

- Thiazides are substituted sulfonamides and may cross-react with sulfonamide antibiotics
- Urticaria
- Morbilliform eruptions
- Erythema multiforme
- Vasculitis
- Toxic epidermal necrolysis

Nonsteroidal anti-inflammatory drugs

- Morbilliform eruptions
- Bullous fixed drug eruptions

- Vasculitis
- Pseudoporphyria – blistering, erosions and scarring on dorsa of hands, and bridge of nose

Coumadin

- Sharply – demarcated, erythematous, purpuric plaques which become necrotic and form an eschar
- Lesions occur between days 3 and 10 of anticoagulant therapy
- Thrombosis due to a relative drop in circulating protein C levels

Pathogenesis

- Molecular characteristics
  1. Increases in molecular size and complexity are associated with increased immunologic reactions
  2. Small molecules form stable bonds with tissue macromolecules forming haptens
- Environmental/other factors
  1. Viral infections can alter the host response, increasing the frequency of reactions (e.g. mononucleosis or HIV plus ampicillin-induced morbilliform eruptions)
  2. Light exposure with photoallergic reactions (e.g. tetracyclines)
  3. Associated diseases: systemic lupus erythematosus predisposes to developing reactions
  4. Genetic factors: deficiency in epoxide hydrolase, an enzyme required for metabolism of a toxic epoxide derived from aromatic anticonvulsants such as phenytoin, carbamazepine and phenobarbital
- Nonimmunologic methods
  1. Drugs may release mast cell mediators directly, causing urticaria (e.g. opiates, curare, radiocontrast media)
  2. Drugs may activate complement in the absence of antibody
  3. Drugs may alter the pathway of arachidonic acid metabolism (e.g. aspirin)
  4. Individual metabolic variation (e.g. defect in clearing reactive intermediate metabolites with thiazides and sulfonamides)
- Type 1 immunologic reactions:
  1. Mediated by IgE
  2. Result in varying degrees of urticaria, pruritus, bronchospasm and anaphylaxis

3. Immediate reactions occur within minutes after exposure
4. Accelerated reactions occur hours or days after drug exposure
5. Production of IgE directed against the drug or drug–hapten complex
6. Drug molecules in general are usually small enough so that they cannot initiate an immune reaction by themselves but require a carrier protein
7. Re-exposure to drug plus antibodies of IgE cause mast cells to release histamine, slow reacting substance of anaphylaxis (SRS-A), eosinophil chemotactic factor of anaphylaxis, neutrophil chemotactic factors and platelet activating factor
8. Examples: penicilloyl polylysin
- Type 2 immunologic reactions (cytotoxic antibody reaction):
  1. Mediated by cytotoxic antibodies
  2. Specific antigens combine with endogenous tissue components which, when combined, act as an antigen, stimulating the formation of antibodies
  3. Antibodies coat the target tissue and stimulate complement activation and tissue destruction
- Type 3 immunologic reactions (immune complex reaction):
  1. Most drug reactions are caused by this type of reaction: serum sickness, possibly erythema multiforme and erythema nodosum
  2. Classic reaction pattern is serum sickness with fever, arthritis, nephritis, neuritis, edema and urticarial or morbilliform eruptions
  3. Symptoms develop >6 days after exposure
  4. Drug or drug–protein complex acts as an antigen, which stimulates antibody production
  5. Sensitization occurs during first exposure with subsequent antibody formation, usually IgG or IgM
  6. When the concentration of antibodies is high enough, there is formation of large immune complexes
  7. Various sizes of immune complex result; size depends upon the rate of antibody production and immune complex clearance rates
  8. Some immune complexes deposit in the peripheral circulation, where they stimulate inflammation and destroy local tissues

9. Products of the complement cascade, especially C5a and C3a, can degranulate mast cells causing urticaria
- Type 4 immunologic reactions (cell-mediated type):
  1. Keratinocytes are activated and express various cytokines
  2. Associated with morbilliform reactions to some oral drugs (e.g. amoxicillin)
  3. Common as the cause of contact dermatitis (e.g. neomycin)
- Fixed drug eruption:
  1. Histology: superficial and deep perivascular infiltrate with lymphocytes, eosinophils, some neutrophils and necrotic keratinocytes in the epidermis
  2. Hypothesis that intercellular adhesion molecule-1 (ICAM-1) plays a role in site restriction

Diagnosis

- Clinical evaluation:
  1. History of taking drug
  2. Alternative explanations for the rash (e.g. viral causes, contact history)
  3. Timing of drug exposure with flow chart
  4. Removal of the offending agent
  5. Response to rechallenge
- Laboratory tests:
  1. Drug levels
  2. Complete blood count with differential
  3. Liver function tests
  4. Specific drug evaluations:
     a. Penicillin: skin tests
     b. Radioallergosorbent test (RAST) measures specific serum IgE against specific drug
- Histology:
  1. Sparse mixed inflammatory cell infiltrate with eosinophils
  2. Slight vacuolar alteration
  3. Scattered dyskeratotic keratinocytes
  4. Lichenoid drug eruption resembles lichen planus with eosinophils and a deep infiltrate
  5. Fixed drug eruption shows keratinocyte necrosis, melanophages in the papillary dermis and a superficial and deep infiltrate

Differential diagnosis

- Morbilliform drug eruptions
  1. Viral eruption
  2. Miliaria rubra

3. Graft-versus-host disease
4. Kawasaki syndrome
- Urticaria
  1. Insect bites
  2. Vasculitis
- Erythema multiforme
  1. Urticaria
  2. Kawasaki syndrome
- Erythema nodosum
  1. Ecchymoses
  2. Vasculitis
- Photosensitive eruptions
  1. Sunburn
  2. Contact dermatitis
  3. Eczema
- Lupus-like reactions
  1. Systemic lupus erythematosus

Treatment

- Discontinue offending drug
- Supportive therapy as indicated by clinical picture
- Corticosteroids early (prednisone 1–2 mg/kg per day)
- Antihistamines
- Topical antipruritic agents
- Baths, with or without additives (e.g. oatmeal)
- Intravenous immunoglobulins for toxic epidermal necrolysis
- If patient is at risk for anaphylaxis or severe reaction, a medical alert bracelet is warranted
- Consider desensitization if drug is necessary

Prognosis

- Resolution with cessation of drug
- Some pigmentation or scarring can be permanent

References

Barbaud AM, Bene M-C, Schmutz J-L, et al. Role of delayed cellular hypersensitivity and adhesion molecules in amoxicillin-induced morbilliform rashes. Arch Dermatol 1997; 133: 481–6

Callot V, Roujeau J-C, Bagot M, et al. Drug-induced pseudolymphoma and hypersensitivity syndrome. Arch Dermatol 1996; 132: 1315–21

Carroll MC, Yueng-Yue KA, Esterly NB, Drolet BA. Drug-induced hypersensitivity syndrome in pediatric patients. Pediatrics 2001; 108: 485–93

Caumes E, Guermonprez G, Lecomte C, et al. Efficacy and safety of desensitization with sulfmethoxazole and trimethoprim in 48 previously hypersensitive patients infected with human immunodeficiency virus. Arch Dermatol 1997; 133: 465–9

Chosidow O, Bourgault I, Roujeau J-C. Drug rashes. What are the targets of cell-mediated cytotoxicity? Arch Dermatol 1994; 130: 627–9

Gonzalez E, Gonzalez S. Drug photosensitivity, idiopathic photodermatoses, and sunscreens. J Am Acad Dermatol 1996; 35: 871–85

Halevy S, Shai A. Lichenoid drug eruptions. J Am Acad Dermatol 1993; 29: 249–55

Hawfield W, Goodrich R, Warren S, Morrell D. Trauma-induced cutaneous pigmentation from tetracycline: a case report. Pediatr Dermatol 2004; 21: 164–6

Hebert AA, Sigman ES, Levy ML. Serum sickness-like reactions from cefaclor in children. J Am Acad Dermatol 1991; 25: 805–8

Huang Y-L, Hong H-S, Wang Z-W, Kuo T-T. Fatal sodium valproate-induced hypersensitivity syndrome with lichenoid dermatitis and fulminant hepatitis. J Am Acad Dermatol 2003; 49: 316–19

Kaur S, Sarkar R, Thami G, Kanwar AJ. Anticonvulsant hypersensitivity syndrome. Pediatr Dermatol 2002; 19: 142–5

Lee WM. Drug-induced hepatotoxicity. N Engl J Med 1995; 333: 1118–27

Levy ML, Barron KS, Eichenfield L, Honig PJ. Naproxen-induced pseudoporphyria: a distinctive photodermatitis. J Pediatr 1990; 117: 660–4

Litt JZ. Drug Eruption Reference Manual, 9th edn. Parthenon Publishing: New York, 2003

Ming ME, Bhawan J, Stefanato CM, et al. Imipramine-induced hyperpigmentation: four cases and a review of the literature. J Am Acad Dermatol 1999; 40: 159–66

Morelli JG, Tay Y-K, Rogers M, et al. Fixed drug eruptions in children. J Pediatr 1999; 134: 365–7

Nigen S, Knowles SR, Shear NH. Drug eruptions – approaching the diagnosis of drug-induced skin diseases. J Drugs Dermatol 2003; 3: 278–99

Sehgal VN, Srivastava G, Sardana K. Erythroderma/exfoliative dermatitis: a synopsis. Int J Dermatol 2004; 43: 39–47

Shapiro LE, Shear NH. Drug interactions: proteins, pumps, and p-450s. J Am Acad Dermatol 2002; 47: 467–84

Shapiro LE, Knowles SR, Shear NH. Comparative safety of tetracycline, minocycline and doxycycline. Arch Dermatol 1997; 133: 1224–30

Stern RS, Wintroub BU. Cutaneous reactions to drugs. In Fitzpatrick's Dermatology in General Medicine, 5th edn. Freedberg IM, Eisen AZ, Wolff K, et al., eds. McGraw Hill: New York, 1999: 1633–42

Tristani-Firouzi P, Petersen MJ, Saffle JR, et al. Treatment of toxic epidermal necrolysis with intravenous immunoglobulin in children. J Am Acad Dermatol 2002; 47: 548–52

14

PIGMENTARY DISORDERS

LINES OF BLASCHKO

- A form of mosaicism with two or more genetically distinct cell lines arising from a postzygotic somatic mutation (see Table 17.1)
- Follow segmental and linear skin lines which are V-shaped or a circling pattern on the chest and a linear distribution on the extremities
- Should not be confused with dermatomes, which are areas of the skin innervated by sensory nerves
- Can be hypopigmented (e.g. hypomelanosis of Ito), hyperpigmented (e.g. linear and whorled hypermelanosis), or verrucous (e.g. epidermal nevus), depending upon the type of defect

References

Bolognia JL, Orlow SJ, Glick SA. Lines of Blaschko. J Am Acad Dermatol 1994; 31: 157–90

Danarti R, Bittar M, Happle R, Konig A. Linear atrophoderma of Moulin: postulation of mosaicism for a predisposing gene. J Am Acad Dermatol 2003; 49: 492–8

Duran-McKinster C, Moises C, Rodriguez-Jurado R, et al. Streptococcal exanthem in a Blaschkolinear pattern: clinical evidence for genetic mosaicism in hypomelanosis of Ito. Pediatr Dermatol 2002; 19: 423–5

Happle R, Assim A. The lines of Blaschko on the head and neck. J Am Acad Dermatol 2001; 44: 612–15

Kabbash C, Laude TA, Weinberg JM, Silverberg NB. Lichen planus in the lines of Blaschko. Pediatr Dermatol 2002; 19: 541–5

Nehal KS, DeBenito R, Orlow SJ. Analysis of 54 cases of hypopigmentation and hyperpigmentation along the lines of Blaschko. Arch Dermatol 1996; 132: 1167–70

Rott HD. Extracutaneous analogies of Blaschko lines. Am J Med Genet 1999; 85: 338–41

HYPERPIGMENTED DISORDERS

Postinflammatory hyperpigmentation

Major points

- Most common cause of increased pigmentation in childhood
- Follows an inflammatory process or traumatic injury to the epidermis, especially following atopic dermatitis, contact dermatitis, or lichen planus (Figure 14.1)
- Lesions usually localized and follow the distribution of the resolving skin disorder
- More common in dark skin types

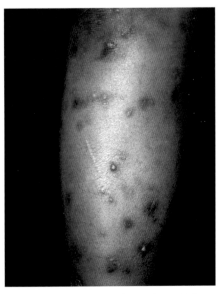

Figure 14.1 Postinflammatory hyperpigmentation following insect bites

Pathogenesis

- Histology: aberrant delivery of melanin to the surrounding keratinocytes and deposition of pigment in the dermal melanophages

Diagnosis

- Clinical presentation

Differential diagnosis

- Café au lait macule
- Becker nevus
- Nevus spilus

Treatment

- No treatment is very effective
- Hydroquinone 2-4% BID may decrease epidermal hyperpigmentation slowly

Prognosis

- After inflammation is resolved, hyperpigmentation fades slowly over many months

References

Ruiz-Maldonado R, Orozco-Covarrubias ML. Postinflammatory hypopigmentation and hyperpigmentation. Semin Cutan Med Surg 1997; 16: 36–43

Generalized hyperpigmentation

Major points

- Widespread accentuation of normal areas of melanin pigmentation all over the body with marked increases in skin creases of palms and soles and mucous membranes
- Generalized hyperpigmentation should be differentiated from normal variation or from sun exposure
- Causes:
  1. Endocrine abnormalities (e.g. Addison disease, Cushing syndrome, acromegaly, melanotropin-stimulating hormone (MSH) excess) (Figure 14.2)
  2. Certain drugs (e.g. heavy metals, phenothiazines, antimalarials)
  3. Hemochromatosis
  4. Chronic renal disease
  5. Chronic hepatic disease
  6. Scleroderma
  7. AIDS

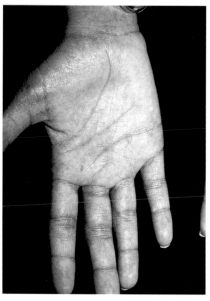

Figure 14.2   Generalized hyperpigmentation caused by Addison disease with accentuation of palmar creases

Pathogenesis

- Etiology depends upon cause of pigmentation
- Melanogenic action of increased pituitary peptides (e.g. MSH in Addison disease)

Diagnosis

- Clinical presentation
- Histology: increased melanin in melanocytes and some melanophages in the dermis

Differential diagnosis

- See Causes (above)

Treatment

- Depends upon the cause of hyperpigmentation
- Discontinuance of medication or treatment of disease does not always improve hyperpigmentation

Prognosis

- Generally permanent, unless caused by a medicine which can be discontinued

References

Fulk CS. Primary disorders of hyperpigmentation. J Am Acad Dermatol 1984; 10: 1–16

Oelkers W. Adrenal insufficiency. N Engl J Med 1996; 335: 1206–12

Congenital nevocellular nevi

Synonym: congenital nevomelanocytic nevi, congenital melanocytic nevi

Major points

- Lesions are apparent at birth or within 1 year of birth (Figure 14.3)
- Surface can be smooth, pebbly, verrucous or lobular
- Pigmentation is usually uniform, medium or dark brown but may have dark brown speckles or black areas. In dark skin, congenital nevocellular nevi (CNN) tend to be more heavily pigmented
- Size ranges from small (2 mm to 1.5 cm) to medium (1.5–19.9 cm) to large (>20 cm) and can cover a large portion of the skin surface
- Except for size, the overall appearance is similar to that of acquired nevi
- Some have coarse long hairs
- Familial tendency has been reported
- CNN of the head or neck (usually large in size) may be associated with leptomeningeal melanocytosis, manifesting as hydrocephalus, seizures, mental retardation, or melanoma, and carries a poor prognosis
- Melanoma arises in ~5–15% in the reported literature

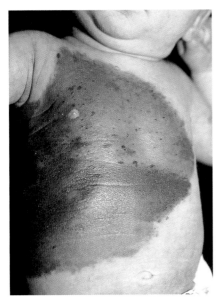

Figure 14.3 Large congenital nevocellular nevus – with variation in color

- Other tumors developing in CNN: schwannoma, neuroid tumor, lipoma, rhabdomyosarcoma, neurofibroma and others

Pathogenesis

- CNN form *in utero* between 8 weeks and 6 months
- Histology: nests, sheets or single nevus cells in the dermis, epidermis and sometimes into subcutaneous tissues with features of neuroid appearance, epithelioid cells and/or spindle cells; involvement around appendageal and neurovascular structures is common

Diagnosis

- Usually clinical, but biopsy might be indicated to confirm the diagnosis in unusual cases

Differential diagnosis

- Mongolian spot
- Café au lait macule
- Lentigo
- Acquired nevocellular nevus
- Nevus sebaceus
- Smooth muscle hamartoma
- Becker nevus

Treatment

- Ulceration, nodules or markedly varied pigmentation suggests the possibility of melanoma and should be biopsied
- Treatment is dependent on perceived risk of melanoma, cosmetic and functional considerations. There is some controversy amongst experts whether excision versus watching is advised
- Excision if indicated; goal is to remove as much of the CNN as possible while preserving function and cosmesis
- Management of extensive CNN should be individualized on a case-by-case basis
- Dermabrasion and other destructive methods may be cosmetically helpful but are controversial

Prognosis

- CNN usually expand in direct proportion to growth of the anatomic site and can actually enlarge. They often darken with time and develop hair; rarely they may become lighter in color

- Incidence of melanoma in CNN is unknown, but ranges from 5 to 15%. In large CNN, half of the cases of melanoma arise before age 5 years
- Prognosis for patients who develop melanoma in a giant CNN is poor, because of early metastasis or late diagnosis

References

DeDavid M, Orlow SJ, Provost N, et al. A study of large congenital melanocytic nevi and associated malignant melanomas: review of cases in the New York University Registry and the world literature. J Am Acad Dermatol 1997; 36: 409–16

Leech SN, Bell H, Leonard N, et al. Neonatal giant congenital nevi with proliferative nodules. Arch Dermatol 2004; 140: 83–8

LoGiudice J, Gosain AK. Pediatric tissue expansion: indications and complications. J Craniofac Surg 2003; 14: 866–72

Management of congenital melanocytic nevi: a decade later. Special Symposium. Pediatr Dermatol 1996; 13: 321–40

Marghoob AA, Borrego JP, Halpern AC. Congenital melanocytic nevi: treatment modalities and management options. Semin Cutan Med Surg 2003; 22: 21–32

Marghoob AA, Schoenbackh SP, Kopf AW, et al Large congenital melanocytic nevi and the risk for the development of malignant melanoma. Arch Dermatol 1996; 132: 170–5

Makkar HS, Frieden IJ. Congenital melanocytic nevi: an update for the pediatrician. Curr Opin Pediatr 2002; 14: 397–403

Shapall S, Frieden I, Chesney M, Newman T. Risk of malignant transformation of congenital melanocytic nevi in blacks. Pediatr Dermatol 1994; 11: 204–8

Zutt M, Kretschmer L, Emmert S, et al. Multicentric malignant melanoma in a giant melanocytic congenital nevus 20 years after dermabrasion in adulthood. Dermatol Surg 2003; 29: 99–101

Acquired melanocytic nevi

Synonyms: pigmented nevi, pigmented moles, melanocytic nevi
Singular: nevus

Major points

- Nevi begin to develop in early childhood as small 1–2 mm pigmented macules
- Lesions slowly enlarge and become papular with age
- Nevi increase in darkening, size and number at puberty
- Most acquired nevi are <0.5 cm in diameter
- The majority of nevi are in sun-exposed areas, particularly the torso, but can be anywhere, including the palms, soles, buttock, scalp
- Types:
  1. Junctional nevus: flat, with nevus cells located at the dermal–epidermal junction
  2. Dermal nevus: dome shaped; nevus cells located within dermis
  3. Compound nevus: slightly elevated dome-shaped hyperpigmented papule with nevus cells at the dermal–epidermal junction and in the dermis
- Dysplastic nevi
  1. Unusually large, variegated in color, often multiple (Figures 14.4 and 14.5)
  2. Common on back and scalp
  3. If numerous, watch for changes of melanoma
- Increased numbers in: atypical mole syndrome, Noonan syndrome, Langer–Giedion syndrome, Turner syndrome, others

Pathogenesis

- Histology: nevus cells at the dermal–epidermal junction, within the dermis, or both
- Nevus cells are thought to arise from the neural crest

Diagnosis

- Clinical presentation

Differential diagnosis

- Congenital nevocelluar nevus
- Folliculitis
- Spitz nevus

Treatment

- Nevi change slowly over months to years; therefore, only observation is warranted
- When indicated, elliptical excision or deep saucerization removal
- Lesion with atypical histology should be excised completely or followed closely for malignant change
- Destructive modes of therapy (e.g. cryotherapy, laser, etc.) not recommended

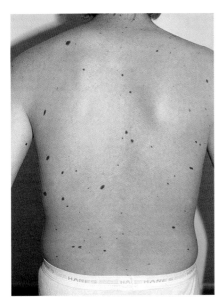

Figure 14.4   Dysplastic nevi – numerous and large nevi

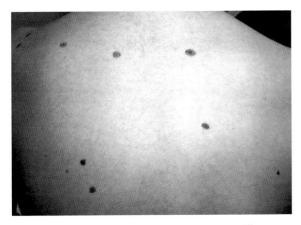

Figure 14.5   Dysplastic nevi – closer view of a different patient. These lesions are all larger than normal and display variegation in color

Prognosis

- Natural course: appearance in childhood, number of lesions peaking in second and third decades then disappearing in seventh to ninth decade
- Majority of CNN are benign, growing in proportion to body growth

References

Bauer J, Garbe C. Acquired melanocytic nevi as risk factor for melanoma development. A comprehensive review of epidemiological data. Pigment Cell Res 2003; 16: 297–306

Drake LA, Ceilley RI, Cornelison RL, et al. Guidelines of care for nevi, II: non-melanocytic nevi, hamartomas, neoplasms, and potentially malignant lesions. J Am Acad Dermatol 1995:32: 104–8

Guidelines of care for nevi, I (nevocellular nevi and seborrheic keratoses). J Am Acad Dermatol 1992; 26: 629–31

Marghoob AA, Orlow SJ, Kopf AW. Syndromes associated with melanocytic nevi. J Am Acad Dermatol 1993; 29: 373–88

Naeyaert JM. Brochez L. Clinical practice. Dysplastic nevi. N Engl J Med 2003; 349: 2233–40

Pope DJ, Sorahan T, Marsen JR, et al. Benign pigmented nevi in children. Arch Dermatol 1992; 128: 1201–6

Salopek TG. The dilemma of the dysplastic nevus. Dermatol Clin 2002; 20: 617–28

Spitz nevus

Synonyms: spindle and epithelioid nevus, benign juvenile melanoma

Major points

- Solitary, reddish brown or dark brown, dome-shaped papule, 0.5–10 mm in size (Figure 14.6)
  1. On face, tends to be reddish brown
  2. On extremities, tends to be brown, mottled or verrucous
- Grows rapidly or slowly for about a year, then stops growing
- Affects children aged 3–13 years, primarily
- No racial or sex predilection
- Solitary lesions most common, but can be agminated or in multiple clusters
- Rare bleeding or pruritus

Pathogenesis

- Presumed to be derived from same progenitor cells giving rise to epidermal melanocytes and nevomelanocytes

Diagnosis

- Histology: nevus cells are large and/or spindle-shaped and slightly pleomorphic with maturation of melanocytes; little or no evidence of upward migration into epidermis

Differential diagnosis

- Pyogenic granuloma
- Hemangioma

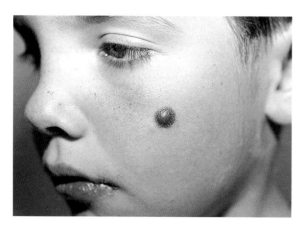

Figure 14.6 Spitz nevus – brown-red papule which appeared quickly on this child's face

- Malignant melanoma
- Juvenile xanthogranuloma
- Mastocytoma
- Acquired intradermal nevus
- Malignant Spitz nevus

Treatment

- Complete excision

Prognosis

- Benign, and do not metastasize
- May persist into adult life, becoming intradermal nevi in some cases
- Some case reports in adults who had 'Spitz nevi' really had melanoma, and therefore in an adult or late teen this diagnosis should be suspect

References

LeBoit PE. 'Safe' Spitz and its alternatives. Pediatr Dermatol 2002; 19: 163–5

Ruiter DJ, van Dijk MC, Ferrier CM. Current diagnostic problems in melanoma pathology. Semin Cutan Med Surg 2003; 22: 33–41

Shimek CM, Golitz LE. The golden anniversary of the Spitz nevus. Arch Dermatol 1999; 135: 333–5

Sordi E, Ferrari A, Piccolo D, Peris K. Pigmented Spitz nevi. Dermatol Surg 2002; 28: 1182–3

Spatz A, Barnhill RL. The Spitz tumor 50 years later: revisiting a landmark contribution and unresolved controversy. J Am Acad Dermatol 1999; 40: 223–8

Spatz A, Calonje E, Handfield-Jones S, Barnhill RL. Spitz tumors in children. Arch Dermatol 1999; 135: 282–5

Su LD, Fullen DR, Sondak VK, et al. Sentinel lymph node biopsy for patients with problematic spitzoid melanocytic lesions: a report on 18 patients. Cancer 2003; 97: 499–507

Blue nevus

Major points

- Acquired or congenital
- Usually solitary
- Blue-gray or blue-black papule, nodule or plaque-like aggregate of dermal melanocytes (Figure 14.7)
- Blue-gray color is an optical effect of dermal melanin seen through overlying skin
- Diameter usually <10 mm, but can range up to 3 cm
- Location usually dorsal hands and feet
- Associated with: lentigines, cardiac myxoma and cutaneous myxomas (Carney complex)

Pathogenesis

- Etiology unknown
- Thought to be ectopic accumulation of melanin-producing melanocytes in the dermis during migration from neural crest to skin
- Origin either Schwann cells, endoneural cells or melanocytes

Diagnosis

- Typical clinical appearance
- Histology: dermal melanocytes with melanin-containing macrophages

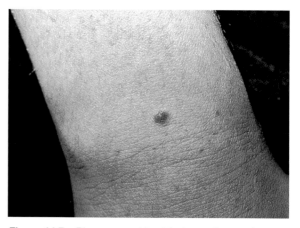

Figure 14.7 Blue nevus – blue-black papule on wrist

Differential diagnosis

- Melanoma
- Nevocellular nevus
- Traumatic tattoo
- Sclerosing hemangioma
- Dermatofibroma
- Carney complex

Treatment

- Surgical excision is advised, because differentiation between blue nevus and melanoma is difficult
- Laser treatment controversial

Prognosis

- Natural evolution has not been studied, but probably benign
- Rare malignant blue nevus found in contiguity with benign blue nevus

References

Carney JA, Stratakis CA. Epithelioid blue nevus and psammomatous melanotic schwannoma: the unusual pigmented skin tumors of the Carney complex. Semin Diag Pathol 1998; 15: 216–24

Hendricks WM. Eruptive blue nevi. J Am Acad Dermatol 1981; 4: 50–3

Hsiao G-H, Hsiao C-W. Plaque-type blue nevus on the face: a variant of Ota's nevus. J Am Acad Dermatol 1994; 30: 849–51

Knoell KA, Nelson KC, Patterson JW. Familial multiple blue nevi. J Am Acad Dermatol 1998; 39: 322–5

Milgraum SS, Cohen ME, Auletta MJ. Treatment of blue nevi with the Q-switched ruby laser. J Am Acad Dermatol 1995; 32: 307–10

Pinto A, Raghavendra S, Lee R, et al. Epithelioid blue nevus of the oral mucosa: a rare histologic variant. Oral Surg Oral Med Oral Pathol Oral Radiol Endodontics 2003; 96: 429–36

Schaffer JV, Bolognia JL. The clinical spectrum of pigmented lesions. Clin Plast Surg 2000; 27: 391–408

Tschen JA, Cartwright J, Font RL. Nonmelanized macromelanosomes in a cellular blue nevus. Arch Dermatol 1989; 125: 809–12

Halo nevus

Synonyms: halo nevomelanocytic nevus, leukoderma acquisitum centrifugum, Sutton nevus

Major points

- Characterized by a pink or brown central nevus surrounded by a halo of depigmentation usually 0.5–5 cm in diameter, often indicating onset of regression of nevus (Figure 14.8)
- Can be associated with acquired or congenital nevi
- More common in children with mean age of 15 years (majority <20 years)
- Multiple lesions common (25–50%)
- Any race
- Common association: vitiligo (18–26%)
- Can be seen with melanoma at distant sites (very rare)

Pathogenesis

- Both humoral and cellular factors may be responsible for nevus destruction

Diagnosis

- Clinical presentation
- Histology: central melanocytic nevus with dermal lymphocytic infiltrate surrounding the nevus, and depigmented zone devoid of epidermal melanocytes

Differential diagnosis

- Vitiligo
- Eczematous eruption around molluscum
- Melanoma (usually adults)

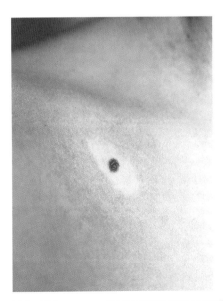

Figure 14.8   Halo nevus – depigmented halo around a typical acquired nevus

Treatment

- Close examination of skin in order to rule out other associated disorders (e.g. vitiligo, dysplastic nevi, melanoma)
- Surgical removal of normal nevus with halo not usually indicated in children because of benign nature

Prognosis

- Central nevus may persist, become less pigmented over time, or disappear with eventual repigmentation

References

Baranda L, Torres-Alvarez B, Moncada B, et al. Presence of activated lymphocytes in the peripheral blood of patients with halo nevi. J Am Acad Dermatol 1999; 41: 567–72

Inamadar AC, Palit A, Athanikar SB, et al. Unusual course of a halo nevus. Pediatr Dermatol 2003; 20: 542–3

Musette P, Bachelez H, Flageul B, et al. Immune-mediated destruction of melanocytes in halo nevi is associated with the local expansion of a limited number of T cell clones. J Immunol 1999; 162: 1789–94

Zeff RA, Freitag A, Grin CM, Grant-Kels JM. The immune response in halo nevi. J Am Acad Dermatol 1997; 37: 620–4

Nevus spilus

Synonym: speckled lentiginous nevus

Major points

- Presents at birth or early childhood as a tan or brown macule which becomes speckled with darker pigmented macules over time (Figure 14.9)

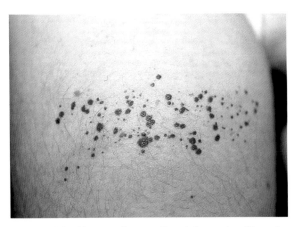

Figure 14.9   Nevus spilus – café au lait macule with nevi

Pathogenesis

- Histology of the light brown area: lentiginous melanocytic hyperplasia. Darker macules/papules demonstrate nests of nevus cells at the dermal–epidermal junction (junctional or compound nevi)

Diagnosis

- Clinical diagnosis

Differential diagnosis

- Becker nevus
- Café au lait macule
- Congenital melanocytic nevus

Treatment

- Observation usually sufficient
- Surgical excision or biopsy is warranted if lesion demonstrates abnormally rapid growth of dark pigment

Prognosis

- Risk of malignant change unknown, but probably very small

References

Casanova D, Bardot J, Aubert JP, et al. Management of nevus spilus. Pediatr Dermatol 1996; 13: 233–8

Cohen LM. Nevus spilus: congenital or acquired? Arch Dermatol 2001; 137: 215–16

Cramer SF. Speckled lentiginous nevus (nevus spilus): the 'roots' of the 'melanocytic garden'. Arch Dermatol 2001; 137: 1654–5

Johr RH, Binder M. Management of nevus spilus–a better way. Pediatr Dermatol 2000; 17: 491–2

Moreno-Arias GA, Bulla F, Vilata-Corell JJ, Camps-Fresneda A. Treatment of widespread segmental nevus spilus by Q-switched alexandrite laser (755 nm, 100 nsec). Dermatol Surg 2001; 27: 841–3

Rhodes AR. Nevus spilus: a potential precursor of cutaneous melanoma worthy of aggressive surgical excision? Pediatr Dermatol 1996; 13: 250–2

Melanoma

Major points

- Rare in children, but has been associated with congenital nevocellular nevi, acquired nevi, or *de novo* (Figures 14.10 and 14.11)

- Change in nevus:
  1. Asymmetry. Irregular pigmentation with darkening of one portion of the nevus, a small dark elevated papule within an otherwise flat papule, or flaking, scaling, ulceration or bleeding
  2. Border irregularity. Lesion appears to be growing in one direction with scalloped edges
  3. Color variation. Appearance of black, dark brown or admixture of red, white and black
  4. Diameter >6 mm; most benign acquired nevi are <6 mm
  5. Symptoms: burning, itching, or tenderness
- Risk factors:
  1. New or changing mole
  2. Age >15 years
  3. Dysplastic nevi, prior melanoma and familial melanoma
  4. Congenital nevocellular nevus
  5. 50 nevi, >2 mm in diameter
  6. 12 nevi, >6 mm in diameter
  7. Light skin color
  8. Marked freckling
  9. Sun sensitivity
  10. Excessive sun exposure
- Associations:
  1. Family history of melanoma
  2. Presence of multiple atypical nevi (atypical mole syndrome)
  3. Xeroderma pigmentosum
  4. Transplacental spread of maternal melanoma

Pathogenesis

- Genetic factors with resultant progressive changes in DNA and inability to repair DNA
- Familial cutaneous malignant melanoma (OMIM no. 15560) can be caused by germline mutations in CDKN2A on chromosome 9p21 and CDK4 on 12q14 and 1p36

Diagnosis

- Clinical features
- Histology: increased numbers of atypical basal melanocytes with atypical nuclei of different sizes, epidermotropism, nest of melanocytes with variation in size and shape, asymmetrical no maturation of melanocytes, signs of regression

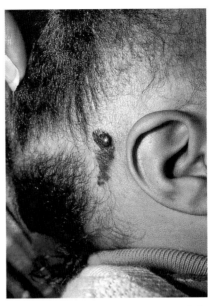

Figure 14.10   Melanoma – arising in a congenital nevus

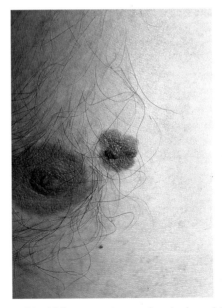

Figure 14.11   Melanoma – changes in color brought this patient to the doctor; it was melanoma *in situ*

Differential diagnosis

- Spitz nevus
- Congenital nevocellular nevus
- Acquired melanocytic nevus
- Blue nevus

- Traumatic hemorrhage (especially under the nails, on the heels, or on the mucous membranes)
- Pyogenic granuloma

Treatment

- Excision with wide margins based on microscopic depth of melanoma cells:
  1. In situ: 2–5 mm excision margin
  2. <1 mm: 1 cm excision margin
  3. 1–2 mm: 1–2 cm excision margin
  4. 2.1–4 mm: 2–3 cm excision margin
  5. >4 mm: 2–3 cm excision margin
- Adjunctive treatments: α-interferon, chemotherapy

Prognosis

- Influenced by depth of the lesion and involvement of lymph nodes
- Five year survival (in general; many factors influence staging): stages I–II: 79%; stage III: 13–69%; stage IV: 6%

References

Arbiser JL. Melanoma. Lessons from metastases. Arch Dermatol 1998; 134: 1027–8

Bevona C, Goggins W, Quinn T, et al. Cutaneous melanomas associated with nevi. Arch Dermatol 2003; 139: 1620–4

de Braud F, Khayat D, Kroon BB, et al. Malignant melanoma. Crit Rev Oncol Hematol 2003; 47: 35–63

Eedy DJ. Surgical treatment of melanoma. Br J Dermatol 2003; 149: 2–12

Handfield-Jones SE, Smith NP. Malignant melanoma in childhood. Br J Dermatol 1996; 134: 607–16

Johnson TM, Hamilton T, Lowe L. Multiple primary melanomas. J Am Acad Dermatol 1998; 39: 422–7

Johnson TM, Yahanda AM, Chang AE, et al. Advances in melanoma therapy. J Am Acad Dermatol 1998; 38: 731–41

Kanzler MH, Swetter SM. Malignant melanoma. Periodic synopsis. J Am Acad Dermatol 2003; 48: 780–3

Monzon J, Liu L, Brill H, et al. CDKN2A mutations in multiple primary melanomas. N Engl J Med 1998; 338: 879–87

Queirolo P, Taveggia P, Gipponi M, Sertoli MR. Sentinel lymph node biopsy in melanoma patients: the medical oncologist's perspective. J Surg Oncol 2004; 85: 162–5

Richardson SK, Tannous ZS, Mihm MC. Congenital and infantile melanoma: review of the literature and report of an uncommon variant, pigment-synthesizing melanoma. J Am Acad Dermatol 2002; 47: 77–90

Saenz NC, Saenz-Badillos J, Busam K, et al. Childhood melanoma survival. Cancer 1999; 85: 750–4

Sahin S, Levin L, Kopf AW, et al. Risk of melanoma in medium-sized congenital melanocytic nevi: a follow-up study. J Am Acad Dermatol 1998; 39: 428–33

Schmid-Wendtner MH, Berking C, Baumert J, et al. Cutaneous melanoma in childhood and adolescence: an analysis of 36 patients. J Am Acad Dermatol 2002; 46: 874–9

Sober AJ, et al. (Task Force). Guidelines of care for primary cutaneous melanoma. J Am Acad Dermatol 2001; 45: 579–86

Wechsler J, Bastuji-Garin S, Spatz A, et al. Reliability of the histopathologic diagnosis of malignant melanoma in childhood. Arch Dermatol 2002; 138: 625–8

Becker nevus

Synonyms: Becker's melanosis, hairy epidermal nevus

Major points

- Male/female ratio >1
- Clinical:
  1. May be present at birth or childhood as a brown patch with smudged borders
  2. Sharply demarcated irregular hyperpigmented patch with or without coarse dark hair (Figure 14.12)
  3. Location characteristically over the shoulder, anterior chest, or scapula, but can be anywhere
  4. Enlarges slowly over ~2 years, then stabilizes
  5. Usual size: 2–20 cm
  6. Asymptomatic
- Rare association: hypoplasia of underlying structures (e.g. hypoplasia of the breast)

Pathogenesis

- Organoid hamartoma of ectoderm and mesoderm
- Increase in expression of testosterone receptors and increased sensitivity to androgens may account for expression of lesion around puberty

Diagnosis

- Clinical presentation
- Histology: slight acanthosis, papillomatosis, hyperpigmented basal cell layer and variable increase in smooth muscle fibers

Differential diagnosis

- Congenital nevocellular nevus
- Smooth muscle hamartoma

Treatment

- No treatment needed
- Pigmented lesion lasers (Q-switched ruby, neodymium : YAG lasers) may improve hyperpigmentation
- Photoprotection decreases darkening from sun exposure
- Bleaching agents with hydroquinone may be helpful
- For hair removal: shaving, depilatories, electrolysis, laser

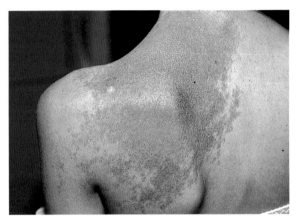

Figure 14.12 Becker nevus – unilateral mottled brown patch with increased hair

Prognosis

- Lesion persists indefinitely
- Benign

References

Chima KN, Janniger CK, Schwartz RA. Becker's melanosis. Cutis 1996; 57: 311–13

Formigon M, Alsina MM, Mascaro JN, Rivera F. Becker's nevus and ipsilateral breast hypoplasia androgen-receptor study in two patients. Arch Dermatol 1992; 128: 992–3

Happle R, Koopman RJ. Becker nevus syndrome. Am J Med Genet 1997; 68: 357–61

Nirde P, Dereure O, Belon C, et al. The association of Becker nevus with hypersensitivity to androgens. Arch Dermatol 1999; 135: 212–14

Freckles (ephelides)

Major points

- 2–3-mm tan-brown macules appearing in sun-exposed areas, particularly on face, upper torso and arms (Figure 14.13)
- Lightly pigmented individuals usually affected
- Tend to fade in winter and increase in summer

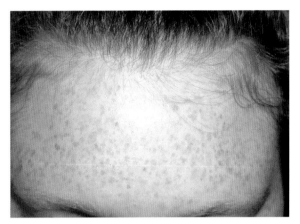

Figure 14.13   Freckles – this young adult has type 1 skin

Pathogenesis

- Caused by sun exposure in light-skinned person with a genetic predispostion
- Histology: hyperpigmentation of basal cell layer
- Melanocytes are large and have more numerous and prominent dendritic processes

Diagnosis

- Clinical presentation

Differential diagnosis

- Lentigines
- Nevocellular nevi

Treatment

- No treatment needed
- Sunscreens and protective clothing can decrease the appearance of new freckles

Prognosis

- Usually permanent but tend to fade with less sun exposure

References

Levine N, Fulk CS, Rubenzik R. Ephelides (freckles). In The Pigmentary System. Nordlund JJ, Boissy RE, Hearing VJ, et al. eds. Oxford University Press: New York, 1998: 849–51

Zhang XJ, He PP, Liang YH, et al. A gene for freckles maps to chromosome 4q32-q34. J Invest Dermatol 2004; 122: 286–90

Lentigo simplex

Plural: lentigines

Major points

- Hyperpigmented macule similar to a freckle, but is darker and does not necessarily show predilection for sun-exposed areas
- Size 2–15 mm in diameter
- Color ranges from brown to black
- Solar lentigines: irregularly shaped, darkly pigmented macules which appear after a severe sunburn; often seen with increased freckles in the same area

Pathogenesis

- Histology: elongation of rete ridges, increase in numbers of melanocytes in basal layer and increased melanin in melanocytes and keratinocytes

Diagnosis

- Clinical presentation

Differential diagnosis

- Junctional nevocellular nevus
- LEOPARD syndrome (multiple lentigines syndrome)
- Peutz–Jeghers syndrome

Treatment

- Laser ablation: carbon dioxide, Q-switched ruby, neodymium : yttrium–aluminum–garnet, and alexandrite

Prognosis

- Persists unless treated

References

Abdelmalek NF, Gerber TL, Menter A. Cardiocutaneous syndromes and associations. J Am Acad Dermatol 2002; 46: 161–83

Arnsmeier SL, Paller AS. Pigmentary anomalies in the multiple lentigines syndrome: is it distinct from LEOPARD syndrome? Pediatr Deramtol 1996; 13: 100–4

Chamlin SL, Williams ML. Pigmented lesions in adolescents. Adolesc Med State Art Rev 2001; 12: 195–212

Chong W-S, Klanwarin W, Giam Y-C. Generalized lentiginosis in two children lacking systemic associations: case report and review of the literature. Pediatr Dermatol 2004; 21: 139–45

Cognetta AB Jr, Stolz W, Katz B, et al. Dermatoscopy of lentigo maligna. Dermatol Clin 2001; 19: 307–18

Fulk CS. Primary disorders of hyperpigmentation. J Am Acad Dermatol 1984; 10: 1–16

O'Neill JF, James WD. Inherited patterned lentiginosis in blacks. Arch Dermatol 1989; 125: 1231–5

Rahman SB, Bhawan J. Lentigo. Intern J Dermatol 1996; 35: 229–38

Smith SR, O'Grady TC. Reticulated ephelides: 'inkspots' revisited. Arch Dermatol 1996; 132: 353–4

Tanzi EL, Lupton JR, Alster TS. Lasers in dermatology: four decades of progress. J Am Acad Dermatol 2003; 49:1–31

Café au lait macules

Major points

- Discrete brown macules (Figure 14.14)
- Appear at birth or during childhood
- Size 1 mm to >20 cm
- May involve any skin surface
- Neurofibromatosis: >6 macules greater than 0.5 cm in diameter if <15 years old, and 1.5 cm if >15 years (Figure 14.15)

Pathogenesis

- Histology: increased numbers of melanocytes and increased melanin in melanocytes and keratinocytes

Diagnosis

- Clinical presentation

Differential diagnosis

- Neurofibromatosis
- McCune–Albright syndrome
- LEOPARD syndrome
- Epidermal nevus

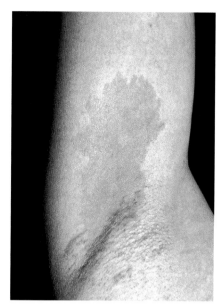

Figure 14.14   Café au lait macule – associated with neurofibromatosis

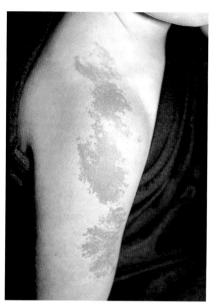

Figure 14.15   Café au lait macules in a linear distribution, not associated with neurofibromatosis

- Nevocellular nevus
- Lentigo/lentigines

Treatment

- None usually needed
- On the face, treatment with a pigmented laser may be temporarily helpful but may need multiple treatments

Prognosis

- Lesions tend to be stable in size and distribution

References

Goldberg Y, Dibbern K, Klein J, et al. Neurofibromatosis type 1 – an update and review for the primary pediatrician. Clin Pediatr 1996; 35: 545–61

Karabiber H, Sasmaz S, Turanli G, Yakinci C. Prevalence of hypopigmented maculae and café-au-lait spots in idiopathic epileptic and healthy children. J Child Neurol 2002; 17: 57–9

Landau M, Krafchik BR. The diagnostic value of café au lait macules. J Am Acad Dermatol 1999; 40: 877–90

Okazaki M, Yoshimura K, Suzuki Y, et al. The mechanism of epidermal hyperpigmentation in cafe-au-lait macules of neurofibromatosis type 1 (von Recklinghausen's disease) may be associated with dermal fibroblast-derived stem cell factor and hepatocyte growth factor. Br J Dermatol 2003; 148: 689–97

McCune–Albright syndrome

Major points

- Triad of findings:
  1. Large irregularly shaped café au lait macules, usually on trunk; may be present at birth, usually evident in infancy
  2. Precocious puberty (especially females)
  3. Polyostotic fibrous dysplasia – usually onset at <10 years of age
- Other findings:
  1. Endocrine abnormalities (e.g. acromegaly, hyperthyroidism, autonomous adrenal hyperplasia)
  2. Ovarian cysts
  3. Facial asymmetry

Pathogenesis

- Activating missense mutation in gene for alpha subunit of GS, the G protein that stimulates cyclic adenosine monophosphate formation
- Somatic mutation of GS alpha gene in early embryogenesis produces a mosaic of normal and mutant-bearing tissues
- Manifestions and severity depend on number and location of abnormal cells
- Gene locus: 20q13.2

- Gene: GNAS1, stimulatory G protein, alpha subunit (Gsa; activating mutations)

Diagnosis

- Clinical presentation

Differential diagnosis

- Neurofibromatosis
- Proteus syndrome

Treatment

- See Café au lait macules

Prognosis

- Depends upon endocrine and bony involvement
- Lesions are static

References

de Sanctis C, Lala R, Matarazzo P, et al. Pubertal development in patients with McCune-Albright syndrome or pseudohypoparathyroidism. J Pediatr Endocrinol Metab 2003; 16 (Suppl 2): 293–6

Landau M, Krafchik BR. The diagnostic value of café au lait macules. J Am Acad Dermatol 1999; 40: 877–90

Levine MA. Clinical implications of genetic defects in G proteins: oncogenic mutations in G alpha s as the molecular basis for the McCune–Albright syndrome. Arch Med Res 1999; 30: 522–31

Lumbroso S, Paris F, Sultan C. McCune–Albright syndrome: molecular genetics. J Pediatr Endocrinol Metab 2002; 15 (Suppl 3): 875–82

Roth JG, Esterly NB. McCune–Albright syndrome with multiple bilateral café au lait spots. Pediatr Dermatol 1991; 8: 35–9

Shenker A, Weinstein LS, Moran A, et al. Severe endocrine and nonendocrine manifestations of the McCune–Albright syndrome associated with activating mutations of stimulatory G protein GS. J Pediatr 1993; 123: 509–18

Weinstein LS, Shenker A, Gejman PV, et al: Activating mutations of the stimulatory G protein in the McCune–Albright syndrome. N Engl J Med 1991; 325: 1688–95

Melasma

Major points

- Common acquired hypermelanosis in teenage and adult women

- Increased macular pigmentation in sun-exposed areas (Figure 14.16)
- Symmetric, patchy, facial melanosis
- Often associated with pregnancy or oral contraceptives

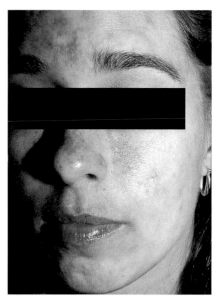

Figure 14.16   Melasma – can be caused by oral contraceptives

- Female/male ratio >1
- More common in Latinos and Asians

Pathogenesis

- Increase in number and activity of melanocytes
- Histology: increase in epidermal and/or dermal melanin

Diagnosis

- Clinical presentation

Differential diagnosis

- Postinflammatory hyperpigmentation
- Phytophotocontact dermatitis

Treatment

- Discontinuation of oral contraceptives
- Topical sunscreens
- Bleaching creams with hydroquinone 2–4% BID for <6 months
- Cover-up makeup

Prognosis

- Exacerbated by sun exposure
- Chronic condition which may wax and wane

References

Grimes PE. Melasma. Etiologic and therapeutic consideration. Arch Dermatol 1995; 131: 1453–7

Guevara IL, Pandya AG. Safety and efficacy of 4% hydroquinone combined with 10% glycolic acid, antioxidants, and sunscreen in the treatment of melasma. Int J Dermatol 2003; 42: 966–72

Mongolian spot

Synonym: congenital dermal melanocytosis

Major points

- Clinical
  1. Blue-gray macules with indistinct margins (Figure 14.17)
  2. Common in Asians and Blacks, occasionally in Whites
  3. Locations – lumbosacral area most common; aberrant lesions can be on face, extremities and torso
  4. Size ranges from a few centimeters to >20 cm.
  5. Can be multiple or single

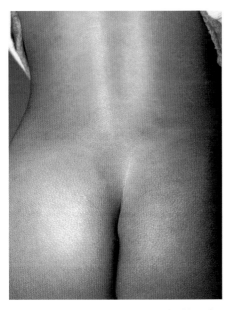

Figure 14.17   Mongolian spot in the typical location on the lumbar back

Pathogenesis

- Dermal pigmentation appears gray-blue because of decreased reflectance in longer wavelength region compared with surrounding area

Diagnosis

- Clinical presentation
- Histology: dermal melanocytes with fully melanized melanosomes

Differential diagnosis

- Bruises
- Congenital nevocellular nevus

Treatment

- Opaque cosmetics
- Q-switched ruby laser

Prognosis

- Natural course of lumbosacral macules is to fade in childhood
- Aberrant lesions stay indefinitely and tend not to fade

References

Bashiti HM, Blair JD, Triska RA, Keller L. Generalized dermal melanocytosis. Arch Dermatol 1981; 117: 791–3

Cordova A. The mongolian spot. Clin Pediatr 1981; 20: 714–22

Fulk CS. Primary disorders of hyperpigmentation. J Am Acad Dermatol 1984; 10: 1–16

Hori Y, Takayama O. Circumscribed dermal melanoses. Classification and histologic features. Dermatol Clin 1988; 6: 315–26

Leung AK, Kao CP. Extensive mongolian spots with involvement of the scalp. Pediatr Dermatol 1999; 16: 371–2

Smalek JE. Significance of mongolian spots. J Pediatr 1980; 97: 504–5

Stanford DG, Georgouras KE. Dermal melanocytosis: a clinical spectrum. Aust J Dermatol 1996; 37: 19–25

Van Gysel D, Oranje AP, Stroink H, Simonsz HJ. Phakomatosis pigmentovascularis. Pediatr Dermatol 1996; 13: 33–5

Nevus of Ota/nevus of Ito

Synonyms for nevus of Ota: oculodermal melanocytosis, nevus fuscoceruleus ophthalmomaxillaris

Synonym for nevus of Ito: nevus fuscoceruleus acromiodeltoideus

Major points

- Clinical
  1. Sporadic inheritance
  2. More common in Asians and Blacks
  3. Female/male ratio >1
  4. Characterized by unilateral, blue-black macules intermingled with small brown macules, giving a mottled appearance (Figure 14.18)
  5. Location of nevus of Ota: skin innervated by V1 and V2; mucosa, conjunctiva, tympanic membrane may be involved
  6. Location of nevus of Ito: unilateral pigmentation over supraclavicular, deltoid and scapular regions
  7. Half the lesions present at birth; remainder appear at puberty

Pathogenesis

- Histology: melanocytes widely scattered in reticular dermis with melanosomes singly dispersed and fully melanized

Diagnosis

- Clinical presentation

Differential diagnosis

- Congenital nevocellular nevus
- Mongolian spot

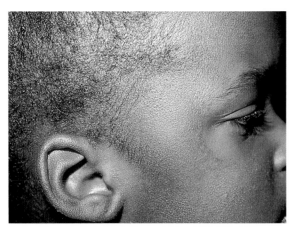

Figure 14.18 Nevus of Ota – dark gray patch around the eye (published in An Illustrated Dictionary of Dermatologic Syndromes by SB Mallory and S Leal-Khouri)

Treatment

- Q-switched ruby laser – may require multiple treatments
- Cosmetic camouflage

Prognosis

- Tends to enlarge and darken with time
- Very rarely, melanoma arises within the lesion
- Glaucoma arises in 10%

References

Fulk CS. Primary disorders of hyperpigmentation. J Am Acad Dermatol 1984; 10: 1–16

Hirayama T, Suzuki T. A new classification of Ota's nevus based on histopathological features. Dermatologica 1991; 183: 169–72

Kono T, Chan HH, Ercocen AR, et al. Use of Q-switched ruby laser in the treatment of nevus of Ota in different age groups. Lasers Surg Med 2003; 32: 391–5

Lee CS, Lim HW. Cutaneous diseases in Asians. Dermatol Clin 2003; 21: 669–77

Leung AK, Kao CP, Lee TK. Mongolian spots with involvement of the temporal area. Int J Dermatol 2001; 40: 288–9

Liesegang TJ. Pigmented conjunctival and scleral lesions. Mayo Clin Proc 1994; 69: 151–61

Watanabe S, Takahashi H. Treatment of nevus of Ota with the Q-switched ruby laser. N J Engl J Med 1994; 331: 1745–50

Incontinentia pigmenti

Synonym: Block–Sulzberger syndrome

Major points

- X-linked dominant disorder characterized by linear rows of blisters in first year of life, followed by swirling hyperpigmentation which follow Blaschko lines
- Four stages which can overlap:
  1. Bullous stage (age birth to ~1 year) – linear rows of blisters following Blaschko lines on extremities and occasionally trunk; lesions can recur or new lesions can develop
  2. Verrucous stage (~3 months to 3 years) – linear, verrucous lesions develop usually on extremities
  3. Hyperpigmented stage (1 year to 20 years) – whorls of dirty-brown to slate-gray

hyperpigmentation mainly on the trunk following Blaschko lines; fades in adolescence (Figure 14.19)
4. Hypopigmented stages (adulthood) – streaks of hairless atrophic hypopigmentation on the extremities; often subtle

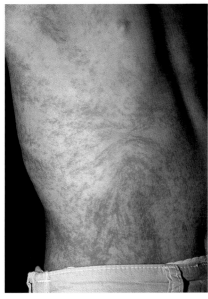

Figure 14.19   Incontinentia pigmenti (stage 3) – whorling pigmentation following Blaschko lines

- Associated manifestations:
  1. Dental (65–80%) – anodontia, hypodontia and others
  2. Hair (38–50%) – thin or sparse hair, patches of alopecia (especially vertex), woolly hair nevus
  3. CNS (10–31%) – seizures, mental retardation, hemiplegia and others
  4. Eye (35–40%) – strabismus, abnormalities of developing retinal vessels
  5. Skeletal (14%) – chondrodystrophy, cleft lip and/or palate, clubfoot, contractures, hemiatrophy and others
  6. Nails (7–40%) – onychogryphosis, pitting, ridging, subungual keratotic tumors and others
  7. Breast – unilateral aplasia
  8. Eosinophilia (up to 65%) in infancy

Pathogenesis

- X-linked dominant disorder, usually lethal in male

- Gene locus Xq28. Gene: NEMO (nuclear factor κB essential modulator IKK-gamma)

Diagnosis

- Clinical diagnosis but confirmed with biopsy of skin in early life
- Histology:
  1. Bullous stage: numerous eosinophils with spongiosis in the epidermis
  2. Verrucous stage: eosinophilic dyskeratosis, hyperkeratosis, acanthosis, papillomatosis
  3. Pigmented stage: melanin in dermis or in dermal macrophages
  4. Hypopigmented stage: absence of skin appendages; mild epidermal atrophy; melanocytes decreased or normal

Differential diagnosis

- Bullous stage:
  1. Herpes simplex
  2. Bullous impetigo
  3. Other bullous disorders (see Chapter 6)
- Verrucous stage:
  1. Linear epidermal nevus
  2. Warts
- Pigmented stage:
  1. Epidermal nevus
  2. Linear and whorled hypermelanosis
- Hypopigmented stage:
  1. Anetoderma
  2. Goltz syndrome

Treatment

- Symptomatic treatment
- Skin in neonatal period – topical care and topical antibiotics
- Other organ systems should be examined as indicated by specialists: ophthalmology, audiology, neurology, dental, genetics

Prognosis

- Watch for seizures early in life (which often improve with time) with referral to neurologist if indicated; magnetic resonance imaging (MRI) or computerized tomography (CT) scan do not need to be routinely ordered
- Birth defects (e.g. alopecia, eye abnormalities) are permanent
- Pigmentary changes improve with age

References

Hadj-Rabia S, Froidevaux D, Bodak N, et al. Clinical study of 40 cases of incontinentia pigmenti. Arch Dermatol 2003; 139: 1163–70

Happle R. A fresh look at incontinentia pigmenti. Arch Dermatol 2003; 139: 1206–8

Hennel SJ, Ekert PG, Volpe JJ, Inder TE. Insights into the pathogenesis of cerebral lesions in incontinentia pigmenti. Pediatr Neurol 2003; 29: 148–50

Shah SN, Gibbs S, Upton CJ, et al. Incontinentia pigmenti associated with cerebral palsy and cerebral leukomalacia: a case report and literature review. Pediatr Dermatol 2003; 20: 491–4

Zvulunov A, Esterly NB. Neurocutaneous syndromes associated with pigmentary skin lesions. J Am Acad Dermatol 1995; 32: 915–35

Erythema dyschromicum perstans

Synonym: ashy dermatosis

Major points

- Idiopathic, acquired, generalized, macular, blue-gray hyperpigmentation
- Clinical features
  1. Common in Latin Americans
  2. Sporadic
  3. Healthy individuals from childhood to adolescence
  4. May begin as erythematous macules which fade and becomes slate-gray or ashy or may begin *de novo* as gray macules (Figure 14.20)
  5. Lesions slowly enlarge and coalesce

Pathogenesis

- Pathogenesis unknown
- Histology: increased melanin in dermis and epidermis with vacuolization of basal cell layer

Diagnosis

- Clinical presentation

Differential diagnosis

- Mongolian spots
- Postinflammatory hyperpigmentation
- Lichen planus

Treatment

- None very effective

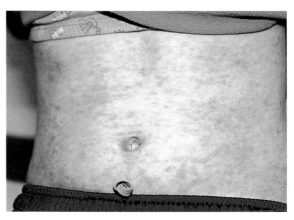

Figure 14.20   Erythema dyschromicum perstans – slate-gray macules with indistinct borders

Prognosis

- Usually static once process stops

References

Meffert JJ. Erythema dyschromicum perstans: a case report and review. Cutis 2002; 70: 62

Metin A, Calka O, Ugras S. Lichen planopilaris coexisting with erythema dyschromicum perstans. Br J Dermatol 2001; 145: 522–3

Osswald SS, Proffer LH, Sartori CR. Erythema dyschromicum perstans: a case report and review. Cutis 2001; 68: 25–8

Pandya AG, Guevara IL. Disorders of hyperpigmentation. Dermatol Clin 2000; 18: 91–8

Silverberg NB, Herz J, Wagner A, Paller AS. Erythema dyschromicum perstans in prepubertal children. Pediatr Dermatol 2003; 20: 529–30

Acanthosis nigricans

Major points

- Clinical manifestations:
  1. Brownish-black, velvety thickening of the skin with increased skin markings (Figure 14.21)
  2. Prominent in axillae, posterior neck, sides of the neck, groin, antecubital, popliteal surfaces and the umbilical area
  3. May have soft papillomas (skin tags) or warty nodules on the affected skin
  4. Rarely may affect mucocutaneous skin: eyelids, conjunctivae, lips, oral cavity, vulva

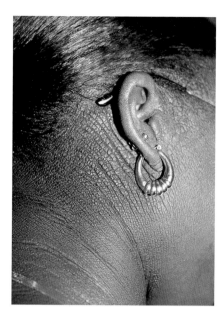

Figure 14.21   Acanthosis nigricans – typical velvety, dark appearance on the neck

- Epidemiology:
  1. Male/female ratio =1
  2. Occurs most commonly during puberty, or in early adulthood
  3. Peak prevalence in childhood is age ~12 years
  4. Strong association with obesity: 66% prevalence in adolescents weighing >200% of their ideal body weight
- Benign acanthosis nigricans (AN)
  1. Rare autosomal dominant genodermatosis
  2. Associated with multiple melanocytic nevi
  3. Presents at birth or early childhood
- Obesity-associated AN
  1. Most common form
  2. Clinical course of skin lesions follows weight gain and loss
- Acral AN
  1. Occurs in healthy individuals
  2. Distribution over dorsal hands and feet
- Syndromic AN – syndromes with associated insulin resistance
  1. Lawrence–Seip syndrome (lipodystrophy and AN)
  2. Leprechaunism
  3. Polycystic ovary disease
  4. Crouzon syndrome
  5. Others

- Malignancy-associated AN
  1. Rare in children
  2. Sudden onset and rapid spread of skin involvement
  3. Associated with internal malignancy (e.g. gastric cancer, Wilms tumor)
- Medication-induced AN – e.g. nicotinic acid, diethylstilbestrol (DES), corticosteroids, estrogens, oral contraceptives

Pathogenesis

- Hyperinsulinemia is implicated in pathogenesis
  1. Usually caused by underlying insulin resistance in obesity or syndromes
  2. Excess insulin binds to receptors on keratinocytes and fibroblasts, leading to increased proliferation of epidermal cells
- Tumor product with insulin-like activity or transforming growth factor (TGF-α) activity is implicated in malignant AN
- Histology: hyperkeratosis and epidermal papillomatosis; areas of acanthosis alternating with atrophy

Diagnosis

- Clinical features
- Evaluate for underlying endocrine abnormality or malignancy if indicated

Differential diagnosis

- Confluent and reticulate papillomatosis
- Retained keratin

Treatment

- Directed at correcting underlying disease
  1. Weight loss
  2. Correction of underlying endocrine dysfunction
  3. Discontinue offending drug
  4. Treat underlying malignancy
- If mild AN, may not require treatment
- Topical emollients, keratolytics, topical retinoid (e.g. tretinoin 0.1% cream once daily for 2 weeks) or low-dose systemic retinoids

Prognosis

- Clinical course tends to follow exacerbation or resolution of underlying disorder
- Obesity-associated AN may improve with weight loss

References

Brockow K, Steinkraus V, Rinninger F, et al. Acanthosis nigricans: a marker for hyperinsulinemia. Pediatr Dermatol 1995; 12: 323–6

Hermanns-Le T, Hermanns JF, Pierard GE. Juvenile acanthosis nigricans and insulin resistance. Pediatr Dermatol 2002; 19: 12–14

Panidis D, Skiadopoulos S, Rousso D, et al. Association of acanthosis nigricans with insulin resistance in patients with polycystic ovar`y syndrome. Br J Dermatol 1995; 132: 936–41

Schroeder B. Early diagnosis, presenting complaints, and management of hyperandrogenism in adolescents. Curr Wom Health Rep 2001; 1: 124–30

Schwartz RA, Janniger CK. Childhood acanthosis nigricans. Cutis 1995; 55: 337–9

Torley D, Bellus GA, Munro CS. Genes, growth factors and acanthosis nigricans. Br J Dermatol 2002; 147: 1096–101

Uyttendaele H, Koss T, Bagheri B, et al. Generalized acanthosis nigricans in an otherwise healthy young child. Pediatr Dermatol 2003; 20: 254–6

Confluent and reticulated papillomatosis

Synonym: Gougerot and Carteaud syndrome

Major points

- Distinctive clinical disorder of adolescents and young adults
- Female/male ratio >1
- Blacks/Whites ratio >1
- Presents with brown hyperkeratotic papules coalescing into plaques with reticulate periphery (Figure 14.22)
- Location: chest, inframammary area, neck, shoulders, interscapular back and epigastric area

Pathogenesis

- Unknown etiology
- Considered a variant of acanthosis nigricans or a disorder of keratinization
- May be related to endocrine abnormalities or host reponse to *Pityrosporum orbiculare*

Diagnosis

- Clinical findings
- Histology: similar to acanthosis nigricans with undulating hyperkeratosis, papillomatosis and mild acanthosis with basal hyperpigmentation

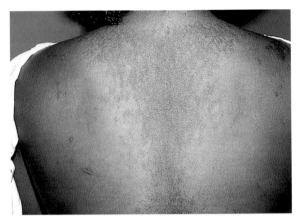

Figure 14.22   Confluent and reticulated papillomatosis – lesions can resemble tinea versicolor but a scraping for hyphae is negative, and it does not respond to antifungal therapy

Differential diagnosis

- Tinea versicolor
- Acanthosis nigricans

Treatment

- Oral minocycline 100 mg BID
- Variable success with topical therapy: salicylic acid, selenium sulfide, antifungals, 5-fluorouracil, calcipotriene, retinoids
- Oral retinoids if minocycline is ineffective

Prognosis

- Benign persistent course with recurrences

References

Bowman PH, Davis LS. Confluent and reticulated papillomatosis: response to tazarotene. J Am Acad Dermatol 2003; 48(5 Suppl): S80–1

Hirokawa M, Matsumoto M, Iizuka H. Confluent and reticulated papillomatosis: a case with concurrent acanthosis nigricans associated with obesity and insulin resistance. Dermatology 1994; 188: 148–51

Jang HS, Oh CK, Cha JH, et al. Six cases of confluent and reticulated papillomatosis alleviated by various antibiotics. J Am Acad Dermatol 2001; 44: 652–5

Mutasim DF. Confluent and reticulated papillomatosis without papillomatosis. J Am Acad Dermatol 2003; 49: 1182–4

Shimizu S, Han-Yaku H. Confluent and reticulated papillomatosis responsive to minocycline. Dermatology 1997; 194: 59–61

HYPOPIGMENTED DISORDERS

Vitiligo

Major points

- Common, sometimes heritable, acquired loss of pigment in interfollicular melanocytes
- Affects ~1–2% of all races
- Types
    1. Generalized – most common type; macules are symmetrical involving extensor surfaces of distal digits, knees, elbows and periorificial areas; mucosal involvement common (Figure 14.23)
    2. Segmental – unilateral macules with dermatomal or segmental configuration which remains stable and is unlikely to be associated with autoimmune diseases; trigeminal area most common (Figure 14.24)
    3. Focal – an isolated macule or a few scattered macules
    4. Universal – widespread vitiligo; often associated with multiple endocrinopathy syndrome
- Clinical:
    1. Onset at any age from birth to 81 years, with majority of cases beginning in childhood
    2. Macules are chalky white, round or oval, with fairly distinct often scalloped margins measuring several millimeters to many centimeters without any epidermal changes
    3. Trichrome vitiligo: presence of a band of lighter skin which interfaces between white and normal color displaying three colors: white, light tan and normal skin color (Figure 14.25)
    4. Lesions begin as small areas and enlarge over time with coalescence, which can be extensive
    5. Can exhibit Koebner phenomenon with involvement after injury
    6. Associated with poliosis, prematurely gray hair, halo nevi and alopecia areata
- Generalized vitiligo can be associated with various autoimmune disorders: thyroid disease, diabetes mellitus, Addison disease, pernicious anemia, multiple autoantibodies, hypoparathyroidism
- Ocular involvement: iritis, retinal pigmentary abnormalities, chorioretinitis; visual acuity usually normal
- Rare syndromes:
    1. Vogt–Koyanagi–Harada syndrome: rare multisystem disease characterized by aseptic

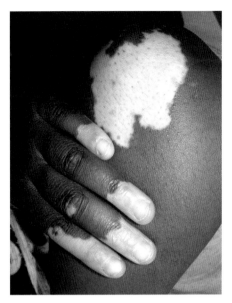

Figure 14.23   Vitiligo classically on the fingertips, knees and elbows

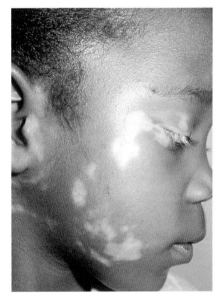

Figure 14.24   Vitiligo – acquired depigmented patches in a segmental distribution

meningoencephalitis, vitiligo, poliosis, uveitis, dysacousia
    2. Alezzandrini syndrome: characterized by unilateral facial vitiligo, poliosis (white patches of hair), ipsilateral pigmentary retinitis with gradual visual loss, and deafness

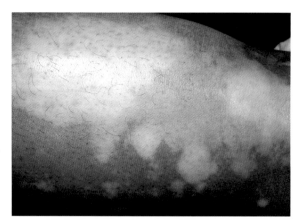

Figure 14.25   Vitiligo – trichrome color change

Pathogenesis

- Generalized vitiligo is a polygenic disorder; up to 30% have a family member affected
- Segmental vitiligo is not inherited
- Theories for mechanism of destruction of melanocytes: autoimmune, neurochemical, or self-destruction (toxic)

Diagnosis

- Clinical presentation. Wood's lamp examination may be helpful to identify lesions in light-skinned individuals
- Histology: loss of melanocytes; lymphocytes may be present in upper dermis in evolving macules

Differential diagnosis

- Postinflammatory hypopigmentation
- Pityriasis alba
- Tinea versicolor
- Tuberous sclerosis
- Nevus depigmentosus
- Chemical leukoderma (phenolic compounds)
- Lupus erythematosus
- Melanoma-associated leukoderma
- Piebaldism
- Waardenburg syndrome
- Leprosy

Treatment

- Education about disease is most helpful
- Sunscreens to vitiliginous areas to avoid sunburn

- Repigmentation (slow and requires commitment from patient and parents):
  1. Topical corticosteroids (mid-strength to ultra-potent) 1–2 times a day
  2. Psoralen (oral or topical) plus UVA light (PUVA)
  3. UVB light, 2–3 times per week
  4. Success depends upon presence of follicular melanocytes
- Surgical techniques with micrografts from uninvolved skin can be used only if patches are stable (non-progressive)
- Depigmentation with monobenzylether of hydroquinone 20% should be reserved for only those patients who have lost a large percentage of color and have no hope of repigmenting naturally
- Psychosocial factors should be addressed
- Cover-up cosmetics (e.g. Dermablend®) or temporary dyes

Prognosis

- Natural course of generalized vitiligo is unpredictable, but most vitiligo is slowly progressive. Spontaneous regression rare. Treatment can repigment some areas (face responds best)
- Segmental vitiligo is usually stable but can respond to treatment

References

Drake LA, Dinehart SM, Farmer ER, et al. Guidelines of care of vitiligo. J Am Acad Dermatol 1996; 35: 620–6

Gauthier Y, Cario Andre M, Taieb A. A critical appraisal of vitiligo etiologic theories. Is melanocyte loss a melanocytorrhagy? Pigment Cell Res 2003; 16: 322–32

Herane MI. Vitiligo and leukoderma in children. Clin Dermatol 2003; 21: 283–95

Hoffman MD, Dudley C. Suspected Alezzandrini's syndrome in a diabetic patient with unilateral retinal detachment and ipsilateral vitiligo and poliosis. J Am Acad Dermatol 1992; 26: 496–8

Majumder PP, Nordlund JJ, Nath SK. Pattern of familial aggregation of vitiligo. Arch Dermatol 1993; 129: 994–8

Ongenae K, Van Geel N, Naeyaert JM. Evidence for an autoimmune pathogenesis of vitiligo. Pigment Cell Res 2003; 16: 90–100

Schaffer JV, Bolognia JL. The treatment of hypopigmentation in children. Clin Dermatol 2003; 21: 296–310

Tsukamoto K, Osada A, Kitamura R, et al. Approaches to repigmentation of vitiligo skin: new treatment with ultrasonic abrasion, seed-grafting and psoralen plus ultraviolet A therapy. Pigment Cell Res 2002; 15: 331–4

Albinism

Synonym: oculocutaneous albinism

Major points

- General
  1. Albinism includes a group of genetic disorders with dilution or absence of ocular and cutaneous pigmentation
  2. All races affected
  3. Lack of pigment is caused by an abnormal maturation of melanosomes
- Types of oculocutaneous albinism (OCA):
  1. OCA 1A (tyrosinase-negative OCA)
     a. Marked hypopigmentation of the skin and eyes (Figure 14.26)
     b. Skin varies from pink to milky white
     c. Hair white
     d. Eyes are pale blue with a pink or red reflex which can be seen through the iris
     e. Severe photophobia caused by lack of pigment
     f. Associated ocular abnormalities: decreased visual acuity, nystagmus and strabismus
  2. OCA 1B (minimal pigment OCA, yellow OCA)
     a. Hair begins white but may progress to dark blonde or brown in adolescence
     b. Irides progressively darken
     c. Skin can tan minimally
     d. Nevi and freckles may develop
     e. Temperature-sensitive variant: darkly pigmented hair on the arms and legs, and lightly pigmented hair centrally
  3. OCA 2 (tyrosinase-positive OCA)
     a. Dilution of pigment of hair and iris but not complete loss
     b. Skin color paler than in relatives
     c. Hair white or light blonde
     d. With maturity, pigment increases and nevi and freckles can develop
     e. Photophobia and nystagmus are present, but not as severe as in OCA 1A
     f. More common in African-Americans
  4. OCA 3 (rufous OCA)
     a. Red hair and lighter skin

Pathogenesis

- OCA 1: mutation of the tyrosinase gene (chromosome 11p1)
  1. Complete loss with phenotype OCA 1A; reduced activity (5–10% of normal) results in OCA 1B
- OCA 2: mutation of the P gene (chromosome 15q11.2-12), membrane transporter gene
- OCA 3: mutation of TYRP1 gene affecting melanin synthesis; chromosome 9p23

Diagnosis

- Clinical presentation
- Genetic testing
- Electron microscopy can determine the stages of melanosomes

Differential diagnosis

- Prader–Willi syndrome
- Angelman syndrome
- Homocystinuria
- Apert syndrome
- Vitiligo (generalized)
- Phenylketonuria

Treatment

- Photoprotection is most important to reduce risk of cutaneous malignancies
- Ophthalmological evaluation and follow-up

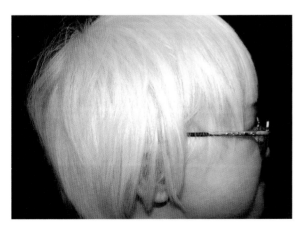

Figure 14.26 Albinism – type 1 oculocutaneous albinism

Prognosis

- Cutaneous squamous cell carcinoma and basal cell carcinoma along with other signs of photoaging are common in unprotected skin

References

King RA. Albinism. In The Pigmentary System. Nordlund JJ, Boissy RE, Hearing VJ, et al. eds). Oxford University Press: New York, 1998: 553–75

Oetting WS, Fryer JP, Shriram S, King RA. Oculocutaneous albinism type 1: the last 100 years. Pigment Cell Res 2003; 16: 307–11

Oetting WS. The tyrosinase gene and oculocutaneous albinism type 1 (OCA1): a model for understanding the molecular biology of melanin formation. Pigment Cell Res 2000; 13: 320–5

Orlow SJ. Albinism: an update. Semin Cutan Med Surg 1997; 16: 24–9

Sarangarajan R, Boissy RE. Tyrp1 and oculocutaneous albinism type 3. Pigment Cell Res 2001; 14: 437–44

Tomita Y. The molecular genetics of albinism and piebaldism. Arch Dermatol 1994; 130: 355–8

Waardenburg syndrome

Major points

- Waardenburg syndrome type I
  1. Depigmented patches of the skin and hair
  2. Heterochromia irides
  3. Deafness
  4. Dystopia canthorum
  5. Broad nasal root
  6. Synophrys (confluence of the medial eyebrows)
  7. Hypoplasia of the nasal alae
  8. Gene/gene locus: PAX 3 gene (transcription factor for melanocyte proliferation and migration from the neural crest)/2q35
  9. Autosomal dominant
- Waardenburg syndrome type II
  1. Similar to type I except without dystopia canthorum
  2. Gene/gene locus: MITF gene (microphthalmia-associated transcription factor)/3p14.1-12.3 and others
  3. Autosomal dominant
- Waardenburg syndrome type III (Klein–Waardenburg syndrome)

  1. Similar to type I with limb abnormalities
  2. Gene/gene locus: PAX 3 gene/2q35
  3. Autosomal dominant
- Waardenburg syndrome type IV
  1. Similar to type I with Hirschsprung disease
  2. Gene/gene locus: endothelin B receptor gene/20q13.2-q13.3
  3. Autosomal recessive

References

da Silva EO. Waardenburg I syndrome: a clinical and genetic study of two large Brazilian kindreds and literature review. Am J Med Genet 1991; 40: 65–74

Mollaaghababa R, Pavan WJ. The importance of having your SOX on: role of SOX10 in the development of neural crest-derived melanocytes and glia. Oncogene 2003; 22: 3024–34

Read AP, Newton VE. Waardenburg syndrome. J Med Genet 1997; 34: 656–65

Shanske A, Ferreira JC, Leonard JC, et al. Hirschsprung disease in an infant with a contiguous gene syndrome of chromosome 13. Am J Med Genet 2001; 102: 231–6

Shibahara S, Takeda K, Yasumoto K, et al. Microphthalmia-associated transcription factor (MITF): multiplicity in structure, function, and regulation. Symposium Proceedings. J Invest Dermatol 2001; 6: 99–104

Piebaldism

Major points

- Clinical features
  1. Symmetrical well-demarcated patches of depigmented skin and hair with V-shape on forehead and frontal scalp, patches on anterior chest and abdomen, and extremities around elbows and knees with sparing of hands and feet (Figure 14.27)
  2. No progressive loss of pigment
  3. No extracutaneous findings except in a few families with deafness
  4. 80–90% of patients have a white forelock

Pathogenesis

- Defective cell proliferation and migration of melanocytes during embryogenesis caused by mutation in c-KIT gene which is responsible for melanocytic proliferation; chromosome 14q12

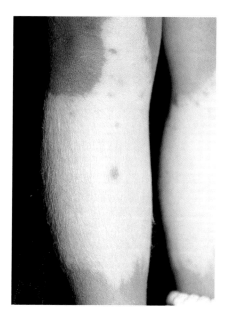

Figure 14.27 Piebaldism – symmetrical congenital depigmentation with thumbprint hypermelanotic macules within the depigmented patches

Diagnosis

- Clinical diagnosis
- Confirmed by genetic analysis with mutations on c-KIT gene
- Histology: melanocytes are absent from white patches

Differential diagnosis

- Waardenburg syndrome
- Vitiligo

Treatment

- Cosmetic covering
- Sun protection of the white patches

Prognosis

- White patches stable and may develop actinic keratoses

References

Boissy RE, Nordlund JJ. Molecular basis of congenital hypopigmentary disorders in humans: a review. Pigment Cell Res 1997; 10: 12–24

Richards KA, Fukai K, Oiso N, Paller AS. A novel KIT mutation results in piebaldism with progressive depigmentation. J Am Acad Dermatol 2001; 44: 288–92

Spritz RA. Molecular basis of human piebaldism. J Invest Dermatol 1994; 103: 137S–140S

Spritz RA. Piebaldism, Waardenburg syndrome, and related disorders of melanocyte development. Semin Cutan Med Surg 1997; 16: 15–23

Syrris P Malik NM, Murday VA, et al. Three novel mutations of the proto-oncogene KIT cause human piebaldism. Am J Med Genet 2000; 95: 79–81

Tomita Y. The molecular genetics of albinism and piebaldism. Arch Dermatol 1994; 130: 355–8

Hermansky–Pudlak syndrome

Major points

- Tyrosinase-positive albinism
- Bleeding diathesis with epistaxis, gingival bleeding or bleeding after surgical procedures
- Autosomal recessive; more common in Puerto Ricans and Dutch
- Ceroid storage disease affecting lungs, gut, platelets
- Gene/gene locus: HPS1 (transmembrane protein)/chromosome 10q2 and others

References

Gahl WA, Brantly M, Kaiser-Kupfer MI, et al. Genetic defects and clinical characteristics of patients with a form of oculocutaneous albinism (Hermansky–Pudlak syndrome). N Engl J Med 1998; 338: 1258–64

Huizing M, Boissy RE, Gahl WA. Hermansky-Pudlak syndrome: vesicle formation from yeast to man. Pigment Cell Res 2002; 15: 405–19

Huizing M, Gahl WA. Disorders of vesicles of lysosomal lineage: the Hermansky–Pudlak syndromes. Curr Mol Med 2002; 2: 451–67

Starcevic M, Nazarian R, Dell'Angelica EC. The molecular machinery for the biogenesis of lysosome-related organelles: lessons from Hermansky–Pudlak syndrome. Semin Cell Dev Biol 2002; 13: 271–8

Vanhooteghem O, Courtens W, Andre J, et al. Hermansky–Pudlak syndrome: a case report and discussion. Pediatr Dermatol 1998; 15: 374–7

Phenylketonuria

Major points

- Caused by absence of hepatic phenylalanine hydroxylase (PAH) with build-up of phenylalanine

- If untreated, phenylketonuria results in mental retardation and pigment dilution
- Most patients have blonde hair, blue eyes, fair skin, photosensitivity, mousy body odor and neurologic disturbances
- When treated, skin coloration reverts to normal
- Autosomal recessive
- Gene/gene locus: phenylalanine hydroxylase/12q24.1 and others

References

Beasley MG, Costello PM, Smith I. Outcome of treatment in young adults with phenylketonuria detected by routine neonatal screening between 1964 and 1971. Q J Med 1994; 87: 155–60

Erlandsen H, Patch MG, Gamez A, et al. Structural studies on phenylalanine hydroxylase and implications toward understanding and treating phenylketonuria. Pediatrics 2003; 112: 1557–65

Mineroff AD. Phenylketonuria. In The Pigmentary System. Nordlund JJ, Boissy RE, Hearing VJ, King RA, Ortonne JP, eds. Oxford University Press: New York, 1998: 590–1

Zschocke J. Focus on the molecular genetics of phenylketonuria. Hum Mutat 2003; 21: 331–2

Hypomelanosis of Ito

Synonym: incontinentia pigmenti achromians

Major points

- Hypopigmented streaks and whorls, mainly on the trunk, following the lines of Blaschko (Figure 14.28)
- Present at birth or becomes apparent during early life
- Macular pigmentation tends to be stable over time or may fade
- Inheritance sporadic or autosomal dominant
- Female/male ratio: 2.5–1
- Other cutaneous findings: aplasia cutis, fibromas, follicular keratosis, angiomas, generalized or focal hypertrichosis, and abnormalities in the teeth, hair, nails and sweat glands
- Extracutaneous findings (30%): mainly CNS, musculoskeletal and ocular system involvement
- Other findings: limb-length discrepancies, facial hemiatrophy, scoliosis, abnormal facies, genitourinary abnormalities, cardiac abnormalities

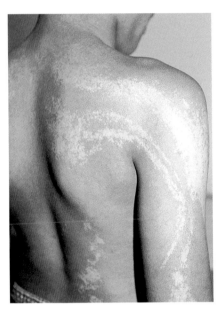

Figure 14.28   Hypomelanosis of Ito – hypopigmented streaks following Blaschko lines

Pathogenesis

- Mosaicism caused by two distinct germ lines formed during embryogenesis

Diagnosis

- Clinical presentation
- Histology: hypopigmented areas show normal or reduced number of melanocytes with reduction in number of melanosomes

Differential diagnosis

- Goltz syndrome
- Vitiligo
- Nevus depigmentosus
- Incontinentia pigmenti (stage 4)
- Epidermal nevi
- Lichen striatus
- Segmental vitiligo

Treatment

- Cosmetic cover-up is rarely needed

Prognosis

- Majority of children are normal, but in the first 2 years of life children should be observed for developmental delay and CNS abnormalities

- Neurologic and ocular examinations may be indicated
- Hypopigmentation may fade or be stable

References

Duran-McKinster C, Moises C, Rodriguez-Jurado R, et al. Streptococcal exanthem in a blaschkolinear pattern: clinical evidence for genetic mosaicism in hypomelanosis of Ito. Pediatr Dermatol 2002; 19: 423–5

Kuster W, Ehrig T, Happle R. In The Pigmentary System. Nordlund JJ, Boissy RE, Hearing VJ, et al. eds. Oxford University Press: . New York, 1998: 594–601

Kuster W, Konig A. Hypomelanosis of Ito: no entity, but a cutaneous sign of mosaicism. Am J Med Genet 1999; 85: 346–50

Nehal KS, DeBenito R, Orlow SJ. Analysis of 54 cases of hypopigmentation and hyperpigmentation along the lines of Blaschko. Arch Dermatol 1996; 132: 1167–70

Ruggieri M, Pavone L. Hypomelanosis of Ito: clinical syndrome or just phenotype? J Child Neurol 2000; 15: 635–44

Ruiz-Maldonado R, Roussaint S, Tamayo L, et al. Hypomelanosis of Ito: diagnostic criteria and report of 41 cases. Pediatr Dermatol 1992; 9: 1–10

Nevus depigmentosus (nevus achromicus)

Major points

- Single, well-circumscribed, hypopigmented patch, sometimes following the lines of Blaschko or in a segmental unilateral distribution (Figure 14.29)
- Border of lesion may be serrated or jagged
- Lesions present at birth or within the first years of life
- Usual locations: trunk and proximal extremities
- Male/female ratio = 1
- Rare associated findings: hemihypertrophy, seizures and mental retardation

Pathogenesis

- Hypothesis: functional defect of melanocytes and morphologic abnormalities of melanosomes

Diagnosis

- Clinical examination
- Under Wood's light examination, lesions show off-white accentuation, in contrast to vitiligo, which is bright white

Figure 14.29   Nevus depigmentosus – congenital hypopigmented well-defined patch

- Electron microscopy: defect in transfer of pigment between the melanocyte and keratinocyte with a decreased number of melanosomes in the keratinocytes; number of melanocytes normal

Differential diagnosis

- Nevus anemicus
- Segmental vitiligo
- Hypopigmented macules of tuberous sclerosis
- Hypomelanosis of Ito
- Pityriasis alba
- Postinflammatory hypopigmentation

Treatment

- Usually none needed
- Camouflage makeup such as Dermablend® or Covermark®

Prognosis

- Stable in size and distribution throughout life

References

Alkemade H, Juhlin L. Unilateral lentiginosis with nevus depigmentosus on the other side. J Am Acad Dermatol 2000; 43: 361–3

Dippel E, Utikal J, Feller G, et al. Nevi flammei affecting two contralateral quadrants and nevus depigmentosus: a new type of phacomatosis pigmentovascularis? Am J Med Genet 2003; 119A: 228–30

Lee HS, Chun YS, Hann SK. Nevus depigmentosus: clinical features and histopathologic characteristics in 67 patients. J Am Acad Dermatol 1999; 40: 21–6

Postinflammatory hypopigmentation

Major points

- Partial loss of cutaneous melanin in affected area of skin resulting from an inflammatory process (Figures 14.30 and 14.31)
- Appears as a hypochromic macule or patch in distribution of previous inflammation

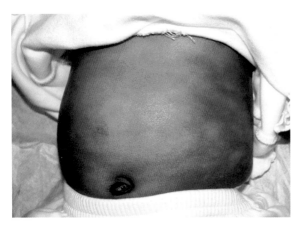

Figure 14.30   Postinflammatory hypopigmentation from eczema in a baby. The color reverted to normal after therapy

- More easily seen in dark skin
- Trauma and inflammation are thought to cause dysfunction of melanocytes
- Wood's lamp examination enhances hypopigmented areas in light skin and helps distinguish between depigmentation and hypopigmentation

Pathogenesis

- Histology can help to establish the cause of hypopigmentation

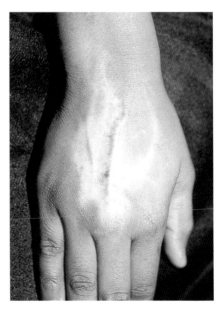

Figure 14.31   Postinflammatory hypopigmentation caused by a steroid injection for a cyst

Diagnosis

- Clinical presentation with history of inflammation

Differential diagnosis

- Tinea corporis
- Tinea versicolor
- Seborrheic dermatitis

Treatment

- Treat underlying cause of inflammation

Prognosis

- Can improve with treatment or remain static

References

Herane MI. Vitiligo and leukoderma in children. Clin Dermatol 2003; 21: 283–95

Ruiz-Maldonado R, Orozco-Covarrubias ML. Postinflammatory hypopigmentation and hyperpigmentation. Semin Cutan Med Surg 1997; 16: 36–43

15

COLLAGEN VASCULAR DISEASES

DERMATOMYOSITIS

Major points

- Affects three children per million per year in the USA
- Bimodal distribution: peaks at 5–9 years of age and again in teenage years
- Equal gender distribution at 5–9 years of age; 10 : 1 female predominance in early teenage years
- Skin manifestations:
  1. Heliotrope rash – violaceous, periorbital erythema with swelling
  2. Gottron papules – scaly, erythematous papules overlying metacarpal–phalangeal joints or interphalangeal joints (Figure 15.1)
  3. Erythematous malar rash and over neck, upper back and arms (shawl sign)
  4. Scaly, erythematous patches of the elbows, knees and cheeks
  5. Nails: periungual telangiectasias and cuticular overgrowth
  6. Poikiloderma
  7. Calcinosis cutis – usually occurs late in the course of disease, occurs much more frequently in children than adults; incidence can be reduced with aggressive treatment
- Noncutaneous manifestations:
  1. Symmetric, progressive, proximal muscle weakness (Gower sign)
  2. Muscle pain
  3. Constitutional symptoms: fever, weight loss, fatigue
  4. Dysphagia
  5. Nasal speech, hoarseness

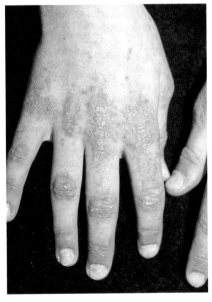

Figure 15.1 Dermatomyositis – typical Gottron papules over the knuckles

  6. Abdominal pain
  7. Arthritis and tenosynovitis
  8. Pulmonary disease (diffuse interstitial fibrosis, secondary aspiration and infection)
  9. Cardiac disease: heart block, arrythmias, pericarditis
  10. Gastrointestinal disease (mucosal ulceration)
  11. Calcinosis around joints and in intermuscular fascial planes
- Differs from adult dermatomyositis in that malignancy is extremely rare (work-up for malignancy is unnecessary)

Pathogenesis

- Etiology unknown
- Presumed autoimmune disorder
- May be multifactorial: infectious, genetic and environmental etiologies have been implicated

Diagnosis

- Criteria (Bohan and Peter)
  1. Characteristic rash, plus three of the four following:
     a. Symmetric proximal muscle weakness
     b. Elevated muscle enzymes (aldolase, creatine kinase, lactate dehydrogenase, transaminases (AST/ALT)
     c. Muscle biopsy (chronic inflammation with or without necrosis)
     d. Abnormal electromyogram (EMG)
- Magnetic resonance imaging (MRI) is useful in determining areas of muscle involvement:
  1. Identifies areas of edema and inflammation
  2. Used to identify appropriate muscle biopsy site
  3. Used to follow disease course

Differential diagnosis

- Systemic lupus erythematosus
- Photosensitive eruption (e.g. drug-induced dermatitis)
- Postinfectious myositis
- Other myopathies

Treatment

- Systemic corticosteroids – most cases respond to corticosteroid therapy
  1. Oral prednisone taper over several months
  2. High-dose intravenous pulse methylprednisolone (IVMP)
- Methotrexate is second-line agent of choice with recalcitrant disease
- If no response or there are intolerable adverse effects, other therapies to consider: cytoxan, hydroxychloroquine, azathioprine, cyclosporine, intravenous immunoglobulins (IVIG) and plasmapheresis
- Sun protection and sun avoidance
- Physical therapy to prevent contractures
- Early aggressive therapy is successful in minimizing long-term sequelae, including calcinosis

Prognosis

- With successful treatment, prognosis is good – overall mortality <7%
- Most children will completely recover after a single course (lasting months to years)
- ~25% will have disease with repeated acute exacerbations or persistence despite treatment
- Causes of mortality: myocarditis, progressive myositis, bowel perforation, aspiration pneumonia
- Causes of morbidity:
  1. Calcinosis may occur in up to 40%
  2. Joint contractures
  3. Cutaneous and gastrointestinal ulcers
  4. Residual muscle weakness and disability
- Cutaneous features can persist for years despite resolution of all other features of the disease

References

Drake LA, Dinehart SM, Farmer ER, et al. Guidelines of care for dermatomyositis. American Academy of Dermatology. J Am Acad Dermatol 1996; 34: 824–9

Fisler RE, Liang MG, Fuhlbrigge RC, et al. Aggressive management of juvenile dermatomyositis results in improved outcome and decreased incidence of calcinosis. J Am Acad Dermatol 2002; 47: 505–11

Pachman LM, Hayford JR, Chung A, et al. Juvenile dermatomyositis at diagnosis: Clinical characteristics of 79 children. J Rheumatol 1998; 25: 1198–204

Pachman LM. Juvenile dermatomyositis: immunogenetics, pathophysiology, and disease expression. Rheum Dis N Amer 2002; 28: 579–602

Ruperto N, Ravelli A, Murry KJ, et al. Paediatric Rheumatology International Trials Organization (PRINTO). Pediatric Rheumatology Collaborative Study Group (PRCSG). Preliminary core sets of measures for disease activity and damage assessment in juvenile systemic lupus erythematosus and juvenile dermatomyositis. Rheumatology 2003; 42: 1452–9

Santmyire-Rosenberger B, Dugan EM. Skin involvement in dermatomyositis. Curr Opin Rheumatol 2003; 15: 714–22.

Uzel G, Pachman LM. Cytokines in juvenile dermatomyositis pathophysiology: potential and challenge. Curr Opin Rheumatol 2003; 15: 691–7

SYSTEMIC LUPUS ERYTHEMATOSUS

Major points

- Incidence is ~5–10 per 100 000
- Disease shows a female predominance after puberty

- Black, Hispanic and Asian children have increased frequency of disease
- 25% of patients with systemic lupus erythematosus (SLE) have onset in the first two decades of life
- 80% of adolescents with SLE have cutaneous findings
- Cutaneous manifestations (presenting sign in 25%):
  1. Photosensitive eruption – malar or 'butterfly' rash, erythema with scale (Figure 15.2)
  2. Discoid lesions – round, sharply demarcated, erythematous lesions with adherent scale, follicular plugging, telangiectasias and scarring
  3. Telangiectasias – cuticular and other locations
  4. Livedo reticularis
  5. Scarring or nonscarring alopecia
  6. Nasal or oral ulcerations (particularly the hard palate)
  7. Vasculitis, erythema nodosum, lupus panniculitis can also occur
- Systemic symptoms:
  1. Arthritis, arthralgias
  2. Fever, malaise, weight loss, lymphadenopathy, muscle weakness
  3. Raynaud phenomenon
  4. Pulmonary and cardiac disease
  5. CNS involvement (neuropsychiatric)
  6. Renal disease (extent of involvement related to prognosis)

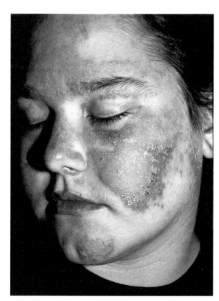

Figure 15.2 Systemic lupus erythematosus with butterfly rash

- Association with complement deficiencies, such as C2 deficiency

Pathogenesis

- Autoimmune disorder
- Genetic predisposition
- Many factors potentially contribute: viral, hormonal, environmental and immunogenetic
- Histology: vacuolar change of epidermal cells with a perivascular lymphohistiocytic infiltrate
- Direct immunofluorescence (DIF): granular deposition of IgG, with or without IgM, and complement at the dermal–epidermal junction and around hair follicles; IgA may occasionally be seen
- Circulating antibodies can be detected

Diagnosis

- American College of Rheumatology (ACR) criteria require four of the following 11 for diagnosis:
  1. Malar rash
  2. Discoid rash
  3. Photosensitivity
  4. Oral ulcers
  5. Arthritis: peripheral, nonerosive, involving two or more joints
  6. Serositis: pleuritis or pericarditis
  7. Renal disorder: proteinuria or cellular casts
  8. Neurologic disorder
  9. Hematologic disorder: anemia, leukopenia, lymphopenia, thrombocytopenia
  10. Immunologic disorder: positive antiphospholipid antibody, anti-DNA, or anti-Sm antibody; false positivity for syphilis
  11. Positive antinuclear antibody(ANA)
- Complement levels (C3 and C4) are low – levels may be used to monitor disease activity
- Biopsies may be performed: skin, renal or liver, as indicated

Differential diagnosis

- Dermatomyositis
- Juvenile rheumatoid arthritis
- Fifth disease
- Drug-induced lupus-like reactions (e.g. isoniazid, hydralazine, procainamide, D-penicillamine, minocycline)

Treatment

- High-dose systemic corticosteroids – continuous or pulsed

- Immunosuppressive agents:
  1. Azathioprine (Imuran®), cyclophosphamide (Cytoxan®), methotrexate, chlorambucil, mycophenolate mofetil
  2. Usually reserved for patients with severe systemic involvement (including renal and/or CNS disease)
  3. Combination with steroid therapy is effective and decreases steroid dose needed
- Topical corticosteroids for cutaneous lesions
- Oral hydroxychloroquine – for photosensitive cutaneous lesions
- Sun protection and avoidance
- Renal transplantation for end-stage renal disease

Prognosis

- Early diagnosis and aggressive treatment can improve prognosis
- Dependent on the degree of systemic involvement
- Frequently a more severe disease in children than in adults (renal and CNS disease common)
- Worst prognosis in children with diffuse proliferative glomerulonephritis and hypertension in the first 6 months of disease
- Infection is the cause of most deaths, especially in patients on chronic corticosteroid therapy

References

Barnett NK, Wright DA. Connective tissue diseases and arthritides. In Pediatric Dermatology, 3rd edn. Mosby: New York, 2003: 943–50

Dall'Era M, Davis JC. Systemic lupus erythematosus. How to manage, when to refer. Postgrad Med 2003; 114: 31–7, 40

DeSilva TN, Kress DW. Management of collagen vascular diseases in childhood. Clin Dermatol 1998; 16: 579–92

Drake LA, Dinehart SM, Farmer ER, et al. Guidelines of care for cutaneous lupus erythematosus. American Academy of Dermatology. J Am Acad Dermatol 1996; 34: 830–6

Gibson LE, Specks U, Homburger H. Clinical utility of ANCA tests for the dermatologist. Int J Dermatol 2003; 42: 859–69

Gill JM, Quisel AM, Rocca PV, Walters DT. Diagnosis of systemic lupus erythematosus. Am Fam Physician 2003; 68: 2179–86

Hamasaki K, Mimura T, Kanda H, et al. Systemic lupus erythematosus and thrombotic thrombocytopenic purpura: a case report and literature review. Clin Rheumatol 2003; 22: 355–8

Lyon VB, Nocton JJ, Drolet BA, Esterly NB. Necrotic facial papules in an adolescent: C2 deficiency with eventual development of lupus erythematosus. Pediatr Dermatol 2003; 20: 318–22

Mevorach D. Systemic lupus erythematosus and apoptosis: a question of balance. Clin Rev Allergy Immunol 2003; 25: 49–60

Ruperto N, Ravelli A, Murray KJ, et al. Paediatric Rheumatology International Trials Organization (PRINTO). Pediatric Rheumatology Collaborative Study Group (PRCSG). Preliminary core sets of measures for disease activity and damage assessment in juvenile systemic lupus erythematosus and juvenile dermatomyositis. Rheumatology 2003; 42: 1452–9

NEONATAL LUPUS ERYTHEMATOSUS

See Chapter 2

DISCOID LUPUS ERYTHEMATOSUS

Major points

- Characterized by the presence of discoid skin lesions without systemic involvement
  1. Some children with discoid lupus erythematosus (DLE) may progress to SLE; this transition seems to be more frequent and more severe in children and teens
  2. Discoid lesions may also be seen as a cutaneous manifestation of SLE
- Uncommon in children; <5% of patients with DLE develop disease before age 16 years
- Clinical presentation:
  1. Erythematous, sharply demarcated, scaly round plaques sometimes with telangiectasias (Figures 15.3 and 15.4)
  2. Lesions may be hyperpigmented or hypopigmented
  3. Adnexal involvement with follicular plugging and scarring alopecia
  4. Localized to sun-exposed areas – often over nose and malar eminences
  5. Most frequent locations: face, hands, ears and scalp
     a. Localized DLE – involvement limited to head
     b. Disseminated DLE – involvement below neck

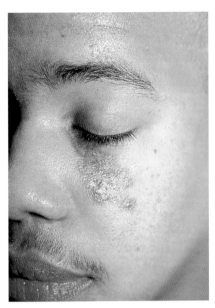

Figure 15.3 Discoid lupus erythematosus – typical erythematous, scaly, atrophic plaque with central atrophy

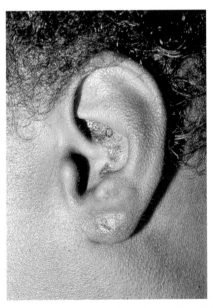

Figure 15.4 Discoid lupus erythematosus – keratotic papules in the ear, a common location

6. Results in atrophic, dyschromic scars
- Low incidence of photosensitivity as compared to DLE in adults
- Lack of female predominance as compared to other autoimmune diseases

Pathogenesis

- Autoimmune disorder
- Histology: inflammatory, mononuclear infiltrate involving upper and lower dermis and interface, perivascular and periadnexal areas; thickened basement membrane zone; keratinocyte damage; follicular plugging
- DIF: granular deposits at the dermal–epidermal junction
  1. Negative DIF does not rule out the diagnosis
  2. Scarred, burned-out lesions may no longer contain immunoreactants
- Predominance of activated T cells
- Sun exposure has been implicated in the development and exacerbation

Diagnosis

- Characteristic clinical findings
- Skin biopsy for histologic examination and DIF

Differential diagnosis

- Polymorphous light eruption
- Trauma
- Factitial dermatitis
- Sarcoidosis

Treatment

- Sun protection and avoidance
- Topical corticosteroids
- Intralesional corticosteroids
- Systemic therapy: hydroxychloroquine, systemic corticosteroids, dapsone

Prognosis

- Scarring, atrophy and dyspigmentation are common
- May progress to SLE

References

Cherif F, Mebazaa A, Mokni M, et al. Childhood discoid lupus erythematosus: a Tunisian retrospective study of 16 cases. Pediatr Dermatol 2003; 20: 295–8

George PM, Tunnessen WW. Childhood discoid lupus erythematosus. Arch Dermatol 1993; 129: 613–17

McMullen EA, Armstrong KD, Bingham EA, Walsh MY. Childhood discoid lupus erythematosus: a report of two cases. Pediatr Dermatol 1998; 15: 439–42

SCLERODERMA

Synonyms: systemic sclerosis, progressive systemic sclerosis

Major points

- Childhood cases account for 3% of all cases of scleroderma
- Female/male ratio >1
- Raynaud phenomenon occurs in 90% overall and may precede onset of disease
- Clinical subcategories:
  1. Diffuse disease – trunk and proximal portions of extremities
  2. Limited disease – only face and distal extremities involved
  3. CREST syndrome – Calcinosis, Raynaud phenomenon, Esophageal dysmotility, Sclerodactyly, Telangiectasia (rare in children)
- Clinical findings:
  1. Skin: generalized sclerotic changes, tightening, induration, occasional pruritus; progression to fibrosis and contractures; may be preceded by edema or rarely, an erythematous phase (Figure 15.5)
  2. Nailfold capillary dilatation and dropout
  3. Raynaud phenomenon
  4. Sclerodactyly
  5. Distal fingertip pitting from infarction
  6. Pulmonary disease: most commonly restrictive lung disease, interstitial lung disease
  7. Esophageal disease: symptoms of gastroesophageal reflux from esophageal dysmotility
  8. Renal disease
  9. Cardiac disease
  10. Myositis, arthritis, arthralgias, muscle atrophy

Pathogenesis

- Most evidence supports an immunologic (autoimmune) mechanism
- Histology: dense sclerosis of the dermis with excessive collagen deposition and trapping of adnexal structures
  1. Early phases: dense lymphocytic infiltrate at the interface between the deep dermis and the subcutaneous fat

Diagnosis

- Characteristic clinical findings
- Autoantibodies:
  1. ANA (22–100% in children)
  2. Anti-Scl 70 (40% in children)
  3. Anticentromere antibodies common in CREST syndrome, less common in systemic sclerosis (rarely found in children)

Differential diagnosis

- Scleredema
- Scleromyxedema
- Eosinophilic fasciitis
- Mixed connective tissue disease
- Chronic graft versus host disease
- Drug or chemical exposure

Treatment

- Early treatment to prevent irreversible organ tissue fibrosis
- Systemic therapies:
  1. Systemic corticosteroids
  2. D-Penicillamine
  3. Methotrexate
  4. PUVA - Psoralen+UVA
  5. Cyclophosphamide
  6. Cyclosporine
- Cutaneous treatment:
  1. Bland emollients (e.g. petrolatum)
  2. Avoidance of extreme temperatures (especially cold)
  3. Physical therapy to prevent joint contractures

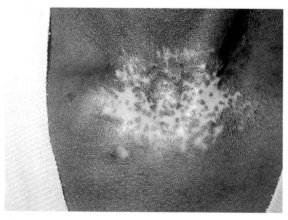

Figure 15.5   Scleroderma – depigmented, sclerotic patch with retained follicular pigmentation

- Raynaud phenomenon:
  1. Cold protection and avoidance
  2. Avoidance of smoking
  3. Calcium channel blockers (e.g. nifedipine)
  4. Nitroglycerin patch to fingertips for temporary relief
  5. IV infusion of prostaglandin E_1 and prostacyclin for nonhealing ulcers or debilitating disease
- Gastroesophageal disease with reflux esophagitis:
  1. Proton pump inhibitors (e.g. omeprazole)
  2. Head of bed elevation, light meals
- Pulmonary disease: cyclophosphamide
- Renal disease (with malignant hypertension):
  1. Angiotensin-converting enzyme (ACE)-inhibitors (e.g. captopril)
  2. Hemodialysis

Prognosis

- Slow progression for years with organ failure and death (similar to adults)
- Young males and patients with significant cardiac, pulmonary, or renal disease have worse prognosis
- Interstitial lung disease is the most common cause of mortality

References

Atamas SP, White B. The role of chemokines in the pathogenesis of scleroderma. Curr Opin Rheumatol 2003; 15: 772–7

Black CM. Scleroderma and fasciitis in children. Curr Opin Rheumatol 1995; 7: 442–6

Drake LA, Dinehart SM, Farmer ER, et al. Guidelines of care for scleroderma and sclerodermoid disorders. J Am Acad Dermatol 1996; 35: 609–14

Harris ML, Rosen A. Autoimmunity in scleroderma: the origin, pathogenetic role, and clinical significance of autoantibodies. Curr Opin Rheumatol 2003; 15: 778–84

Leask A, Denton CP, Abraham DJ. Insights into the molecular mechanism of chronic fibrosis: the role of connective tissue growth factor in scleroderma. J Invest Dermatol 2004; 122: 1–6

Murray KJ, Laxer RM. Scleroderma in children and adolescents. Rheum Dis Clin North Am 2002; 28: 603–24

Vancheeswaran R, Black CM, David J, et al. Childhood-onset scleroderma: is it different from adult-onset disease? Arth Rheum 1996; 39: 1041–9

MORPHEA

Synonym: localized scleroderma

Major points

- Sclerodermatous patches limited to skin (Figures 15.6 and 15.7)
- Progression to systemic involvement is exceedingly rare
- Self-limited disorder, lasting ~3–5 years
- Often an unsolicited history of trauma to the area
- Clinical course: superficial erythema and inflammation of skin followed by hardening of the area and subdermal structures; loss of hair and anhidrosis; hypo- or hyperpigmentation; may affect muscle or bone if extensive or over a joint
- Linear scleroderma
  1. Most frequent type in children
  2. Usually unilateral along part of an extremity, but may affect thorax, abdomen, or buttocks
  3. Linear lesions are initially erythematous plaques, gradually lose their color centrally and become white, shiny, atrophic or thickened with sclerosis
  4. May cause joint contractures, muscle wasting, or limb growth failure if over a joint

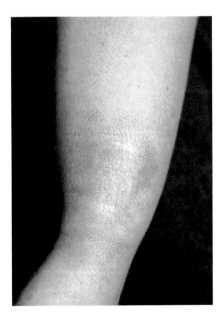

Figure 15.6   Morphea – hyperpigmented, sclerotic plaque on extremity

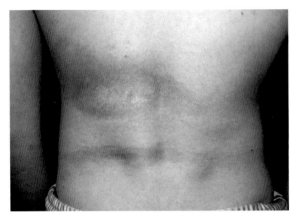

Figure 15.7 Morphea – two large plaques on the back. He later developed a large plaque on one leg

- En coup de sabre
    1. Ivory sclerotic plaque with peripheral hyperpigmentation appears on forehead and scalp (resembling a saber cut) (Figure 15.8)
        a. May cause alopecia of the scalp, eyebrows, eyelashes
        b. May affect nose, cheek, chin and neck
        c. Ranges in severity from minor indentation to severe hemifacial atrophy
    2. May have CNS involvement (e.g. seizures, intracranial calcification, intracranial aneurysm), tongue atrophy, tooth growth abnormalities, uveitis
    3. Parry-Romberg syndrome (progressive facial hemiatrophy) considered by some authors to be a variant of en coup de sabre type
- Plaque morphea
    1. Oval patches or plaques involving the skin and subcutaneous tissue
    2. Most common on trunk, may be seen on extremities, head and neck
    3. Erythematous or hyperpigmented plaques, several centimeters in diameter; central clearing with a violaceous border; later a white center that becomes shiny, firm and waxy
    4. Plaques tend to have no hair or sweating
    5. May see plaque morphea and linear lesions in the same patient
- Generalized morphea
    1. Large plaques in different anatomic locations (>4 plaque lesions in ≥2 body sites)
    2. Lesions similar to plaque morphea with generalized involvement

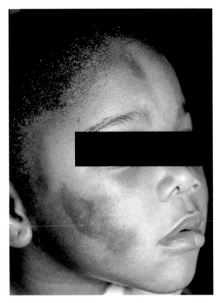

Figure 15.8 Morphea (en coup de sabre) – hyperpigmented, sclerotic indentation on the forehead and cheek

Pathogenesis

- Thought to be an autoimmune disorder
- Early inflammation with edema and increased vascularity; progressing to sclerosis and abnormal collagen formation; ultimately resulting in atrophy
- Trauma and *Borrelia burgdorferi* infection have been implicated as triggers
- Histology:
    1. Early: dermal edema with swelling and degeneration of collagen fibrils, lymphocytic infiltrate around dermal vessels and appendages
    2. Late: progressive dermal thickening and condensation of collagen – with bundles densely packed and aligned parallel to the dermal – epidermal junction with loss of appendages

Diagnosis

- Clinical findings
- Skin biopsy may be performed to aid in diagnosis but not always necessary
- Laboratory studies: none specific but may be helpful in following the course; ANA, complete blood count (CBC) with differential, immunoglobulins, rheumatoid arthritis factor
- Consider work-up for other collagen vascular diseases as indicated by history and physical

examination; extensive disease may be more likely to have immunologic abnormalities

- MRI/ultrasound – useful if there is CNS or eye involvement or to determine depth of lesions

Differential diagnosis

- Postinflammatory hyperpigmentation
- Erythema dyschromicum perstans
- Lichen sclerosus
- Traumatic scars
- Eosinophilic fasciitis
- Scleredema of Buschke

Treatment

- Systemic therapy:
  1. Low-dose methotrexate
  2. Systemic corticosteroids (oral or IV pulse)
  3. Oral calcitriol (vitamin D analog)
  4. PUVA (not recommended for <11 years)
  5. D-Penicillamine
- Topical therapy:
  1. Potent topical steroids
  2. Emollients
  3. Topical calcipotriene
- Physical therapy/occupational therapy for joint involvement
- Psychological support as needed

Prognosis

- Lesions tend to have an active, progressive phase for several years then slowly resolve spontaneously with softening of skin
- Progression exceedingly rare to systemic involvement
- Potential sequelae include: residual hyperpigmentation, skin atrophy, limb atrophy, joint contractures and psychological sequelae

References

Cunningham BB, Landells ID, Langman C, et al. Topical calcipotriene for morphea/linear scleroderma. J Am Acad Dermatol 1998; 39: 211–15

Drake LA, Dinehart SM, Farmer ER, et al. Guidelines of care for scleroderma and sclerodermoid disorders. J Am Acad Dermatol 1996; 35: 609–14

Hawk A, English JC 3rd. Localized and systemic scleroderma. Semin Cutan Med Surg 2001; 20: 27–37

Jablonska S, Blaszczyk M. Scleroderma and sclerotic skin conditions: unapproved treatments. Clin Dermatol 2002; 20: 634–7

Murray KJ, Laxer RM. Scleroderma in children and adolescents. Rheum Dis Clin North Am 2002; 28: 603–24

Nelson AM. Localized scleroderma including morphea, linear scleroderma and eosinophilic fasciitis. Curr Prob Pediatr 1996; 26: 318–24

Sehgal VN, Srivastava G, Aggarwal AK, et al. Localized scleroderma/morphea. Int J Dermatol 2002; 41: 467–75

LICHEN SCLEROSUS

Synonyms: lichen sclerosus et atrophicus

Major points

- Female/male ratio is 10 : 1
- Some clinical overlap seen between morphea and LS
- Clinical findings:
  1. Ivory or white, shiny macules or papules that coalesce into homogeneous hypo- or depigmented plaques; affected area is sharply demarcated from surrounding skin (Figures 15.9 and 15.10)
  2. Commonly encircles the vulvar and perianal areas in a 'figure of eight' pattern
  3. Extragenital involvement on the trunk, forearm, neck and face
  4. Other cutaneous findings: vesicles, bullae (which are occasionally hemorrhagic), ulcerations, excoriations
  5. Symptoms: pruritus, dysuria, painful defecation, and anal and vulvar bleeding
  6. In males, major symptom may be phimosis

Pathogenesis

- Inflammatory disorder of unknown etiology
- Familial cases have been reported
- LS in children has been associated with trauma
- Histology: homogenized collagen with a band-like lymphocytic infiltrate underlying a normal or atrophic epidermis

Diagnosis

- Characteristic clinical findings
- Skin biopsy may be helpful in uncertain cases

Differential diagnosis

- Morphea
- Trauma, including sexual abuse

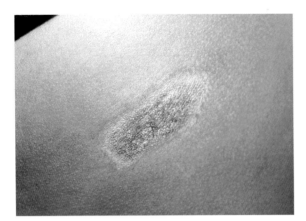

Figure 15.9   Lichen sclerosus – hypopigmented, atrophic plaque

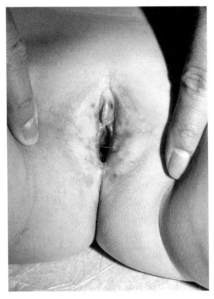

Figure 15.10   Lichen sclerosus – involving the vulva

- Vitiligo
- Postinflammatory hypopigmentation

Treatment

- Topical corticosteroids:
  1. Potent topical corticosteroids (e.g. 0.05% betamethasone ointment) BID for short period of time, usually 2–4 weeks; then tapered to once daily; may need to use intermittently for symptoms
  2. Taper to low-potency steroids when disease under control

- Proper perineal hygiene
- Nonocclusive underwear
- Avoid trauma (e.g. bicycle riding)
- Antimicrobial treatment for secondary bacterial or yeast infections
- Topical tacrolimus or pimecrolimus (off label) BID

Prognosis

- Two-thirds of pre-pubertal girls will have clearing or improvement of lesions at puberty (childhood form has better prognosis than adult form)
- Potential complications of persistent lesions: scarring and labial atrophy; constriction of the vaginal introitus or urethral meatus
- Squamous cell carcinoma is a rare complication of LS in adults

References

Fischer G, Rogers M. Treatment of childhood vulvar lichen sclerosus with potent topical corticosteroids. Pediatr Dermatol 1997; 14: 235–8

Helm KF, Gibson LE, Muller SA. Lichen sclerosus et atrophicus in children and young adults. Pediatr Dermatol 1991; 8: 97–101

Neill SM, Tatnall FM, Cox NH. British Association of Dermatologists. Guidelines for the management of lichen sclerosus. Br J Dermatol 2002; 147: 640–9

Sahn EE, Bluestein EL, Olivia S. Familial lichen sclerosus et atrophicus in childhood. Pediatr Dermatol 1994; 11: 160–3

Tasker GL, Wojnarowska F. Lichen sclerosus. Clin Exp Dermatol 2003; 28: 128–33

Warrington SA, de San Lazaro C. Lichen sclerosus et atrophicus and sexual abuse. Arch Dis Child 1996; 75: 512–16

VASCULITIS

Major points

- Group of disorders characterized by inflammation of blood vessel walls
- Cutaneous manifestations: purpura, petechiae, ecchymosis, erythematous macules, papules, nodules, urticaria, livedo reticularis, necrosis, ulceration, vesicles, pustules, bullae, pyoderma gangrenosum-like lesions, erythema nodosum-like lesions (Figure 15.11)

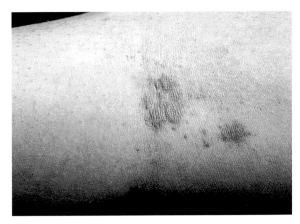

Figure 15.11   Vasculitis – associated with systemic lupus erythematosus

- Most common vasculitis in childhood is Henoch–Schönlein purpura (see below)
- Tends to be more self-limited in children than adults
- Classified by the size of vessel affected (small, medium or large vessel)
  1. Large-vessel vasculitis
     a. Giant cell (temporal) arteritis
     b. Takayasu arteritis
  2. Medium-vessel vasculitis
     a. Kawasaki disease (see Chapter 11)
     b. Classic polyarteritis nodosa (PAN)
  3. Small-vessel vasculitis (leukocytoclastic vasculitis)
     a. Henoch–Schönlein purpura
     b. Cutaneous leukocytoclastic vasculitis
     c. Microscopic polyarteritis nodosa
     d. Wegener granulomatosis
     e. Churg–Strauss syndrome
     f. Essential cryoglobulinemic vasculitis
- Major types of vasculitis seen in children:
  1. Henoch–Schönlein purpura (see below)
  2. Polyarteritis nodosa
     a. Constitutional symptoms: malaise, fever, weight loss
     b. Hypertension
     c. Skin findings: purpuric papules with or without necrosis, livedo reticularis, tender subcutaneous nodules
     d. Systemic involvement: musculoskeletal, renal, nervous system, gastrointestinal (GI) tract most commonly affected

  3. Takayasu arteritis
     a. Granulomatous inflammation of the aorta and its main branches causing stenosis and aneurysms
     b. In children, thoracic and abdominal aorta most commonly affected
     c. 'Pulseless' disease – diminished or no pulses in the arms and blood pressure discrepancies between arms
     d. Lacks skin lesions
  4. Wegener granulomatosis
     a. Granulomatous inflammation involving the respiratory tract (sinuses, nasal passages, pharynx, lungs) and kidneys (glomerulonephritis)
     b. Common clinical presentation: malaise, fever, sinusitis, epistaxis and hematuria
     c. May have necrotizing lesions of the skin, CNS, or gut

Pathogenesis

- May be triggered by a variety of agents: infection, drugs and malignancy (Table 15.1)
- Infectious vasculitis: bacterial, rickettsial, mycobacterial, spirochetal, fungal, viral
- Immune-mediated vasculitis can be categorized as:
  1. T-cell-mediated inflammation (e.g. Takayasu arteritis)
  2. Antibody-mediated inflammation:
     a. Immune complex deposition in vessel walls (e.g. IgA immune complex deposition in Henoch–Schönlein purpura)
     b. Direct binding of antibodies to vessel wall antigens (e.g. Kawasaki disease)
     c. Activation of leukocytes by leukocyte-specific antigens (e.g. antineutrophilic cytoplasmic autoantibodies (ANCA))

Diagnosis

- Clinical findings – look for evidence of infection, drug history, environmental/allergen exposure and systemic manifestations on history and physical examination
- Skin biopsy to confirm diagnosis
- Directed biopsies of specific organs to evaluate visceral disease
- Laboratory studies: ANA, cryoglobulins, hepatitis B and C antibodies, ANCA, complement levels, IgA–fibronectin aggregates

---

Table 15.1   Common causes and associated underlying diseases in leukocytoclastic vasculitis

Infections
Streptococcal and neisserial bacterial infections
Hepatitis B
Cytomegalovirus
Epstein–Barr virus

Medications and drugs
Sulfa antibiotics
Thiazides, phenothiazines, sulfonylureas and other
  sulfa-related drugs
Quinidine
Phenytoin
Injected illicit drugs
Allopurinol
Radiographic contrast media
Nonsteroidal anti-inflammatory agents

Autoimmune diseases
Lupus erythematosus
Rheumatoid arthritis
Giant cell arteritis
Wegener granulomatosis
Mixed connective tissue disease
Sjögren syndrome
Inflammatory bowel disease

Dysproteinemias
Cryoglobulinemia
Monoclonal and polyclonal gammopathies

Malignancies
Myeloma
Leukemia
Lymphoma

Food products
Food dyes and preservatives

Adapted from Schachner and Hansen, Pediatric Dermatology, 3rd edn. Mosby, New York 2003; 823

- Imaging studies as indicated: chest X-ray, CT scans, angiography or magnetic resonance angiography – if there are bruits or ischemic symptoms
- Further work-up determined by extent of systemic disease

Differential diagnosis

- Coagulopathies (e.g. thrombocytopenia, disseminated intravascular coagulation (DIC), platelet dysfunction)
- Occlusive disorders

Treatment

- Should be directed toward symptoms and prevention of visceral disease
- Infection must be ruled out before starting immunosuppressive therapy
- Removal of causative agents: e.g. infectious pathogen, drug, malignancy (rare in childhood)
- Corticosteroids
- Immunosuppressive agents (e.g. azathioprine or cyclophosphamide)

Prognosis

- Dependent on disease severity and presence/extent of systemic involvement

References

Crowson AN, Mihm MC Jr, Magro CM. Cutaneous vasculitis: a review. J Cutan Pathol 2003; 30: 161–73

Fiorentino DF. Cutaneous vasculitis. J Am Acad Dermatol 2003; 48: 311–40

Ozen S. The spectrum of vasculitis in children. Best Pract Res Clin Rheumatol 2002; 16: 411–25

Weyard CM, Goronzy JJ. Medium- and large-vessel vasculitis. N Engl J Med 2003; 349: 160–9

HENOCH–SCHÖNLEIN PURPURA

Synonyms: anaphylactoid purpura

Major points

- Leukocytoclastic vasculitis characterized by palpable purpura, joint pain, abdominal pain and renal disease (i.e. glomerulonephritis)
- Incidence is 14 per 100 000 per year in children
- Male/female ratio is ~1.5 : 1
- Peak incidence between 2 and 5 years
- Often a history of a recent upper respiratory infection (66–75%) – viral or streptococcal infection
- Cutaneous findings:
  1. Palpable purpura (but may be only macular) (Figure 15.12)
  2. Distribution is usually symmetric over buttocks and lower extremities but can occur on upper extremities over extensor surfaces (elbows, knees), trunk and face
  3. Petechiae, maculopapular erythematous rash, ulcers, vesicles and bullae (which may become hemorrhagic) and edema

4. Younger children <3 years age have more scalp, periorbital and acral edema
- Extracutaneous findings:
  1. Joint symptoms – arthralgias and/or arthritis
  2. Colicky abdominal pain from GI involvement: bleeding, melena, hematemesis, hemorrhage and intussusception (ileoileal)
  3. Renal involvement – glomerulonephritis
- Acute hemorrhagic edema of childhood
  1. Shares many features with Henoch–Schönlein purpura – once considered a variant, but is likely to be a distinct entity
  2. Age usually <2 years; has been reported at birth
  3. Clinical findings:
     a. Abrupt onset of fever and tender edema of the face, eyelids, ears, scrotum and acral extremities
     b. Purpuric, ecchymotic lesions on face and extremities (usually sparing the trunk)
     c. Circinate, medallion-like pattern
     d. No other associated systemic symptoms other than fever; good general health
  4. Pathogenesis: small-vessel vasculitis thought to be a hypersensitivity reaction to an infectious agent or following immunization

a. Has been reported following staphylococcal or streptococcal infection, upper respiratory infection, otitis, urinary tract infection, conjunctivitis, or adenovirus
     b. IgA is variably present
  5. Diagnosis:
     a. Characteristic clinical findings
     b. Skin involvement only – renal and GI systems should be evaluated to rule out involvement
     c. Laboratory studies: leukocytosis, thrombocytosis, eosinophilia, elevated erythrocyte sedimentation rate (ESR)
  6. No treatment is usually necessary
  7. Antibiotics for associated infection

Pathogenesis

- IgA immune complex-mediated small-vessel vasculitis
- Thought to be triggered by a preceding respiratory infection; considered a hypersensitivity reaction
- Histology: leukocytoclastic vasculitis of capillaries in upper dermis with perivascular neutrophils, nuclear debris and extravasated erythrocytes; IgA deposition in vessels on DIF
- Distribution of lesions has been suggested to be gravity dependent (predilection for buttock and lower extremities in older children)
- Henoch–Schönlein purpura nephropathy is caused by mesangial IgA deposition

Diagnosis

- Characteristic cutaneous findings in the presence of joint swelling and abdominal pain
- Skin biopsy and DIF (important for diagnosis) – leukocytoclastic vasculitis; DIF demonstrates perivascular IgA, C3 and fibrin deposits
- About half the patients have elevated serum IgA; circulating IgA-containing immune complexes may be present
- Urinalysis to establish renal status
- Abdominal ultrasound examination for abdominal pain to evaluate for intussusception
- Guaiac stool for frank or occult blood

Differential diagnosis

- Other vasculitis
- Septic vasculitis

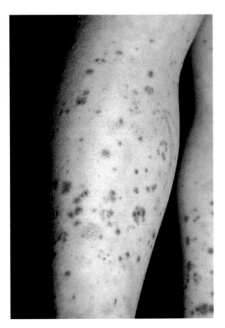

Figure 15.12   Henoch–Schönlein purpura with palpable purpura on lower legs

Treatment

- Supportive, bed rest
- Elevation of swollen areas
- Nonsteroidal anti-inflammatory medications (NSAIDs) for joint symptoms
- Corticosteroids for GI symptoms
- High-dose pulse steroids or immunosuppressive agents (e.g. cyclophosphamide or azathioprine) for progressive renal disease

Prognosis

- Generally considered benign and self-limited in the pediatric age group
  1. More severe disease in adults
  2. Resolution usually in 2–4 weeks; may relapse for several months (up to 40% of patients); can rarely become chronic (up to years)
- Long-term morbidity and mortality rates due to renal failure
  1. End-stage renal disease occurs in 5% of patients
  2. Risk factors for renal involvement: purpura affecting the upper part of the trunk, fever, elevated ESR, recent history of upper respiratory infection
- Recurrence after a 1-year asymptomatic period can occur in 10% of patients

References

Al-Sheyyab M, El-Shanti H, Ajlouni S, et al. The clinical spectrum of Henoch–Schönlein purpura in infants and young children. Eur J Pediatr 1995; 154: 699–701

Ballinger S. Henoch–Schönlein purpura. Curr Opin Rheumatol 2003; 15: 591–4

Fervenza FC. Henoch–Schönlein purpura nephritis. Int J Dermatol 2003; 42: 170–7

Gonggryp LA, Todd G. Acute hemorrhagic edema of childhood (AHE). Pediatr Dermatol 1998; 15: 91–6

Nussinovitch M, Prais D, Finkelstein Y, et al. Cutaneous manifestations of Henoch–Schönlein purpura in young children. Pediatr Dermatol 1998; 15: 426–8

Magro CM, Crowson AN. A clinical and histologic study of 37 cases of immunoglobulin-A associated vasculitis. Am J Dermatopathol 1999; 21: 234–40

Manzoni APD, Viecili JB, Benvenuto de Andrade C, et al. Acute hemorrhagic edema of infancy: a case report. Int J Dermatol 2004; 43: 48–51

Piette WW. What is Schönlein–Henoch purpura, and why should we care? Arch Dermatol 1997; 133: 515–18

Saulsbury FT. Hemorrhagic bullous lesions in Henöch–Schonlein purpura. Pediatr Dermatol 1998; 15: 357–9

PURPURA FULMINANS

Major points

- Heterogeneous group of disorders characterized by acute onset, rapidly progressing, purpuric lesions which develop into extensive areas of skin necrosis, hemorrhage and peripheral gangrene (Figure 15.13)
- Development of disseminated intravascular coagulation (DIC) is a defining feature
- Occurs in three clinical settings:
  1. Acute infectious purpura fulminans (most common)
     a. In the setting of overwhelming sepsis
     b. Majority of cases due to meningococcal sepsis (*Neisseria meningitidis*); develops in 15–25% of those with meningococcemia
     c. Occurs rarely with other pathogens: *Streptococcus pneumoniae*, group B streptococcus (in neonates), *Haemophilus influenzae* type b and others
  2. Homozygous protein C or protein S deficiency
     a. Seen in neonatal period

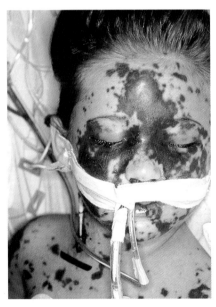

Figure 15.13 Purpura fulminans – associated with sepsis

3. Idiopathic purpura fulminans (uncommon)
   a. Postinfectious–after a relatively benign antecedent infection (e.g. varicella or group A streptococcal infection)
   b. Unknown etiology–after noninfectious condition (e.g. cutaneous hypersensitivity reaction, or stomatitis)
   c. Differs from acute infectious form in that organ involvement other than skin usually does not occur, extremities are spared, and there is lower mortality (circulatory collapse not initially present)
- Cutaneous lesions:
  1. Early skin discomfort followed by erythema with or without edema and petechiae
  2. Rapid evolution into painful, indurated, well-demarcated purpuric papules and plaques with erythematous borders
  3. Late vesicles and bullae in necrotic areas, hemorrhagic necrosis, and eschar formation
  4. Gangrene of subcutaneous tissues, muscle and/or bone
- Extracutaneous clinical features:
  1. Epiphyseal growth plate necrosis; may lead to limb shortening
  2. Shock, thrombotic hemorrhage of multiple vascular beds and organ systems (e.g. adrenal glands, lungs and kidney), and multi-organ dysfunction are common

Pathogenesis

- Cutaneous lesions caused by widespread dermal vascular thrombosis
- Laboratory evidence of a consumptive coagulopathy (DIC)
  1. Prolonged prothrombin time (PT) and partial thromboplastin time (PTT)
  2. Decreased fibrinogen levels
  3. Elevated fibrin degradation products (e.g. D-dimers)
  4. Reduced protein C, protein S and antithrombin III levels
- Histology: dermal vascular thrombosis and secondary hemorrhagic necrosis

Diagnosis

- Characteristic clinical course
- Laboratory studies: CBC with platelet count, PT, PTT, fibrinogen, fibrin

degradation products, protein C and S, antithrombin III

Differential diagnosis

- Thrombotic thombocytopenic purpura
- Hemolytic uremic syndrome
- Coumadin (warfarin) necrosis

Treatment

- Acute infectious purpura fulminans:
  1. Treat underlying infection and shock with supportive measures and IV antibiotics
  2. Fresh-frozen plasma or prothrombin complex concentrate – for protein C, protein S and antithrombin III replacement
  3. Blood components as necessary: packed red blood cells, platelets, cryoprecipitate
  4. Vitamin K
  5. Consultation of surgical and nutritional services
  6. Local skin care: topical antibiotics and debridement as needed
- Idiopathic purpura fulminans
  1. Fresh-frozen plasma or prothrombin complex concentrate for replacement of coagulation products
  2. Heparin anticoagulation: full-dose heparin for at least 2 weeks after skin lesions cease to develop
  3. Protein C concentrate if indicated
  4. Antibiotic coverage until culture results are negative – to cover Gram-positive cocci, meningococci, Gram-negative bacilli
  5. Local skin care using topical antibiotics and debridement as needed
- Neonatal purpura fulminans
  1. Acute setting:
     a. Initiate therapy immediately
     b. Fresh-frozen plasma or prothrombin complex concentrate – replace protein C and S
     c. Alternative: protein C concentrate, advantage of avoiding blood volume overload
  2. Long-term treatment:
     a. Low-dose oral anticoagulants plus replacement therapy
     b. Topical nitroglycerin may be applied to poorly perfused extremities
     c. Protein C concentrates for protein C deficiency

Prognosis

- Can be fatal, especially in cases of acute infectious purpura fulminans
  1. Meningococcemia with purpura fulminans carries a 20–60% mortality rate
  2. Idiopathic purpura fulminans has lower mortality rate (~15%)
- High morbidity related to loss of digits, limbs, or areas of skin

References

Baselga E, Drolet BA, Esterly NB. Purpura in infants and children. J Am Acad Dermatol 1997; 37: 673–705

Darmstadt GL. Acute infectious purpura fulminans: pathogenesis and medical management. Pediatr Dermatol 1998; 15: 169–83

Esmon CT. The protein C pathway. Chest 2003; 124 (3 Suppl): 26S–32S

Ilan Y, Naparstek Y. Henoch Schönlein purpura in children and adults: is it one entity? Semin Arthritis Rheum 2002; 32: 139–40

Levin M, Eley BS, Louis J, et al. Postinfectious purpura fulminans caused by an autoantibody directed against protein C. J Pediatr 1995; 127: 355–63

Manco-Johnson MJ, Nuss R, Key N, et al. Lupus anticoagulant and protein S deficiency in children with postvaricella purpura fulminans or thrombosis. J Pediatr 1996; 128: 319–23

Pathan N, Faust SN, Levin M. Pathophysiology of meningococcal meningitis and septicaemia. Arch Dis Child 2003; 88: 601–7

Wheeler JS, Anderson BJ, De Chalain TM. Surgical interventions in children with meningococcal purpura fulminans – a review of 117 procedures in 21 children. J Pediatr Surg 2003; 38: 597–603

PIGMENTED PURPURA

Synonym: primary (idiopathic) capillaritis

General

- Group of closely related, chronic, benign conditions with similar histologic and clinical manifestations
  1. Clinical: nonpalpable petechiae and hemosiderotic eruptions; old and new petechiae can be seen at the same examination (Figure 15.14)

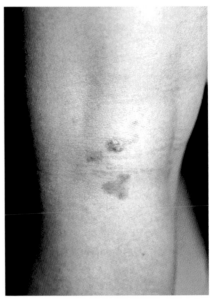

Figure 15.14   Pigmented purpura with cayenne pepper red dots and hemosiderin deposition

  2. Histology: perivascular lymphocytic infiltrate, extravasation of red blood cells, deposit of hemosiderin (mostly inside macrophages), narrowing of the lumen of small vessels, and endothelial swelling
- Unknown etiology
- Includes:
  1. Schamberg progressive pigmented purpura (see below)
  2. Lichen aureus (see below)
  3. Purpura annularis telangiectodes of Majocchi
  4. Pigmented purpuric lichenoid dermatitis of Gougerot and Blum
  5. Eczematoid-like purpura of Coucas and Kapetanakis

References

Kim HJ, Skidmore RA, Woosley JT. Pigmented purpura over the lower extremities. Purpura annularis telangiectodes of Majocchi. Arch Dermatol 1998; 134: 1477–80

Pock L, Capkova S. Segmental pigmented purpura. Pediatr Dermatol 2002; 19: 517–19

Reinhold U, Seiter S, Ugurel S, Tilgen W. Treatment of progressive pigmented purpura with oral bioflavonoids and ascorbic acid: an open pilot study in 3 patients. J Am Acad Dermatol 1999; 41: 207–8

Satoh T, Yokozeki H, Nishioka K. Chronic pigmented purpura associated with odontogenic infection. J Am Acad Dermatol 2002; 46: 942–4

Weston WL, Orchard D. Vascular reaction. In Pediatric Dermatology, 3rd edn. Schachner LA, Hansen RC, eds. Mosby: New York, 2003: 821–2

Schamberg disease

Synonym: Schamberg progressive pigmented purpura

Major points

- Most common of the pigmented purpuras
- Common cause of chronic petechiae in children
- Clinical findings:
  1. Asymptomatic nonpalpable purpura and petechiae with orange to brown patches; old and new petechiae can be seen within a patch
  2. Usually affects the legs but can be seen elsewhere (e.g. trunk)
  3. Usually bilateral but may be asymmetric or unilateral, especially in adolescents
- Chronic course, often lasts months to years

Pathogenesis

- Etiology unknown
- Benign chronic capillaritis; capillary fragility leads to red cell extravasation
- Histology: mild perivascular infiltrate, mainly lymphocytes, extravasated red blood cells, and macrophages containing hemosiderin deposits involving the papillary and upper dermis; focal parakeratosis and spongiosis of epidermis

Diagnosis

- Characteristic clinical findings
- Biopsy helpful

Differential diagnosis

- Vasculitis
- Cutaneous T-cell lymphoma
- Pityriasis lichenoides

Treatment

- Treatment is difficult and often ineffective
- Mid-strength topical steroids
- Therapies that have been reported to be effective without serious side-effects: combination therapy with oral bioflavinoids and ascorbic acid; pentoxifylline

Prognosis

- Benign but chronic course
- Petechiae and pigmentation may last for months to years

References

Hersh CS, Shwayder TA. Unilateral progressive pigmentary purpura (Schamberg's disease) in a 15-year-old boy. J Am Acad Dermatol 1991; 24: 651

Kano Y, Hirayama K, Orihara M, Shiohara T. Successful treatment of Schamberg's disease with pentoxifylline. J Am Acad Dermatol 1997; 36: 827–30

Reinhold U, Seiter S, Ugurel S, Tilgen W. Treatment of progressive pigmented purpura with oral bioflavonoids and ascorbic acid: an open pilot study in 3 patients. J Am Acad Dermatol 1999; 41: 207–8

Torrelo A, Requena C, Mediero IG, Zambrano A. Schamberg's purpura in children: a review of 13 cases. J Am Acad Dermatol 2003; 48: 31–3

Lichen aureus

Synonym: lichen purpuricus

Major points

- Type of pigmented purpura
- Male/female ratio = 1
- Onset at any age (17% of cases occur in children)
- Clinical findings:
  1. Yellow-gold (aureus), gold-brown, or burnt-orange papules or macules; isolated or coalescing into patches of 1–20 cm in diameter; with scattered petechiae (Figure 15.15)
  2. Solitary or multiple lesions
  3. Unilateral, bilateral, or rarely a segmental or zosteriform distribution
  4. Occurs more often on the legs, arms, trunk; reported on the abdomen and face
  5. Usually asymptomatic, but rarely is pruritic, painful, or accompanied by a burning sensation

Pathogenesis

- Etiology unknown
- Benign chronic capillaritis; capillary fragility leads to red cell extravasation

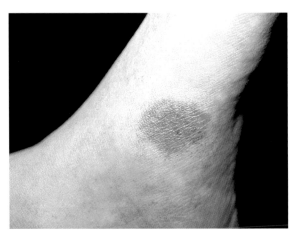

Figure 15.15   Lichen aureus – yellow-brown persistent patch

- Sporadic cases associated with drug consumption or asymptomatic infection (e.g. lower urinary tract infection, otitis, tonsillitis)
- Histology: lymphohistiocytic band-like infiltrate, sometimes perivascular, in papillary dermis, extravasated erythrocytes, and hemosiderin deposits; overlying epidermis is normal

Diagnosis

- Characteristic clinical findings
- No associated laboratory abnormalities
- Biopsy helpful

Differential diagnosis

- Bruising
- Drug eruption
- Dermatitis artefacta

Treatment

- Largely unresponsive to treatment (topical or systemic)
- Topical steroids useful in rare instances
- PUVA has been used successfully in those >11 years of age

Prognosis

- Chronic course
- Tends to resolve spontaneously in months to years (variable)

References

Aoki M, Kawana S. Lichen aureus. Cutis 2002; 69: 145–8

Gelmetti C, Cerri D, Grimalt R. Lichen aureus in childhood. Pediatr Dermatol 1991; 8: 280–3

Ling TC, Goulden V, Goodfield MJ. PUVA therapy in lichen aureus. J Am Acad Dermatol 2001; 45: 145–6

Patrizi A, Neri I, Marini R, et al. Lichen aureus with uncommon clinical features in a child. Pediatr Dermatol 1996; 13: 173

Rubio FA, Robayna G, Herranz P, et al. Abdominal lichen aureus in a child. Pediatr Dermatol 1997; 14: 411

16

VASCULAR AND LYMPHATIC DISEASES

VASCULAR DISORDERS

General

- Vascular birthmarks are one of the most common forms of congenital lesions
- Occur in 1–2% of children surveyed in the newborn nursery

Hemangioma of infancy

Synonym: strawberry hemangioma

General

- Benign growth of endothelial cells which appears at birth or within the first 2 months of life, and slowly involutes over 5–10 years
- Female/male ratio is 5 : 1
- Premature babies <1500 g are more commonly affected
- 50% on head and neck
- Multiple lesions are seen in 15–30% of cases

Major points

- At birth, skin may appear normal in color and texture or have a precursor lesion (Figure 16.1)
- Precursor lesions:
  1. Faint hypopigmentation resembling nevus anemicus
  2. Small telangiectatic patch
  3. Area of erythema resembling a capillary malformation
  4. Skin ulceration
  5. Bruise-like area

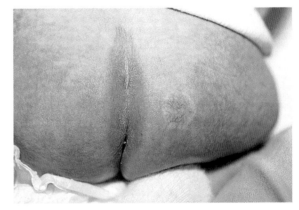

Figure 16.1 Superficial hemangioma – early, with halo from vasoconstriction

- Growth phase:
  1. Begins within first 2 months with a quickly growing, red vascular plaque (Figures 16.2–16.7)
  2. Grows for 6–15 months
  3. Followed by stabilization period where growth plateaus and begins to develop a white surface
  4. After this plateau period, hemangioma begins to involute
  5. Fully developed hemangiomas of infancy are present at birth in about 5% of cases
- Involution: virtually all undergo spontaneous involution
  1. Some leave no trace of previous lesion
  2. Abnormal skin is often left behind: telangiectasias, atrophy, hypopigmentation, anetoderma (Figures 16.8 and 16.9)
  3. Fifty per cent involute by 5 years, 70% involute by 7 years and 90% involute by 9 years

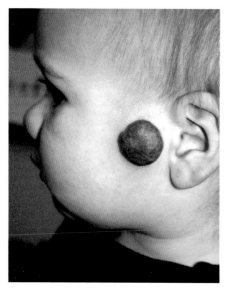

Figure 16.2   Hemangioma – typical vascular nodule on the face

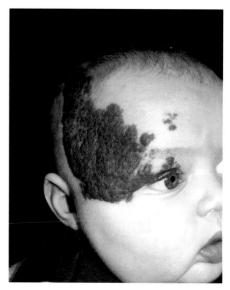

Figure 16.4   Hemangioma – segmental vascular plaque associated with closure of the eyelid. This child required oral steroids to keep the eyelid open

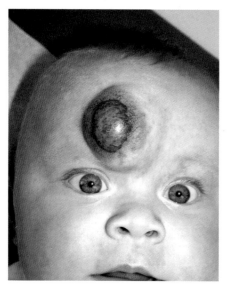

Figure 16.3   Superficial and deep hemangioma – typical vascular nodule on the forehead

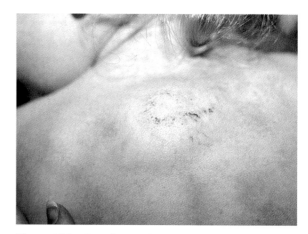

Figure 16.5   Deep hemangioma – deep purple tumor with telangiectasias on the surface

- Clinical subtypes:
  1. Superficial hemangiomas are most common and constitute 50–60% of all hemangiomas
  2. Deep hemangiomas (previously called 'cavernous hemangiomas') are deep bluish swellings with a telangiectatic surface

  3. Mixed hemangiomas have both superficial and deep components
  4. Disseminated neonatal hemangiomatosis – numerous small hemangiomas (1 mm to 2 cm) with high risk of internal involvement (e.g. liver, gastrointestinal tract and/or brain) and heart failure (Figure 16.10)
- Complications
  1. Ulceration may occur in the growth phase, especially around the mouth or in the diaper

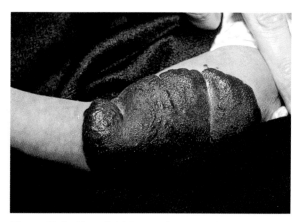

Figure 16.6 Superficial hemangioma – typical vascular plaque with papular surface

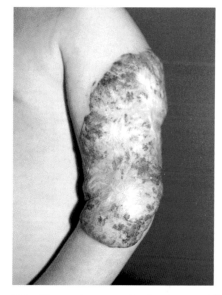

Figure 16.8 Hemangioma – residual scar at age $2^1/_2$ years with crinkly surface changes (same child as Fig 16.6)

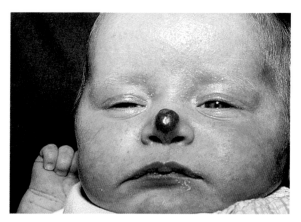

Figure 16.7 Cyrano nose – hemangioma involving the nasal tip

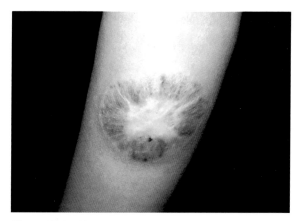

Figure 16.9 Hemangioma – residual scar at age 4 years in another patient

area; heals slowly and can last for months (Figure 16.11)

2. Bleeding is rarely a problem, although frequently expressed by parents as a concern
   a. If bleeding should occur, direct pressure to the area for several minutes will usually stop the bleeding. If it does not stop, surgical intervention may be warranted
3. Kasabach–Merritt syndrome
   a. Sudden growth of the lesion, tenseness, tenderness and a purpuric appearance
   b. Decreased platelets
   c. Petechiae and purpura
   d. Average age: 6 weeks
   e. Histology: tufted angioma, or Kaposiform hemangioendothelioma

4. PHACES syndrome: Posterior fossa brain malformations (e.g. Dandy–Walker malformation), Hemangiomas (especially large, plaque-like facial lesions), Arterial anomalies, Coarctation of the aorta or other cardiac defects, Eye abnormalities, Sternal cleft or supra-umbilical raphe (Figure 16.12)
5. Sacral hemangioma: associated with tethered cord (Figure 16.13)
6. Airway compromise: usually associated with large hemangiomas in the beard distribution (Figure 16.14)

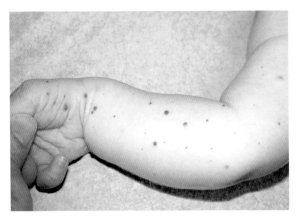

Figure 16.10   Diffuse neonatal hemangiomatosis associated with liver hemangiomatosis

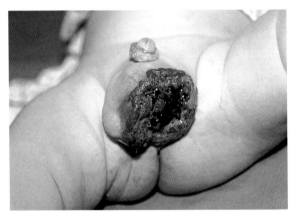

Figure 16.11   Ulcerated hemangiomas often occur in the diaper area

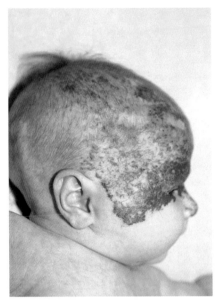

Figure 16.12   PHACES syndrome – associated with Dandy–Walker malformation

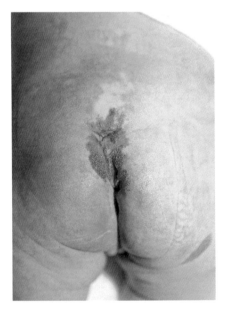

Figure 16.13   Sacral hemangioma – associated with tethered cord

Pathogenesis

- Etiology unknown, but it is thought that angiogenic factors are involved (overexpression of basic fibroblast growth factor, vascular endothelial growth factor, proliferating cell nuclear antigen, type IV collagenase, etc.)
- Proliferation of endothelial cells
- Embryologically blastogenic factors play a role
- Skin biopsy is rarely needed; however, it can differentiate soft tissue tumors (e.g. Kaposiform hemangioendothelioma, myofibromatosis, rhabdomyosarcoma)
- Endothelia of hemangiomas express GLUT1, a glucose transporter normally restricted to endothelia with blood–tissue barrier function, as in brain and placenta as well as other immunohistochemical markers resembling placental tissue

Diagnosis

- Typical clinical appearance in 95% of cases
- For atypical lesions, diagnostic tests may be helpful:
  1. Platelet count to evaluate for Kasabach–Merritt syndrome

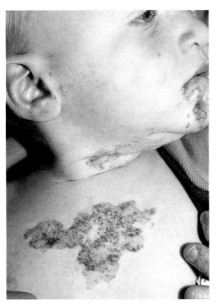

Figure 16.14 Hemangiomas in the beard area and chest can be associated with tracheal hemangiomas

2. Ultrasound: may be helpful in hepatic hemangiomas, but also useful with large facial hemangiomas to differentiate extent of lesion and possible structural brain abnormalities
3. Magnetic resonance imaging (MRI) can distinguish between hemangiomas and venous malformations, and determine structural brain abnormalities

Differential diagnosis

- Capillary malformation
- Venous malformation
- Arteriovenous malformation
- Pyogenic granuloma
- Nasal glioma
- Spitz nevus
- Dermoid cyst
- Blue nevus
- Myofibromatosis
- Rhabdoid tumor

Treatment

- Parent education: discussion of natural history of hemangiomas; serial photographs helpful; anticipatory guidance on how to handle comments and queries from strangers, family members

- Periodic re-evaluation, particularly in growth and involutional phases
- Therapy should be individualized based on size of lesion, location, presence of complications and age of patient
- Watchful waiting is treatment for majority of hemangiomas of infancy
- Surgery may be indicated when the child is 3–5 years of age, and occasionally earlier
- Indications for treatment:
  1. Life-threatening illness
  2. Loss of vision, amblyopia (hemangioma around the eye should always be followed by an ophthalmologist)
  3. Respiratory distress or stridor
  4. Kasabach–Merritt syndrome
  5. Hepatic hemangiomatosis
  6. Cardiac failure
  7. Skin ulceration
  8. Bleeding
  9. Permanent disfigurement, particularly large hemangiomas on face, nose, lips, ear
- Medical treatment
  1. Intralesional corticosteroids – triamcinolone 3–5 mg/kg per treatment (maximum 20 mg)
  2. Systemic corticosteroids: prednisone 2–5 mg/kg per day given BID initially then once daily for several months until stablization, then tapered
  3. Interferon-α (subcutaneous) – initial dose of 1–3 million U/m^2 per day and increased as tolerated until hemangioma or symptoms have improved. Side-effect: spastic diplegia in ~10%
  4. Pressure occlusion on an extremity with Ace wrap or Jobst stocking, making sure that the distal portion does not develop necrosis
- Surgical excision
  1. Not necessary in majority of cases
  2. May be indicated for small, easily excisable lesions on face or pedunculated hemangiomas likely to leave significant fibrofatty residua after involution
- Flash-lamp pumped pulsed dye laser
  1. Decreases telangiectasias on surface, and those left over after lesion has resolved
  2. Ulcerated hemangiomas may heal more quickly and less painfully
  3. Other lasers (argon, copper vapor, Nd-YAG, krypton, KTP) may be useful in certain cases

- Cryosurgery with cryoprobe
- Radiation
  1. Generally should be avoided, but may be indicated in severe, uncontrollable hemangiomas
- Embolization may be attempted in selected lesions which have life-threatening consequences
- Photography is very helpful in documenting progression and resolution

Prognosis

- Depends upon location, complications, results after involution, psychological effects
- Early on, it can be difficult to predict the ultimate size, rate of involution, and results; however, a physician knowledgable about hemangiomas would be a good source of information

References

Barlow CF, Priebe CJ, Mulliken JB, et al. Spastic diplegia as a complication of interferon alfa-2a treatment of hemangiomas of infancy. J Pediatr 1998; 132: 527–30

Bennett ML, Fleischer AB, Chamlin SL, Frieden IJ. Oral corticosteroid use is effective for cutaneous hemangiomas. Arch Dermatol 2001; 137: 1208–13

Boon LM, MacDonald DM, Mulliken JB. Complications of systemic corticosteroid therapy for problematic hemangioma. Plast Reconstr Surg 1999; 104: 1616–23

Bronzetti G, Giardini A, Patrizi A, et al. Ipsilateral hemangioma and aortic arch anomalies in posterior fossa malformations, hemangiomas, arterial anomalies, coarctation of the aorta and cardiac defects and eye abnormalities (PHACE) anomaly: report and review. Pediatrics 2004; 113: 412–15

Ceisler EJ, Santos L, Blei F. Periocular hemangiomas: what every physician should know. Pediatr Dermatol 2004; 21: 1–9

Drolet BA, Esterly NB, Frieden IJ. Hemangiomas in children. N Engl J Med 1999; 341: 173–81

Elsas FJ, Lewis AR. Topical treatment of periocular capillary hemangioma. J Pediatr Ophthalmol Strabismus 1994; 31: 153–6

Enjolras O, Riche MD, Merland JJ, et al. Management of alarming hemangiomas in infancy: a review of 25 cases. Pediatrics 1990; 85: 491–7

Esterly NB. Cutaneous hemangiomas, vascular stains and malformations, and associated syndromes. Curr Probl Dermatol 1995; 7: 65–108

Frieden IJ, Eichenfield LF, Esterly NB, et al. Guidelines of care for hemangiomas of infancy. J Am Acad Dermatol 1997; 37: 631–7

Frieden IJ, Reese V, Cohen D. PHACE Syndrome. Arch Dermatol 1996; 132: 307–11

Herron MD, Coffin CM, Vanderhooft SL. Tufted angiomas: variability of the clinical morphology. Pediatr Dermatol 2002; 19: 394–401

Metry DW, Dowd CF, Barkovich J, Frieden IJ. The many faces of PHACE syndrome. J Pediatr 2001; 139: 117–23

Metry DW, Hebert AA. Benign cutaneous vascular tumors of infancy. When to worry, what to do. Arch Dermatol 2000; 136: 905–14

Mulliken JB, Young AE. Vascular Birthmarks: Hemangiomas and Malformations. WB Saunders: Philadelphia, 1988

North PE, Waner M, Mizeracki A, et al. A unique microvascular phenotype shared by juvenile hemangiomas and human placenta. Arch Dermatol 2001; 137: 559–70

Wananukul S, Nuchprayoon I, Seksarn P. Treatment of Kasabach–Merritt syndrome: a stepwise regimen of prednisolone, dipyridamole, and interferon. Int J Dermatol 2003; 42: 741–8

Wong S-N, Tay YK. Tufted angioma: a report of five cases. Pediatr Dermatol 2002; 19: 388–93

Vascular malformations

General

- Malformation denotes an abnormal structure resulting from an aberration in embryologic development
- They do not resolve on their own and are always present at birth, although they might not be noticeable at birth
- They can involve veins, arteries, capillaries and occasionally lymphatic channels

Major points

- Capillary malformations (port wine stains, nevus flammeus)
  1. Most common type of vascular malformation
  2. Commonly occurs on the face, usually unilaterally, but can be anywhere on the body
  3. Noticeable at birth as pink, red or deep purple, macular patch which blanches with pressure (Figures 16.15 and 16.16)
  4. Involvement of first portion of fifth cranial nerve (V1) involving upper eyelid can be associated with glaucoma (~45%). An ophthalmologist should be consulted

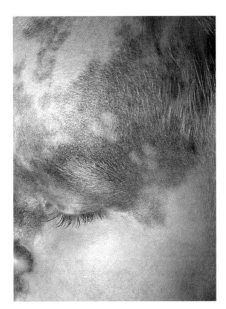

Figure 16.15   Capillary malformation (port wine stain), which is flat and pink in an infant

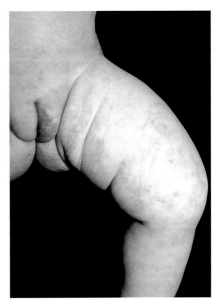

Figure 16.17   Venous malformation – notice purple varicosities

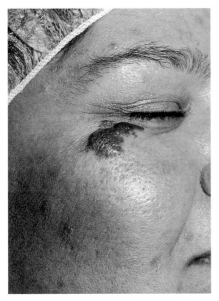

Figure 16.16   Capillary malformation in an adult, raised with dark red-purple papules

5. Small risk of glaucoma occurs in V2; V3 has no risk of glaucoma
- Venous malformations
  1. Appears as blue or purple, grouped, subcutaneous nodules with enlarged neighboring veins (Figure 16.17)

2. Hyperhidrosis overlying the malformation is common
3. Symptoms
   a. Usually asymptomatic
   b. May develop pressure on other nearby structures
   c. Pain may be caused by slow flow and clot formation
   d. Complications usually later in life
4. Varicosities (varicose veins) commonly occur
5. Complications:
   a. Glaucoma is associated with lesions in V1 and V2 distribution
6. Blue rubber bleb syndrome (OMIM no. 112200)
   a. Multiple venous malformations of the skin and gastrointestinal (GI) tract
   b. Blue or purple soft rubbery nodules which can be easily compressed
   c. Nocturnal pain in the lesions common
   d. Bleeding in the GI tract from the lesions may cause melena and anemia
   e. Other organs may be involved
   f. Autosomal dominant; chromosome 9p21; gene: receptor tyrosine kinase TIE2
7. Maffucci syndrome (OMIM no. 166000)
   a. Diffuse asymmetric enchondromatosis and multiple venous malformations

b. Soft blue subcutaneous nodules which progressively enlarge
c. Hard nodules appear on long bones, hands, fingers and feet
d. Gross deformity may occur
e. Enchondromas can transform into chondrosarcoma (~15%)
f. Gene map locus 3p22-p21.1; gene: PTH/PTHRP type I receptor

Pathogenesis

- Vascular ectasias rather than a proliferative process; progressive vascular dilatation of pre-existing blood vessels caused by either a defect in vascular walls or abnormalities of supporting structure of surrounding dermis
- Arterial malformations are high-flow lesions that can cause right-to-left shunting with subsequent heart failure
  1. Doppler testing can reveal shunting
  2. Listen to the lesion with a stethoscope for a bruit

Diagnosis

- Clinical presentation
- May need further testing: MRI if not straightforward or complications arise

Differential diagnosis

- Hemangioma of infancy
- Lymphatic malformation

Treatment

- Pulsed dye laser (577–585 nm)
- Surgery may be warranted in lesions with persistent pain, or bleeding
- Sclerotherapy by interventional radiologist for symptomatic deep venous malformations
- Treatment for tenderness with warm packs and oral aspirin

Prognosis

- Persist into adult life, becoming darker purple, raised and thickened with cobblestone appearance
- Small angiomatous nodules may appear within the lesion
- Prognosis depends upon location, size and extent

References

Bedocs PM, Gould JW. Blue rubber-bleb nevus syndrome: a case report. Cutis 2003; 71: 315–18

Cantatore JL, Kriegel DA. Laser surgery: an approach to the pediatric patient. J Am Acad Dermatol 2004; 50: 165–84

Enjolras O, Ciabrini D, Mazoyer E, et al. Extensive pure venous malformations in the upper or lower limb: a review of 27 cases. J Am Acad Dermatol 1997; 36: 219–25

Enjolras O. Vascular tumors and vascular malformations: are we at the dawn of a better knowledge? Pediatr Dermatol 1999; 16: 238–41

Ertem D, Acar Y, Kotiloglu E, et al. Blue rubber bleb nevus syndrome. Pediatrics 2001; 107: 418–20

Gabikian P, Clatterbuck RE, Gailloud P, Rigamonti D. Developmental venous anomalies and sinus pericranii in the blue rubber-bleb nevus syndrome. Case report. J Neurosurg 2003; 99: 409–11

McClean K, Hanke CW. The medical necessity for treatment of port-wine stains. Dermatol Surg 1997; 23: 663–7

Michel S, Landthaler M, Hohenleutner U. Recurrence of port-wine stains after treatement with flashlamp-pumped pulsed dye laser. Br J Dermatol 2000; 143: 1230–4

Nguyen CM, Yohn JJ, Huff C, et al. Facial port wine stains in childhood: prediction of the rate of improvement as a function of the age of the patient, size and location of the port wine stain and the number of treatments with the pulsed dye (585 nm) laser. Br J Dermatol 1998; 138: 821–5

Requena L, Sangueza OP. Cutaneous vascular anomalies. Part I. Hamartomas, malformations, and dilatation of preexisting vessels. J Am Acad Dermatol 1997; 37: 523–49

Sheu M, Fauteux G, Chang H, et al. Sinus pericranii: dermatologic considerations and literature review. J Am Acad Dermatol 2002; 46: 934–41

Sturge–Weber syndrome

Major points

- Facial capillary malformation including the V1 distribution (upper eyelid and forehead), accompanied by ipsilateral leptomeningeal angiomatosis (Figure 16.18)
- Glaucoma is usual but not invariably present
- Vascular malformation may be unilateral with a sharp midline cut-off, or may be bilateral and extensive
- Seizures are the most frequent neurological manifestation

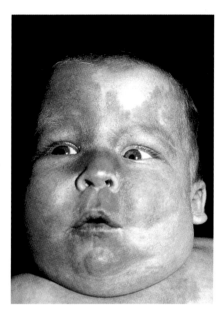

Figure 16.18 Sturge–Weber syndrome – associated with glaucoma, mental retardation and seizures

- Mental retardation common
- Other neurological abnormalities: hemiplegia, hemisensory defects, homonymous hemianopsia
- Other eye findings: buphthalmos, blindness
- Other skin findings: overgrowth of soft tissue and underlying bone of the face

Pathogenesis

- Etiology unknown
- Vascular malformation of vessels of brain, eye and skin
- Histology: increase in dilated venules, mainly in upper reticular dermis

Diagnosis

- MRI or computerized tomography (CT) scan can identify abnormal vasculature and extent of cortical calcifications
- Eye examination demonstrates glaucoma

Differential diagnosis

- Capillary malformation without internal involvement
- Other vascular malformations

Treatment

- Glaucoma should be followed by an ophthalmologist and may require surgery

- Seizures and mental retardation should be followed by pediatrician and/or neurologist

Prognosis

- Lesions are static or progressive

References

Bebin EM, Gomez MR. Prognosis in Sturge–Weber disease: comparison of unihemispheric and bihemispheric involvement. J Child Neurol 1988; 3:181–4

Dahan D, Fenichel GM, El-Said R. Neurocutaneous syndromes. Adolesc Med State Art Rev 2002; 13: 495–509

Eerola I, Boon LM, Mulliken JB, et al. Capillary malformation–arteriovenous malformation, a new clinical and genetic disorder caused by RASA1 mutations. Am J Hum Genet 2003; 73: 1240–9

Enjolras O, Riche MC, Merland JJ. Facial port-wine stains and Sturge–Weber syndrome. Pediatrics 1985; 76: 48–51

Klippel–Trenaunay syndrome

Major points

- Cutaneous capillary and venous malformations, congenital varicosities, and hypertrophy of involved limb (Figures 16.19 and 16.20)
- Occasionally with an arteriovenous fistula (Parkes–Weber syndrome)
- Involved limb hypertrophied, with enlargement of muscles, thickened skin and excess subcutaneous fat
- Lymphedema can be present
- Venous thrombosis common
- Female/male ratio = 1
- Single lower limb is most common area involved, but bilateral lower limbs or upper limbs may be involved
- Lesions present at birth
- Sporadic

Pathogenesis

- Etiology of overgrowth of tissues unknown but may be secondary to oversupply of blood to the subcutaneous tissues

Diagnosis

- Clinical presentation

Differential diagnosis

- Vascular malformation without internal involvement

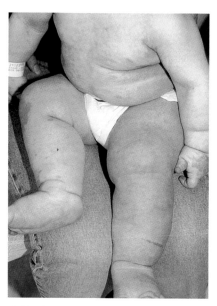

Figure 16.19   Klippel–Trenaunay syndrome demonstrating hypertrophy of the limb with a capillary malformation

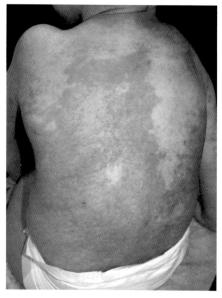

Figure 16.20   Klippel–Trenaunay syndrome with extensive vascular malformation of the back as well as the extremities

Treatment

- Superficial component can be treated with pulsed dye laser
- If there is leg length discrepancy, orthopedic referral
- Possible embolization if complications arise

Prognosis

- Variable: may be static or progressive in hypertrophy
- May have increased leg length discrepancy

References

Aelvoet GE, Jorens PG, Roelen LM. Genetic aspects of the Klippel–Trenaunay syndrome. Br J Dermatol 1992; 126: 603–7

Bird LM, Jones MC, Kuppermann N, Huskins WC. Gram-negative bacteremia in four patients with Klippel–Trenaunay–Weber syndrome. Pediatrics 1996; 98: 739–41

Dogan R, Faruk Dogan O, Oc M, et al. A rare vascular malformation, Klippel–Trenaunay syndrome. Report of a case with deep vein agenesis and review of the literature. J Cardiovasc Surg 2003; 44: 95–100

Eerola I, Boon LM, Mulliken JB, et al. Capillary malformation–arteriovenous malformation, a new clinical and genetic disorder caused by RASA1 mutations. Am J Hum Genet 2003; 73: 1240–9

Marler JJ, Fishman SJ, Upton J, et al. Prenatal diagnosis of vascular anomalies. J Pediatr Surg 2002; 37: 318–26

Requena L, Sangueza OP. Cutaneous vascular anomalies. Part I. Hamartomas, malformations, and dilatation of preexisting vessels. J Am Acad Dermatol 1997; 37:,523–49

Cutis marmorata telangiectatica congenita

Major points

- Malformation of blood vessels characterized by blue-violet, reticulated, marbled, cutaneous, vascular pattern present at birth, often with atrophy of involved tissues
- Unresponsive to warming
- Often segmental, involving one limb (frequently the leg) with a sharp cut-off at the midline (89%) or may be generalized (11%)
- Reticulated pattern frequently indented, atrophic, or may have ulcerations (Figure 16.21)
- Purplish color accentuated by crying, vigorous movement, or cold temperatures
- Telangiectasias often seen within area
- Associated with various congenital anomalies in 50% of patients (usually minor):
  1. Hypertrophy or atrophy of involved limb
  2. Other vascular anomalies

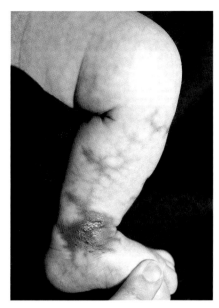

Figure 16.21 Cutis marmorata telangiectatica congenita – reticulated, atrophic, vascular pattern on an extremity

3. Macrocephaly
4. Glaucoma (if face involved)
5. Persistent ductus arteriosus
6. Congenital nevus
7. Mental retardation
- Sporadic inheritance

Pathogenesis

- Etiology unknown, but thought to be ectasia of veins and possibly of capillaries from vasospasm *in utero*
- Histology: dilated capillaries and veins in all layers of dermis and subcutaneous fat

Diagnosis

- Clinical presentation

Differential diagnosis

- Cutis marmorata (normal variant)
- Klippel–Trenaunay syndrome
- Sturge–Weber syndrome
- Diffuse phlebectasia (appears later and is progressive)

Treatment

- Treatment is usually not needed
- If lesions persist, pulsed dye laser

Prognosis

- Gradual improvement in first 2 years
- Some lesions do not resolve completely

References

Devillers ACA, de Waard-van der Spek FB, Oranje AP. Cutis marmorata telangiectatica congenita. Clinical features in 35 cases. Arch Dermatol 1999; 135: 34–8

Fujita M, Darmstadt GL, Dinulos JG. Cutis marmorata telangiectatica congenita with hemangiomatous histopathologic features. J Am Acad Dermatol 2003; 48: 950–4

Happle R. Dohi Memorial Lecture. New aspects of cutaneous mosaicism. J Dermatol 2002; 29: 681–92

Mazereeuw-Hautier J, Carel-Caneppele S, Bonafe JL. Cutis marmorata telangiectatica congenita: report of two persistent cases. Pediatr Dermatol 2002; 19: 506–9

Requena L, Sangueza OP. Cutaneous vascular anomalies. Part I. Hamartomas, malformations, and dilatation of preexisting vessels. J Am Acad Dermatol 1997; 37: 523–49

Glomuvenous malformations

Synonyms: glomus tumors, glomangiomas

Major points

- Present as single or multiple, purple papules, nodules or plaques scattered over body (Figure 16.22)
- Size ranges from 5 mm to large plaques
- Usually asymptomatic but may be painful
- Congenital large plaques have been reported
- Lesions progressively enlarge slowly with time
- Usually sporadic but may be inherited – autosomal dominant with incomplete penetrance and variable expressivity

Pathogenesis

- Abnormality of glomulin gene mapped to chromosome 1p21
- Uncontrolled growth of glomus cells

Diagnosis

- Clinical diagnosis with histologic confirmation
- Histology: nonencapsulated tumors with vascular spaces lined by one or two layers of glomus cells

Differential diagnosis

- Venous malformation
- Varicosities

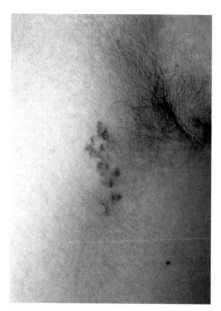

Figure 16.22   Glomuvenous malformation – typical purple intermittently painful vascular plaque

Treatment

- Surgical excision
- Large lesions may be difficult, and usually do not respond to pulsed dye laser

Prognosis

- Slowly progressive enlargement; can develop pain

References

Brouillard P, Boon LM, Mulliken JB, et al. Mutations in a novel factor, glomulin, are responsible for glomuvenous malformations ('glomangiomas'). Am J Hum Genet 2002; 70: 866–74

Brouillard P, Vikkula M. Vascular malformations: localized defects in vascular morphogenesis. Clin Genet 2003; 63: 340–51

Enjolras O, Mulliken JB. Vascular tumors and vascular malformations. New issues. Adv Dermatol 1997; 13: 375–423

Nevus anemicus

Major points

- Uncommon congenital vascular lesion which appears lighter than surrounding skin as a pale macule; no pigment involved

- Female/male ratio = 1
- Circumscribed, pale macule with irregular margins (Figure 16.23)
- Sometimes surrounded by satellite pink macules
- Location anywhere on body, but most often seen on upper chest
- Not accentuated by Wood's lamp examination

Pathogenesis

- Pharmacologic anomaly responding to catecholamines rather than an anatomic one
- Vascular structures are histologically normal

Diagnosis

- With diascopy, lesion is indistinguishable from blanched surrounding skin
- Friction, cold or heat accentuates normal surrounding skin but does not induce erythema within the lesion

Differential diagnosis

- Nevus depigmentosus
- Vitiligo
- Hypopigmented macules of tuberous sclerosis

Treatment

- Not needed, but camouflage make-up may be desired

Prognosis

- Static

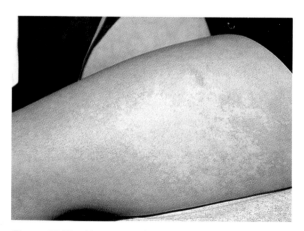

Figure 16.23   Nevus anemicus – vasoconstricted patch unchanged by rubbing

References

Eichenfield L, Larralde M. Neonatal skin and skin disorders. In Pediatric Dermatology, 3rd edn. Schachner LA, Hansen RC, eds. Mosby: Edinburgh, 2003: 221

Requena L, Sangueza OP. Cutaneous vascular anomalies. Part I. Hamartomas, malformations, and dilatation of preexisting vessels. J Am Acad Dermatol 1997; 37: 523–49

Nevus simplex (salmon patch)

Major points

- Benign, erythematous, macular patch on newborn's glabellar region (Figure 16.24)
- Tends to disappear or lighten signficantly in first year of life
- On face, colloquially called 'angel's kiss'
- On posterior neck, known as 'stork bite'
- 25–40% of newborns of all races have pink–red macular lesions on face, usually in midline glabella (salmon patch), or in occipital or nuchal regions

Pathogenesis

- Thought to represent persistence of fetal circulatory patterns

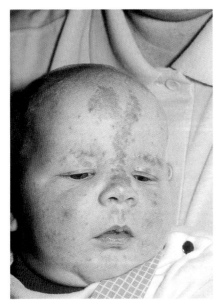

Figure 16.24   Salmon patch (nevus simplex) – typical glabellar distribution which improved in the first year of life

Diagnosis

- Clinical presentation

Differential diagnosis

- Capillary malformation

Treatment

- None needed
- If persistent, pulsed dye laser

Prognosis

- Nuchal lesions persist through life unchanged
- Sacral lesions persist through life, and are rarely associated with underlying anomalies
- Facial lesions usually lighten within the first years of life

References

Frieden I, Enjolras O, Esterly NB. Vascular lesions. In Pediatric Dermatology, 3rd edn. Schachner LA, Hansen RC, eds. Churchill Livingstone: New York, 2003: 833–62

Angiokeratoma

Major points

- Acquired, hyperkeratotic, superficial vascular abnormality with ectasia of pre-existing blood vessels in the papillary dermis
- Location usually lower extremities
- Presents either at birth or appears early in life as flat red, purple or blue patch (Figure 16.25)
- Slowly enlarges with time and becomes progressively verrucous or scaly
- Satellite lesions frequent
- Lesions bleed with trauma
- Types of angiokeratomas:
    1. Solitary angiokeratoma
        a. Small, warty, purple-black papule usually on lower extremities
        b. Thought to be caused by injury, trauma or chronic irritation
        c. Thrombosis may occur
    2. Angiokeratoma circumscriptum
        a. Large, solitary, hyperkeratotic, vascular, verrucous plaques
        b. Usually present at birth
        c. Occurs in bands, streaks or linear arrangements
        d. Commonly on extremity

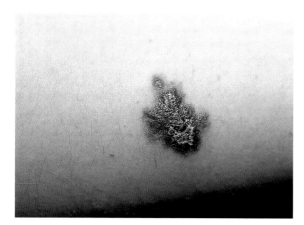

Figure 16.25   Angiokeratoma – purple-red, hyperkeratotic plaque

3. Angiokeratoma of Mibelli
   a. Several red-purple papules with hyperkeratotic surface on dorsal hand or foot, particularly fingers and toes
   b. Appears in childhood or adolescence
   c. More common in females
   d. May be associated with cold injury, acrocyanosis or chilblains
   e. Autosomal dominant
4. Angiokeratoma of Fordyce
   a. Multiple red-purple 2–4-mm papules on scrotum or vulva
   b. Most common in elderly patients
5. Angiokeratoma corporis diffusum
   a. Cutaneous manifestation of Fabry disease, an X-linked recessive disorder caused by the deficiency of lysosomal hydrolase α-galactosidase A
   b. Multiple lesions appear in late childhood
   c. Small, punctuate, dark, red-purple papules 1–2 mm in size usually more prominent on the lower trunk and legs
   d. Enlarge and become more prominent with time
   e. Neutral glycosphingolipids (trihexosylceramide) accumulates within lysosomes of endothelial cells, fibroblasts, and other cells throughout the body resulting in renal, cardiac, ocular and neurological abnormalities
   f. Can also be seen in fucosidosis, galactosidosis and other rare enzymatic deficiencies

Pathogenesis

- Etiology unknown
- Histology: thickened epidermis with hyperkeratosis, dilated capillaries and venules in papillary and reticular dermis. In Fabry disease, vacuolization of endothelial cells and smooth muscle cells as well as other cells
- Electron microscopy: lipid deposits in endothelial cells, pericytes and other cells which have characteristic lamellar structure

Diagnosis

- Clinical presentation
- Biopsy often needed for confirmation

Differential diagnosis

- Hemangioma of infancy
- Vascular malformation
- Angiomas
- Pyogenic granuloma

Treatment

- Excision
- CO_2 laser
- Enzyme replacement for Fabry disease

Prognosis

- Static or progressive

References

Kiyohara T, Kumakiri M, Kawasaki T, et al. Linear acral pseudolymphomatous angiokeratoma of children (APACHE): further evidence that APACHE is a cutaneous pseudolymphoma. J Am Acad Dermatol 2003; 48 (2 Suppl): 15–7

Mohrenschlager M, Braun-Falco M, Ring J, Abeck D. Fabry disease: recognition and management of cutaneous manifestations. Am J Clin Dermatol 2003; 4: 189–96

Schiller PI, Itin PH. Angiokeratomas: an update. Dermatology 1996; 193: 275–82

LYMPHATIC MALFORMATIONS

General

- Term used to describe localized or diffuse malformations of cutaneous, subcutaneous, or submucous lymphatic vessels

Lymphangioma circumscriptum

Major points

- Most common variant of cutaneous lymphatic malformations
- Present at birth but may not be apparent, and may be noticed in childhood as a solitary soft tissue swelling
- Superficial lymphatic malformations are characterized by clear vesicles on the surface of the skin, grouped in plaques (Figure 16.26)
- Often small areas of bleeding within lymphatic channels from abnormal blood vessels which run parallel to abnormal lymph channels
- Verrucous surface sometimes seen
- Often involves deeper tissues
- Location can be anywhere but has a predilection for axilla, shoulder, neck, tongue and proximal parts of extremities
- Usually asymptomatic, but may ooze lymph fluid

Pathogenesis

- Congenital malformation of lymphatics with formation of large cisterns that lie in subcutaneous tissue and communicate with superficial lymphatic system by dilated dermal lymphatics
- Histology: dilated lymph vessels lined by flat endothelial cells situated beneath the epidermis and within the reticular dermis
- Deeper involvement is common, with individual lymph channels arranged in clusters
- Erythrocytes may be seen within some channels

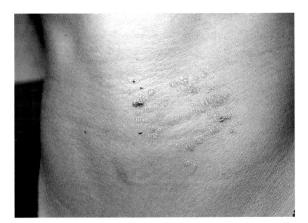

Figure 16.26 Lymphangioma circumscriptum – clear vesicles with some hemorrhage into the vesicles

Diagnosis

- Clinical presentation
- Biopsy may be indicated, especially in deeper lesions without characteristic clinical features

Differential diagnosis

- Herpes simplex
- Hemangioma
- Kaposi sarcoma
- Warts
- Molluscum contagiosum

Treatment

- Surgical excision frequently results in recurrences because of interconnecting lymphatic channels
- Surgery should depend upon severity of signs and symptoms
- CO_2 laser can ablate superficial component, but often recurs
- Sclerotherapy by interventional radiologists for macrocystic lesions followed by surgery in some cases

Prognosis

- Static or slowly progressive

References

Axt-Fliedner R, Hendrik HJ, Schwaiger C, et al. Prenatal and perinatal aspects of a giant fetal cervicothoracal lymphangioma. Fetal Diagn Ther 2002; 17: 3–7

Giguere CM, Bauman NM, Smith RJ. New treatment options for lymphangioma in infants and children. Ann Otol Rhinol Laryngol 2002; 111: 1066–75

Hilliard RI, McKendry JBJ, Phillips MJ. Congenital abnormalities of the lymphatic system: a new clinical classification. Pediatrics 1990; 86: 988–94

McAlvany JP, Jorizzo JL, Zanolli D, et al. Magnetic resonance imaging in the evaluation of lymphangioma circumscriptum. Arch Dermatol 1993; 129: 194–7

Mulliken JB, Fishman SJ, Burrows PE. Vascular anomalies Curr Probl Surg 2000; 37: 517–84

Ryan TJ, Mortimer PS, Jones RL. Lymphatics of the skin, neglected but important. Inter J Dermatol 1986; 25: 411–19

Macrocystic lymphatic malformations

Major points

- Abnormal lymphatic channels in deeper portions of the lymphatic system

- Characterized by subcutaneous painless nodules covered by normal skin
- Usually asymptomatic, but may be painful when pressed or bumped
- Cystic hygroma occurs around neck, axillae and inguinal regions with prominent deep component (Figure 16.27)
  1. Presents at birth or early childhood as a large cystic mass; demonstrated by transillumination
  2. Cystic hygromas of posterior neck associated with Turner or Noonan syndrome, hydrops fetalis and other congenital malformations

Pathogenesis

- Histology: irregular, dilated and interconnecting lymphatic vessels with multilocular cystic cavities in subcutaneous fat
- Some lymph channels contain smooth muscle bundles in walls

Diagnosis

- Clinical presentation
- Biopsy may be needed

Differential diagnosis

- Lipoma
- Epidermal cyst
- Tumors

Treatment

- Surgical removal of bulk of lesion is usually indicated; high rate of recurrence
- Sclerosing agents by interventional radiology

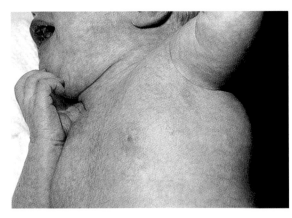

Figure 16.27   Cystic hygroma – congential deep swelling under arm

Prognosis

- Static or slowly progressive
- Painful if traumatized

References

Gallagher PG, Mahoney MJ, Gosche JR. Cystic hygroma in the fetus and newborn. Semin Perinatol 1999; 23: 341–56

Requena L, Sangueza OP. Cutaneous vascular anomalies. Part I. Hamartomas, malformations, and dilatation of preexisting vessels. J Am Acad Dermatol 1997; 37: 523–49

Weintraub AS, Holzman IR. Neonatal care of infants with head and neck anomalies. Otolaryngol Clin North Am 2000; 33: 1171–89

Lymphedema

Major points

- Malformation or destruction of lymphatic channels and subsequent swelling of tissues
- Primary lymphedema
  1. Congenital lymphedema (Figure 16.28)
  2. Milroy disease: congenital, autosomal dominant
  3. Idiopathic
     a. Lymphedema praecox appears between ages of 10 and 25 years
     b. Lymphedema tardum (after age 35 years)
- Secondary lymphedema
  1. Infection
  2. Surgical destruction
  3. Malignant infiltration
  4. Fibrosis (radiation, stasis)
- Female/male ratio >1
- Swelling of limb or limbs is gradual and painless
- Swelling improves when feet are elevated overnight
- Soft, pitting edema of distal extremities

Pathogenesis

- Malformation of lymphatic channels with aplasia, hypoplasia or varicosities of lymphatic channels
- Milroy disease: gene map locus 5q35.3; FLT4 gene, which encodes the vascular endothelial growth factor receptor-3
- Lymphedema praecox: gene map locus 16q24.3; forkhead family transcription factor gene MFH1 (FOXC2)

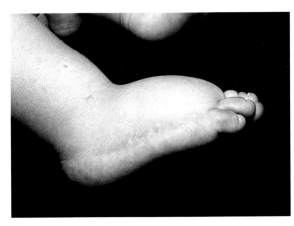

Figure 16.28   Congenital lymphedema – swelling of the feet and legs

Diagnosis

- Clinical presentation
- Lymphoscintigraphy with radioisotopic preparations can differentiate lymphedema from other causes of edema
- MRI of area involved
- Abdominal MRI may be needed to rule out extensive involvement or tumor
- Secondary causes should be ruled out

Differential diagnosis

- Lipodystrophy
- Panniculitis
- Myxedema

Treatment

- Minimize edema to prevent progression
- Prevent secondary complications (e.g. cellulitis) and further destruction of lymphatic channels
- Elastic garments (e.g. Jobst stockings) with pressures of >20 mmHg should be worn during the day
- Lymphedema pumps with sequential chambers

Prognosis

- Progressive or stable
- In Turner syndrome, lymphedema can resolve

References

Araujo JA, Curbelo JG, Mayol AL, et al. Effective management of marked lymphedema of the leg. Int J Dermatol 1997; 36: 389–92

Evans AL, Brice G, Sotirova V, et al. Mapping of primary congenital lymphedema to the 5q35.3 region. Am J Hum Genet 1999; 64: 547–55

Irrthum A, Karkkainen MJ, Devriendt K, et al. Congenital hereditary lymphedema caused by a mutation that inactivates VEGFR3 tyrosine kinase. Am J Hum Genet 2000; 67: 295–301

Makhoul IR, Sujov P, Ghanem N, Bronshtein M. Prenatal diagnosis of Milroy's primary congenital lymphedema. Prenat Diagn 2002; 22: 823–6

Veraart JCJM, Neumann HAM. Effects of medical elastic compression stockings on interface pressure and edema prevention. Dermatol Surg 1996; 22: 867–71

Wu JJ, Wagner AM. Verruciform xanthoma in association with Milroy disease and leaky capillary syndrome. Pediatr Dermatol 2003; 20: 44–7

ACQUIRED LESIONS

Pyogenic granuloma

Major points

- Common vascular tumor in childhood and pregnancy, accounting for 0.5% of pediatric nodules
- No racial or sex predilection
- A misnomer: neither bacterial (pyogenic) nor granulomatous in origin
- Commonly occurs between 1 and 4 years of age
- Location: face and neck most common but can occur anywhere
- Begins as small (5–8 mm) vascular papules
- Rapidly enlarges over several weeks to a dull red, dome-shaped, smooth, nontender papule (Figure 16.29)
- Usually solitary
- Rarely, multiple grouped satellite lesions develop around the original lesion
- Often pedunculated with a collarette of scale
- Surface becomes crusted and bleeds easily

Pathogenesis

- Etiology unknown
- Trauma may play a role
- May represent an inflammatory repair mechanism with granulation tissue and blood vessels

Diagnosis

- Histology: hemangioma-like proliferation of capillaries with flattened epidermis and epidermal collarette

Differential diagnosis

- Hemangioma of infancy
- Telangiectasia (spider angioma)
- Traumatized wart or molluscum
- Irritated melanocytic nevi
- Spitz nevus
- Amelanotic melanoma
- Eccrine poroma (on sole of the foot)
- Solitary glomus tumor
- Bacillary angiomatosis (seen in HIV-positive male patients)

Treatment

- Shave excision with curettage and electrodesiccation or surgical excision
- Pulsed dye laser may be effective in small lesions, but may require multiple treatments

Prognosis

- Small risk of recurrence after removal
- Untreated lesions tend to enlarge slowly, ulcerate and bleed

References

Frieden I, Enjolras O, Esterly NB. Vascular Lesions. In Pediatric Dermatology, 3rd edn. Schachner LA, Hansen RC, eds. Churchill Livingstone: New York, 2003: 833–62

Fleming AN, Smith PJ. Vascular cell tumors of the hand in children. Hand Clin 2000; 16: 609–24

Morelli JG. Use of lasers in pediatric dermatology. Dermatol Clin 1998; 16: 489–95

Pagliai KA, Cohen BA. Pyogenic granuloma in children. Pediatr Dermatol 2004; 21: 10–13

Livedo reticularis

Major points

- Mottled, reddish-blue macular discoloration of skin forming net-like pattern (Figure 16.30)
- Pattern is persistent, but darkens when environment is cold, and lightens when skin is warmed
- Idiopathic livedo reticularis

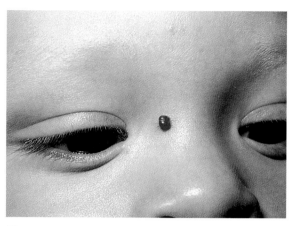

Figure 16.29 Pyogenic granuloma – typical bleeding, friable, vascular papule

1. Most often seen in women
2. Symmetrical diffuse mottling, usually on extremities
3. Numbness and tingling common
4. Painful ulceration uncommon
- Secondary causes:
  1. Intravascular obstruction
     a. Hematologic stasis: paralysis, emboli, cryoglobulinemia, anticardiolipin antibody syndrome
     b. Vessel wall disease: anticardiolipin antibody syndrome, polyarteritis nodosa, lupus erythematosus, dermatomyositis, syphilis, tuberculosis
     c. Drugs: amantadine, quinine, quinidine

Pathogenesis

- Thought to be due to slow venous drainage at margins of areas of skin richly supplied by arterial cones
- Increased viscosity and low flow rates in superficial venous plexus caused by cold
- Deoxygenation occurs and bluish pattern becomes more pronounced

Diagnosis

- Clinical presentation
- Rule out causes

Differential diagnosis

- Cutis marmorata (physiologic)
- Congenital abnormalities of blood vessels

- Congenital heart disease
- Cutis marmorata telangiectatica congenita
- Angioma serpiginosum
- Erythema ab igne

Treatment

- Usually persistent despite treatment of underlying disorder
- Avoidance of cold

Prognosis

- Persistent or progressive

References

Abrahamian LM, Berke A, Van Voohees AS. Type 1 diabetes mellitus associated with livedo reticularis: case report and review of the literature. Pediatr Dermatol 1991; 8: 46–50

Asherson RA, Cervera R. Unusual manifestations of the antiphospholipid syndrome. Clin Rev Allergy Immunol 2003; 25: 61–78

Gibson GE, Su WP, Pittelkow MR. Antiphospholipid syndrome and the skin. J Am Acad Dermatol 1997; 36: 970–82

Quintero-Del-Rio AI. Antiphospholipid antibodies in pediatrics. Curr Rheumatol Rep 2002; 4: 387–91

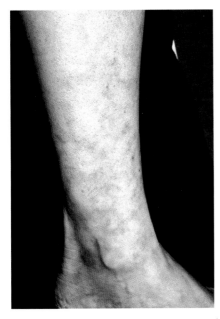

Figure 16.30   Livedo reticularis – reticulated vascular pattern associated with collagen vascular disease (anticardiolipin antibodies)

Spider angioma

Synonyms: telangiectasia, nevus araneus

Major points

- Most common type of telangiectasia in childhood
- Benign fixed pinpoint vascular punctum (0.5–4 mm) with radiating, tiny capillaries resembling legs of a spider
- Central vascular papule is a superficial arteriole which feeds into web of surrounding telangiectasias, occasionally pulsing
- Occurs either as single lesions or in crops
- Most common on sun-exposed areas, such as face and arms
- Occurs in 10–15% of normal adults and children
- More common in northern Europeans

Pathogenesis

- Etiology unknown
- Genetic predisposition
- Sun or trauma may play a role
- Histology: ascending arteriole which ends in a thin-walled ampulla just beneath the epidermis with radiating arterial branches in the papillary dermis

Diagnosis

- Clinical presentation
- Diascopy (pressure with a glass slide) results in disappearance of lesion

Differential diagnosis

- Multiple telangiectasias

Treatment

- Pulsed dye laser
- Light electrodesiccation of central feeder vessel
- Treatment does not prevent new lesions in other areas
- Recurrence rare

Prognosis

- Natural history has not been well studied, but most lesions are persistent; some may spontaneously disappear

References

Geronemus RG. Treatment of spider telangiectases in children using the flashlamp-pumped pulsed dye laser. Pediatr Dermatol 1991; 8: 61–3

Requena L, Sangueza OP. Cutaneous vascular anomalies. Part I. Hamartomas, malformations, and dilatation of preexisting vessels. J Am Acad Dermatol 1997; 37: 523–49

Telangiectasias

Major points

- Abnormal permanent dilatation of venules and occasionally capillaries and arterioles of subpapillary plexus (Figure 16.31)
- Telangiectases may be seen in:
  1. Collagen vascular diseases
  2. Mastocytosis
  3. Trauma
  4. Sun damage
  5. Radiodermatitis
  6. Poikiloderma
  7. Ataxia telangiectasia
  8. Essential or benign telangiectasias

Pathogenesis

- Histology: capillaries are dilated within papillary dermis, affecting venous portion of capillary loop

Diagnosis

- Clinical presentation
- Diascopy causes disappearance of lesion

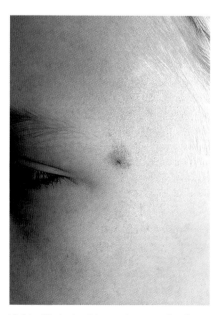

Figure 16.31   Typical spider angioma on the face

Differential diagnosis

- Spider angioma

Treatment

- Pulsed dye laser
- Light electrodesiccation of the central feeder vessels
- Treatment does not prevent new lesions in other areas
- Sunscreens may prevent new lesions

Prognosis

- Persistent unless treated
- Recurrence is occasionally seen

References

Abrahmian LM, Rothe MJ, Grant-Kels JM. Primary telangiectasia of childhood. Int J Dermatol 1992; 31: 307–13

Gold MH, Eramo L, Prendiville JS. Hereditary benign telangiectasia. Pediatr Dermatol 1989; 6: 194–7

Goldman MP, Bennett RG. Treatment of telangiectasia: a review. J Am Acad Dermatol 1987; 17: 167–82

Gonzalez E, Gange RW, Momtaz KT. Treatment of telangiectases and other benign vascular lesions with the 577 nm pulsed dye laser. J Am Acad Dermatol 1992; 27: 220–6

Marchuk DA, Srinivasan S, Squire TL, Zawistowski JS. Vascular morphogenesis: tales of two syndromes. Hum Mol Genet 2003; 12: R97–112

Generalized essential telangiectasias

Major points

- More common in females in late teens to adults and made worse in pregnancy
- Rarely involve conjunctivae and oral mucosa
- No bleeding diathesis or associated internal disease (e.g. liver disease)

Pathogenesis

- Etiology unknown
- Histology: dilated horizontal subpapillary venous plexus

Diagnosis

- Clinical presentation

Differential diagnosis

- Hereditary hemorrhagic telangiectasia
- Collagen vascular diseases

Treatment

- Pulsed dye or other vascular laser

Prognosis

- Persistent and can be progressive

References

Abrahmian LM, Rothe MJ, Grant-Kels JM. Primary telangiectasia of childhood. Int J Dermatol 1992; 31: 307–13

Gold MH, Eramo L, Prendiville JS. Hereditary benign telangiectasia. Pediatr Dermatol 1989; 6: 194–7

Hereditary hemorrhagic telangiectasia

Synonym: Osler–Weber–Rendu syndrome

Major points

- Characterized by telangiectases involving the skin, mucous membranes and internal organs (especially GI tract, lungs)
- Dark red, slightly elevated, central punctum with radiating vessels which can become matted with age
- In childhood, epistaxis from telangiectasias in nose
- Location most prominent on palms, soles, lips, tongue, palate, nasal mucous membranes and under nails
- GI involvement: bleeding is frequent and melena and anemia are common
- Lungs: arteriovenous fistulas or other venous malformations
- Other organs: kidney, spleen, bladder, liver, meninges and brain
- Autosomal dominant

Pathogenesis

- Histology: dilated thin-walled post-capillary venules, closely apposing overlying epidermis, lined by one layer of flattened endothelial cells
- Perivascular connective tissue is abnormal and is thought to be responsible for telangiectasias and hemorrhage
- Gene locus/gene: OWR1-9q34.1/ENG (endoglin); OWR2- 12q11-q14/ACVRL1 (activin A receptor-like kinase-1)

Diagnosis

- Clinical presentation
- Evaluation of GI tract and lungs

Differential diagnosis

- Essential telangiectasias

Treatment

- Pulsed dye laser or other vascular laser
- Electrocautery

Prognosis

- Slow progression of cutaneous, gastrointestinal and pulmonary lesions with bleeding, anemia
- Arteriovenous fistula in lungs can develop

References

Azuma H. Genetic and molecular pathogenesis of hereditary hemorrhagic telangiectasia. J Med Invest 2000; 47: 81–90

Begbie ME, Wallace GM, Shovlin CL. Hereditary haemorrhagic telangiectasia (Osler–Weber–Rendu syndrome): a view from the 21st century. Postgrad Med J 2003; 79: 18–24

Guttmacher AE, Marchuk DA, White RI. Hereditary hemorrhagic telangiectasia. N Engl J Med 1995; 333: 918–24

Peery WH. Clinical spectrum of hereditary hemorrhagic telangiectasia. Am J Med 1987; 82: 989–97

Swanson DL, Dahl MV. Embolic abscesses in hereditary hemorrhagic telangiectasia. J Am Acad Dermatol 1991; 24: 580–3

van den Driesche S, Mummery CL, Westermann CJ. Hereditary hemorrhagic telangiectasia: an update on transforming growth factor beta signaling in vasculogenesis and angiogenesis. Cardiovasc Res 2003; 58: 20–31

17

TUMORS, CYSTS AND GROWTHS

BLASCHKO LINES

See Chapter 14 for definition
Lesions that follow Blaschko lines (Table 17.1)

Epidermal nevus

Major points

- Hamartoma of cutaneous elements
- No racial predilection
- Sporadic, with a few cases in families
- 60% present at birth; 95% present by age 7 years
- Types:
  1. Nevus verrucosus – most common type
     a. Hyperpigmented, warty plaque measuring 2 to >10cm (Figure 17.1)
     b. Usually solitary

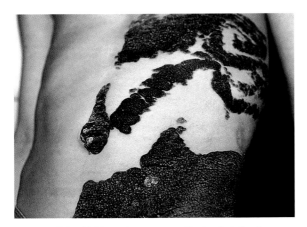

Figure 17.1 Epidermal nevus – on the body following Blaschko lines (published in An Illustrated Dictionary of Dermatologic Syndromes by SB Mallory and S Leal-Khouri)

Table 17.1 Disorders which follow Blaschko lines/segmental disorders

Nevoid/hamartomas
Epidermal nevus/ILVEN
Nevus sebaceus
Nevus comedonicus
Porokeratotic eccrine ostial and dermal duct nevus
Nevus lipomatosus
CHILD syndrome

Pigmented lesions
Incontinentia pigmenti
Hypomelanosis of Ito
Nevus depigmentosus
Linear and whorled nevoid hypermelanosis
Segmental vitiligo
Tuberous sclerosis with leukodermic macules
Café au lait macules (McCune–Albright syndrome)
Congenital nevus

Vascular lesions
Angiokeratoma circumscriptum
Verrucous hemangioma
Glomuvenous malformations
Venous malformations
Angioma serpiginosum
Lymphangioma circumscriptum
Unilateral nevoid telangiectasia

Other
Lichen striatus
Linear lichen planus
Focal dermal hypoplasia (Goltz syndrome)
Conradi–Hünermann syndrome (X-linked dominant)
Menkes syndrome (female carriers)
X-linked hypohidrotic ectodermal dysplasia (female carriers)
Oral–facial–digital syndrome, type 1
Linear porokeratosis
Linear keratosis follicularis

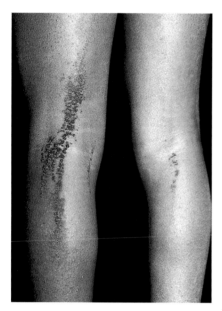

Figure 17.2   Epidermal nevus – on the legs following Blaschko lines

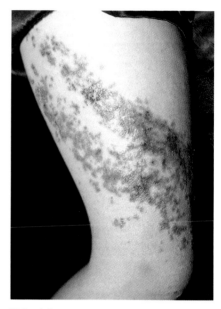

Figure 17.3   Inflammatory linear verrucous epidermal nevus – scaly, erythematous streaks following Blaschko lines on the leg

c.   Linear or oval in shape
d.   Most common on extremities, but can be anywhere
e.   Does not continue to grow after age 7 years except in proportion to the child

2. Nevus unius lateris (systematized epidermal nevus)
a.   Extensive lesions which can be unilateral or bilateral (Figure 17.2)
b.   Can continue to expand into adolescence, following Blaschko lines
c.   Associated with underlying systemic deformities in 30% of patients (called 'epidermal nevus syndrome' with CNS, skeletal, cardiovascular, ocular abnormalities)

3. Ichthyosis hystrix
a.   Extensive lesions following Blaschko lines
b.   Histology: epidermolytic hyperkeratosis

4. Inflammatory linear verrucous epidermal nevus (ILVEN)
a.   Erythematous scaly linear plaque/plaques (Figure 17.3)
b.   Small or large
c.   Intensely pruritic
d.   Often in groin
e.   More common in females (4 : 1)

Pathogenesis

*   Mosaicism arising from somatic mutations early in embryogenesis. Two distinct cell lines result and migrate along developmental lines (Blaschko lines) producing patchy and linear abnormalities
*   If epidermal nevus has histology of epidermolytic hyperkeratosis and if the gonads are involved in the somatic mutation, offspring may be affected with widespread epidermolytic hyperkeratosis

Diagnosis

*   Histology:
1.   Papillomatous hyperplasia of the epidermis with or without epidermolytic hyperkeratosis
2.   Inflammation in the dermis may be seen in the inflammatory types

Differential diagnosis

*   Nevus verrucosus
1.   Nevus sebaceus
2.   Seborrheic keratosis
3.   Verrucae
*   Inflammatory linear verrucous epidermal nevus
1.   Psoriasis
2.   Linear lichen planus
3.   Lichen simplex chronicus
4.   Darier disease

Treatment

- Solitary epidermal nevi usually require no treatment
- Surgery must include upper levels of dermis in order to prevent recurrences
- Other techniques which may be effective for removal: CO_2 laser, dermabrasion, chemical peels, liquid nitrogen
- Pruritus in ILVEN may be improved with potent topical or intralesional steroids, pulsed dye laser or short contact dithranol

Prognosis

- Lesions persist unless fully removed

References

Alam, M, Arndt KA. A method for pulsed carbon dioxide laser treatment of epidermal nevi. J Am Acad Dermatol 2002; 46; 554–6

Boyce S, Alster TS. CO_2 laser treatment of epidermal nevi: long-term success. Dermatol Surg 2002; 28: 611–14

Grebe TA, Rimsza ME, Richter SF, et al. Further delineation of the epidermal nevus syndrome: two cases with new findings and literature review. Am J Med Genetics 1993; 47: 24–30

Happle R, Rogers M. Epidermal nevi. Adv Dermatol 2002; 18: 175–201

Ivker R, Resnick SD, Skidmore RA. Hypophosphatemic vitamin D-resistant rickets, precocious puberty, and the epidermal nevus syndrome. Arch Dermatol 1997; 133: 1557–61

Paller AS, Syder AJ, Chan Y-M, et al. Genetic and clinical mosaicism in a type of epidermal nevus. N Engl J Med 1994; 331: 1408–15

Prayson RA, Kotagal P, Wyllie E, Bingaman W. Linear epidermal nevus and nevus sebaceus syndrome. Arch Pathol Lab Med 1999; 123: 301–5

Rogers M, McCrossin I, Commens C. Epidermal nevi and the epidermal nevus syndrome. J Am Acad Dermatol 1989; 20: 476–88

Nevus sebaceus

Synonym: nevus sebaceus of Jadassohn, organoid nevus

Major points

- Congenital hamartoma of skin and adnexae, predominantly sebaceous glands, abortive hair follicles and ectopic apocrine glands
- Sporadic in occurrence; familial cases have been reported
- No racial or sexual predilection
- Incidence 0.3% of the population
- Solitary oval or linear hairless plaque on the scalp, head or neck (Figure 17.4)

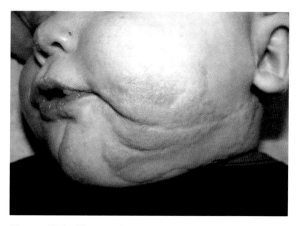

Figure 17.4 Nevus sebaceus – extensive, yellowish plaque on the face following Blaschko lines

- Surface smooth, velvety or wart-like with a yellowish color
- Size ranges from 0.5 to >6 cm; can be extensive
- In childhood, the lesions flatten and become less apparent; thought to be caused by the reduction of maternal hormones and sebaceous glands
- At puberty, most plaques thicken and become verrucous (Figure 17.5)
- Development of hamartomatous tumors within the lesion usually after puberty
  1. Tumors: syringocystadenoma papilliferum, trichoblastoma, hidradenoma, basal cell carcinoma, others
  2. Malignant tumors such as squamous cell carcinoma, apocrine carcinoma and other adnexal carcinomas are rare before age 40 years
  3. Detected by development of a papule with ulceration within the lesion
- Extensive lesions may be associated with multiple systemic manifestations in the nevus sebaceus syndrome (Schimmelpenning syndrome): seizures, mental retardation, arteriovenous malformations of the brain, skeletal abnormalities, ophthalmologic abnormalities

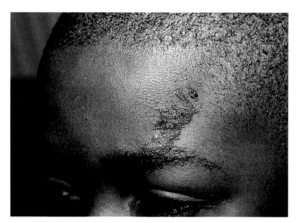

Figure 17.5 Nevus sebaceus – verrucous plaque on the forehead of an 11-year-old

Pathogenesis

- Complex hamartoma of pilosebaceous follicles, epidermis and adenexal structures that are under hormonal control

Diagnosis

- Histology:
  1. Early: small underdeveloped sebaceous glands and hair follicles
  2. Childhood: small, immature ectopic appendageal structures
  3. Puberty: hyperplasia and maturation of the sebaceous glands. Hair follicles remain rudimentary; fully developed apocrine glands occur

Differential diagnosis

- Epidermal nevus
- Aplasia cutis
- Congenital triangular alopecia
- Cutaneous infection (e.g. staphylococcal, streptococcal, herpes simplex)

Treatment

- Full-thickness surgical excision around the time of puberty is recommended
- If excision will result in a worse cosmetic defect, then observation may be reasonable
- CO_2 laser is a second choice for destruction of the lesion in a difficult area; however, recurrences may occur

Prognosis

- Lesions persist throughout life
- Potential in adulthood to develop nodules or skin tumors

References

Cribier B, Scrivener Y, Grosshans E. Tumors arising in nevus sebaceus: a study of 596 cases. J Am Acad Dermatol 2000; 42: 263–8

LeSueur BW, Silvis NG, Hansen RC. Basal cell carcinoma in children: report of 3 cases. Arch Dermatol 2000; 136: 370–2

Oranje AP, Przyrembel H, Meradji M, et al. Solomon's epidermal nevus syndrome (type: linear nevus sebaceus) and hypophosphatemic vitamin D-resistant rickets. Arch Dermatol 1994; 130: 1167–71

Rogers M, McCrossin I, Commens C. Epidermal nevi and the epidermal nevus syndrome. J Am Acad Dermatol 1989; 20: 476–88

Santibanez-Gallerani A, Marshall D, Duarte AM, et al. Should nevus sebaceus of Jadassohn in children be excised? A study of 757 cases, and literature review. J Craniofac Surg 2003; 14: 658–60

Turner CD, Shea CR, Rosoff PM. Basal cell carcinoma originating from a nevus sebaceus on the scalp of a 7-year-old boy. J Pediatr Hematol Oncol 2001; 23: 247–9

Nevus comedonicus

Major points

- Presents at birth or early childhood
- Dilated follicular orifices on top of papules, closely set and usually linear (Figure 17.6)
- Site: face, neck, upper arms and chest
- Usually solitary
- If systematized (rare), developmental defects of the CNS, eyes, bone and skin can be associated
- Usually asymptomatic, but individual papules and cysts within plaques may become inflamed, resembling acne vulgaris

Pathogenesis

- Considered to be a variant of epidermal nevus, a hamartoma of abnormal hair follicle infundibula

Diagnosis

- Clinical diagnosis
- Histology: multiple dilated follicles filled with keratinous plugs

Differential diagnosis

- Acne vulgaris
- Nevus sebaceus

Treatment

- Topical retinoids
- Keratolytic agents: 12% ammonium lactate lotion (LacHydrin), tretinoin
- Surgical excision

Prognosis

- Persistent

References

Beck MH, Dave VK. Extensive nevus comedonicus. Arch Dermatol 1980; 116: 1048–50

Cestari TF, Rubim M, Valentini BC. Nevus comedonicus: case report and brief review of the literature. Pediatr Dermatol 1991; 8: 300–5

Patrizi A, Neri I, Fiorentini C, Marzaduri S. Nevus comedonicus syndrome: a new pediatric case. Pediatr Dermatol 1998; 15: 304–6

Seo YJ, Piao YJ, Suhr KB, et al. A case of nevus comedonicus syndrome associated with neurologic and skeletal abnormalities. Int J Dermatol 2001; 40: 648–50

Vasiloudes PE, Morelli JG, Weston WL. Inflammatory nevus comedonicus in children. J Am Acad Dermatol 1998; 38: 834–6

CYSTS

Epidermal cyst

Major points

- Slow-growing, firm, ballotable round dermal nodule (Figure 17.7)
- Range in size from 0.5 to 15 cm
- Neonates:
  1. Can be seen anywhere
  2. If present in the midline (face, nose) and associated with pits or cysts, may indicate intracranial connection
- Adolescents:
  1. Solitary cysts with acne vulgaris
  2. Multiple cysts in childhood or adolescents might suggest Gardner syndrome
- Ruptured epidermal cysts become markedly inflamed; caused by keratin inciting a foreign body reaction

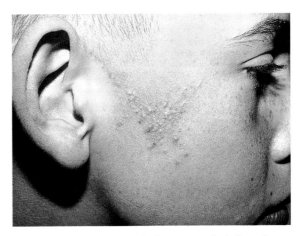

Figure 17.6   Nevus comedonicus – note the inflamed open and closed comedones

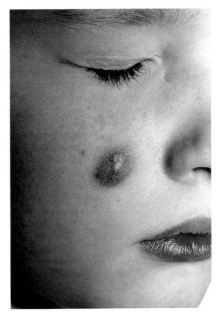

Figure 17.7   Epidermal cyst – inflamed tender ruptured cyst on the cheek

Pathogenesis

- Epidermal cysts result from the proliferation of surface epidermal cells within the dermis producing keratin. They arise from cells of the follicular infundibulum, or from implantation of epidermal cells into the dermis through trauma, or from trapping of epidermal cells along embryonal fusion planes

Diagnosis

- Easy to diagnose if there is a central punctum from which keratinous material can be expressed
- Clinically difficult to distinguish between epidermal and dermoid cysts without a biopsy

Differential diagnosis

See Table 17.2

Treatment

- Surgical excision with removal of the entire cyst wall

Prognosis

- Cysts persist and slowly enlarge over time
- If traumatized, the cyst wall can break, extruding keratinous material into the surrounding dermis, causing marked inflammation

References

Knight PJ, Reiner CB. Superficial lumps in children. Pediatrics 1983; 72: 147–53

Pariser RJ. Benign neoplasms of the skin. Med Clin North Am 1998; 82: 1285–307

Table 17.2   Benign skin papules, nodules and cysts in infants and children

Epidermal cyst
Dermoid cyst
Pilomatrixoma
Nasal glioma
Encephalocele
Branchial cleft cyst
Milia
Eruptive vellus hair cysts
Fibroma
Neurofibroma
Lipoma
Panniculitis
Juvenile xanthogranuloma
Mastocytoma
Lymphangioma
Granuloma annulare
Syringoma
Trichoepithelioma
Dermatofibroma
Keloid
Calcinosis cutis
Osteoma cutis
Foreign body granuloma

Vasiloudes PE, Morelli JG, Weston WL. Plantar epidermal cysts in children. Arch Dermatol 1997; 133: 1465

Zuber TJ. Minimal excision technique for epidermoid (sebaceous) cysts. Am Fam Physician 2002; 65: 1409–12, 1417–18, 1420

Milia

Major points

- A milium (plural, milia) is a 1–2 mm superficial white globoid papule within the epidermis or upper dermis
- Consists of a tiny ball of keratin with a thin cyst wall
- Common on the face of newborns, and within scars (especially in epidermolysis bullosa)
- Milia on the palate of newborns called Epstein pearls

Pathogenesis

- Etiology unknown
- Milia are thought to be derived from pilosebaceous follicles

Diagnosis

- Clinical diagnosis
- Histology: identical to an epidermal cyst, differing only in size

Differential diagnosis

- Molluscum contagiosum
- Keratosis pilaris

Treatment

- Lesions can be easily expressed with a comedone extractor after incision with a surgical blade or needle

Prognosis

- Superficial milia can spontaneously extrude; deeper ones may be persistent

References

Bridges AG, Lucky AW, Haney G, Mutasim DF. Milia en plaque of the eyelids in childhood: case report and review of the literature. Pediatr Dermatol 1998; 15: 282–4

Cairns ML, Knable AL. Multiple eruptive milia in a 15-year-old boy. Pediatr Dermatol 1999; 16: 108–10

Girardi M, Federman GL, McNiff JM. Familial multiple basaloid follicular hamartomas: a report of two affected sisters. Pediatr Dermatol 1999; 16: 281–4

Langley RGB, Walsh NMG, Ross JB. Multiple eruptive milia: report of a case, review of the literature, and a classification. J Am Acad Dermatol 1997; 37: 353–6

Stefanidou MP, Panayotides JG, Tosca AD. Milia en plaque: a case report and review of the literature. Dermatol Surg 2002; 28: 291–5

Dermoid cyst

Major points

- Manifest at birth (40%) or before age 5 years (70%)
- Solitary, soft round subcutaneous cyst which is freely moveable within the dermis (Figure 17.8)
- Sinus opening or hairs may be associated
- Size usually 1–4 cm
- Location usually on the forehead, most common in the lateral third of the eyebrow or midline nasal bridge. Also seen on the anterior or lateral neck, sternum, scrotum, perineal raphe and sacral areas
- In the periorbital area, may cause proptosis or eyelid displacement
- Most dermoid cysts are superficial, but up to 45% may have intracranial connections to extradural or intradural compartments often indicated by a sinus pit
- Usually asymptomatic; rarely recurrent infections with cellulitis or abscess; pressure erosion of the bone may occur

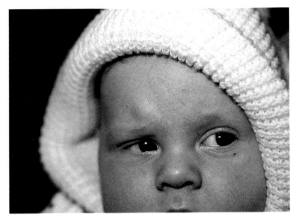

Figure 17.8   Dermoid cyst – above the eyebrow of an infant

Pathogenesis

- Caused by the sequestration of epithelium along the planes of closure of embryonic clefts

Diagnosis

- Biopsy should not be performed unless it is certain there is no intracranial connection
- Histology: an encapsulated cyst with a wall composed of keratinizing, stratified squamous epithelium with hair follicles, sebaceous glands, eccrine and aprocrine glands; within the cyst are lipids, keratin and hair

Differential diagnosis

See Table 17.2

Treatment

- Simple excision
- Midline lesions of the face should be evaluated with an MRI looking for intracranial connections
- Surgery by a pediatric neurosurgeon is essential for lesions with intracranial connections in order to avoid ascending infection
- Dermoid cysts located along the lateral eyebrows rarely have intracranial connections and do not require MRI

Prognosis

- Excellent if completely excised

References

Ackerman LL, Menezes AH, Follett KA. Cervical and thoracic dermal sinus tracts. A case series and review of the literature. Pediatr Neurosurg 2002; 37: 137–47

Brownstein MH, Helwig EB. Subcutaneous dermoid cysts. Arch Dermatol 1973; 107: 237–9

Drolet BA. Cutaneous signs of neural tube dysraphism. PediatrClin North Am 2000; 47: 813–23

Paller AS, Pensler JM, Tomita T. Nasal midline masses in infants and children. Arch Dermatol 1991; 127: 362–6

Pilomatrixoma

Synonym: calcifying epithelioma of Malherbe

Major points

- Firm, freely movable slowly growing papule/nodule usually <1 cm (can be up to 5 cm) (Figure 17.9)

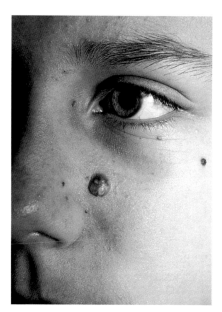

Figure 17.9 Pilomatrixoma – enlarging hard cyst on the cheek

- Overlying skin may have a bluish hue
- Usually solitary; multiple lesions have been reported
- Location: common on the face of a child but can be seen anywhere
- May feel rock-hard
- Slight female predominance
- No racial predilection
- Sporadic; familial cases reported
- If cyst ruptures to the surface, it may drain chalky calcium-containing material
- If ruptured under the skin, it may be very inflamed and painful

Pathogenesis

- Benign hyperplasia of the cells of hair matrix
- Cyst composed of elements of normal hair cortex
- Characteristic calcium phosphate deposition within the cyst
- Not usually associated with underlying disease

Diagnosis

- Histology: two populations of cells: irregular islands of basophilic cells at the periphery, and pale shadow cells containing no nuclei
  1. Within cyst: keratin, foreign body reaction, calcification and sometimes ossification

2. Cyst is irregular in shape, with connective tissue capsule

Differential diagnosis

See Table 17.2

Treatment

- Surgical excision

Prognosis

- Persistent
- Natural history: slow enlargement over months

References

Ahmad M, Khan IU, Khan AH, et al. Pilomatricoma: a retrospective study. Int J Dermatol 1992; 31: 703–5

Cambiaghi S, Ermacora E, Brusasco A, et al. Multiple pilomatricomas in Rubinstein–Taybi syndrome: a case report. Pediatr Dermatol 1994; 11: 21–5

Demircan M, Balik E. Pilomatricoma in children: a prospective study. Pediatr Dermatol 1997; 14: 430–2

Julian CG, Bowers PW. A clinical review of 209 pilomatricomas. J Am Acad Dermatol 1998; 39: 191–5

Kopeloff I, Orlow SJ, Sanchez MR. Multiple pilomatricomas: report of two cases and review of the association with myotonic dystrophy. Cutis 1992; 50: 290–2

Mencia-Gutierrez E, Gutierrez-Diaz E, Garcia-Suarez E, Ricoy JR. Eyelid pilomatricomas in young adults: a report of 8 cases. Cutis 2002; 69: 23–6

Yencha MW. Head and neck pilomatricoma in the pediatric age group: a retrospective study and literature review. Int J Pediatr Otorhinolaryngol 2001; 57: 123–8

Eruptive vellus hair cysts

Major points

- Multiple small, discrete, soft 1–4 mm skin-colored or hyperpigmented papules (Figure 17.10)
- Location: lower chest and upper abdomen in a follicular pattern is typical; other areas can be involved
- Occasional umbilication
- Asymptomatic
- Ages usually 4–18 years
- No systemic associations
- No sexual or racial predilection
- Autosomal dominant and familial cases have been reported

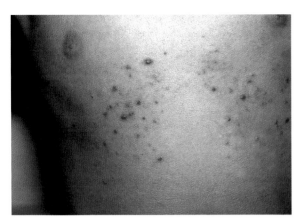

Figure 17.10 Eruptive vellus hair cysts – typical mid-chest follicular papules resembling comedones

Pathogenesis

- Defect in the development of vellus hair follicles which predispose to follicular occlusion at the infundibular level
- Relation to steatocystoma multiplex has been suggested, because the cyst wall can contain sebaceous glands

Diagnosis

- Clinical diagnosis
- Biopsy may be necessary to confirm the diagnosis
- Histology: small mid-dermal cysts lined by squamous epithelium; cysts contain lamellar keratin and tiny nonpigmented vellus hair shafts

Differential diagnosis

- Epidermoid cysts
- Syringomas
- Steatocystoma multiplex
- Acne
- Viral exanthems
- Molluscum contagiosum

Treatment

- Topical keratolytics (e.g. lactic acid, tretinoin cream) may hasten resolution
- Excision or other destructive measures may be needed for larger lesions

Prognosis

- Lesions may spontaneously resolve over months to years
- New lesions can continue to form

References

Mahendran R, Pollock B, Clark S. Multiple asymptomatic papules in a child. Pediatr Dermatol 2003: 20: 451–2

Ohtake N, Kubota Y, Takayama O, et al. Relationship between steatocystoma multiplex and eruptive vellus hair cysts. J Am Acad Dermatol 1992; 26: 876–8

Reep MD, Robson KJ. Eruptive vellus hair cysts presenting as multiple periorbital papules in a 13 year old boy. Pediatr Dermatol 2002; 19: 26–7

FAT

Lipoma

Major points

- Common, benign, asymptomatic, well-demarcated nodule with a doughy consistency
- Size: 1 cm to >15 cm
- If a lesion compresses a nerve, it may be painful
- Location often on neck and trunk but can be anywhere
- Usually solitary but may be multiple

Pathogenesis

- Benign mesenchymal tumor of unknown etiology

Diagnosis

- Histology: well-circumscribed sheets of mature, uniform adipocytes with thin strands of fibrous tissue intersecting the sheets of adipocytes

Differential diagnosis

See Table 17.2

Treatment

- Surgical excision if indicated

Prognosis

- Most lipomas are asymptomatic and stable
- Trauma or ischemia can cause necrosis of lipomas with pain, and later dystrophic calcification

References

McAtee-Smith J, Hebert AA, Rapini RP, Goldberg NS. Skin lesions of the spinal axis and spinal dysraphism. Arch Pediatr Adolesc Med 1994; 148: 740–8

Salam GA. Lipoma excision. Am Fam Physician 2002; 65: 901–4

Sanchez MR, Colomb FM, Moy JA, Petozkin JR. Giant lipoma: case report and review of the literature. J Am Acad Dermatol 1993; 28: 266–8

Trapp CF, Baker EJ. Mobile encapsulated lipomas. Cutis 1992; 49: 63–4

Zvijac JE, Sheldon DA, Schurhoff MR. Extensive lipoma causing suprascapular nerve entrapment. Am J Orthop 2003; 32: 141–3

Nevus lipomatosus

Major points

- Presents at birth or childhood
- Multiloculated yellowish or skin-colored plaque of rubbery papules and nodules
- Location usually in lumbosacral area or thighs but may be anywhere
- Size usually several centimeters or larger
- Asymptomatic
- No underlying associations

Pathogenesis

- Rare, benign hamartoma of mature fat cells

Diagnosis

- Histology: mature, polypoid fat with the appearance of an acrochordon (skin tag)

Differential diagnosis

- Goltz syndrome (focal dermal hypoplasia)
- Encephalocraniocutaneous lipomatosis

Treatment

- None usually needed
- Surgical excision
- Liposuction

Prognosis

- Benign with no malignant potential

References

Bergonse FN, Cymbalista NC, Nico MM, et al. Giant nevus lipomatosus cutaneus superficiails: case report and review of the literature. J Dermatol 2000; 27: 16–19

Inoue M, Ueda K, Hashimoto T. Nevus lipomatosus cutaneus superficialis with follicular papules and hypertrophic pilo-sebaceous units. Int J Dermatol 2002; 41: 241–3

Knuttel R, Silver EA. A cerebriform mass on the right buttock. Dermatol Surg 2003; 29: 780–1

Lane JE, Clark E, Marzec T. Nevus lipomatosus cutaneus superficialis. Pediatr Dermatol 2003; 20: 313–14

Anetoderma

Synonym: macular atrophy

Major points

- Multiple oval depressions or slightly bulging papules with wrinkled surface (Figure 17.11)
- Herniates inward with fingertip pressure
- Location: mainly upper trunk and upper arms, but can be anywhere
- May or may not be preceded by inflammation
- Secondary anetoderma may develop after certain cutaneous processes such as syphilis, leprosy, lupus and others

Pathogenesis

- Results from increased degradation or reduced synthesis of elastic tissue
- Histology:
  1. Perivascular infiltrate of lymphocytes (predominantly helper T cells)
  2. Scattered macrophages, giant cells with some elastophagocytosis
  3. In established lesion, elastic fibers are sparse in superficial dermis and almost completely absent in mid-dermis

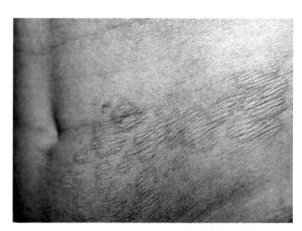

Figure 17.11   Anetoderma – note wrinkly skin overlying slightly raised plaques

Diagnosis

- Clinical diagnosis

Differential diagnosis

- Connective tissue nevus
- Nevus lipomatosis

Treatment

- None known to help

Prognosis

- Stable or may increase in number

References

Colditz PB, Dunster KR, Joy GJ, et al. Anetoderma of prematurity in association with electrocardiographic electrodes. J Am Acad Dermatol 1999; 41: 479–81

Ghomrasseni S, Dridi M, Gogly B, et al. Anetoderma: an altered balance between metalloproteinases and tissue inhibitors of metalloproteinases. Am J Dermatopathol 2002; 24: 118–29

Karrer S, Szeimies R-M, Stolz W, Landthaler M. Primary anetoderma in children: report of two cases and literature review. Pediatr Dermatol 1996; 13: 382–5

Prizant TL, Lucky AW, Frieden IJ, et al. Spontaneous atrophic patches in extremely premature infants. Arch Dermatol 1996; 132: 671–4

Sparsa A, Piette JC, Wechsler B, et al. Anetoderma and its prothrombotic abnormalities. J Am Acad Dermatol 2003; 49: 1008–12

Thomas JE, Mehregan DR, Holland J, Mehregan DA. Familial anetoderma. Int J Dermatol 2003; 42: 75–7

Piezogenic pedal papules

Major points

- Common entity found in 10–20% of the general population
- More common in women
- Asymptomatic skin-colored papules seen along the sides of the plantar surface only when weight-bearing (Figure 17.12)
- Occasionally painful
- Often seen in runners

Pathogenesis

- Caused by herniations of subcutaneous fat into the dermis on the sides of the feet caused by weight bearing

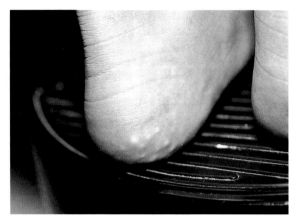

Figure 17.12 Piezogenic pedal papules – herniations of fat which are more pronounced when standing

- Histology: thickened dermis, loss of normal small fat compartments in the lower dermis and subcutis with many protrusions of enlarged fat lobules into the dermis caused by degeneration of the thin fibrous septa

Diagnosis

- Clinical diagnosis

Differential diagnosis

- Lipomas
- Connective tissue nevus
- Plexiform neurofibroma

Treatment

- Special orthotic heel cups for severely painful lesions

Prognosis

- Usually stable unless there is chronic stress on the feet, in which case it may progress

References

Boni R, Dummer R. Compression therapy in painful piezogenic pedal papules. Arch Dermatol 1996; 132: 127–8

Van Straaten EA, Van Langen IM, Oorthuys JWE, Oosting J. Piezogenic papules of the feet in healthy children and their possible relation with connective tissue disorders. Pediatr Dermatol 1991; 8: 277–9

Woodrow SL, Brereton-Smith G, Handfield-Jones S. Painful piezogenic pedal papules: response to local electro-acupuncture. Br J Dermatol 1997; 136: 628–30

Panniculitis

Major points

- Panniculitis is a term used to describe a group of diseases with inflammation in the subcutaneous fat (see Table 17.3)
- Presents with erythematous or violaceous, painful, subcutaneous nodules (Figures 17.13 and 17.14)
- Size usually 1–4 cm
- Common location: lower legs, symmetrical, but nodules may be anywhere
- Usually do not ulcerate
- Recurrent crops
- Lesions involve over a few weeks, and erythema is replaced with hyperpigmentation
- Erythema nodosum – most common type of panniculitis (see Table 17.4)

Pathogenesis

- Inflammation of fat; etiology depends upon type of panniculitis

Diagnosis

- Histology: degeneration and necrosis of lipocytes with an infiltrate of polymorphonuclear leukocytes and lymphocytes within the lobules of fat or in the septae

Differential diagnosis

- Epidermal cyst (ruptured)
- Cellulitis

Treatment

- Bed rest if lesions occur on legs
- Withdrawal of offending agent (e.g. drugs)
- Nonsteroidal anti-inflammatory agents
- Oral steroids may be indicated, particularly in cases of vasculitis

Prognosis

- Course variable, depending upon the type of panniculitis
- May spontaneously resolve or persist with new lesions occurring in crops

References

Aronson IK, Zeitz HJ, Variakojis D. Panniculitis in childhood. Pediatr Dermatol 1988; 5: 216–30

Table 17.3 Types of panniculitis

Neonatal panniculitis
Sclerema neonatorum
Subcutaneous fat necrosis of the neonate

Physical panniculitis
Cold-induced (popsicle panniculitis)
Traumatic
Chemical-induced
Factitial
Post-steroid injection

Systemic diseases with panniculitis
Systemic lupus erythematosus
Pancreatitis
Sarcoidosis
Renal failure
Lymphoma
Leukemia
Infections
α_1-antitrypsin deficiency

Vasculitis
Nodular vasculitis
Polyarteritis nodosa
Cutaneous polyarteritis nodosa
Superficial migratory thrombophlebitis

Septal panniculitis without vasculitis
Erythema nodosum
Scleroderma panniculitis
Eosinophilic fasciitis
Eosinophilic myalgia syndrome

Idiopathic lobular panniculitis (Weber–Christian disease)

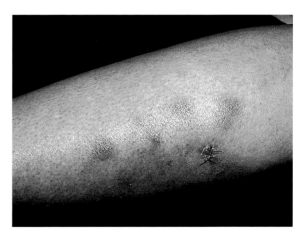

Figure 17.13 Panniculitis associated with Crohn disease

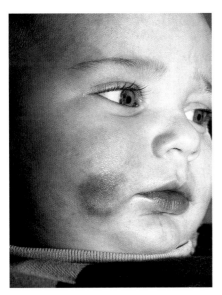

Figure 17.14   Popsicle panniculitis – caused by sucking on a cold popsicle

Eberhard BA, Ilowite NT. Panniculitis and lipodystrophy. Curr Opin Rheumatol 2002; 14: 566–70

McBean J, Sable A, Maude J, Robinson-Bostom L. Alpha1-antitrypsin deficiency panniculitis. Cutis 2003; 71: 205–9

Ruiz-Maldonado R, Parrilla FM, Luz Orozco-Covarrubias M, et al. Edematous, scarring vasculitic panniculitis: a new multisystemic disease with malignant potential. J Am Acad Dermatol 1995; 32: 37–44

Sutra-Loubet C, Carlotti A, Guillemette J, Wallach D. Neutrophilic panniculitis. J Am Acad Dermatol 2004; 50: 280–5

Table 17.4   Major etiologies of erythema nodosum
Drug-induced Sulfonamides Bromides Oral contraceptives
Bacterial infections Streptococcal infections *Yersinia enterocolitica* *Mycoplasma pneumoniae* Leprosy Leptospirosis Tularemia *Bartonella henselae* (cat scratch disease)
Fungal infections Coccidioidomycosis Blastomycosis Histoplasmosis Dermatophytosis
Viral infections/other infections Paravaccinia Infectious mononucleosis Hepatitis B Psittacosis Tuberculosis
Other diseases Sarcoidosis Ulcerative colitis Crohn disease Lymphoma Leukemia Behçet syndrome

CONNECTIVE TISSUE

Fibromatoses

General

- Two broad groups: superficial (fascial) fibromatoses, and deep (musculoaponeurotic) fibromatoses
- Benign proliferations of myofibroblasts

Major points

- Infantile digital fibromatosis
  1. Most common fibrous proliferation in the first year of life
  2. Solitary, smooth, dome-shaped nodule on the distal digital phalanx, which is either skin-colored or red (Figure 17.15)
  3. Size reaches 1–3 cm
  4. Multiple tumors common
  5. Fingers affected commonly (86%)
  6. No sex predilection
  7. Can spontaneously involute
  8. May need to be surgically excised, but there is a high recurrence rate
- Infantile myofibromatosis
  1. Seen at birth or early life
  2. Multiple cutaneous nodules with underlying tumors in the muscle, bone and visceral organs
  3. Lesions are firm, skin-colored to red-purple nodules ranging in size from 0.5 to 7 cm
  4. If limited to skin and bones, does not require treatment unless there is functional

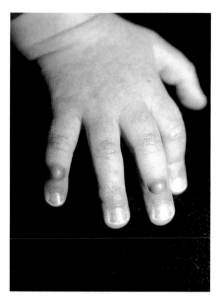

Figure 17.15   Infantile digital fibromatosis – painless, firm papules on an infant's fingers

impairment. More aggressive types may require chemotherapy or radiation and may be fatal
- Plantar fibromatosis
  1. Firm, nontender nodule on mid-plantar surface of foot present at birth
  2. Uncomfortable when child walks
  3. Requires excision when symptomatic; recurrence is uncommon if completely excised
- Knuckle pads
  1. Solitary or multiple thickenings over the metacarpophalangeal or proximal interphalangeal joints (Figure 17.16)
  2. Require no treatment

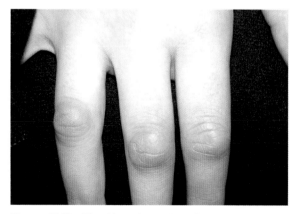

Figure 17.16   Knuckle pads on all the fingers

- Fibrous hamartoma of infancy
  1. Solitary (or multiple) nodules usually located on the shoulder, arm or axilla
  2. Present at birth or shortly after
  3. Treat with excision; recurrence is uncommon
- Juvenile hyaline fibromatosis
  1. Very rare triad of fibrous growths on the head and neck, flexion contractures and gingival hyperplasia
  2. Skull and encephalic abnormalities
  3. Autosomal recessive
  4. Relentless progression

Pathogenesis

- Etiology is unknown, but fibromatoses are characterized by a proliferation of fibrous/myofibrous tissue

Diagnosis

- Histology is essential
  1. Infantile digital fibromatosis: perinuclear cytoplasmic inclusions seen with trichrome stain (may represent actin microfilaments) within a proliferation of fibrous tissue
  2. Infantile myofibromatosis: spindle-shaped fibroblasts in whorls and interlacing bundles
  3. Fibrous hamartoma of infancy: distinctive tracts of fibroblasts, fat and small blue cells within the lesion
  4. Juvenile hyaline fibromatosis: hyalinized collagen with fibroblast proliferation

Differential diagnosis

- Knuckle pads: Gottron papules (dermatomyositis), acanthosis nigricans
- Infantile myofibromatosis: soft tissue sarcomas, hemangioendotheliomas, fibrosarcomas, lipomas, fibrous histiocytomas, lipoblastomas, neurofibromas, rhabdomyosarcomas
- Infantile digital fibroma/fibrous hamartoma of infancy: sarcoma

Prognosis

- Deeper variants can behave aggressively and become infiltrative but do not metastasize

References

Bellman B, Wooming G, Landsman L, et al. Infantile myofibromatosis: a case report. Pediatr Dermatol 1991; 8: 306–9

Caylakli F, Cakmak O, Seckin D, et al. Juvenile hyaline fibromatosis: a case report. Int J Pediatr Otorhinolaryngol 2003; 67: 557–61

Counsell SJ, Devile C, Mercuri E, et al. Magnetic resonance imaging assessment of infantile myofibromatosis. Clin Radiol 2002; 57: 67–70

Dickey GE, Sotelo-Avila C. Fibrous hamartoma of infancy: current review. Pediatr Dev Pathol 1999; 2: 236–43

Eich GF, Hoeffel JC, Tschappeler H, et al. Fibrous tumours in children: imaging features of a heterogeneous group of disorders. Pediatr Radiol 1998; 28: 500–9

Gandhi MM, Nathan PC, Weitzman S, Levitt GA. Successful treatment of life-threatening generalized infantile myofibromatosis using low-dose chemotherapy. J Pediatr Hematol Oncol 2003; 25: 750–4

Goldberg NS, Bauer BS, Kraus H, et al. Infantile myofibromatosis: a review of clinicopathology with perspectives on new treatment choices. Pediatr Dermatol 1988; 5: 37–46

Haleem A, Al-Hindi HN, Juboury MA, et al. Juvenile hyaline fibromatosis: morphologic, immunohistochemical, and ultrastructural study of three siblings. Am J Dermatopathol 2002; 24: 218–24

Ikediobi NI, Iyengar V, Hwang L, et al. Infantile myofibromatosis: support for autosomal dominant inheritance. J Am Acad Dermatol 2003; 49 (2 Suppl): S148–50

Kang SK, Chang SE, Choi JH, et al. A case of congenital infantile digital fibromatosis. Pediatr Dermatol 2002; 19: 462–3

Kanwar AJ, Kaur S, Thami GP, Mohan H. Congenital infantile digital fibromatosis. Pediatr Dermatol 2002; 19: 370–1

Keltz M, DiCostanzo D, Desai P, Cohen SR. Infantile (desmoid-type) fibromatosis. Pediatr Dermatol 1995; 12: 149–51

Rahman N, Dunstan M, Teare MD, et al. The gene for juvenile hyaline fibromatosis maps to chromosome 4q21. Am J Hum Genet 2002; 71: 975–80

Keloids

Major points

- Mildly tender, firm papule or nodule arising in site of previous injury (e.g. surgery, ear piercing, cystic acne, burns) and extends beyond the border of the original injury (Figure 17.17)
- Lesions are skin-colored, pink or hyperpigmented

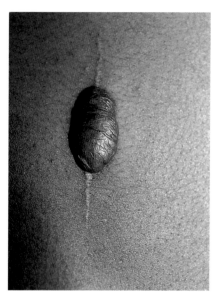

Figure 17.17   Keloid – firm plaque in a scar

- Can be disfiguring
- May be painful, especially when growing
- Common locations are shoulders, chest and earlobes
- More common in dark-skinned teenagers

Pathogenesis

- Caused by unchecked proliferation of fibrous tissue and collagen following an injury to the dermis which invades the surrounding skin

Diagnosis

- Histology: whorls of young fibrous tissue and fibroblasts arranged in a haphazard manner with thick, eosinophilic, acellular bands of collagen and thickening of dermis; mast cells and plasma cells increased in number; elastin usually absent

Differential diagnosis

- Hypertrophic scar
- Fibrosarcoma

Treatment

- Intralesional steroids (e.g. triamcinolone 10–40 mg/ml) given every 2–4 weeks until flattened and not growing
- Larger lesions should be excised with subsequent steroid injections until growth of the lesion has stopped

Prognosis

- Keloids tend to persist and enlarge slowly over time and can recur even when treated

References

Berman B, Bieley HC. Keloids. J Am Acad Dermatol 1995; 33: 117–23

Gold MH. A controlled clinical trial of topical silicone gel sheeting in the treatment of hypertrophic scars and keloids. J Am Acad Dermatol 1994; 30: 506–7

Kelly AP. Pseudofolliculitis barbae and acne keloidalis nuchae. Dermatol Clin 2003; 21: 645–53

Marneros AG, Norris JEC, Olsen JR, Reichenberger E. Clinical genetics of familial keloids. Arch Dermatol 2001; 137: 1429–34

Poocharoen VN, Berman B. New therapies for the management of keloids. J Craniofac Surg 2003; 14: 654–7

Rahban SR, Garner WL. Fibroproliferative scars. Clin Plast Surg 2003; 30: 77–89

Sahl WJ, Clever J. Cutaneous scars: part II. Int J Dermatol 1994; 33: 763–9

Acne keloidalis nuchae

Major points:

- Chronic scarring folliculitis located on posterior neck in young Black men
- Characteristic follicular papules that coalesce into firm plaques and nodules (Figure 17.18)
- Begins with a chronic folliculitis which heals with keloid-like papules
- Can form small to large plaques
- Lesions usually pruritic or painful

Pathogenesis

- Etiology uncertain
- Aggravated by shaving tightly curled hair at the nape of the neck and having the new hair curve back into the skin, causing inflammation at the deep infundibular and isthmic levels of the hair follicle
- Histology:
  1. Early: inflammatory cells in the upper one-third of hair follicle; sebaceous glands diminished
  2. Later: dermal fibrosis and scar formation

Diagnosis

- Clinical diagnosis

Differential diagnosis

- Folliculitis
- Hypertrophic scars
- Pseudofolliculitis barbae

Treatment

- Early treatment essential
- Intralesional steroids or short course of oral steroids for acute inflammation
- Surgical excision followed by intralesional steroids if extensive
- Oral antibiotics (e.g. minocycline, doxycycline) and topical retinoids

Prognosis

- Chronic unless treated

References

Dinehart SM, Herzberg AJ, Kerns BJ, Pollack SV. Acne keloidalis: a review. J Dermatol Surg Oncol 1989; 15: 642–7

Giovannini UM. Treatment of scars by steroid injections. Wound Repair Regeneration 2002; 10: 116–17

Glenn MJ, Bennett RG, Kelly AP. Acne keloidalis nuchae: treatment with excision and second-intention healing. J Am Acad Dermatol 1995; 33: 243–6

Tsao SS, Dover JS, Arndt KA, Kaminer MS. Scar management: keloid, hypertrophic, atrophic, and acne scars. Semin Cutan Med Surg 2002; 21: 46–75

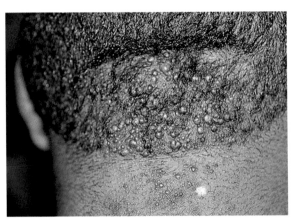

Figure 17.18 Acne keloidalis nuchae – typically seen at the nape of the neck

Hypertrophic scars

Major points

- Firm, slightly raised, flat, pink or red nodule or plaque in the area of previous injury or inflammation but stays within the site of original injury

Pathogenesis

- Caused by unchecked proliferation of fibrous tissue following an injury to the dermis

Diagnosis

- Histology: whorls of young fibrous tissue and fibroblasts arranged in a haphazard manner with marked thickening of the dermis

Differential diagnosis

- Keloid
- Basal cell carcinoma
- Skin appendage tumors
- Dermatofibroma

Treatment

- Intralesional steroids (e.g. triamcinolone 10–40 mg/ml) given every 2–4 weeks until flattened
- Silicone gel sheeting worn continuously for several months

Prognosis

- Hypertrophic scars can flatten with time, but are usually stable after 1 year

References

Brissett AE, Sherris DA. Scar contractures, hypertrophic scars, and keloids. Fac Plast Surg 2001; 17: 263–72

Gold MH. A controlled clinical trial of topical silicone gel sheeting in the treatment of hypertrophic scars and keloids. J Am Acad Dermatol 1994; 30: 506–7

Nemeth AJ. Keloids and hypertrophic scars. J Dermatol Surg Oncol 1993; 19: 738–46

Sahl WJ, Clever J. Cutaneous scars: part II. Intern J Dermatol 1994; 33: 763–9

Shaffer JJ, Taylor SC, Cook-Bolden F. Keloidal scars: a review with a critical look at therapeutic options. J Am Acad Dermatol 2002; 46 (2 Suppl): S63–97

Striae distensae

Major points

- Visible scars with linear, smooth bands of atrophic skin (Figure 17.19)
- Begin as reddish streaks, then turn purple, and finally white

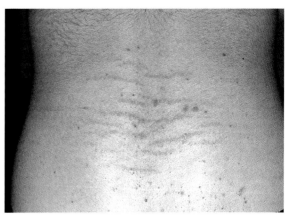

Figure 17.19   Striae distensae ('stretch marks') occur commonly in teens on the lower back, inner thighs and breasts

- Most common sites: thighs, buttocks, breasts in girls, lower back in boys

Pathogenesis

- Histology: thin overlying epidermis, fine dermal collagen bundles arranged in straight parallel lines, some inflammation, and elastolysis; late stages show dermal collagen in thin eosinophilic bundles, oriented in straight lines
- Pathogenesis unknown, probably relates to changes in extracellular matrix components
- Causes: puberty, obesity, corticosteroids, pregnancy, increased adrenocortical function, genetic factors

Diagnosis

- Clinical inspection

Differential diagnosis

- Ehlers–Danlos syndrome
- Marfan syndrome
- Child abuse

Treatment

- Usually no treatment is necessary
- Pulsed dye laser can improve redness in early lesions
- Discontinuance of steroids, if this is a precipitating factor
- Emollients (e.g. petrolatum, cocoa butter)

Prognosis

- Lesions are permanent

References

Di Lernia V, Bonci A, Cattania M, Bisighini G. Striae distensae (rubrae) in monozygotic twins. Pediatr Dermatol 2001; 18: 261–2

Garcia Hidalgo L. Dermatological complications of obesity. Am J Clin Dermatol 2002; 3: 497–506

Jabbour SA. Cutaneous manifestations of endocrine disorders: a guide for dermatologists. Am J Clin Dermatol 2003; 4: 315–31

McDaniel DH. Laser therapy of stretch marks. Dermatol Clin 2002; 20: 67–76

Dermatofibroma

Synonym: fibrous histiocytoma

Major points

- Common, benign, asymptomatic papule or papules ranging from 0.5 mm to 1 cm, commonly found on the lower legs, but may occur anywhere (Figure 17.20)

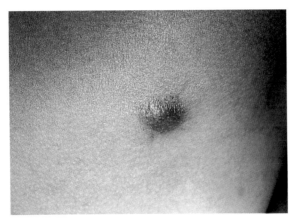

Figure 17.20   Dermatofibroma – firm brown papule commonly seen on the lower legs

- Usually solitary but may be multiple
- Color varies: yellow, red, purple or dark brown with rim of brown pigment and variation in color
- Palpation: firm or hard; feels like a pea which is fixed to the skin surface and freely movable over the subcutis
- Lateral pressure produces a 'dimple sign' with an overlying depression in the center of the papule

Pathogenesis

- Cause unknown but thought to be the result of trauma, insect bites, or viral infection

Diagnosis

- Clinical features characteristic
- Histology: whorling fascicles of spindle cells; edges are poorly defined. A Grenz zone of normal tissue lies above the lesion in the papillary dermis; epidermis is acanthotic

Differential diagnosis

- Nevocellular nevus
- Melanoma
- Xanthoma
- Prurigo nodularis
- Seborrheic keratosis
- Dermatofibrosarcoma protuberans

Treatment

- None usually needed
- Excision if painful or large

Prognosis

- Lesions are benign and usually stable
- Can resolve, leaving hypo- or hyperpigmentation

References

Bouyssou-Gauthier M-L, Labrousse F, Longis B, et al. Dermatofibrosarcoma protuberans in childhood. Pediatr Dermatol 1997; 14: 463–5

Curco N, Jucgla A, Bordas X, Moreno A. Dermatofibroma with spreading satellitosis. J Am Acad Dermatol 1992; 27: 1017–18

Holst VA, Junkins-Hopkins JM, Elenitsas R. Cutaneous smooth muscle neoplasms: clinical features, histologic findings, and treatment options. J Am Acad Dermatol 2002; 46: 477–90

Kutzner H. Expression of the human progenitor cell antigen CD34 (HPCA-1) distinguishes dermatofibrosarcoma protuberans from fibrous histiocytoma in formalin-fixed, paraffin-embedded tissue. J Am Acad Dermatol 1993; 28: 613–17

Lew W, Lim HS, Kim YC. Cutaneous metastatic malignant fibrous histiocytoma. J Am Acad Dermatol 2003; 48 (2 Suppl): S39–40

Niiyama S, Katsuoka K, Happle R, Hoffmann R. Multiple eruptive dermatofibromas: a review of the literature. Acta Derm Venereol 2002; 82: 241–4

Neurofibroma

Major points

- Presents as a skin-colored papule or nodule, soft to palpation ranging in size from 0.5 to >3 cm
- Upon pressure to the lesion, the neurofibroma pushes into the skin giving the sensation that one is pushing a button through a buttonhole
- Some lesions are pedunculated
- Usually solitary unless seen in the context of neurofibromatosis (see Chapter 20)
- Variants such as plexiform neurofibroma can be seen in neurofibromatosis

Pathogenesis

- Hyperplasia of nerve elements arising in nerves, composed of Schwann cells, fibroblasts and endothelial cells

Diagnosis

- Biopsy often needed for confirmation
- Histology: Schwann cells, fibroblasts, endothelial cells, mast cells, perineural fibroblasts and axons arranged haphazardly in a matrix containing collagen and myxoid ground substance; circumscribed but not encapsulated

Differential diagnosis

- Dermal nevus
- Skin tag (acrochordon)
- Dermatofibroma

Treatment

- Usually no treatment needed
- Simple excision if indicated

Prognosis

- Small neurofibromas not associated with neurofibromatosis tend to remain stable or slowly enlarge with time

- Those associated with neurofibromatosis tend to enlarge slowly

References

DeBella K, Szudek J, Friedman JM. Use of the National Institutes of Health criteria for diagnosis of neurofibromatosis 1 in children. Pediatrics 2000; 105: 608–14

Johnson NS, Saal HM, Lovell AM, Schorry EK. Social and emotional problems in children with neurofibromatosis type 1: evidence and proposed interventions. J Pediatr 1999; 134: 767–72

Kandt RS. Tuberous sclerosis complex and neurofibromatosis type 1: the two most common neurocutaneous diseases. Neurol Clin 2003; 21: 983–1004

Riccardi VM. Of mass and men. Neurofibromas and histogenesis [Editorial]. Arch Dermatol 2000; 136: 1257–8

Viskochil DH. It takes two to tango: mast cell and Schwann cell interactions in neurofibromas. J Clin Invest 2003; 112: 1791–3

Corns and calluses

Synonym: clavus (multiple: clavi)

Major points

- Hyperkeratotic plaque seen over pressure or frictional areas typically on the feet
- When pared with a blade, there is a central translucent core, without thrombosed capillaries (as seen in warts)
- Corns can be hard, soft, vascular, or neurovascular
- Hard corns are usually over the dorsal interphalangeal joints, on the plantar surface underlying the metatarsal heads, or on the great toe
- Soft corns arise interdigitally, typically in the fourth web space

Pathogenesis

- Corns are caused by ill-fitting footwear with pointed toes causing crowding in the shoe toe box, or from the digits pressing on each other

Diagnosis

- Clinical features

Differential diagnosis

- Verruca vulgaris
- Verruca plantaris

- Glomus tumors
- Eccrine poroma

Treatment

- Pare with scalpel blade
- Salicylic acid plasters and other keratolytics used in combination with paring
- Obtain shoes that fit better

Prognosis

- Lesions are stable or progressive unless underlying cause is addressed

References

Smith M. Environmental and sports-related skin diseases. In Dermatology. Bolognia JL, Jorizzo JL, Rapini R, eds. Mosby: London, 2003: 1399

Connective tissue nevus

Major points

- Connective tissue nevi (CTN) are hamartomas of either collagen or elastin or an abnormality in ground substance plus structural components of connective tissue
- Male/female ratio = 1
- Sporadic or autosomal dominant inheritance
- Usually present at birth or in early childhood
- Characteristic firm, nontender, irregularly shaped, or oval skin-colored plaque (Figure 17.21)
- Common locations: trunk, buttocks, or extremities

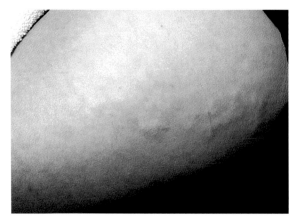

Figure 17.21   Connective tissue nevus – skin-colored plaque

- Surface of plaque has a pebbled appearance (termed peau d'orange, 'skin of an orange')
- Solitary lesions usually measure 2–10 cm, whereas clustered lesions usually are 4–5 mm
- Associations:
  1. Tuberous sclerosis: shagreen plaques
  2. Buschke–Ollendorff syndrome (dermatofibrosis lenticularis disseminata) shows multiple small CTN and osteopoikilosis (bony dysplasia of the long bones, pelvis, hands and feet)

Pathogenesis

- Hamartoma with various amounts of collagen, elastin and adipose tissue without increase in fibroblasts

Diagnosis

- Often requires biopsy for confirmation
- Biopsy should be a small wedge biopsy including lesional and nonlesional skin in order to compare normal and abnormal dermal tissues

Differential diagnosis

- Smooth muscle hamartoma
- Plexiform neurofibroma
- Neurofibroma
- Amyloidosis
- Colloid millium
- Nevus lipomatosus

Treatment

- Reassurance to parents of benign nature
- Surgical excision

Prognosis

- Most solitary CTN are benign and not associated with other syndromes

References

Chang SE, Kang SK, Kim ES, et al. A case of congenital mucinous nevus: a connective tissue nevus of the proteoglycan type. Pediatr Dermatol 2003; 20: 229–31

Crivellato E. Disseminated nevus anelasticus. Int J Dermatol 1986; 25: 171–3

DePadova-Elder S, Mols-Kowalczewski BL, Lambert WC. Multiple connective tissue nevi. Cutis 1988; 42: 222–4

Uitto J, Santa Cruz DJ, Eisen AZ. Connective tissue nevi of the skin. J Am Acad Dermatol 1980; 3: 441–61

Yeh SW, Magalhaes AM, Vasconcellos MR, et al. Zosteriform connective tissue nevus: a case report. Int J Dermatol 2003; 42: 720–2

Smooth muscle hamartoma

Major points

- Lesions are solitary, skin-colored or hyperpigmented, infiltrative patches or plaques with accentuation of hair follicles (Figure 17.22)

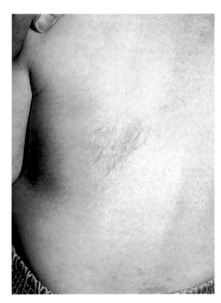

Figure 17.22 Smooth muscle hamartoma – with overlying hypertrichosis

- Size usually 1–5 cm
- Hypertrichosis develops in two-thirds of lesions
- Often overlooked in infancy
- Rarely acquired in later life
- Common location in lumbosacral area (67%)
- No associated systemic abnormalities
- When firmly stroked, fasciculation of the skin causes the appearance of goosebumps or cobblestones (pseudo-Darier sign) from the stimulation of aberrant arrector pili muscles
- Slight male predominance

Pathogenesis

- Some authors think smooth muscle hamartoma and Becker nevus are hamartomas of a single

spectrum, with varying increases of epidermis, smooth muscle and hair appendages

Diagnosis

- Histology: numerous smooth muscle fibers oriented haphazardly within the dermis

Differential diagnosis

- Mastocytoma
- Connective tissue nevus
- Plexiform neurofibroma
- Congenital nevus
- Becker nevus

Treatment

- None needed
- Seldom requires excision

Prognosis

- Lesion is benign and stable

References

D'Addario SF, Morgan M, Talley L, Smoller BR. h-Caldesmon as a specific marker of smooth muscle cell differentiation in some soft tissue tumors of the skin. J Cutan Pathol 2002; 29: 426–9

Grau-Massanes M, Raimer SS, Colome-Grimmer M, et al. Congenital smooth muscle hamartoma presenting as a linear atrophic plaque: case report and review of the literature. Pediatr Dermatol 1996; 13: 222–5

Gualandri L, Cambiaghi S, Ermacora E, et al. Multiple familial smooth muscle hamartomas. Pediatr Dermatol 2001; 18: 17–20

Holst VA, Junkins-Hopkins JM, Elenitsas R. Cutaneous smooth muscle neoplasms: clinical features, histologic findings, and treatment options. J Am Acad Dermatol 2002; 46: 477–90

INFILTRATIONS

Juvenile xanthogranuloma

Major points

- Most common non-Langerhans cell histiocytosis of childhood
- Sporadic in occurrence
- No sexual or racial predilection
- Usually appear in early infancy, between 1 and 4 years

- One lesion (25% of cases) to hundreds of firm, reddish-yellow papules/nodules; size 1–10 mm (Figure 17.23)
- Continues to develop lesions over 2 years
- Telangiectasias on surface are common
- Occasional superficial erosions
- Types:
  1. Disseminated micronodular juvenile xanthogranuloma (JXG): small papular lesions (<6 mm) are most common
  2. Patients who have larger nodules tend to have fewer lesions
  3. Solitary giant JXG (4–10 cm)
  4. Clustered variant
  5. Generalized lichenoid variant
- Typical locations: face, neck, scalp, but trunk and extremities can be involved
- Extracutaneous sites (very rare): eyes, lungs, pericardium, spleen, liver, testes, meninges
  1. Rarely symptomatic except eye involvement
  2. Eye involvement more common in disseminated micronodular variant. Usually unilateral and can be confused with retinoblastoma
- Numerous associations. Most are probably coincidental except JXG associated with neurofibromatosis and juvenile chronic myelogenous leukemia

Pathogenesis

- Cause unknown
- May be a reactive histiocytic process rather than a neoplasia
- Blood lipid levels normal

Diagnosis

- Histology:
  1. Early lesions show accumulation of macrophages without lipid droplets
  2. Well-developed lesions demonstrate granulomatous infiltrate with foamy lipid-laden macrophages and Touton giant cells
  3. No Birbeck granules on electron microscopy or S-100 protein present

Differential diagnosis

- Mastocytoma
- Spitz nevus
- Benign cephalic histiocytosis

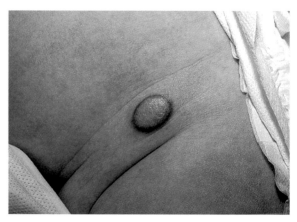

Figure 17.23   Juvenile xanthogranuloma – yellow papule with red halo

- Langerhans cell histiocytosis
- Tuberous xanthoma
- Papular xanthoma (Figure 17.24)
- Multicentric reticulohistiocytosis

Treatment

- None is necessary except in ulcerated or large lesions where surgical intervention may be warranted

Prognosis

- Excellent, with complete involution within 6 months in 30%
- Spontaneous involution in the remainder by 3–6 years
- Residual pigmentation or atrophy may occur

References

Chang MW. Update on juvenile xanthogranuloma: unusual cutaneous and systemic variants. Semin Cutan Med Surg 1999; 18: 195–205

Chang MW, Frieden IJ, Good W. The risk of intraocular juvenile xanthogranuloma: survey of current practices and assessment of risk. J Am Acad Dermatol 1996; 34: 445–9

Freyer DR, Kennedy R, Bostrom BC, et al. Juvenile xanthogranuloma: forms of systemic disease and their clinical implications. J Pediatr 1996; 129: 227–37

Piraccini BM, Fanti PA, Iorizzo M, Tosti A. Juvenile xanthogranuloma of the proximal nail fold. Pediatr Dermatol 2003; 20: 307–8

Zelger B, Burgdorf WH. The cutaneous 'histiocytoses'. Adv Dermatol 2001; 17: 77–114

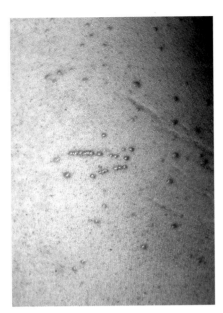

Figure 17.24   Eruptive xanthomas – in a patient with elevated triglycerides and diabetes

Zvulunov A, Barak Y, Metzker A. Juvenile xanthogranuloma, neurofibromatosis, and juvenile chronic myelogenous leukemia. Arch Dermatol 1995; 131: 904–8

Mastocytosis

Major points

- Group of disorders characterized by the infiltration of mast cells into the tissues, particularly the skin
- Usually begins in childhood and distinct from adult mastocytosis which tends to have a poor prognosis
- No sex predilection
- More common in Whites
- Sporadic occurrence; however, a familial form exists
- Onset between birth and 2 years in the majority of cases, with fewer presenting later in childhood
- Types of mastocytosis: solitary mastocytoma, urticaria pigmentosa, diffuse mastocytosis, telangiectasia macularis eruptiva perstans, systemic mastocytosis and mast cell leukemia
  1. In pediatrics, the following account for >95% of cases of mastocytosis: solitary mastocytoma, urticaria pigmentosa and diffuse mastocytosis

- Solitary mastocytoma
  1. Usually solitary, but occasionally several lesions
  2. New lesions develop for several months after the first lesion appears, but tend not to continue to develop past 1 year
  3. Most common on neck, arms and trunk, but can be anywhere
  4. Typical oval to round 1–5 cm slightly brownish yellow nodule which feels thickened or rubbery with a pebbly surface
  5. Darier sign: urtication can be demonstrated by stroking the lesion with a typical wheal and flare
  6. History of bulla formation, generalized pruritus, flushing, colicky abdominal pain, diarrhea
  7. Symptoms often resolve within 2 years, even when the lesion persists
  8. Most plaques have flattened or disappeared by age 10 years
- Urticaria pigmentosa (UP)
  1. Most common form of mastocytosis
  2. Predominantly a disease of infants and young children
  3. Symptoms begin between 3 and 9 months
  4. Numerous 5 mm to 2 cm reddish brown to yellowish brown slightly elevated nodules, predominantly on the trunk, but can be anywhere; generally has fewer lesions (Figure 17.25)
  5. Darier sign is positive in most lesions (Figure 17.26)
  6. May be associated with dermatographism
  7. New lesions may continue to develop for many years
  8. Bullae may develop within the lesions
  9. Pruritus is often the only symptom
  10. History of bulla formation, generalized pruritus, flushing, colicky abdominal pain, diarrhea
- Diffuse cutaneous mastocytosis (DCM)
  1. Rare in childhood
  2. Neonates born with erythematous, thickened doughy feeling skin which appears lichenified
  3. Severe widespread bullae may occur
  4. Systemic involvement is prominent with flushing, diarrhea, vomiting, abdominal pain, respiratory distress, shock; can be fatal

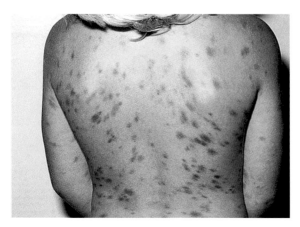

Figure 17.25 Mastocytosis – typical urticaria pigmentosa with numerous brown-yellow papules

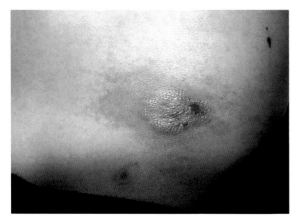

Figure 17.26 Mastocytosis – Darier sign can be elicited by rubbing a lesion of mastocytosis

- Telangiectasia eruptiva macularis perstans (TMEP)
  1. Seen in <1% of cases of mastocytosis
  2. Appears as tan to brown macules and patchy erythema with telangiectasias
  3. Mainly in teens or adults
- Systemic mastocytosis
  1. More common in widespread disease of UP and DCM
  2. Skeletal system may show evidence of involvement on X-ray (e.g. lytic, cystic or sclerotic lesions), but in most cases of UP and DCM these lesions resolve
  3. Involvement of other systems: lungs, liver, spleen, kidney and heart with hepatosplenomegaly, anemia, bone pain, failure to thrive

- Malignant mast cell disease
  1. Involvement of hematopoietic and reticuloendothelial systems
  2. Occurs in 30% of adults with mastocytosis; very rare in children
  3. One reported case of acute lymphoblastic leukemia associated with UP in a child
- Mastocytosis syndrome
  1. Results from massive release of vasoactive mediators from mast cells
  2. Can be caused by any mast cell degranulator (see Table 17.5)
  3. Symptoms: flushing, tachycardia, diarrhea, projectile vomiting, abdominal pain, respiratory distress (wheezing), hypotension, severe pruritus and potential shock
  4. Should be treated immediately

Pathogenesis

- Thought to represent a reactive hyperplasia of normal mast cells, rather than a neoplasia

Table 17.5   Mast cell degranulators

Drugs
Aspirin
Nonsteroidal anti-inflammatory drugs (e.g. ibuprofen, naproxen)
Alcohol
Caffeine
Codeine
Morphine
Narcotics
Polymyxin B (can be in topical antibiotics)
Radiographic dyes
Some anesthetics

Physical stimuli
Hot baths
Exercise
Rubbing the skin
Cold stress (entering a cold lake or exiting a swimming pool)
Hot spicy foods (also in some candies)

Other
Snake venom
Shellfish
Emotional stress
Insect bites

- Normal mast cells help protect the body by surveillance of environmental antigens
  1. Found in skin, respiratory tract, GI tract, genitourinary tract and adjacent to neurovascular bundles
  2. Receptors on mast cells have a high affinity for Fc portion of IgE antibody with subsequent degranulation
- Soluble mediators released from keratinocytes may cause accumulation of mast cells in the upper dermis
- Patients with mastocytosis do not have an increase in allergies

Diagnosis

- With a solitary mastocytoma or UP, clinical appearance and typical Darier sign will usually make the diagnosis
- Histology: dense infiltration of normal-appearing mast cells in the upper dermis
  1. Biopsy should not be performed on a recently stroked lesion, because the mast cells have degranulated and will not be seen with Giemsa stain
- Mast cells contain active mediators: histamine, heparin, tryptase, chymase, acid hydrolases, prostaglandin D_2 (PGD_2), leukotriene C_4, platelet-activating factor and tumor necrosis factor-α
- Routinely, no laboratory tests are necessary. However, in some patients, the following tests may be monitored (depending upon symptoms): complete blood count, serum chemistry profiles, radiologic skeletal survey, bone marrow aspiration
- In diffuse disease, the following may be helpful in following the disease: serum or urinary histamine levels, urinary *N*-methylhistamine, *N*-methylimidazoleacetic acid (metabolites of histamine)
- Other markers of mast cell degranulation: PGD_2, tryptase and heparin
- Skeletal survey or technetium bone scan may be indicated for bone pain

Differential diagnosis

- Solitary mastocytoma/urticaria pigmentosa
  1. Juvenile xanthogranuloma
  2. Spitz nevus
  3. Nodular scabies

  4. Congenital nevus
- Diffuse cutaneous mastocytosis
  1. Histiocytosis
  2. Bullous erythema multiforme
  3. Staphylococcal scalded skin syndrome
  4. Epidermolysis bullosa
  5. Infiltrative leukemias
- TMEP
  1. Telangiectasias
  2. Urticaria
  3. Ephiledes

Treatment

- No treatment of a solitary mastocytoma is usually needed
- Excision of a solitary mastocytoma is reserved for severely symptomatic lesions only
- Antihistamines may relieve pruritus (H1 blockers with or without H2 blockers)
- Oral disodium chromoglycate for GI symptoms
- Topical application of high-potency steroid ointments under occlusion may be helpful in isolated lesions or TMEP, with reduction of symptoms
- Intralesional steroids may reduce symptoms in individual lesions
- Systemic steroids are not effective
- Topical antibiotics, if used on the lesions, should not contain polymyxin B; mupirocin is recommended
- Psoralen with ultraviolet A light can be used in children aged >11 years for extensive disease
- Symptoms of mastocytosis syndrome (e.g. hypotension, wheezing, shock) should be treated aggressively with intravenous fluids, antihistamines, epinephrine, corticosteroids and vasopressors
- Parents of children should always carry a list of potential drugs which can degranulate mast cells to avoid complications (Table 17.5)
- Some children with extensive disease would benefit from an identification bracelet and a syringe of epinephrine kept nearby (e.g. EpiPen®)

Prognosis

- Solitary mastocytoma resolves with few sequelae; bullae rarely scar
- Urticaria pigmentosa in childhood spontaneously resolves. A small number of patients with more

systemic manifestations will continue into adulthood, and have a more guarded prognosis

- Diffuse cutaneous mastocytosis with early onset of blisters has a poor prognosis. Without blisters, the prognosis is better. Eventually, the skin improves in symptoms and texture
- Malignant mast cell disease with infiltration of bone marrow and other organs has a very poor prognosis
- Severe symptoms should be treated in the emergency room

References

Almahroos M, Kurban AK. Management of mastocytosis. Clin Dermatol 2003; 21: 274–7

Caken H, Ciftci A, Kisaarslan AF, et al. A child with systemic mastocytosis who had a facial appearance resembling an aged man. Pediatr Dermatol 2002; 19: 184–5

Golkar L, Bernhard JD. Mastocytosis. Lancet 1997; 349: 1379–85

Heide R, Tank B, Oranje AP. Mastocytosis in childhood. Pediatr Dermatol 2002; 19: 375–81

Longley J, Duffy TP, Kohn S. The mast cell and mast cell disease. J Am Acad Dermatol 1995; 32: 545–61

Murphy M, Walsh D, Drumm B, Watson R. Bullous mastocytosis: a fatal outcome. Pediatr Dermatol 1999; 16: 452–5

Shah PY, Sharma V, Worobec AS, et al. Congenital bullous mastocytosis with myeloproliferative disorder and c-*kit* mutation. J Am Acad Dermatol 1998; 39: 119–21

Tharp MD. Understanding mast cells and mastocytosis. J Invest Dermatol 1997; 108: 698–9

Tharp MD, Chan IJ. Mastocytosis. Adv Dermatol 2003; 19: 207–36

Valent P, Akin C, Sperr WR, et al. Diagnosis and treatment of systemic mastocytosis: state of the art. Br J Haematol 2003; 122: 695–717

Valent P, Akin C, Sperr WR, et al. Mast cell proliferative disorders: current view on variants recognized by the World Health Organization. Hematol Oncol Clin North Am 2003; 17: 1227–41

Calcinosis cutis

Major points

- Presents with firm, stony 1–30-mm papules or plaques which may have an erythematous border (Figure 17.27)

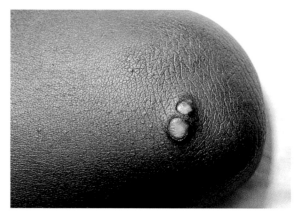

Figure 17.27 Calcinosis cutis – rock-hard, white papules on an elbow

- May be tender and ulcerate, discharging gritty material
- Distribution can be anywhere, but most common on the extremities, face and scrotum
- With extensive calcinosis, complications of contractures, pain and suppuration with or without superinfection may occur
- Dystrophic calcinosis cutis
  1. Most common form of calcinosis cutis
  2. Caused by deposition of calcium salts within previously damaged tissues with no metabolic abnormalities
  3. Localized forms arise in acne scars, ulcers, foreign body granulomas, subcutaneous fat necrosis of the newborn, neonatal heel sticks, cysts, lipomas and pilomatrixomas
  4. Widespread calcification is seen in systemic sclerosis, CREST syndrome, dermatomyositis, pseudoxanthoma elasticum, systemic lupus erythematosus and Ehlers–Danlos syndrome
  5. Iatrogenic causes: extravasation of intravenous calcium salts, electroencephalogram leads and electromyogram leads
- Idiopathic calcinosis cutis
  1. No evidence of local tissue injury or systemic metabolic disorder
  2. Localized
     a. Idiopathic calcinosis circumscripta
     b. Solitary congenital calcified nodule of the ear
     c. Idiopathic calcinosis of the scrotum or vulva

3. Generalized
   a. Milia-like idiopathic calcinosis cutis, seen in Down syndrome
- Metastatic calcinosis cutis
  1. Occurs with abnormal metabolism of calcium and/or phosphorous: chronic renal failure, vitamin D intoxication, sarcoidosis, parathyroid neoplasms, tumors
  2. Calcinosis is rarely seen in the skin, but more commonly in kidney, lung, gastric mucosa, eyes and arteries

Pathogenesis

- Precipitation or deposition of hydroxyapatite crystals of calcium phosphate within cutaneous tissues
- Etiology not understood, but unidentified local factors may promote calcification within tissues
- Calcium deposits tend to occur in areas of damaged tissue or elastic fibers

Diagnosis

- Radiographs reveal radio-opaque densities in areas of calcification
- Laboratory abnormalities are found only in metastatic form
- Histology: calcium deposits in the dermis or subcutaneous tissues with or without a foreign body reaction

Differential diagnosis

- Osteoma cutis
- Myositis ossificans
- Pilomatrixoma

Treatment

- Excision of isolated lesions may be indicated
- Correcting a metabolic disorder usually does not resolve the calcinosis, but may stop progression

Prognosis

- Lesions rarely resolve spontaneously
- Superficial lesions may self-extrude through the skin

References

Ahn SK, Kim KT, Lee SH, et al. The efficacy of treatment with triamcinolone acetonide in calcinosis cutis following extravasation of calcium gluconate: a preliminary study. Pediatr Dermatol 1997; 14: 103–9

Evans MJ, Blessing K, Gray ES. Subepidermal calcified nodule in children: a clinicopathologic study of 21 cases. Pediatr Dermatol 1995; 12: 307–10

Kotsuji T, Imakado S, Iwasaki N, et al. Milia-like idiopathic calcinosis cutis in a patient with translocation Down syndrome. J Am Acad Dermatol 2001; 45: 152–3

Lai CH, Farah R, Mallory SB. Congenital calcinosis cutis of the ear. J Am Acad Dermatol 2003; 49: 122–4

Ostrov BE, Goldsmith DP, Eichenfield AH, Athreya BH. Hypercalcemia during the resolution of calcinosis universalis in juvenile dermatomyositis. J Rheumatol 1991; 18: 1730–4

Rodriguez-Cano L, Garcia-Patos V, Creus M, et al. Childhood calcinosis cutis. Pediatr Dermatol 1996; 13: 114–17

Touart DM, Sau P. Cutaneous deposition diseases. Part II. J Am Acad Dermatol 1998; 39: 527–44

Walsh JS, Fairley JA. Calcifying disorders of the skin. J Am Acad Dermatol 1995; 33: 693–706

Osteoma cutis

Major points

- Present as multiple or solitary, hard, raised 1–5-cm nodules with surrounding normal or erythematous skin
- Lesions commonly seen on the face
- Usually asymptomatic; may be painful or tender
- Superficial lesions may become inflamed and extrude bony particles
- Primary ossification:
  1. Albright hereditary osteodystrophy (AHO)
     a. Includes: pseudohypoparathyroidism and pseudopseudohypoparathyroidism
     b. Heterogeneous disorder with multiple areas of subcutaneous ossification which are present at birth or may occur later
     c. Lesions may occur anywhere and range in size from pinpoint to 5 cm
     d. Other associated abnormalities: short stature, round facies, multiple skeletal abnormalities (curvature of the radius and shortened metacarpals and metatarsals), short broad nails, basal ganglia calcification, hypothyroidism, mental retardatiion, defective teeth and cataracts
     e. Dimpling sign seen over knuckles caused by the shortened metacarpals
     f. Inherited disorder: autosomal dominant or X-linked dominant

g. Pseudohypoparathyroidism is characterized by a low serum calcium, hyperphosphatemia, and no response to parathyroid hormone (PTH), no renal diseases or other cause

h. Pseudopseudohypoparathyoidism has normal calcium and phosphorus levels and no response to PTH

i. Progression to pseudohypoparathyroidism with hypocalcemia and seizures may occur, and patients need to be monitored closely

2. Other forms of primary osteoma cutis:
   a. Widespread osteomas present since birth or early life without AHO
   b. Single, large, plaque-like osteomas present since birth on the scalp or extremities
   c. Single, small osteomas arising in later life with or without epidermal elimination
   d. Multiple miliary osteomas of the face: multiple 0.1–0.4-cm bluish white papules on the face. Most common in women with longstanding acne who have taken tetracycline or minocycline

- Secondary ossification (also called metaplastic osteoma cutis)
  1. Associated with neoplasms, cysts, inflammatory processes (e.g. dermatomyositis, scleroderma), scarring, metabolic conditions, trauma and pre-existing cutaneous mineralization

Pathogenesis

- AHO: gene locus: 20q13.2
  1. Gene: GNAS1; partial deficiency of the protein which couples hormone receptors to stimulate adenylate cyclase, which causes multiple hormone resistance
- Secondary forms: hypothesized to follow inflammatory process or other insult

Diagnosis

- Histology: proliferation of bony tissue with spicules of bone within the dermis and subcutaneous tissue, calcification, lamellae, lacunae, osteoblasts, osteocytes and rarely bone marrow formation

Differential diagnosis

- Calcinosis cutis
- Subungual exostosis of the finger or toe (Figure 17.28)

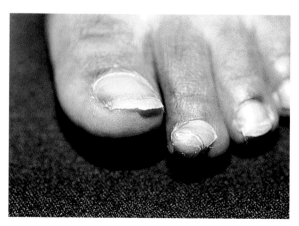

Figure 17.28   Exostosis – bony nodule on the tip of the toe requiring surgical excision

- Calcifying epithelioma
- Pilomatrixoma

Treatment

- Surgical excision of larger or painful lesions
- Isotretinoin may aggravate osteoma formation
- Close follow-up of patients with AHO is important, with routine checking of calcium, phosphorous and thyroid hormone

Prognosis

- Persists indefinitely, but occasionally extrudes spontaneously

References

Altman JF, Nehal KS, Busam KJ, Halpern AC. Treatment of primary miliary osteoma cutis with incision, curettage, and primary closure. J Am Acad Dermatol 2001; 44: 96–9

Bergonse FN, Nico MM, Kavamura MI, Sotto MN. Miliary osteoma of the face: a report of 4 cases and review of the literature. Cutis 2002; 69: 383–6

Chan I, Hamada T, Hardman C, et al. Progressive osseous heteroplasia resulting from a new mutation in the GNAS1 gene. Clin Exp Dermatol 2004; 29: 77–80

Izraeli S, Metzker A, Horev G, et al. Albright hereditary osteodystrophy with hypothyroidism, normocalcemia, and normal Gs protein activity: a family presenting with congenital osteoma cutis. Am J Med Genet 1992; 43: 764–7

Miller ES, Esterly NB, Fairley JA. Progressive osseous heteroplasia. Arch Dermatol 1996; 132: 787–91

Moritz DL, Elewski B. Pigmented postacne osteoma cutis in a patient treated with minocycline: report and review of the literature. J Am Acad Dermatol 1991; 24: 851–3

Prendiville JS, Lucky W, Mallory SB, et al. Osteoma cutis as a presenting sign of pseudohypoparathyroidism. Pediatr Dermatol 1992; 9: 11–18

GROWTHS

Steatocystoma multiplex

Major points

- Uncommon cause of cysts in childhood
- Appears as asymptomatic, multiple, firm, skin-colored or yellowish papules several millimeters to 1–3 cm in size (Figure 17.29)

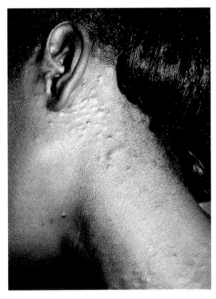

Figure 17.29 Steatocystoma multiplex – numerous yellowish papules on the neck

- When punctured, a characteristic oily or creamy fluid is discharged
- Common areas are axillae, chest and arms, but may appear anywhere
- Usually begins in adolescence or early adulthood
- Male/female ratio = 1
- Autosomal dominant or sporadic
- Can be associated with pachyonychia congenita type 2

Pathogenesis

- Etiology unknown

Diagnosis

- Histology: flattened sebaceous gland lobules and folded cyst walls within the cyst

Differential diagnosis

See Table 17.2

Treatment

- Because lesions are usually numerous, surgical excision is difficult
- Inflamed lesions can be excised or treated with incision and drainage

Prognosis

- Lesions persist indefinitely

References

Ahn SK, Swang SM, Lee SH, Lee WS. Steatocystoma multiplex localized only in the face. Int J Dermatol 1997; 36: 372

Cho S, Chang SE, Choi JH, et al. Clinical and histologic features of 64 cases of steatocystoma multiplex. J Dermatology 2002; 29: 152–6

Kaur T, Kanwar AJ. Steatocystoma multiplex in four successive generations. J Dermatol 2003; 30: 559–61

Kaya TI, Ikizoglu G, Kokturk A, Tursen U. A simple surgical technique for the treatment of steatocystoma multiplex. Int J Dermatol 2001; 40: 785–8

Ohtake N, Kubota Y, Takayama O, et al. Relationship between steatocystoma multiplex and eruptive vellus hair cysts. J Am Acad Dermatol 1992; 26: 876–8

Sato K, Shibuya K, Taguchi H, et al. Aspiration therapy in steatocystoma multiplex. Arch Dermatol 1993; 129: 35–7

Syringomas

Major points

- Appear at puberty as 1–2-mm skin-colored to yellowish papules (Figure 17.30)
- Location: most common around eyes, lids, upper cheeks, axillae and abdomen
- Female/male ratio >1
- May be autosomal dominant

Pathogenesis

- Thought to be a benign hyperplasia of the cells of the eccrine sweat ducts

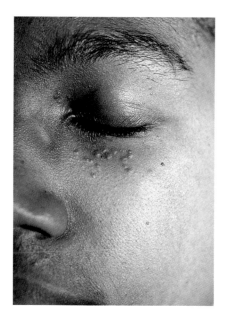

Figure 17.30 Syringomas – multiple, familial skin-colored papules around the eyes, a typical location

Diagnosis

- Histology: numerous small eccrine ducts in the dermis with surrounding fibrosis; some ducts bulge out to form small comma-like excrescences (tadpole appearance)

Differential diagnosis

See Table 17.2

Treatment

- Difficult to treat
- Electrocautery somewhat helpful

Prognosis

- Lesions persist and may become numerous

References

Goyal S, Martins CR. Multiple syringomas on the abdomen, thighs, and groin. Cutis 2000; 66: 259–62

Guitart J, Rosenbaum MM, Requena L. 'Eruptive syringoma': a misnomer for a reactive eccrine gland ductal proliferation? J Cutan Pathol 2003; 30: 202–5

Karma P, Benedetto AV. Intralesional electrodesiccation of syringomas. Dermatol Surg 1997; 23: 921–4

Nguyen DB, Patterson JW, Wilson BB. Syringoma of the moustache area. J Am Acad Dermatol 2003; 49: 337–9

Pruzan DL, Esterly NB, Prose NS. Eruptive syringoma. Arch Dermatol 1989; 125: 1119–20

Trichoepithelioma

Major points

- Presents in late childhood and adolescence
- Appears as solitary or numerous 2–8-mm skin-colored papules on the face, usually around the nose and mid-face (Figure 17.31)
- Fine telangiectasias on the surface
- May be seen on other parts of the body, especially the scalp, neck and upper trunk
- Multiple lesions are seen in Spiegler-Brooke syndrome (OMIM no. 605041), an autosomal dominant disorder; gene map locus 16q12-q13; gene CYLD
- Solitary lesions are not inherited

Pathogenesis

- Benign tumor with follicular germinative differentiation

Diagnosis

- Histology: multiple horn cysts and basophilic tumor islands in mid-dermis; can be difficult to distinguish from basal cell carcinoma

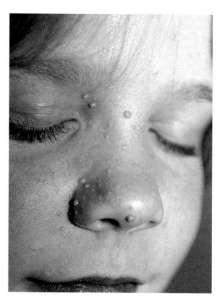

Figure 17.31 Trichoepithelioma – multiple, skin-colored, asymptomatic, slow-growing papules on the face

Differential diagnosis

- Basal cell carcinoma
- Pilomatricoma
- Nevocellular nevus
- Syringoma
- Acne vulgaris

Treatment

- Surgical excision; recurrence common unless completely removed

Prognosis

- Gradually increase in number and size, then stabilize
- Lesions do not resolve spontaneously

References

Centurion SA, Schwartz RA, Lambert WC. Trichoepithelioma papulosum multiplex. J Dermatol 2000; 27: 137–43

Johnson SC, Bennett RG. Occurrence of basal cell carcinoma among multiple trichoepitheliomas. J Am Acad Dermatol 1993; 28: 322–6

Matt D, Xin H, Vortmeyer AO, et al. Sporadic trichoepithelioma demonstrates deletions at 9q22.3. Arch Dermatol 2000; 136: 657–60

Puig L, Nadal C, Fernandez-Figueras MT, et al. Brooke-Spiegler syndrome variant: segregation of tumor types with mixed differentiation in two generations. Am J Dermatopathol 1998; 20: 56–60

Requena L, Farina MC, Robledo M, et al. Multiple hereditary infundibulocystic basal cell carcinomas: a genodermatosis different from nevoid basal cell carcinoma syndrome. Arch Dermatol 1999; 135: 1227–35

Shaffelburg M, Miller R. Treatment of multiple trichoepithelioma with electrosurgery. Dermatol Surg 1998; 24: 1154–6

TUMORS/MALIGNANCIES

Basal cell carcinoma

Major points

- Appear on the face or upper body as a skin-colored papule with telangiectasias on the surface
- Seen in light-skinned individuals (skin types 1–3) with increased sun exposure
- If left untreated, basal cell carcinoma is slow growing and may ulcerate
- Rare in childhood and should suggest a syndrome: basal cell nevus syndrome (see Chapter 20), xeroderma pigmentosum (see Chapter 12), or Bazex syndrome

Pathogenesis

- Malignant growth arising from basal cells in patient with chronic sun exposure and genetic susceptibility
- For basal cell nevus syndrome: gene locus/gene: 9q22/PTCH1 gene

Diagnosis

- Biopsy necessary
- Histology: solid masses of basal cells with a large nucleus and little cytoplasm

Differential diagnosis

- Pilomatricoma
- Nevocellular nevus
- Trichoepithelioma
- Syringoma
- Acne vulgaris
- Tuberous sclerosis (angiofibromas)

Treatment

- Excision
- Radiation should be avoided in childhood
- Prophylactic avoidance of sun, use of sunscreens

Prognosis

- Chronic slow progression of individual lesions
- Rarely metastasize, but may be disfiguring if orbit or nasal area invaded

References

Comstock J, Hansen RC, Korc A. Basal cell carcinoma in a 12-year-old boy. Pediatrics 1990; 86: 460–2

Drake LA, Ceilley RI, Comelison RL, et al. (Committee on Guidelines of Care) Guidelines of care for basal cell carcinoma. J Am Acad Dermaol 1992; 26: 117–20

Gaspari AA, Sauder DN. Immunotherapy of basal cell carcinoma: evolving approaches. Dermatol Surg 2003; 29: 1027–34

Ledwig PA, Paller AS. Congenital basal cell carcinoma. Arch Dermatol 1991; 127: 1066–7

Orozco-Covarrubias M, Tamayo-Sanchez L, Duran-McKinster C, et al. Malignant cutaneous tumors in children: twenty years of experience at a large pediatric hospital. J Am Acad Dermatol 1994; 30: 243–9

Strayer SM, Reynolds PL. Diagnosing skin malignancy: assessment of predictive clinical criteria and risk factors. J Fam Pract 2003; 52: 210–18

Tsao H. Update on familial cancer syndromes and the skin. J Am Acad Dermatol 2000; 42: 939–69

Wong CS, Strange RC, Lear JT. Basal cell carcinoma. Br Med J 2003; 327: 794–8

Leukemia cutis

Major points

- Primary (specific) lesions are caused by direct invasion of leukemic cells; appear as multiple, brown-red or violaceous papules and nodules (Figure 17.32)
- Acute lymphocytic leukemia (ALL) is the most common form of childhood leukemia
  1. Peak incidence is 4 years of age
  2. Petechiae are seen in 50% of cases at the time of presentation
- Acute nonlymphocytic leukemia has myelocytic or monocytic differentiation
  1. Leukemia cutis is more common in acute monoblastic leukemia and congenital leukemias (50%)
  2. Congenital leukemia often presents with 'blueberry muffin lesions' which show on histology dermal erythropoiesis

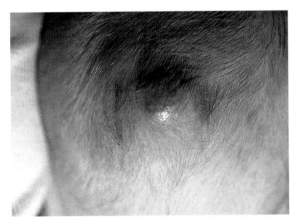

Figure 17.32 Leukemia cutis – large, firm, quickly growing nodule on the scalp of an infant who had acute lymphocytic leukemia

3. Other presentations:
   a. Gingival hypertrophy
   b. Soft tissue mass, most common in the deep soft tissues of the head and neck
4. More common in children with Fanconi anemia, Down syndrome, Bloom syndrome, ataxia telangiectasia, Wiscott–Aldrich syndrome and neurofibromatosis

- Chronic lymphocytic leukemia is rare in childhood
- Chronic nonlymphocytic leukemia
  1. Accounts for <5% of leukemias in childhood
  2. Adult form, seen in teenagers with Philadelphia chromosome
  3. Juvenile form is seen most commonly in neurofibromatosis
- Nonspecific or secondary lesions which may suggest the diagnosis:
  1. Erythematous plaques or nodules, purpura, petechiae, ecchymoses, erythema nodosum, pyoderma gangrenosum, diffuse erythroderma, Sweet syndrome

Pathogenesis

- Uncontrolled replication of immature bone marrow cells

Diagnosis

- Histology of a lesion of primary leukemia cutis reveals a diffuse infiltrate of leukemic cells around blood vessels and in between collagen bundles

Differential diagnosis

- Congenital lesions: congenital infections (cytomegalovirus toxoplasmosis, other viral infections)
- Tumors
- Granuloma annulare
- Cysts

Treatment

- Refer to pediatric oncologist
- Treatment of leukemia cures skin manifestations

Prognosis

- Prognosis depends upon type of leukemia

References

Baselga E, Drolet BA, Esterly NB. Purpura in infants and children. J Am Acad Dermatol 1997; 37: 673–705

Buescher L, Anderson PC. Circinate plaques heralding juvenile chronic myelogenous leukemia. Pediatr Dermatol 1990; 7: 122–5

Chang HY, Wong KM, Bosenberg M, et al. Myelogenous leukemia cutis resembling stasis dermatitis. J Am Acad Dermatol 2003; 49: 128–9

Grundy RG, Martinez A, Kempski H, et al. Spontaneous remission of congenital leukemia: a case for conservative treatment. J Pediatr Hematol Oncol 2000; 22: 252–5

Maher-Wiese VL, Wenner NP, Grant-Kels JM. Metastatic cutaneous lesions in children and adolescents with a case report of metastatic neuroblastoma. J Am Acad Dermatol 1992; 26: 620–8

Millot F, Robert A, Bertrand Y, et al. Cutaneous involvement in children with acute lymphoblastic leukemia or lymphoblastic lymphoma. Pediatrics 1997; 100: 60–4

Pui C-H. Childhood leukemias. N Engl J Med 1995; 332: 1618–30

Lymphoma

Major points

- Lymphomas are the third most common malignancy in childhood, after leukemia and CNS tumors
- Presents as an infiltrative plaque, nodule or asymptomatic scaly dermatitis
- Most common in adults, but can be seen in children
- Cutaneous T-cell lymphoma (CTCL) (See Chapter 3)
  1. Presents with a scaly eczematous dermatitis (patch or plaque stage), poikiloderma vasculare atrophicans, or tumor nodules
  2. Indolent T-helper cell lymphoma which affects the skin primarily with late spread to lymph nodes, bone marrow and viscera
  3. Sézary syndrome manifests as a diffuse erythroderma with circulating abnormal T cells
- Hodgkin lymphoma:
  1. Occurs in adolescence; rarely before age 5 years
  2. Usual presentation is painless lymphadenopathy in the neck
  3. Male/female ratio >1
  4. Skin manifestations rare (e.g. papules, tumors, ulcerated nodules), but seen in advanced disease which has failed aggressive chemotherapy and radiation

5. Secondary signs: pruritus, acquired ichthyosis and herpes zoster
- B-cell lymphomas:
  1. Painless enlarging lymphadenoathy most common
  2. Rapidly growing and poorly differentiated
  3. Cutaneous lesions: papules or nodules which may ulcerate and form arcuate lesions
  4. Common location: scalp

Pathogenesis

- Anaplasia of B or T cells

Diagnosis

- Biopsy of tissue confirms and differentiates the diagnosis

Differential diagnosis

- Pseudolymphoma
- Persistent insect bite reaction
- Granuloma annulare
- Lymphomatoid papulosis
- Follicular mucinosis

Treatment

- Depends upon type of lymphoma
- CTCL is treated with psoralen plus ultraviolet light A (PUVA) or topical nitrogen mustard or, for a single plaque, ultrapotent steroids

Prognosis

- Depends upon the type of lymphoma
- CTCL has a good prognosis, but requires life-long observation and therapy

References

Burg G, Kempf W, Haeffner AC, et al. Cutaneous lymphomas. Curr Prob Dermatol 1997; 9: 137–204

Jones D, Duvic M. The current state and future of clonality studies in mycosis fungoides. J Invest Dermatol 2003; 121: ix–x

Maher-Wiese VL, Wenner NP, Grant-Kels JM. Metastatic cutaneous lesions in children and adolescents with a case report of metastatic neuroblastoma. J Am Acad Dermatol 1992; 26: 620–8

Orozco-Covarrubias ML, Tamayo-Sanchez L, Duran-McKinster C, et al. Malignant cutaneous tumors in children. J Am Acad Dermatol 1994; 30: 243–9

Querfeld C, Rosen ST, Kuzel TM, Guitart J. Cutaneous T-cell lymphomas: a review with emphasis on new treatment approaches. Semin Cutan Med Surg 2003; 22: 150–61

Sandlund JT, Downing JR, Crist WM. Non-Hodgkin's lymphoma in childhood. N Engl J Med 1996; 334: 1238–48

Shani-Adir A, Lucky AW, Prendiville J, et al. Subcutaneous panniculitic T-cell lymphoma in children: response to combination therapy with cyclosporine and chemotherapy. J Am Acad Dermatol 2004; 50 (2 Suppl): S18–22

Thorley-Lawson DA, Gross A. Persistence of the Epstein–Barr virus and the origins of associated lymphomas. N Engl J Med 2004; 350: 1328–37

Zackheim HS, Vonderheid EC, Ramsay DL, et al. Relative frequency of various forms of primary cutaneous lymphomas. J Am Acad Dermatol 2000; 43: 793–6

Histiocytosis

Major points

- Histiocytoses includes a group of benign and fatal disorders which may be manifested in a variety of ways
- Langerhans cell histiocytosis (LCH) was traditionally separated into the following groups, but these are now included under the heading of LCH:
  1. Eosinophilic granuloma (localized bony lesions)
  2. Hand–Schuller–Christian disease (multiple organ involvement with skull defects, diabetes insipidus and exophthalmos)
  3. Letterer–Siwe disease (visceral lesions in lungs, lymph nodes, liver, spleen, bone marrow and skin)
- Letterer–Siwe disease is most common
  1. Peak incidence occurs between 1 and 4 years, but can occur at any age
  2. Discrete yellow-brown scaly papules which coalesce in the seborrheic areas (e.g. diaper area, postauricular area, scalp, etc.) and may show petechiae (Figure 17.33)
  3. Other involvement
     a. Bone lesions: lytic lesions (typical in skull), proptosis, mastoid involvement and others
     b. Lymph nodes
     c. Bone marrow (pancytopenia)
     d. Liver enlargement

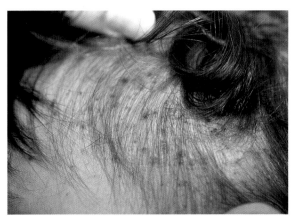

Figure 17.33   Langerhans cell histiocytosis – keratotic hemorrhagic papules resembling seborrheic dermatitis

     e. Spleen enlargement
     f. Lungs
     g. GI tract
     h. Thymic enlargement
     i. Endocrine glands (diabetes insipidus, anterior pituitary involvement with growth hormone deficiency)
     j. CNS involvement rare (intracranial hypertension, seizures)
- Other forms of histiocytosis:
  1. Self-healing reticulohistiocytosis presents with papules and nodules that frequently ulcerate at birth (Figure 17.34)
  2. Benign cephalic histiocytosis: 2–5-mm yellow-red papules on the face and neck in a child <1 year of age (non-Langerhans cell histiocytosis)

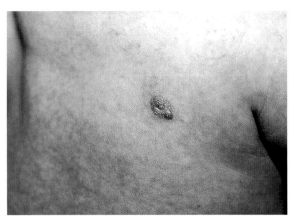

Figure 17.34   Self-healing histiocytosis – isolated congenital papule

Pathogenesis

- Clonal neoplastic disorder of Langerhans cells (monocyte/macrophage which contains Birbeck granules; expresses CD1 glycoprotein)

Diagnosis

- Biopsy necessary for confirmation of diagnosis
- Histology: histiocytes with clear or eosinophilic cytoplasm and indented nuclei, macrophages, lymphocytes and other cells; stains positive for CD1a and S100 protein
- Electron microscopy demonstrates Birbeck granules in LCH

Differential diagnosis

- Seborrhea
- Eczema
- Scabies
- Irritant diaper dermatitis
- Mastocytosis
- Juvenile xanthogranuloma

Treatment

- Refer to pediatric hematologist/oncologist
- Therapy depends upon the extent of involvement of disease and location of infiltrates
- In milder cases, observation may be indicated
- For extensive disease, chemotherapy (e.g. corticosteroids, vinblastine or etoposide)
- Skin lesions may respond to topical steroids, topical nitrogen mustard or PUVA

Prognosis

- Depends upon age of patient at diagnosis (younger patients have poorer prognosis), extent of disease and rate of disease progression

References

Bhatia S, Nesbit ME, Egeler RM, et al. Epidemiologic study of Langerhans cell histiocytosis in children. J Pediatr 1997; 130: 774–84

Egeler RM, D'Angio GJ. Langerhans cell histiocytosis. J Pediatr 1995; 127: 1–11

Kilborn TN, Teh J, Goodman TR. Paediatric manifestations of Langerhans cell histiocytosis: a review of the clinical and radiological findings. Clin Radiol 2003; 58: 269–78

Seward JL, Malone JC, Callen JP. Generalized eruptive histiocytosis. J Am Acad Dermatol 2004; 50: 116–20

Shani-Adir A, Chou P, Morgan E, Mancini AJ. A child with both Langerhans and non-Langerhans cell histiocytosis. Pediatr Dermatol 2002; 19: 419–22

Snow JL, Su WPD. Histiocytic disease. J Am Acad Dermatol 1995; 33: 111–16

Willman CL, Busque L, Griffith BB, et al. Langerhans'-cell histiocytosis (histiocytosis X) – a clonal proliferative disease. N Engl J Med 1994; 331: 154–60

Rhabdomyosarcoma

Major points

- Most common malignant soft-tissue tumor in childhood
- Causes 5% of childhood solid malignancies
- Peak ages: 1–5 years and adolescence
- Predilection for the head and neck region, genitourinary tract, the retroperitoneum and soft tissues of the extremities
- Local signs of destruction may occur with progression of the lesion
- May spread by local extension or lymphatic/hematogenous metastases
- Sporadic inheritance

Pathogenesis

- Malignant tumor of striated muscles

Diagnosis

- Histology: composed of small round cells, spindle or polygonal cells or large pleomorphic cells; variants: embryonal (including botryoid variant), alveolar, pleomorphic
- Immunoperoxidase stains positive for vimentin, desmin, myoglobin and muscle actin

Differential diagnosis

- Epidermal cyst
- Lymphangioma
- Leukemia cutis
- Other tumors
- Infectious (fasciitis)

Treatment

- Refer to hematologist/oncologist
- Radiation and combination chemotherapy followed by surgical excision

Prognosis

- Determined by extent and location of disease

References

Brecher AR, Reyes-Mugica M, Kamino H, Chang MW. Congenital primary cutaneous rhabdomyosarcoma in a neonate. Pediatr Dermatol 2003; 20: 335–8

Pisick E, Skarin AT, Salgia R. Recent advances in the molecular biology, diagnosis and novel therapies for various small blue cell tumors. Anticancer Res 2003; 23: 3379–96

Herzog CE, Stewart JM, Blakely ML. Pediatric soft tissue sarcomas. Surg Oncol Clin North Am 2003; 12: 419–47

Sebire NJ, Malone M. Myogenin and MyoD1 expression in paediatric rhabdomyosarcomas. J Clin Pathol 2003; 56: 412–16

Neuroblastoma

Major points

- Second most common solid tumor malignancy in childhood
- Usually presents before age 5 years with an enlarging mass in the upper abdomen or retroperitoneal space
- Cutaneous lesions are uncommon outside the neonatal period
- Metastatic disease occurs early and frequently
- Cutaneous metastases appear as multiple 2 mm to 2 cm bluish papules or nodules scattered over the body ('blueberry muffin' appearance) which tend to blanch centrally and develop an erythematous halo 2–3 minutes after stroking, which lasts about 1 hour, resulting from local tumor catecholamine release causing vasoconstriction
- Metastatic cutaneous lesions common on the trunk and extremities, but can be anywhere on the body
- Bilateral periorbital ecchymoses, described as 'raccoon eyes' (from orbital metastases)
- Heterochromia irides
- Nonspecific signs and symptoms include: fever, weight loss, flushing, sweating, joint pains and others
- Occurrence is usually sporadic but may be autosomal dominant
- Male/female ratio = 1

Pathogenesis

- Tumor of primitive neural crest cells of the sympathetic nervous system in the adrenal medulla, sympathetic side chain, visceral ganglia, paraganglia, bladder, or genitalia. Tumors can be seen anywhere these cells migrate

Diagnosis

- Histology: dermal or subcutaneous infiltrate of small blue cells with large nuclei, mitoses, hemorrhage
- Staging important to determine treatment and prognosis
- Laboratory findings: elevated levels of urinary catecholamines or their metabolites (vanillylmandelic acid and homovanillic acid)

Differential diagnosis

- Leukemia cutis
- Sarcomas
- Lymphoma
- Child abuse ('raccoon eyes')
- Congenital infections (TORCH and other 'blueberry-muffin' syndromes)
- Vascular tumors
- Histiocytosis

Treatment

- Refer to pediatric oncologist and pediatric surgeon

Prognosis

- Staging, classification and prognosis determined by tumor burden, nodal involvement and distant metastases
  1. Stages I and II have 60–80% 2-year survival rate
  2. Stages III and IV have 7–13% 2-year survival rate
  3. Stage IV-S has 60–90% survival rate

References

Dominey AM, Hawkins H, Levy ML. Congenital cutaneous and subcutaneous nodules. Pediatr Dermatol 1992; 9: 301–3

Lee KL, Ma JF, Shortliffe LD. Neuroblastoma: management, recurrence, and follow-up. Urol Clin North Am 2003; 30: 881–90

Maher-Wiese VL, Wenner NP, Grant-Kels JM. Metastatic cutaneous lesions in children and adolescents with a case report of metastatic neuroblastoma. J Am Acad Dermatol 1992; 26: 620–8

Matthay KK. Neuroblastoma: a clinical challenge and biologic puzzle. Cancer J Clin 1995; 45: 179–92

Moore SW, Satge D, Sasco AJ, et al. The epidemiology of neonatal tumours. Report of an international working group. Pediatr Surg Int 2003; 19: 509–19

Weinstein JL, Katzenstein HM, Cohn SL. Advances in the diagnosis and treatment of neuroblastoma. Oncologist 2003; 8: 278–92

18

HAIR DISORDERS

Major points

- Alopecia: general term for sparseness of hair
- Loss of 25–50% of scalp hair is necessary for diffuse loss to be clinically noticeable in most people
- Scalp has ~100 000–150 000 hairs
- Anagen and telogen hairs randomly distributed
- Growth rate 0.3–0.4 mm/day (1 cm/month)
  a. Depends upon site (vertex faster than temples)
- Normal hair growth is cyclical
  1. Anagen phase
     a. Active growth phase
     b. Lasts ~2–6 years
     c. 80–90% of scalp hairs
     d. Shiny, white sheath near proximal end
     e. Pigmented bulb
  2. Catagen phase
     a. Transitional phase
     b. 5% of scalp hairs
     c. Lasts few days to 2 weeks
  3. Telogen phase
     a. Resting phase
     b. Lasts ~100 days (2–4 months)
     c. 10–15% of scalp hairs
     d. Club-shaped root
     e. Depigmented terminal bulbs

Diagnosis

- Classification of non-scarring alopecia (See Table 18.1)
- Evaluation of hair loss in childhood (See Table 18.2)

References

Ahmad W, Panteleyev A, Christiano AM. Molecular basis of congenital atrichia in humans and mice. Cutis 1999; 64: 269–76

Messenger AG. The control of hair growth: an overview. J Invest Dermatol 1993; 101: 4S–9S

Miller J, Djabali K, Chen T, et al. Atrichia caused by mutations in the vitamin D receptor gene is a phenocopy of generalized atrichia caused by mutations in the hairless gene. J Invest Dermatol 2001; 117: 612–17

Milner Y, Sudnik J, Filippi M, et al. Exogen, shedding phase of the hair growth cycle: characterization of a mouse model. J Invest Dermatol 2002; 119: 639–44

Paus R, Christoph T, Muller-Rover S. Immunology of the hair follicle: a short journey into terra incognita. Invest Dermatol Symp Proc 1999; 4: 226–34

Paus R, Cotsarlelis G. The biology of hair follicles. N Engl J Med 1999; 341: 491–7

Shapiro J, Price VH. Hair regrowth. Therapeutic agents. Dermatol Clin 1998; 16: 341–56

Sperling LC. Evaluation of hair loss. Curr Prob Dermatol 1996; 8: 97–136

Table 18.1   Types of non-scarring hair loss
Telogen effluvium
Anagen effluvium
Alopecia areata
Androgenetic alopecia
Hair shaft abnormalities
Trauma
Infectious disorders (e.g. dermatophytes, syphilis)
Systemic disease (e.g. thyroid disease, systemic lupus erythematosus, iron deficiency anemia)
Intoxications (e.g. vitamin A, bismuth)
Nutritional deficiencies (e.g. zinc, biotin)
Medications

Tobin DJ, Slominski A, Botchkarev V, Paus R. The fate of hair follicle melanocytes during the hair growth cycle. Invest Dermatol Symp Proc 1999; 4: 323–32

Table 18.2   Evaluation of hair loss in childhood

History

Duration of loss
Rate of shedding
Breakage versus falling out from roots
Drug intake
Hair care
Trauma
General health, developmental history
Family history of hair disorders
Symptoms (pruritus, etc.)
Pregnancy

Physical examination

Scalp examination: scarring versus nonscarring
Hair texture, length, color
Pattern and distribution of loss; diffuse versus
  patchy
Tips tapered versus broken ends
General hair distribution
Teeth, nails, sweating abnormalities
Mentation
Other anomalies

Useful procedures

Hair pull: 30–50 hairs grasped between thumb and
  forefinger with firm, steady traction applied along
  the lengths of the hairs; 2–5 telogen hairs –
  normal; >6 hairs extracted considered abnormal
Hair pluck: forcefully extracting ~50 hairs from the
  scalp by clamping hairs about 1 cm from skin
  surface with a rubber coated hemostat and pulling
Microscopic examination: anagen versus telogen
  hairs
KOH preparation
Fungal, bacterial cultures
Scalp biopsy
Laboratory evaluation: complete blood count,
  thyroxine, thyroid stimulating hormone, rapid
  plasma reagin, serum iron,
dehydroepiandrosterone sulfate, free testosterone

CONGENITAL ALOPECIA: LOCALIZED

Occipital alopecia

Major points

- Normal process
- Common disorder in first year
- Well-defined patch of alopecia with broken hairs over occiput (Figure 18.1)

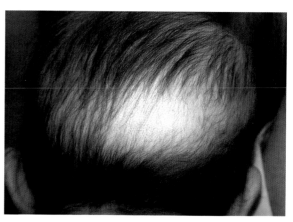

Figure 18.1   Occipital alopecia – this common patchy hair loss occurs in infants in the first year of life

Pathogenesis

- Lanugo hairs on posterior scalp shed at ~8–12 weeks of age, then replaced with normal anagen hairs

Diagnosis

- Clinical diagnosis

Differential diagnosis

- Alopecia areata
- Hair shaft disorders

Treatment

- None needed

Prognosis

- Excellent

References

Olsen EA. Hair loss in childhood. In Disorders of Hair Growth. Olsen EA, ed. McGraw-Hill: New York, 1994: 139–88

Patchy alopecia

Major points

- Aplasia cutis congenita: irregularly shaped erosion which leads to scarring or oval patch covered by membrane (see Chapter 2)
- Melanocytic nevus: associated with hyper- or hypotrichosis
- Hemangioma of infancy: after resolution, may have localized alopecia
- Nevus sebaceus: linear or oval patch of alopecia with yellowish papules (see Chapter 17)
- Epidermal or organoid nevi: linear, grouped, verrucous papules
- Temporal triangular alopecia (Figure 18.2)
    1. Well-circumscribed triangular or lance-shaped area of alopecia at the temple
    2. Appears at 2–5 years of age; unilateral (80%) or bilateral
    3. Vellus hairs present; occasionally a few terminal hairs
    4. Erroneously thought to be from forceps delivery
- Cranial meningoceles, encephaloceles, heterotopic brain tissue: can be surrounded by collar of thick hair (called 'hair collar sign')
- Birth trauma (forceps) from pressure on hair follicles
- Rare syndromes with patchy hair loss
    1. Conradi–Hünermann syndrome
    2. Goltz syndrome

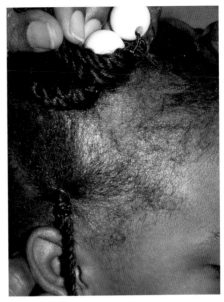

Figure 18.3   This type of hair loss resembles triangular alopecia but is caused by styling practices where the hair is pulled tightly into braids

    3. Hallerman–streiff syndrome
    4. CHILD syndrome
- Causes of scarring alopecia (Table 18.4)

References

Armstrong DKB, Burrows D. Congenital triangular alopecia. Pediatr Dermatol 1996; 13: 394–6

Elmer KB, George RM. Congenital triangular alopecia: a case report and review. Cutis 2002; 69: 255–6

Garcia-Hernandez MJ, Rodriguez-Pichardo A, Camacho F. Congenital triangular alopecia (Brauer nevus). Pediatr Dermatol 1995; 12: 301–3

Trakimas C, Sperling LC, Skelton HG, et al. Clinical and histologic findings in temporal triangular alopecia. J Am Acad Dermatol 1994; 31: 205–9

CONGENITAL ALOPECIA: DIFFUSE

Early-onset diffuse alopecia

Major points

- Causes:
    1. Metabolic disorders/nutritional deficiencies
        a. Acrodermatitis enteropathica (zinc deficiency)

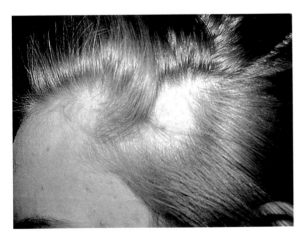

Figure 18.2   Triangular alopecia – congenital and familial patch of alopecia usually over one or both temples

b. Biotin deficiency
c. Essential fatty acid deficiency
d. Amino acid disorders
2. Congenital alopecia universalis
3. Loose anagen syndrome
4. Hair shaft defects
5. Genetic syndromes
a. KID syndrome
b. Trichorhinophalangeal syndrome

References

Ahmad W, Panteleyev AA, Christiano AM. The molecular basis of congenital atrichia in humans and mice: mutations in the hairless gene. Invest Dermatol Symp Proc 1999; 4: 240–3

Cambiaghi S, Barbareschi M. A sporadic case of congenital hypotrichosis simplex of the scalp: difficulties in diagnosis and classification. Pediatr Dermatol 1999; 16: 301–4

Carrington PR, Chen H, Altick JA. Trichorhinophalangeal syndrome, type I. J Am Acad Dermatol 1994; 31: 331–6

Ludecke H-J, Wagner MJ, Nardmann J, et al. Molecular dissection of a contiguous gene syndrome: localization of the genes involved in the Langer–Giedion syndrome. Hum Mol Genet 1995; 4: 31–6

Nardmann J, Tranebjaerg L, Horsthembke B, Ludecke H-J. The tricho-rhino-phalangeal syndromes: frequency and parental origin of 8q deletions. Hum Genet 1997; 99: 638–43

Roberts JL, Whiting DA, Henry D, et al. Marie Unna congenital hypotrichosis: clinical description, histopathology, scanning electron microscopy of a previously unreported large pedigree. Invest Dermatol Symp Proc 1999; 4: 261–7

Zlotogorski A, Hochberg Z, Mirmirani P, et al. Clinical and pathologic correlations in genetically distinct forms of atrichia. Arch Dermatol 2003; 139: 1591–6

Ectodermal dysplasia (hypohidrotic/anhidrotic)

Synonym: anhidrotic ectodermal dysplasia, Christ–Siemens–Touraine syndrome

Major points

- Presents at birth
- Hair-fine, sparse, light and twisted terminal hairs and eyebrows; may thicken at puberty (Figure 18.4)
- Sweat glands – partial or complete absence with heat intolerance; sweat pores absent on visual inspection of fingertips

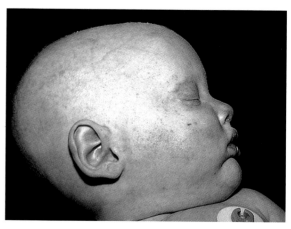

Figure 18.4 Hypohidrotic ectodermal dysplasia – newborn with absence of hair

- Teeth – hypodontia, anodontia, and conical incisors
- Nails – normal or brittle, thin, ridged
- Characteristc facies
  1. Thick, everted lips
  2. Frontal bossing
  3. Large, pointed ears
  4. Saddle nose
  5. Maxillary hypoplasia
- Other findings
  1. Frequent bronchitis and pneumonia
  2. Recurrent otitis media, impacted cerumen
  3. Hoarse voice
  4. Failure to thrive (20%)
  5. Unexplained fever in infancy and childhood
  6. Poorly developed mucous glands in respiratory and gastrointestinal tract
  7. Periorbital hyperpigmentation
  8. Skin – soft, dry, finely wrinkled
  9. X-linked recessive
  10. Increased frequency of atopic dermatitis

Pathogenesis

- Gene locus: Xq12-q13.1
- Gene: ectodysplasin-A (ED1)

Diagnosis

- Clinical presentation

Differential diagnosis

- Other (Figure 18.5)

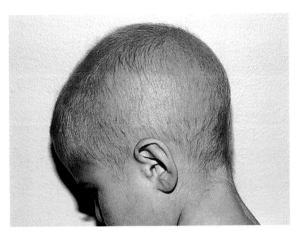

Figure 18.5 Isolated scalp hypotrichosis – with no other ectodermal defects

Treatment

- Environmental control for temperature stability: air conditioning or specialized cooling units
- Dental consultation for abnormal teeth, with dentures and dental implants
- Hair appliances (wigs) if necessary
- Treatment of infections as needed
- National Foundation for Ectodermal Dysplasias (www.nfed.org)

Prognosis

- Good with close supervision
- Increased mortality in infancy

References

Aswegan AL, Josephson KD, Mowbray R, et al. Autosomal dominant hypohidrotic ectodermal dysplasia in a large family. Am J Med Genet 1997; 72: 462–7

Azon-Masoliver A, Ferrando J. Loose anagen hair in hypohidrotic ectodermal dysplasia. Pediatr Dermatol 1996; 13: 29–32

Cambiaghi S, Restano L, Paakkonen K, et al. Clinical findings in mosaic carriers of hypohidrotic ectodermal dysplasia. Arch Dermatol 2000; 136: 217–24

Dahan D, Fenichel GM, El-Said R. Neurocutaneous syndromes. Adolesc Med State Art Rev 2002; 13: 495–509

Hummel P, Guddack S. Psychosocial stress and adaptive functioning in children and adolescents suffering from hypohidrotic ectodermal dysplasia. Pediatr Dermatol 1997; 14: 180–5

Lamartine J. Towards a new classification of ectodermal dysplasias. Clin Exp Dermatol 2003; 28: 351–5

Wisniewski SA, Kobielak A, Trzeciak WH, Kobielak K. Recent advances in understanding of the molecular basis of anhidrotic ectodermal dysplasia: discovery of a ligand, ectodysplasin A and its two receptors. J Appl Genet 2002; 43: 97–107

Ectodermal dysplasia (hidrotic)

Synonym: Clouston syndrome

Major points

- Generalized hypotrichosis (sparse, fine, blond, wiry, brittle hair); hair loss may be progressive
- Nail dystrophy: nails may be white in early childhood; thickened nails; slow growth; paronychial infections (Figure 18.6)
- Hyperkeratosis of the palms and soles with pebbling on the fingertips, which increases with age
- Teeth – normal
- Mild mental retardation or normal mentation
- Sweating normal
- Conjunctivitis
- Blepharitis possible secondary to absence of protection from eyelashes
- More common in French Canadian families
- Autosomal dominant

Pathogenesis

- Gene locus: 13q12
- Gene: GJB6 (gap junction protein) which encodes CX30 (connexin-30)

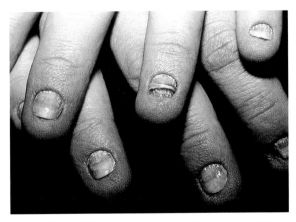

Figure 18.6 Hidrotic ectodermal dysplasia – small nails with pebbling of fingertips in a patient with hypotrichosis

Diagnosis

- Clinical presentation
- Histology: orthohyperkeratosis of palms and soles with normal granular layer
- Abnormal hair with nonspecific narrowing and fraying

Differential diagnosis

- Other ectodermal dysplasias
- Ankyloblepharon ectodermal dysplasia clefting (AEC) syndrome
- Pachyonychia congenita

Treatment

- Hair appliance (wig) if necessary

Prognosis

- Hair and nail abnormalities permanent

References

Chitty LS, Dennis N, Baraitser M. Hidrotic ectodermal dysplasia of hair, teeth, and nails: case reports and review. J Med Genet 1996; 33: 707–10

Hayflick SJ, Taylor T, McKinnon W, et al. Clouston syndrome (hidrotic ectodermal dysplasia) is not linked to keratin gene clusters on chromosomes 12 and 17. J Invest Dermatol 1996; 107: 11–14

Lamartine J, Essenfelder GM, Kibar Z, et al. Mutations in GJB6 cause hidrotic ectodermal dysplasia. Nature Genet 2000; 26: 142–4

Priolo M, Silengo M, Lerone M, Ravazzolo R. Ectodermal dysplasias: not only 'skin' deep. Clin Genet 2000; 58: 415–30

ACQUIRED NON-SCARRING ALOPECIA

Alopecia areata

Major points

- Common disorder
- Incidence: 17 per 100 000 population per year
- 24–50% begins at age <16 years
- Male/female ratio = 1
- Family history found in ~10–20%
- Sudden onset of asymptomatic well-defined oval or round patches of hair loss (Figures 18.7 and 18.8)
- Location

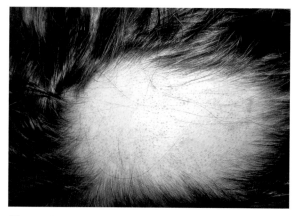

Figure 18.7 Alopecia areata – sudden loss of hair with exclamation point hairs appearing as broken-off hairs along the periphery

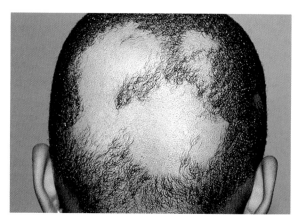

Figure 18.8 Alopecia areata – patchy, smooth hair loss of sudden onset

1. Alopecia areata – patchy hair loss
2. Alopecia totalis – loss of entire scalp hair with retention of other hair
3. Alopecia universalis – loss of all body hair
4. Can occur in any hair-bearing area: scalp, eyebrows, eyelashes, beard, body hair
5. Ophiasis region – along the nape of the neck
- Characteristic exclamation point hairs: hairs that taper as they approach the scalp
- Regrowth hair often depigmented initially
- Nail changes in 10–44%
  1. Fine grid-like pitting, regularly arranged in horizontal or vertical rows
  2. Trachyonychia (rough sandpaper nails)
- Associated with: thyroid disease, vitiligo and other autoimmune disorders

- Increased incidence in Down syndrome
- Atopy seen in 10–22% of cases

Pathogenesis

- Etiology unknown, generally thought to be an autoimmune disorder
- Histology
  1. Perifollicular lymphocytic infiltrate surrounding hair bulbs resembling a 'swarm of bees'
  2. Infiltrate: activated T lymphocytes with macrophages and Langerhans cells
  3. Reduction in anagen : telogen ratio
  4. Miniaturized dystrophic hairs

Diagnosis

- Clinical appearance
- Hair pull test positive in active areas, especially at periphery of patch with increased number of telogen hairs and dystrophic anagen hairs

Differential diagnosis

- Telogen effluvium
- Trichotillomania
- Androgenetic alopecia
- Syphilis (secondary)
- Tinea capitis

Treatment

- Treatments only control the problem
- Treatments should be used for a long time (minimum 3–6 months) because of the chronic nature of the disease
- Patient education and psychological support
- Corticosteroids
  1. Topical: mid- to ultrapotent steroids BID
  2. Intralesional: triamcinolone acetonide 2.5–5 mg/ml administered with 30-gauge needle with multiple intradermal injections of 0.1 ml per site, approximately 1 cm apart; maximum total 3 ml on scalp per visit; repeat every 4–6 weeks until improvement seen
  3. Systemic steroids: recommended for extensive cases with sudden onset; high relapse rate
     a. Prednisone 20–40 mg/day with tapering by 5 mg /week for 4–6 weeks followed by alternate day therapy, and slow tapering with eventual discontinuation

- Topical irritants
  1. Anthralin 0.25–1% cream, applied overnight or as short contact therapy, initially for 30 minutes and gradually increasing to 1 hour. Mild dermatitis is desired for a therapeutic effect
- Topical sensitizers
  1. Squaric acid dibutyl ester (SADBE) or diphenylcyclopropenone (DPCP): sensitization of the skin with resultant contact allergic reaction, followed by repeated treatments of the low-dose agent to maintain a low-grade allergic reaction. Response should be seen after 12 weeks
- Topical minoxidil 2–5% applied BID
- PUVA: psoralen taken orally or applied topically followed by UVA irradiation; administered 2–3 times per week; not recommended for children aged <10 years
- Wig (prosthesis)
- Support group: National Alopecia Areata Foundation

Web site: www.alopeciaareata.com

Prognosis

- Variable and unpredictable
- Course recurrent in ~50%
- Natural history: spontaneous remissions and recurrences
- Limited involvement: prognosis good with growth in 1 year seen in 95%
- 7–10% develop severe chronic form
- Prognosis worse if there is:
  1. Early onset
  2. Ophiasis pattern
  3. Atopy
  4. Nail dystrophy
  5. Long duration
  6. Presence of other autoimmune diseases
  7. Family history
  8. Extensive hair loss

References

Bodemer C, Peuchmaur M, Fraitaig S, et al. Role of cytotoxic T cells in chronic alopecia areata. J Invest Dermatol 2000; 114: 112–16

Cotelless C, Peris K, Caracciolo E, et al. The use of topical diphenylcyclopropenone for the treatment of extensive alopecia areata. J Am Acad Dermatol 2001; 44: 73–6

Freyschmidt-Paul P, Happle R, McElwee KJ, Hoffmann R. Alopecia areata: treatment of today and tomorrow. J Invest Dermatol Symp Proc 2003; 8: 12–17

Hoffmann R. The potential role of cytokines and T cells in alopecia areata. Invest Dermatol Symp Proc 1999; 4: 235–8

Madani S, Shapiro J. Alopecia areata update. J Am Acad Dermatol 2000; 42: 549–66

McElwee KJ, Freyschmidt-Paul P, Sundberg JP, Hoffmann R. The pathogenesis of alopecia areata in rodent models. J Invest Dermatol Symp Proc 2003; 8: 6–11

Olsen E, Hordinshky M, McDonald-Hull S, et al. Alopecia areata investigations assessment guidelines. J Am Acad Dermatol 1999; 40: 242–6

Sehgal VN, Jain S. Alopecia areata: clinical perspective and an insight into pathogenesis. J Dermatol 2003; 30: 271–89

Tosti A, Guidetti MS, Bardazzi R, Misciali C. Long-term results of topical immunotherapy in children with alopecia totalis or alopecia universalis. J Am Acad Dermatol 1996; 35: 199–201

Whiting DA. Histopathologic features of alopecia areata. Arch Dermatol 2003; 139: 1555–9

Telogen effluvium

Major points

- Common type of hair loss
- Sparse diffuse loss of scalp hair (Figure 18.9)
- Hallmark: excessive shedding of telogen hairs caused by altered growth cycle
- Occurs 6 weeks to 4 months after inciting event
- Lasts 6–24 weeks
- Regrowth within 6 months

Pathogenesis

- Abnormally large shift from anagen to telogen hairs within a short period of time
- Instead of 10% hairs in telogen (normal), there are 30–50% in telogen
- Etiologies:
  1. Drugs: anticonvulsants, anticoagulants, angiotensin-converting enzyme (ACE) inhibitors, β-blockers, interferons, lithium, oral contraceptive pills (during or after discontinuation), retinoids, excessive vitamin A
  2. Febrile or systemic illness
  3. Crash diets
  4. Postpartum
  5. Major surgical procedures, anesthesia

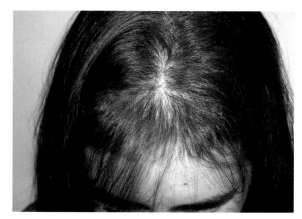

Figure 18.9 Telogen effluvium – caused by severe, febrile illness with obvious regrowth of anagen hairs at the periphery of the scalp

6. Endocrine disorders: hypo- orhyperthyroidism
7. Severe emotional stress
8. Deficiencies: iron, zinc, biotin
9. Physiologic effluvium of the newborn

Diagnosis

- History very helpful
- Hair pull or pluck: increased telogen hairs up to 50% of hairs
- If precipitating factor not found, consider doing: complete blood count (CBC), chemistry profile, serum iron, thyroid studies

Differential diagnosis

- Kwashiorkor
- Acrodermatitis enteropathica
- Celiac disease

Treatment

- Patient education as to cause and prognosis, with reassurance
- Gentle hair care: avoid manipulation, vigorous shampooing, combing, brushing

Prognosis

- Complete regrowth within 6 months if precipitating factor eliminated

References

Ben-Amitai D, Garty BZ. Alopecia in children after cardiac surgery. Pediatr Dermatol 1993; 10: 32–33

Chartier MB, Hoss DM, Grant-Kels JM. Approach to the adult female patient with diffuse nonscarring alopecia. J Am Acad Dermatol 2002; 47: 809–18

Harrison S, Sinclair R. Telogen effluvium. Clin Exp Dermatol 2002; 27: 389–5

Headington JT. Telogen effluvium. Arch Dermatol 1993; 129: 356–63

Pillans PI, Woods DJ. Drug-associated alopecia. Int J Dermatol 1995; 34: 149–58

Rebora A. Telogen effluvium: an etiopathogenetic theory. Int J Dermatol 1993; 32: 339–40

Sperling LC. Hair and systemic disease. Dermatol Clin 2001; 19: 711–26

Anagen effluvium

Major points

- Inhibition of anagen hair-matrix metabolism with resultant hair loss
- Since >80% of scalp hair is normally in anagen, hair loss is marked
- Hairs shed in growing (anagen) phase
- Rapid loss of majority of scalp hair

Pathogenesis

- Chemotherapeutic agents
- Radiation
- Toxins: thallium, boric acid, arsenic, mercury

Diagnosis

- History very helpful
- Hair pull: 'pencil point' dystrophic hairs with proximal tips tapering to a point
- Hair pluck: anagen and telogen hairs

Differential diagnosis

- Telogen effluvium
- Alopecia totalis
- Loose anagen syndrome

Treatment

- Discontinuance of toxic agent or cause

Prognosis

- Excellent if toxic agent removed

References

Botchkarev VA. Molecular mechanisms of chemotherapy-induced hair loss. J Invest Dermatol Symp Proc 2003; 8: 72–5

Duvic M, Lemak NA, Valero V, et al. A randomized trial of minoxdil in chemotherapy-induced alopecia. J Am Acad Dermatol 1996; 35: 74–8

Feldman J, Levisohn DR. Acute alopecia: clue to thallium toxicity. Pediatr Dermatol 1993; 10: 29–31

Pillans PI, Woods DJ. Drug-associated alopecia. Intern J Dermatol 1995; 34: 149–58

Sommer M, Wilson C. Therapeutic approaches to the management of common baldness. Int J Clin Pract 1999; 53: 381–5

Androgenetic alopecia

Synonym: male pattern baldness

Major points

- Most common type of alopecia in adults
- Characterized by progressive pattern of hair loss from scalp (Figure 18.10)
- Patterns:
  1. Bitemporal recession
  2. Frontal thinning
  3. Vertex thinning leaving occipital and temporal margins with hair
  4. Women have diffuse thinning, usually worse centrally; widened parting, with retention of frontal hairline or M-pattern

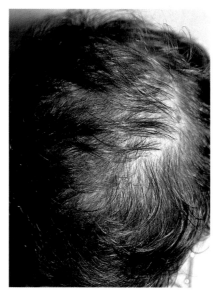

Figure 18.10   Male pattern alopecia in a 14-year-old with a strong genetic history for androgenetic alopecia

- Caused by circulating androgens in genetically susceptible men and women
- Begins between teens and 30 years in both sexes
- Affects 70% of all males in later life and >30% of older women
- Common complaint: thinning
- Inheritance probably polygenic

Pathogenesis

- Gradual transformation of thick scalp hair follicles to smaller follicles over many cycles, resulting in progressively shorter, finer, miniaturized hairs
- Regulated by dihydrotestosterone, which is formed by conversion of testosterone by 5α-reductase
- Histology shows miniaturized follicle with streamer of collapsed connective tissue sheath; increase ratio of telogen to anagen hairs and increase of vellus hairs; mild perifollicular lymphohistiocytic inflammation (nonspecific)

Diagnosis

- Clinical diagnosis
- Family history
- Hair pull test negative

Differential diagnosis

- Virilizing tumors of adrenal or ovary
- Telogen effluvium

Treatment

- Evaluation in teenage girls: free testosterone, dehydroepiandrosterone sulfate, luteinizing hormone, follicle stimulating hormone, prolactin
- Aim of treatment is to retard further thinning
- Topical minoxidil 2 or 5% BID, used for at least 1 year to assess efficacy; must maintain treatment to avoid shedding new growth
- Males: finasteride 1 mg PO daily; response seen as early as 3 months; needs continued treatment (contraindicated in women who may potentially become pregnant)
- Girls:
  1. Oral spironolactone (aldosterone antagonist), 50–200 mg/day
  2. Estrogen

Prognosis

- Slowly progressive

References

Ellis JA, Sinclair R, Harrap SB. Androgenetic alopecia: pathogenesis and potential for therapy. Expert Rev Mol Med 2002; 4: 1–11

Kaufman KD. Androgens and alopecia. Mol Cell Endocrinol 2002; 198: 89–95

Price VH. Androgenetic alopecia in adolescents. Cutis 2003; 71: 115–21

Price VH. Androgenetic alopecia in women. J Invest Dermatol Symp Proc 2003; 8: 24–7

Price VH. Treatment of hair loss. N Engl J Med 1999; 341: 964–73

Trichotillomania

Major points

- Location often frontal or frontoparietal scalp; can occur in scalp, eyebrows, eyelashes, pubic hair
- Irregularly shaped, angular patches with stubbly, broken-off hairs; area is never completely bald (Figures 18.11 and 18.12)
- Begins insidiously as irregular linear or rectangular area of partial hair loss
- Nonscarring
- Occurs in 8 million Americans

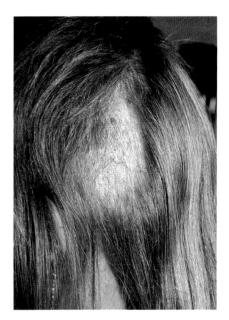

Figure 18.11   Trichotillomania – angular patches of broken-off hairs with areas of normal hair

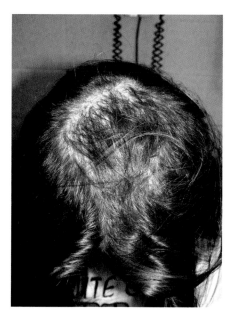

Figure 18.12   Trichotillomania – hair breakage in an unusual pattern on the posterior scalp

- Occurs in all ages >2 years; two-thirds are children, adolescents and young adults
- Two types:
  1. Temporary localized childhood pattern:
     a. Ages 2–6 years
     b. Harmless habit, tends to occur before child falls asleep or when reading, writing, or watching television
     c. No necessary treatment
     d. Good prognosis
  2. Teenage/adult pattern:
     a. Obsessive compulsive disorder
     b. Irresistible urge to pluck hair, either unconscious or semi-conscious
     c. More severe form
     d. Prognosis worse
     e. Most deny doing it
     f. Female/male ratio >1
     g. Often refractory to treatment
     h. Occurs frequently during psychosocial stress
- Other clinical features: focal perifollicular erythema, hemorrhage, excoriations
- Examination of hairs: blunt hair tips
- Concomitant occurrence with alopecia areata has been described

Pathogenesis

- Caused by plucking, pulling, breaking, or twisting one's own hair either consciously or subconsciously
- Histology:
  1. Marked increase in catagen and telogen hairs
  2. Presence of pigment casts
  3. Trichomalacia with abnormally small, distorted, bizarre-shaped hairs
  4. Dilated ostia with empty follicles
  5. Absence of bulbar inflammation

Diagnosis

- Clinical diagnosis
- Confirmed by finding wads of hair or observation of habit
- Histology helpful

Differential diagnosis

- Alopecia areata
- Trichorrhexis nodosa

Treatment

- Supportive
- Psychological evaluation and treatment
- Behavior modification
- Oral anti-obsessive compulsive agents: selective serotonin uptake inhibitors: paroxetine (Paxil®), sertraline (Zoloft®), fluoxetine (Prozac®)
- Topical mild steroid to reduce any inflammation or sense of itching

Prognosis

- Good in childhood type, poor in teenage type if no treatment is given or if problem has been prolonged

References

Hautmann G, Hercogova J, Lotti T. Trichotillomania. J Am Acad Dermatol 2002; 46: 807–21

Khouzam HR, Battista MA, Byers PE. An overview of trichotillomania and its response to treatment with quetiapine. Psychiatry 2002; 65: 261–70

Oranje AP, Peereboom-Wynia JDR, De Raeymaecher DMJ. Trichotillomania in childhood. J Am Acad Dermatol 1986; 15: 614–19

Papadopoulos AJ, Janniger CK, Chodynicki MP, Schwartx RA. Trichotillomania. Int J Dermatol 2003; 42: 330–4

Trueb RM, Cavegn B. Trichotillomania in connection with alopecia areata. Cutis 1996; 58: 67–70

Traction alopecia

Major points

- Common in females with tightly pulled hairstyles, especially Black girls
- Outermost hairs are subject to most tension, so margin of scalp usually affected (Figure 18.3 and 18.13)
- Commonly involves temporal region and frontal scalp
- Scalp surface appears normal, with no scarring
- Insidious onset

Pathogenesis

- Chronic traction of ponytails or braids, with tension on hair shafts or friction from headgear, rubber bands with hair breakage

Diagnosis

- Clinical diagnosis

Differential diagnosis

- Alopecia areata
- Trichotillomania

Treatment

- Gentle hair care (Table 18.3)
- Change hairstyle which includes loose braids, parting hair at different site
- Discontinue rubber bands and manipulation of hair

Prognosis

- Early disease (few months) – hair will recover
- Late disease (years) can cause permanent loss of hair follicles

References

Wilborn WS. Disorders of hair growth in African Americans. In Disorders of Hair Growth. Olsen EA, ed. McGraw-Hill: New York, 1994: 389–407

Traumatic alopecia

Major points

- Sudden onset caused by forceful extraction of hairs or prolonged pressure on scalp during surgery, resulting in focal tissue ischemia
- Clinical features: pain, inflammation, edema, followed by ulceration
- Forcible removal: consider child abuse
- Hair loss usually not permanent

Syndromes with late-onset hypotrichosis

- Ectodermal dysplasias
- Dyskeratosis congenita
- Werner syndrome
- Progeria (Hutchinson–Gilford syndrome)
- Cockayne syndrome
- Rothmund–Thomson syndrome

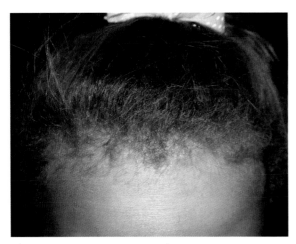

Figure 18.13 Traction alopecia – caused by over-processing extremely curly hair

Table 18.3   Handout for hair care
1. Be gentle
2. Take time with brushing and combing. Brush and comb as little and as gently as possible
3. Use a soft bristle brush or wide-toothed plastic brush
4. Comb: use a wide-toothed, round-tipped comb, bone or plastic; never metal
5. Cream rinse or condition the hair after shampooing, especially if the hair is long. Choose one with protein added
6. If your lifestyle does not include time for gentle combing and brushing, then keeping the hair short might be an option

HAIR SHAFT ABNORMALITIES

Trichorrhexis nodosa

Major points

- Fracture of hair shaft with splaying out and release of individual cortical cells, suggesting the appearance of two brushes being pushed together
- Hairs very fragile and break with trauma
- Common in Black females, whose hairstyles include routine straightening
- Hairs along scalp edge are subject to most tension
- Can be seen with argininosuccinic aciduria (congenital trichorrhexis nodosa), citrullinemia and hypothyroidism

Pathogenesis

- Results from chronic trauma (mechanical or chemical) to hair shafts: traction, twisting, brushing, hot combing, drying, straightening and other chemical treatments

Diagnosis

- Clinical features
- Microscopy of hair shaft

Differential diagnosis

- Other hair shaft abnormalities

Treatment

- Avoid manipulating hair as much as possible (Table 18.3)

Prognosis

- Slow recovery if trauma avoided

References

Lurie R, Hodak E, Ginzburg A, David M. Trichorrhexis nodosa: a manifestation of hypothyroidism. Cutis 1996; 57: 358–9

Quinn CR, Quinn TM, Kelly AP. Hair care practices in African American women. Cutis 2003; 72: 280–9

Trichorrhexis invaginata

Synonym: bamboo hair

Major points

- Characteristic of Netherton syndrome
- Variability of clinical picture
- Hair fragile, short, dull; may affect eyebrows, eyelashes and body hair
- Other features
  1. Ichthyosis linearis circumflexa
  2. Atopic dermatitis
  3. Erythroderma
  4. Secondary colonization with *Staphylococcus aureus*
  5. Increased absorption of topical agents (e.g. tacrolimus)

Pathogenesis

- Microscopy of hair shaft: ball and socket configuration or shallow invagination of distal into proximal shaft, resembling bamboo (Figure 18.14)

Diagnosis

- Clinical features with characteristic microscopy of hair shaft
- Gene locus/gene: chromosome 5q32/ SPINK5 gene encoding the serine protease inhibitor LEKTI

Differential diagnosis

- Atopic dermatitis
- Erythroderma
- Immune deficiencies

Treatment

- Gentle hair care
- Wigs

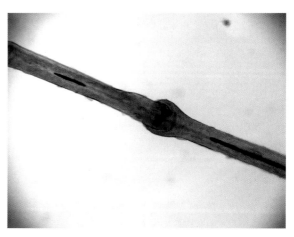

Figure 18.14   Netherton syndrome – bamboo hair (courtesy of Dr Dongshi Li)

- Intermittent topical corticosteroids for atopic dermatitis and scaling
- Emollients

Prognosis

- As hair becomes thicker, it may become slightly less fragile

References

Allen A, Siegfried E, Silverman R, et al. Significant absorption of topical tacrolimus in 3 patients with Netherton syndrome. Arch Dermatol 2001; 137: 747–50

Chavanas S, Bodemer C, Rochat A, et al. Mutations in SPINK5, encoding a serine protease inhibitor, cause Netherton syndrome. Nature Genet 2000; 25: 141–2

Hausser I, Anton-Lamprecht I. Severe congenital generalized exfoliative erythroderma in newborns and infants: a possible sign of Netherton syndrome. Pediatr Dermatol 1996; 13: 183–99

Muller FB, Hausser I, Berg D, et al. Genetic analysis of a severe case of Netherton syndrome and application for prenatal testing. Br J Dermatol 2002; 146: 495–9

Siegel DH. Howard R. Molecular advances in genetic skin diseases. Curr Opin Pediatr 2002; 14: 419–25

Pili torti

Major points

- Twisting of hair shaft on its own axis, usually through an angle of 180°
- Location: scalp, eyebrows, eyelashes
- Onset at birth or early months
- Hair: light in color, spangled, dry, brittle, breaks at different lengths and tends to stand out from scalp (Figure 18.15)
- Autosomal dominant, recessive or sporadic
- Syndromes that show pili torti:
  1. Classic pili torti
     a. May be isolated finding
     b. Can be seen with teeth, nail, eye defects, keratosis pilaris
  2. Björnstad syndrome
     a. Associated with sensorineural deafness
     b. Autosomal dominant
  3. Menkes 'kinky hair' syndrome
     a. Progressive neurodegeneration
     b. Connective tissue abnormalities

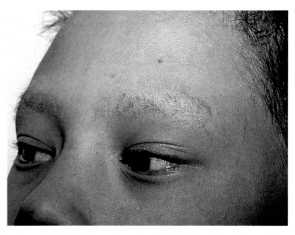

Figure 18.15 Pili torti – twisted hairs involving the scalp and eyebrows

     c. Hair twisted, coarse, sparse, hypopigmented or silvery; fragile, especially in areas of trauma
     d. Untreated disease usually lethal in early years
     e. Gene mutation in copper transporting P type ATPase protein (ATP7A) on chromosome X 13.3; blocks export of dietary copper from GI tract, leading to decreased bioavailability of copper with functional deficiencies of copper-dependent enzymes

Pathogenesis

- Histology of hair shaft: three or four regularly spaced twists, each 0.4–0.9 mm in width, occurring at irregular intervals along the shaft
- Twists almost always through 180° but can be less or more

Diagnosis

- Clinical features with microscopy of hair shaft

Differential diagnosis

- Uncombable hair syndrome
- Other hair shaft abnormalities

Treatment

- Gentle hair care

Prognosis

- Stable; may improve slightly with age

References

Richards KA, Mancini AJ. Three members of a family with pili torti and sensorineural hearing loss: the Bjornstad syndrome. J Am Acad Dermatol 2002; 46: 301–3

Selvaag E. Pili torti and sensorineural hearing loss. A follow-up of Bjornstad's original patients and a review of the literature. Eur J Dermatol 2000; 10: 91–7

Whiting DA. Hair shaft defects. In Disorders of Hair Growth. Olsen EA, ed. McGraw-Hill: New York, 1994: 91–137

Monilethrix

Synonym: beaded hair

Major points

- Beaded hairs on microscopy; nodes have diameter of normal hair, whereas internodes are narrow and are sites of fracture
- Hair usually normal at birth, but replaced by dry, dull, brittle hair which breaks spontaneously
- Scalp has stubbly appearance of hairs (Figure 18.16)
- Follicular keratosis often associated (scalp, face, limbs can have severe involvement)
- Autosomal dominant with high penetrance, but expressivity variable

Pathogenesis

- Characteristic elliptic nodes, 0.7–1 mm apart, with intervening tapered constrictions that are nonmedullated

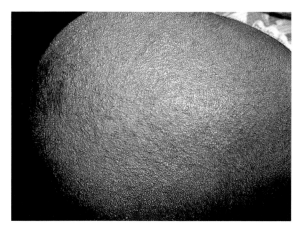

Figure 18.16 Monilethrix – very short hairs with keratotic papules

- Hairs fracture at internodal spaces
- Mutations in human basic hair keratins: hHb1 and hHb6
- Gene map locus 12q13

Diagnosis

- Clinical features with microscopy of hair shaft

Differential diagnosis

- Pseudomonilethrix: artifact caused by hairs pressed between two glass slides
- Other hair shaft anomalies

Treatment

- Gentle hair care

Prognosis

- May improve slightly as hair becomes thicker with age

References

DeBerker DAR, Ferguson DJP, Dawber RPR. Monilethrix: a clinicopathological illustration of a cortical defect. Br J Dermatol 1993; 128: 327–31

Korge BP, Hamm H, Jury CS, et al. Identification of novel mutations in basic hair keratins hHb1 and hHb6 in monilethrix: implications for protein structure and clinical phenotype. J Invest Dermatol 1999; 113: 607–12

Landau M, Brenner S, Metzker A. Medical pearl: an easy way to diagnose severe neonatal monilethrix. J Am Acad Dermatol 2002; 46: 111–12

Smith F. The molecular genetics of keratin disorders. Am J Clin Dermatol 2003; 4: 347–64

Uncombable hair syndrome

Synonyms: spun glass hair, pili trianguli et canaliculi

Major points

- Onset early in childhood
- Hair light silvery-blond, pale, frizzy; stands away from the scalp, cannot be combed flat; often spangled in appearance (Figure 18.17)
- Hair usually normal in length, quantity and strength
- Eyebrows, lashes and body hair normal
- Autosomal dominant, recessive or sporadic

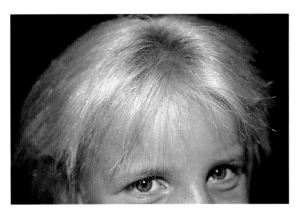

Figure 18.17 Uncombable hair syndrome – spangled hair which is difficult to style

Pathogenesis

- Microscopy of hairs: longitudinal grooving along the shaft or flattened surface with intact cuticle; areas discontinuous and change orientation many times along the shaft
- Cross-sectional microscopy: triangular, or other unusual shapes with longitudinal grooving

Diagnosis

- Clinical diagnosis with characteristic microscopy of hair shaft

Differential diagnosis

- Pili torti
- Loose anagen syndrome

Treatment

- Gentle hair care
- Conditioners helpful
- Hair not particularly fragile

Prognosis

- Good; tends to improve with age, but is always difficult to manage

References

Ang P, Tay YK. What syndrome is this? Uncombable hair syndrome (Pili trianguli et canaliculi). Pediatr Dermatol 1998; 15: 475–6

Hicks J, Metry DW, Barrish J, Levy M. Uncombable hair (cheveux incoiffables, pili trianguli et canaliculi) syndrome: brief review and role of scanning electron microscopy in diagnosis. Ultrastruct Pathol 2001; 25: 99–103

Itin PH, Buhler U, Buchner SA, Guggenheim R. Pili trianguli et canaliculi: a distinctive hair shaft defect leading to uncombable hair. Dermatology 1993; 187: 296–8

Loose anagen syndrome

Major points

- Characterized by actively growing anagen hairs which are loosely anchored and can be easily and painlessly pulled from the scalp
- Mainly blond healthy girls aged 1–9 years
- Parents complain that hair will not grow and seldom needs cutting
- Subtle diffuse or patchy thinning with uneven length of hairs
- Hair appears limp and matted
- Sporadic inheritance; occasionally autosomal dominant

Pathogenesis

- Normal tenacious bond between lower hair shaft and inner root sheath is weak, allowing trivial traction to cause disruption and extraction of hairs

Diagnosis

- Hair pull test (diagnostic) – numerous hair shafts painlessly extracted from scalp
- Microscopy of proximal ends of hairs pulled: anagen hairs without outer root sheaths, with ruffling of hair shaft ('crumpled sock' appearance)

Differential diagnosis

- Uncombable hair syndrome
- Pili torti
- Congenital hypotrichosis

Treatment

- Gentle hair care
- Reassurance

Prognosis

- Can improve with time

References

Boyer JD, Cobb MW, Sperling LC, Rushin JM. Loose anagen hair syndrome mimicking the uncombable hair syndrome. Cutis 1996; 57: 111–12

Chapalain V, Winter H, Langbein L, et al. Is the loose anagen hair syndrome a keratin disorder? A clinical and molecular study. Arch Dermatol 2002; 138: 501–6

Olsen EA, Bettencourt MS, Cote NL. The presence of loose anagen hairs obtained by hair pull in the normal population. Invest Dermatol Symp Proc 1999; 4: 258–60

Tosti A, Piraccini BM. Loose anagen hair syndrome and loose anagen hair. Arch Dermatol 2002; 138: 521–2

Trichothiodystrophy

Synonyms: BIDS, IBIDS, PIBIDS

Major points

- Sulfur-deficient, brittle hair (scalp, eyebrows, eyelashes)
- Neuroectodermal disorder
- Intellectual impairment
- Short stature
- Decreased fertility
- Photosensitivity with impaired DNA repair
- Ichthyosis
- Autosomal recessive

Pathogenesis

- Microscopy of hair shaft: flattened, twisted hair shaft, wavy, irregular, trichoschisis (clean, transverse fractures where there is localized absence of cuticle cells)
- Polarized microscopy: alternating bright and dark bands, resembling a tiger tail
- Sulfur content of hair reduced by 50%
- Gene locus/gene: chromosome 19q13/ mutation in at least two separate genes: ERCC2/XPD, and ERCC3/XPB, which encode the two helicase subunits of transcription/repair vector TFIIH

Diagnosis

- Clinical features with characteristic microscopy of hair shaft

Differential diagnosis

- Other hair shaft abnormalities

Treatment

- Gentle hair care

Prognosis

- Depends upon status of mental capabilities

References

Bergmann E, Egly JM. Trichothiodystrophy, a transcription syndrome. Trends Genet 2001; 17: 279–86

Itin PH, Pittelkow MR. Trichothiodystrophy: review of sulfur-deficient brittle hair syndromes and association with the ectodermal dysplasias. J Am Acad Dermatol 1990; 22: 705–17

Itin PH, Sarasin A, Pittelkow MR. Trichothiodystrophy: update on the sulfur-deficient brittle hair syndromes. J Am Acad Dermatol 2001; 44: 891–920

McCuaig C, Marcoux D, Rasmussen JE, et al. Trichothiodystrophy associated with photosensitivity, gonadal failure, and striking osteosclerosis. J Am Acad Dermatol 1993; 28: 820–6

Sperling LC, DiGiovanna JJ. 'Curly' wood and tiger tails: an explanation for light and dark banding with polarization in trichothiodystrophy. Arch Dermatol 2003; 139: 1189–92

van Brabant AJ, Stan R, Ellis NA. DNA helicases, genomic instability, and human genetic disease. Annu Rev Genomics Hum Genet 2000; 1: 409–59

ACQUIRED SCARRING ALOPECIA

Major points

- End result of inflammatory process affecting pilosebaceous unit, resulting in destruction of tissue and permanent hair loss (See Table 18.4) (Figure 18.18–20)

References

Tan E, Marinka M, Ball N, Shapiro J. Primary cicatricial alopecias: clinicopathology of 112 cases. J Am Acad Dermatol 2004; 50: 25–32

ABNORMALITIES OF INCREASED HAIR

Hypertrichosis

Major points

- Diffuse congenital hypertrichosis
  1. Hypertrichosis lanuginosa
     a. Very rare

Table 18.4   Causes of scarring alopecia

Developmental defects/syndrome

Aplasia cutis congenita
Conradi–Hünermann chondrodysplasia punctata
Incontinentia pigmenti
Ankyloblepharon, ectodermal dysplasia, cleft lip or palate (AEC) syndrome
Epidermolysis bullosa
Hallermann-Streiff syndrome
KID syndrome
Goltz syndrome
Ichthyoses

Infections

Fungal, bacterial, viral (herpes zoster), syphilis

Trauma

Traction
Trichotillomania
Hot-comb alopecia
Radiation
Burns

Inflammatory disorders

Lichen planopilaris: lichen planus localized to follicles; progressive; mild itching; hyperkeratotic follicular papules with erythema and scaling; histology shows lichenoid infiltrate around follicle
Morphea: discrete nontender sclerotic patches with ivory-colored shiny center and violaceous border; can see en coup de sabre pattern on frontal scalp
Scleroderma: generalized progressive systemic sclerosis
Lupus erythematosus: patchy erythema with telangiectases, follicular plugging and central hypo- or depigmentation with peripheral hyperpigmentation; or diffuse
Keratosis pilaris atrophicans: follicular keratinous plugging with erythema
Folliculitis decalvans: recurrent patchy painful folliculitis, mainly of scalp, often associated with *Staphylococcus aureus*
Dissecting cellulitis of scalp: chronic inflammatory disease; painful fluctuant nodules and abscesses interconnected by deep sinus tracts (Figure 18.18)
Alopecia mucinosa: grouped follicular papules and plaques with hair loss: histology shows accumulation of mucin in sebaceous glands with dissolution of cellular attachments; perifollicular and perivascular inflammatory cell infiltrate of lymphocytes, histiocytes and a few eosinophils. (Figure 18.19)

Neoplastic disorders

Acne keloidalis: grouped, small papules typically on nape of neck: caused by shaving of hair and re-entry of curved hairs into skin causing inflammation and keloid formation
Benign tumors: adenexal tumors, hemangiomas
Malignant tumors: leukemias, lymphomas, sarcomas

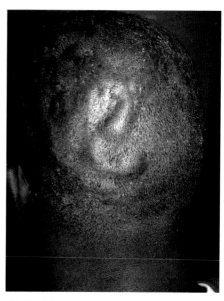

Figure 18.18   Dissecting folliculitis with cysts and tracts which are sterile abscesses

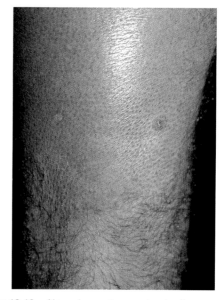

Figure 18.19   Alopecia mucinosa – benign type seen in a teenager

    b. Characterized by retention of lanugo hair
    c. At birth: coat of profuse silky hair up to 10 cm long with accentuation over the spine and ears
    d. Autosomal recessive or dominant
• Prepubertal hypertrichosis

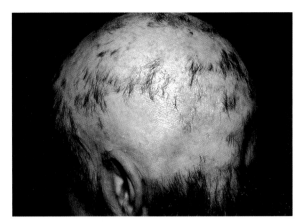

Figure 18.20   Acquired scarring alopecia – lichen planopilaris

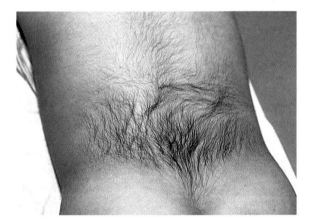

Figure 18.21   Hypertrichosis – familial type on lower back

1. Common
2. Generalized; can present from birth
3. Severity in early childhood varies
4. Profuse terminal hair growth on back and limbs, and also temples, forehead and eyebrows (Figure 18.21)
5. Not clear whether this represents an abnormality or normal range of hair growth seen in some racial groups (e.g. Mediterranean peoples, Indians)
- Drug-induced hypertrichosis (Table 18.5)
- Localized hypertrichosis (see Table 18.5)
  1. Hypertrichosis with spinal fusion abnormalities
     a. Tuft of long hair overlying defect (dimple, sinus tract, lipoma, spinal bifida, occult spinal dysraphism)
     b. Lumbosacral area usually

Table 18.5   Causes of hypertrichosis

Types of congenital circumscribed hypertrichosis
Congenital nevocellular nevus
Congenital Becker nevus
Smooth muscle hamartoma
Nevoid hypertrichosis
Underlying neurofibroma
Hypertrichosis cubiti
Hemihypertrophy
Spinal dysraphism
Anterior cervical hypertrichosis

Congenital syndromes with secondary hypertrichosis
Brachmann-de Lange syndrome
Fetal exposures
  Fetal hydantoin syndrome
  Fetal alcohol syndrome
Lipoatrophic diabetes
Mucopolysaccharidoses
Congenital porphyrias
Rubinstein–Taybi syndrome
Hypomelanosis of Ito

Causes of acquired localized hypertrichosis
Becker nevus
Orthopedic casts and splints
Friction
  Lichen simplex chronicus
  Habitual biting
  Insect bites
  Atopic eczema
Venous malformations, thrombosis
Trichomegaly
  HIV
  Systemic lupus erythematosus
  Linear scleroderma

Causes of acquired generalized hypertrichosis
Infection
Malnutrition
Dermatomyositis
Thyroid abnormalities
Cerebral disturbances
Acrodynia

Pharmacologic causes of hypertrichosis
Phenytoin
Acetazolamide
Streptomycin
Cyclosporin A
Diazoxide
Minoxidil

2. Hypertrichosis with cranial abnormalities ('hair collar' sign)
   a. Peripheral collar of thick dark tuft of hair with an underlying form fruste of a neural tube closure defect and heterotopic brain tissue

Pathogenesis

- Increase in hair growth by conversion of vellus to terminal hairs, or changes in the hair-growth cycle

Diagnosis

- Clinical diagnosis
- Rule out causes of hirsutism, if appropriate

Differential diagnosis

(See Table 18.5)

Treatment

- Depends upon cause of hypertrichosis
- Removal of excess hair: shaving, epilation, chemical depilatories, threading, waxing, electrolysis, laser hair removal

Prognosis

- Depends upon cause of hypertrichosis; usually permanent

References

Miller ML, Yeager JK. Hairy elbows. Arch Dermatol 1995; 131: 858–9

Wendelin DS, Pope DN, Mallory SB. Hypertrichosis. J Am Acad Dermatol 2003; 48: 161–79

Hirsutism

Major points

- Hair in masculine pattern in females on face, chest, upper back, abdomen
- Often associated with other signs of virilization or polycystic ovary syndrome in teens (Figure 18.22)

Pathogenesis

- Abnormality of pituitary, adrenal glands or ovary with increase in male hormones

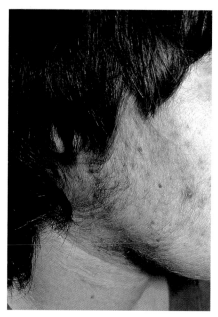

Figure 18.22   Hirsutism caused by polycystic ovary disease in a teenage girl

Diagnosis

- History
- Physical examination
- Laboratory tests: serum testosterone and free testosterone, dehydroepiandrosterone sulfate, cortisol levels, urinary 17-ketosteroids, luteinizing hormone, follicle stimulating hormone, prolactin levels and pelvic ultrasound examination

Differential diagnosis

- Genetic predisposition in some ethnic groups
- Congenital adrenal hyperplasia
- Cushing syndrome
- Hyperprolactinemia
- Ovarian and adrenal tumors

Treatment

- Removal of excess hair: shaving, epilation, chemical depilatories, threading, waxing, electrolysis, laser hair removal
- Oral contraceptives

Prognosis

- Depends upon etiology of hirsutism, usually permanent

References

Shum KW, Cullen DR, Messenger AG. Hair loss in women with hyperandrogenism: four cases responding to finasteride. J Am Acad Dermatol 2002; 47: 733–9

Sperling LC, Heimer WL. Androgen biology as a basis for the diagnosis and treatment of androgenic disorders in women. II. J Am Acad Dermatol 1993; 28: 901–16

Whiting DA. Diagnostic and predictive value of horizontal sections of scalp biopsy specimens in male pattern androgenetic alopecia. J Am Acad Dermatol 1993; 28: 755–63

ABNORMALITIES OF HAIR COLOR

See Table 18.6

Menkes kinky hair syndrome

Major points

- Hair appears lightly pigmented, twisted, sparse
- Microscopic hair examination: pili torti, trichorrhexis nodosa
- General decrease in skin pigmentation
- Progressive severe mental retardation and neurologic defects
- Bony changes resembling scurvy
- Tortuosities of cerebral and systemic vasculature
- Diverticuli of the bladder

Pathogenesis

- Gene/gene locus: ATP7A (copper transporting ATPase enzyme)/Xp 13.3
- Abnormality of a copper binding protein important in cytoplasmic copper transport, causing an inappropriate copper distribution within the cells
- Copper accumulates in fibroblasts and macrophages
- Kinky hair results from a surplus of free sulfhydryl groups and a decrease in copper-dependent disulfide bonds
- Hypopigmentation results from a decrease in tyrosinase, a copper-containing enzyme

Diagnosis

- Clinical presentation
- Low serum copper and ceruloplasm levels
- Genetic testing

Table 18.6   Abnormalities of hair color

Disorders associated with primary reduction of hair color
Oculocutaneous albinism
Chediak–Higashi syndrome
Elejalde syndrome
Griscelli syndrome
Pili torti
Menkes syndrome
Uncombable hair
Phenylketonuria
Homocystinuria
Prader–Willi syndrome

Disorders associated with premature canities (graying)
Autoimmune disease
  Vitiligo
  Alopecia areata
  Pernicious anemia
  Addison disease
  Hypothyroidism
  Hyperthyroidism
Syndromes
  Progeria
  Werner syndrome
  Rothmund–Thomson syndrome
  Dyskeratosis congenita
  Down syndrome
  Cri du chat syndrome
  Böök syndrome

Localized hypopigmentation (poliosis)
Piebaldism
Waardenburg syndrome
Vitiligo
Vogt–Koyanagi–Harada syndrome
Alezzandrini syndrome
Alopecia areata
Tuberous sclerosis
Halo nevus

Differential diagnosis

- Child abuse
- Congenital lipodystrophic diabetes
- Trichothiodystrophy

Treatment

- No effective treatment is available

Prognosis

- Death usually before 1 year of age

- Mildly affected patients can survive to adolescence or adulthood

References

Chelly J, Tumer Z, Tonnesen T, et al. Isolation of a candidate gene for Menkes disease that encodes a potential heavy metal binding protein. Nature Genet 1993; 3: 14–19

Kodama H, Sato E, Yanagawa Y, et al. Biochemical indicator for evaluation of connective tissue abnormalities in Menkes' disease. J Pediatr 2003; 142: 726–8

Menkes JH. Kinky hair disease; twenty five years later. Brain Dev 1988; 10: 77–9

Poulsen L, Horn N, Heilstrup H, et al. X-linked recessive Menkes disease: identification of partial gene deletions in affected males. Clin Genet 2002; 62: 449–57

Shim H, Harris ZL. Genetic defects in copper metabolism. J Nutr 2003; 133 (5 Suppl 1): 1527S–31S

Chediak–Higashi syndrome

Major points

- Hypopigmentation of skin and hair
  1. Hair has a silvery tint because of large melanosome granules in the hair (Figure 18.23)
  2. Loss of iris pigmentation with photophobia

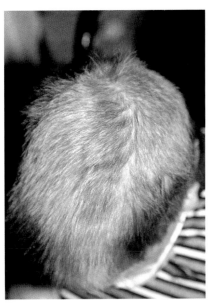

Figure 18.23   Chediak–Higashi syndrome with silvery hair, mental retardation and numerous infections

  3. Visual acuity normal, but strabismus and nystagmus common
- Infections: children usually present with infection and fever in early childhood
  1. Infections of the skin, lungs, and upper respiratory tract with *Staphylococcus aureus*, *Streptococcus* species
  2. Natural killer cell function decreased
- Neurological deterioration is progressive: clumsiness, abnormal gait, paresthesias and other findings
- Accelerated phase: fever, hepatosplenomegaly, lymphadenopathy, pancytopenia; Epstein–Barr virus has been implicated
- Autosomal recessive

Pathogenesis

- Caused by a mutation in the LYST gene on chromosome 1q

Diagnosis

- Clinical presentation
- Giant lysosomal granules are seen in polymorphnuclear leukocytes, melanosomes, and other cells
- Genetic testing

Differential diagnosis

- Elejalde syndrome
- Griscelli syndrome
- Menkes kinky hair syndrome
- Other immunodeficiencies

Treatment

- Supportive treatments with antibiotics
- Bone marrow transplantation early

Prognosis

- Usually fatal before age 10 years, unless patient undergoes successful bone marrow transplant

References

Haddad E, Le Deist F, Blanche S, et al. Treatment of Chediak–Higashi syndrome by allogeneic bone marrow transplantation: report of ten cases. Blood 1995; 85: 3328–33

Shiflett SL, Kaplan J, Ward DM. Chediak–Higashi syndrome: a rare disorder of lysosomes and lysosome related organelles. Pigment Cell Res 2002; 15: 251–7

Ward DM, Shiflett SL, Kaplan J. Chediak–Higashi syndrome: a clinical and molecular view of a rare lysosomal storage disorder. Curr Mol Med 2002; 2: 469–77

Griscelli syndrome

Major points

- Characterized by pigment dilution, hepatosplenomegaly, lymphohistiocytosis, and T and B cell immunodeficiencies
- Immunodeficiency with frequent pyogenic infections, fever, neutropenia, thrombocytopenia
- Hair has a silvery gray tint secondary to the dispersal and clumping of melanin in the hair shaft
- Skin is lighter in color than in siblings and parents
- Neurologic dysfunction with cerebellar and bulbar signs, encephalopathy, seizures, retardation
- Accelerated phase in childhood is usually fatal
- Autosomal recessive
- Gene locus: 15q 21
- Gene: Myosin VA (Type 1), RAB27A (Type 2)

References

Griscelli C, Durandy A, Guy-Grand D, et al. A syndrome associating partial albinism and immunodeficiency. Am J Med 1978; 65: 691–702

Kumar M, Sackey K, Schmalstieg F, et al. Griscelli syndrome: rare neonatal syndrome of recurrent hemophagocytosis. J Pediatr Hematol Oncol 2001; 23: 464–8

Mancini AJ, Chan LS, Paller AS. Partial albinism with immunodeficiency: Griscelli syndrome: report of a case and review of the literature. J Am Acad Dermatol 1998; 38: 295–300

Elejalde syndrome

Major points

- Characterized by silvery hair, severe CNS dysfunction, abnormal inclusions in cells of all tissues
- Neurologic abnormalities
- No immunologic dysfunctions
- Autosomal recessive
- Elejalde syndrome and Griscelli syndrome Type 1 may be the same entity

References

Bahadoran P, Ortonne JP, Ballotti R, de Saint-Basile G. Comment on Elejalde syndrome and relationship with Griscelli syndrome. Am J Med Genet 2003; 116A: 408–9

Duran-McKinster C, Rodriguez-Jurado R, Ridaura C, et al. Elejalde syndrome – a melanolysosomal neurocutaneous syndrome: clinical and morphological findings in 7 patients. Arch Dermatol 1999; 135: 182–6

Elejalde BR, Holguin J, Valencia A, et al. Mutations affecting pigmentation in man: I. Neuroectodermal melanolysosomal disease. Am J Med Genet 1979; 3: 65–80

Ivanovich J, Mallory S, Storer T, et al. 12-year-old male with Elejalde syndrome (neuroectodermal melanolysosomal disease). Am J Med Genet 2001; 98: 313–16

19

NAIL DISORDERS

Agnail

- Hang nail; hard spicules at edge of nail

Alopecia areata

- Shallow pits on surface of nail plate; geometric arrangement giving the appearance of a grid or screen; 60% of patients with alopecia areata have pitting which is reversible (Figure 19.1)

Anonychia

- Absence of nail from birth; associated with nail patella syndrome, ectodermal dysplasias, maternal hydantoin ingestion, Coffin–Siris syndrome and others

Beau's lines

- Uniform transverse grooves across the nail plate usually affecting all nails (Figure 19.2)
- Thumbnails and great toenails more prominent than others
- Grooves move distally with nail growth
- Caused by an arrest in nail plate formation by systemic illness or toxins
- No treatment is needed

Blue nails

- Associated with antimalarial drugs, argyria, bleomycin, congenital pernicious anemia, minocycline and Wilson disease (Figure 19.3)

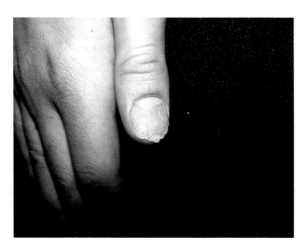

Figure 19.1 Pitting – commonly occurs in alopecia areata and psoriasis

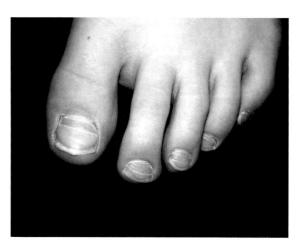

Figure 19.2 Beau's lines – horizontal ridge of all 20 nails following a severe illness

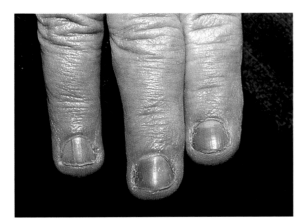

Figure 19.3   Nail pigmentation caused by minocycline

Brachyonychia

- Short nails with width greater than length; associated with Rubinstein–Taybi syndrome, Down syndrome

Clubbing

- Bulbous, fusiform enlargement of distal portion of fingers and toes
- Lovibond's angle >180°
- Associated with cystic fibrosis, cyanotic cardiovascular diseases

Dystrophy

- General term describing nail changes. Examples: trauma, epidermal nevus, lichen striatus, psoriasis, twenty-nail dystrophy and others

Half-and-half nails (Lindsay nails)

- Proximal nail is white (Figure 19.4)
- Distal 20–50% of nail is red, pink, or brown
- Seen in renal failure

Hutchinson sign

- Periungual spread of pigmentation into the proximal and lateral nail folds
- An important indicator of subungual melanoma but not pathognomonic for it

Ingrown nails

- Common problem in infancy, childhood and teens

- Clinical presentations
    1. Congenital hypertrophic lateral nail folds
        a. Presents as a firm red swelling of lateral nail fold with tenderness (Figure 19.5)
        b. Usually disappears spontaneously after several months, but may require surgical intervention
    2. Distal-lateral nail embedding
        a. Caused by uneven cutting of the nail plate with subsequent growth of the plate into an injured lateral nail fold
        b. Painful with exuberant granulation tissue around the edge of the embedded plate
        c. Complications: secondary infection (often *Pseudomonas*) and paronychia

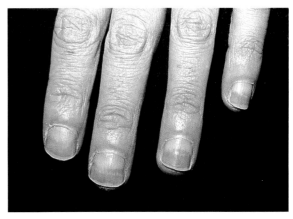

Figure 19.4   Half-and-half nails – proximal nail is white and distal nail is pink; associated with renal disease

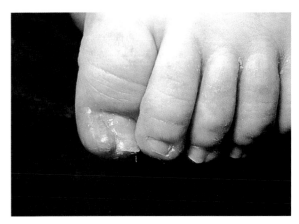

Figure 19.5   Congenital ingrown toenails – erythema and swelling of the lateral nail folds, often bilateral

d. Treatment: subungual packing with sterile cotton in uncomplicated cases with silver nitrate cauterization, oral antibiotics, topical steroid solutions. In complicated cases, surgical removal of the trapped nail plate

e. Rarely, total ungual avulsion may be needed

Koilonychia

- Spoon-shaped or flat nails (Figure 19.6)
- Associated with iron deficiency anemia
- Can be idiopathic or familial

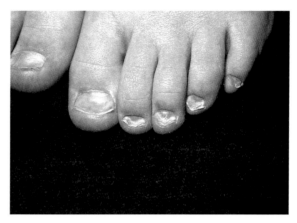

Figure 19.6   Koilonychia – congenital curving of toenails, a common finding in infants and young children

Leukonychia

- White nails (Figure 19.7)
- May be congenital or acquired
- May be totally white, or striped
- May be associated with multiple causes: alopecia areata, hypoalbuminemia, exfoliative dermatitis, Darier disease, pellagra, zinc deficiency

Macronychia

- Large but otherwise normal nail
- Associated with neurofibromatosis, tuberous sclerosis

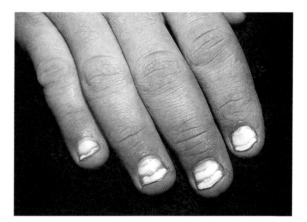

Figure 19.7   Leukonychia – banded type of unknown etiology. This had been present for many years

Malalignment of the great toenails

- Characterized by lateral deviation of the nail plate relative to the axis of the hallux (Figure 19.8)
- Transverse ridging, thickening and gradual tapering towards the distal free edge with dicoloration
- May be discolored from intermittent hemorrhage or microbes
- May be unilateral or bilateral
- Surgical correction may be needed
- Predisposes to paronychia and ingrown nails
- Spontaneous improvement can be seen
- Autosomal dominant

Median nail dystrophy

- Split or canal in nail plate usually just off center from cuticle to free edge (Figure 19.9)

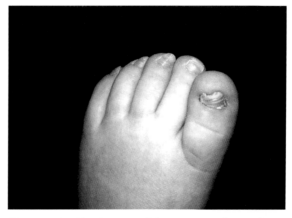

Figure 19.8   Malalignment of the great toenails, causing discomfort

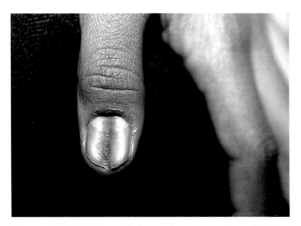

Figure 19.9   Median nail dystrophy – caused by a habit tic

- Caused by trauma or idiopathic; most common on thumb

Mee's lines

- White bands in nail plate which move with plate as it grows
- Associated with arsenic ingestion, cardiac insufficiency, pellagra, renal failure, sickle cell anemia

Micronychia

- Small but otherwise normal nail or nails
- Associated with ectodermal dysplasia, dyskeratosis congenita, nail–patella syndrome

Muehrcke's nails

- Paired white parallel bands seen with hypoalbuminemia
- Bands do not move

Nail–patella syndrome

Synonym: congenital iliac horns syndrome, hereditary osteo-onychodysplasia syndrome
- Onychodystrophy (medial thumbnails most involved) with hypoplasia and splitting with usual sparing of the toenails
- Triangular lunulae
- Absent or rudimentary patellae, with unstable knees

- Elbow dysplasia, subluxation of the radial heads
- Iliac horns (calcifications from the posterior aspect of the ilium)
- Other findings
  1. Renal abnormalities: glomerulonephritis, renal dysplasia, Goodpasture syndrome
  2. Hypoplasia of scapulae
  3. Scoliosis
  4. Cloverleaf pigmentation of irides (Lester iris)
  5. Laxity of skin
  6. Hyperhidrosis
  7. Autosomal dominant
- Gene: LMX1B (LIM-homeobox transcription factor 1β)
- Gene locus: 9q34.1

References

Bongers EM, Gubler MC, Knoers NV. Nail–patella syndrome. Overview on clinical and molecular findings. Pediatr Nephrol 2002; 17: 703–12

Bongers EM, Van Bokhoven H, Van Thienen MN, et al. The small patella syndrome: description of five cases from three families and examination of possible allelism with familial patella aplasia–hypoplasia and nail–patella syndrome. J Med Genet 2001; 38: 209–14

Dreyer SD, Zhou G, Baldini A, et al. Mutations in LMX1B cause abnormal skeletal patterning and renal dysplasia in nail patella syndrome. Nature Genet 1998; 19: 47–50

Ogden JA, Cross GL, Guidera KJ, Ganey TM. Nail patella syndrome. A 55-year follow-up of the original description. J Pediatr Orthop 2002; 11: 333–8

Stratigos AJ, Baden HP. Unraveling the molecular mechanisms of hair and nail genodermatoses. Arch Dermatol 2001; 137: 1465–71

Nevi

- Characterized by longitudinal pigmented bands (Figure 19.10)
- Usually solitary

Onychogryphosis

- Acquired thickening (Figure 19.11)
- Caused by trauma, aging or unknown etiology

Onychoheteropia

- Misplaced nails

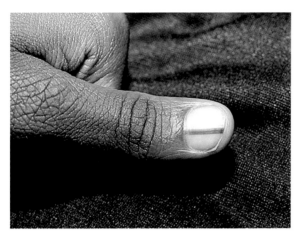

Figure 19.10 Nevus of the nail matrix with linear dark band of pigmentation; because there is no pigment on the proximal nail fold, this is not Hutchinson sign; however, a biopsy of the nail matrix is suggested to rule out malignant melanoma

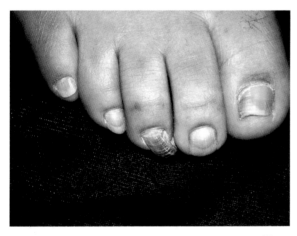

Figure 19.11 Onychogryphosis of the third toenail with onchomycosis of the great toenail

Onycholysis

- Separation of nail plate from nail bed at distal and lateral attachments (Figure 19.12)
- Caused by hypo- or hyperthyroidism, trauma, psoriasis, candidal infections, diabetes, phototoxic reactions to drugs (tetracycline, thorazine), or idiopathic

Onychomadesis

- Separation of entire nail plate (Figure 19.13)

Onychomycosis

- Fungal infection of the nail (See Chapter 9) (Figures 19.14 and 19.15)

Onychophagia

- Nail biting

Onychoschizia

- Splitting of nails into parallel layers, with a lamellar surface so that small pieces flake off

Onychorrhexis

- Excess longitudinal ridging

Pachyonychia congenita

- Type I: Jadassohn–Lewandowsky syndrome
  1. Marked thickening of nails (subungual hyperkeratosis) (Figure 19.16)
  2. Recurrent nail shedding
  3. Plantar and palmar keratoses
  4. Acral bullae
  5. Follicular keratoses on buttocks and extremities
  6. Hyperhidrosis of the palms and soles
  7. Leukoplakia that histologically resembles a white sponge nevus and shows no tendency toward malignant degeneration
  8. Mutation of keratin gene: KRT6A, KRT16 (keratin 6a, keratin 16), gene locus: 17q12-q21, 12q13
- Type II: Jackson-Lawler syndrome
  1. Clinical findings of Type I plus
  2. Bullae of palms and soles
  3. Palmar/plantar hyperhidrosis
  4. Steatocystoma multiplex
  5. Epidermal cysts
  6. Natal teeth
  7. No mucosal lesions
  8. Mutation of gene: KRT6B, KRT17 (keratin 6b, keratin 17)
  9. Gene locus: 17q17-q21, 12q13

Differential diagnosis

- Mucocutaneous candidiasis
- Onychomycosis

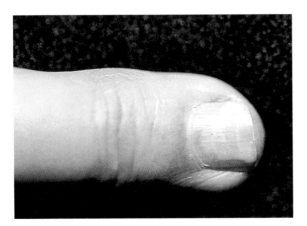

Figure 19.12 Onycholysis – lifting off of the nail plate from the nail bed

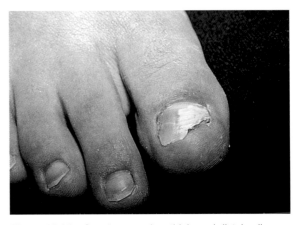

Figure 19.15 Onychomycosis – thickened distal nails with keratotic debris

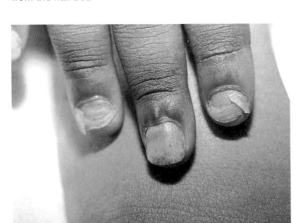

Figure 19.13 Onychomadesis – complete shedding of nails after a severe illness

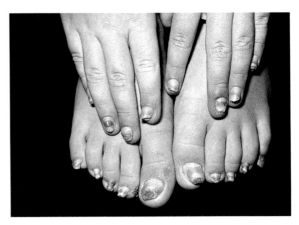

Figure 19.16 Pachyonychia congenita – markedly thick nails

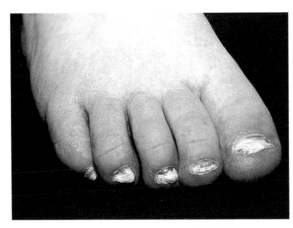

Figure 19.14 Onychomycosis – superficial white discoloration associated with *Trichophyton rubrum* in a child

Treatment

- Surgical removal of nails if severe infections around the nails; keratolytic agents may be helpful

Prognosis

- Chronic thickening of nails with chronic paronychia

References

Feinstein A, Friedman J, Schewach-Millet M. Pachyonychia congenita. J Am Acad Dermatol 1988; 19: 705–11

Paller AS, Moore JA, Scher R. Pachyonychia congenita tarda: a late-onset form of pachyonychia congenita. Arch Dermatol 1991; 127: 701–3

Su WPD, Chun SI, Hammond DE, Gordon H. Pachyonychia congenita: clinical study of 12 cases and review of the literature. Pediatr Dermatol 1990; 7: 33–8

Paronychia

- Infection of periungual tissues
- Common causes: sucking thumb or fingers
- Characterized by painful erythematous induration of proximal or lateral nail folds with fissuring (Figure 19.17)
- Cuticle is obliterated; nail folds round and replaced with granulation tissue
- Pus may be expressed
- Nail dystrophy with wavy undulation may result from inflammation in the proximal nail fold affecting the matrix
- Common organisms: *Staphylococcus, Streptococcus* and *Candida*
- Trauma to the proximal nail fold disrupts the cuticle, and in moist environment, organisms invade
- If multiple fingers and toes are involved, consider predisposing diseases: acrodermatitis enteropathica, mucocutaneous candidiasis, or immunodeficiency syndromes
- Treatment is difficult if predisposing factors are not addressed
  1. Topical combination of steroid and antifungal agents (Mycolog®) used two or three times per day for 4–6 months
  2. Topical clindamycin solution
  3. Drying agents: 4% thymol in chloroform one or two times a day (should not be used in children who put their hands in their mouth)

Pincer nail

- Overcurvature of the nails causing pain and partial strangulation dystrophy of the soft tissues (Figure 19.18)

Polyonychia

- Two or more separate nails on one digit

Pseudomonas nail

- Greenish discoloration under the nail plate with onycholysis (Figure 19.19)

Psoriasis

- Occurs in 15–79% of children with cutaneous signs of psoriasis
- Pitting of the nail plate is most common; rarely can involve all 20 nails (Figure 19.20)
- Other findings: discoloration, onycholysis, distal subungual debris and oil spotting
- Periungual psoriasis can lead to marked nail dystrophy with hyperkeratosis and crumbling of the nail plate

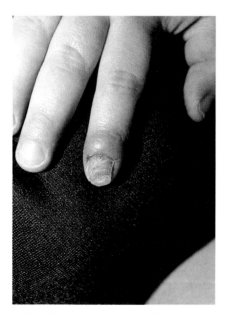

Figure 19.17   Paronychia – inflammation around the nail caused by *Candida albicans*

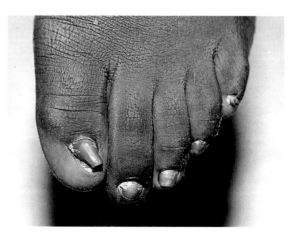

Figure 19.18   Pincer nail causing pain in this teenager

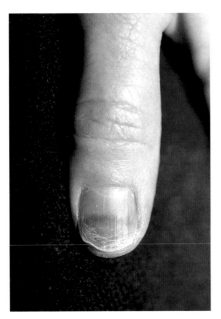

Figure 19.19 *Pseudomonas* infection of the nail bed causing yellow–green discoloration of the nail and the nail bed

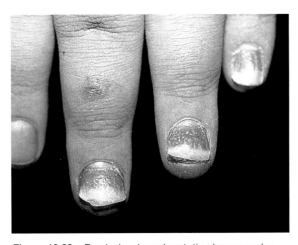

Figure 19.20 Psoriasis – hyperkeratotic plaques under nails with pitting

Pterygium

- Wing-shaped destruction of nail matrix
- Overgrowth of cuticle onto nail eventually destroying the nail, causing scarring
- Associated with dyskeratosis congenita, graft-versus-host disease, Raynaud disease, systemic sclerosis

Racquet nail

- Congenital abnormality of the nail, causing the nail to be broader and shorter
- Most common on the thumb

Red lunulae

- Seen in collagen vascular disease, alopecia areata, congestive heart failure

Splinter hemorrhages

- Associated with subacute bacterial endocarditis, trauma, vasculitis, cirrhosis, trichinosis, scurvy, psoriasis, chronic glomerulonephritis, Darier disease

Terry's nails

- Distal 1–2 mm pink, proximal nail white
- Seen with hypoalbuminemia or hepatic cirrhosis

Trachyonychia

- Uniform roughness of surface of nail plate
- Associated with ichthyosis vulgaris, ectodermal dysplasia, 20-nail dystrophy, others

Traumatic nail injury

- Injury to the nail, nail matrix, nail plate (Figures 19.21 and 19.22)
- Common in childhood
- Can cause permanent dystrophy

Twenty-nail dystrophy

- Acquired dystrophy involving all 20 nails
- Characterized by marked roughness of the nail plates (trachyonychia) with longitudinal grooves, striations, onychorrhexis, distal chipping (Figure 19.23)
- Nails can be either thin or thick
- May be associated with lichen planus
- Cause unknown
- Course variable with improvement in 6 months to 16 years
- Treatment:

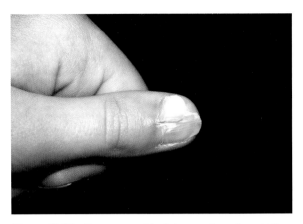

Figure 19.21   Trauma – residual damage to nail caused by slamming the finger in a car door

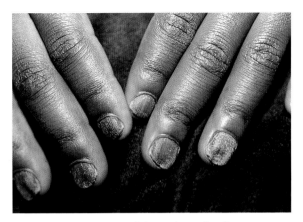

Figure 19.23   Twenty-nail dystrophy – all nails simultaneously developed trachyonychia

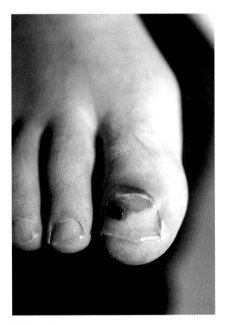

Figure 19.22   Trauma – hemorrhage under the nail from dropping a heavy object on the toe in a patient with hemophilia

1. Potent topical steroids may be of some benefit over 6 months
2. Clear nail lacquers

Whitlow

- Caused by herpes inoculation into finger tip or around nail
- Painful recurrent vesicles around the distal finger or nails

Yellow nails

- Thickened yellow nails
- Associated with chronic lymphedema, pleural effusion, bronchiectasis, chronic bronchitis, rheumatoid arthritis, sinusitis, thyroid disease, psoriasis, pachyonychia congenita, drugs (e.g. tetracycline, penicillamine)

References

Adams BB. Jogger's toenail. J Am Acad Dermatol 2003; 48: S58–9

Carroll LA, Laumann AD. Doxycycline-induced photo-onycholysis. J Drugs Dermatol 2003; 2: 662–3

Cohen PR. Red lunulae: case report and literature review. J Am Acad Dermatol 1992; 26: 292–4

Daniel CR, Piraccini BM, Tosti A. The nail and hair in forensic science. J Am Acad Dermatol 2004; 50: 258–61

Feldman SR, Gammon WR. Unilateral Muehrcke's lines following trauma. Arch Dermatol 1989; 125: 133–4

Jerasutus S, Suvanprakorn P, Kitchawengkul O. Twenty nail dystrophy. Arch Dermatol 1990; 126: 1068–70

Rich P, Scher RK. Nail psoriasis severity index: a useful tool for evaluation of nail psoriasis. J Am Acad Dermatol 2003; 49: 206–12

Saray Y, Seckin D, Gulec AT, et al. Nail disorders in hemodialysis patients and renal transplant recipients: a case–control study. J Am Acad Dermatol 2004; 50: 197–202

20

GENODERMATOSES AND SYNDROMES

ICHTHYOSES

- Heterogeneous group of inherited disorders characterized by the accumulation of scale on the skin surface
- The word ichthyosis comes from the Greek word for fish, referring to the scaliness of the skin
- National organization: www.scalyskin.org (F.I.R.S.T.)

Collodion baby

Major points

- Not specific for any particular ichthyosis
- At birth: taut shiny membrane of skin that resembles plastic wrap (Figure 20.1)
- Membrane often becomes fissured and cracked
- Ectropion

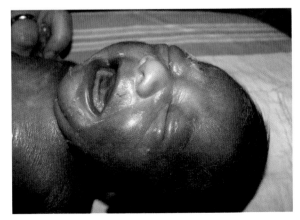

Figure 20.1 Collodion membrane in a neonate

- Eclabium
- Pinnae crumpled
- Tips of fingers often tapered
- Resolves with shedding of membrane
- Hair and nails usually normal

Pathogenesis

- Seen in various types of ichthyosis:
    1. Lamellar ichthyosis
    2. Ichthyosis vulgaris
    3. Congenital ichthyosiform erythroderma (CIE)
    4. Netherton syndrome
    5. Conradi–Hünermann syndrome
    6. Ectodermal dysplasia
    7. Ankyloblepharon ectodermal dysplasia clefting (AEC) syndrome
    8. Gaucher disease type 2
- Caused by retention of or abnormal stratum corneum *in utero*

Diagnosis

- Histology: stratum corneum thickened with orthokeratosis

Differential diagnosis

- Postmaturity desquamation
- Staphylococcal scalded skin syndrome

Treatment

- Emollients (e.g. ointments)
- Increase ambient humidity
- Maintain hygiene to prevent secondary infection
- Surveillance of skin cultures
- Artificial tears for ectropion
- Stabilization of temperature

Prognosis

- Membrane usually shed in 7–10 days
- Outcome depends upon type of ichthyosis

References

Akcakus M, Gunes T, Kurtoglu S, Ozturk A. Collodion baby associated with asymmetric crying facies: a case report. Pediatr Dermatol 2003; 20: 134–6

Buyse L, Graves C, Marks R, et al. Collodion baby dehydration: the danger of high transepidermal water loss. Br J Dermatol 1993; 129: 86–8

DiGiovanna JJ, Robinson-Bostom L. Ichthyosis: etiology, diagnosis, and management. Am J Clin Dermatol 2003; 4: 81–95

Matsumoto K, Muto M, Seki S, et al. Loricrin keratoderma: a cause of congenital ichthyosiform erythroderma and collodion baby. Br J Dermatol 2001; 145: 657–60

Raghunath M, Hennies HC, Ahvazi B, et al. Self-healing collodion baby: a dynamic phenotype explained by a particular transglutaminase-1 mutation. J Invest Dermatol 2003; 120: 224–8

Richard G, Ringpfeil F. Ichthyoses, erythrokeratodermas and related disorders. In Dermatology. Bolognia JL, Jorizzo JL, Rapini RP, eds. Mosby: London, 2003: 775–808

Ichthyosis vulgaris

Major points

- Most common form of ichthyosis
- Incidence: 1 per 300–2000 persons
- Onset 3–12 months of age
- Personal or family history of dry skin or atopy
- Fine white scales, can be dark
- Location: extensor surfaces of the extremities and trunk, with extremities more severely affected (Figure 20.2)
- Margin of scale tends to turn up
- Flexural areas spared
- Hyperlinearity of the palms and keratosis pilaris is common
- Autosomal dominant

Pathogenesis

- Increased adhesiveness of the stratum corneum cells and failure to separate
- Gene locus: 1q21
- Gene: profilaggrin, FLG (filaggrin)

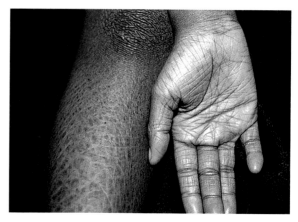

Figure 20.2 Ichthyosis vulgaris associated with hyperlinearity of the palms

Diagnosis

- Clinical presentation
- Histology: absent granular layer and retention hyperkeratosis
- Electron microscopy: abnormally small and crumbly appearing keratohyaline granules

Differential diagnosis

- X-linked ichthyosis in a male
- Sjögren–Larssen syndrome
- Xerosis

Treatment

- Topical keratolytic agents
- α-hydroxyacids
- Moisturize skin with emollients immediately after bathing and frequently through the day

Prognosis

- Life-long disorder with exacerbations in dry (winter) weather

References

Okulicz JF, Schwartz RA. Hereditary and acquired ichthyosis vulgaris. Int J Dermatol 2003; 42: 95–8

Presland RB, Boggess D, Lewis SP, et al. Loss of normal profilaggrin and filaggrin in flaky tail (ft/ft) mice: an animal model for the filaggrin-deficient skin disease ichthyosis vulgaris. J Invest Dermatol 2000; 115: 1072–81

Smack DP, Korge BP, James WD. Keratin and keratinization. J Am Acad Dermatol 1994; 30: 85–102

Williams ML, Elias PM. From basket weave to barrier. Arch Dermatol 1993; 129: 626–9

Zhong W, Cui B, Zhang Y, et al. Linkage analysis suggests a locus of ichthyosis vulgaris on 1q22. J Hum Genet 2003; 48: 390–2

X-linked ichthyosis

Synonym: steroid sulfatase deficiency

Major points

- Incidence: 1 per 2000–6000 males
- Placental steroid sulfatase deficiency syndrome with failure to initiate or progress in labor
- Begins in the first year of life
- Scales large, thick, adherent and dark (dirty appearance) (Figure 20.3)
- Generalized involvement, milder on face
- May involve flexures and neck
- Slightly thickened, scaly palms and soles
- Asymptomatic corneal opacities (50% adult males, some female carriers)
- Cryptorchidism (20%)
- X-linked recessive inheritance (males only)

Pathogenesis

- Cholesterol sulfate in epidermis is built up

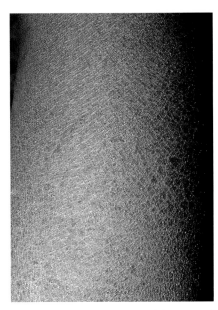

Figure 20.3 X-linked ichthyosis – dark brown scaling on the arms

- Increased adhesiveness of the stratum corneum cells and failure of these cells to separate
- Gene locus: Xp22.32
- Gene: STS (steroid sulfatase)

Diagnosis

- Clinical presentation in a male, often with a positive family history
- Enzyme assay of scale, cultured fibroblasts, keratinocytes or blood leukocytes
- Lipoprotein electrophoresis: rapid mobility of low-density lipoproteins
- Demonstration of gene mutation
- Histology: nondiagnostic; shows retention hyperkeratosis

Differential diagnosis

- Ichthyosis vulgaris
- Sjögren–Larssen syndrome

Treatment

- Topical keratolytic agents: α-hydroxyacids
- Emollients immediately after bathing and frequently through the day
- Increase ambient humidity

Prognosis

- Persistent; worsens in dry weather and may resolve in humid environments
- Risk for testicular carcinoma and hypogonadism

References

Cuevas-Covarrubias SA, Jimenez-Vaca AL, Gonzalez-Huerta LM, et al. Somatic and germinal mosaicism for the steroid sulfatase gene deletion in a steroid sulfatase deficiency carrier. J Invest Dermatol 2002; 119: 972–5

Hernandez-Martin A, Gonzalez-Sarmiento R, De Unamuno P. X-linked ichthyosis: an update. Br J Dermatol 1999; 141: 617–27

Kashork CD, Sutton VR, Fonda Allen JS, et al. Low or absent unconjugated estriol in pregnancy: an indicator for steroid sulfatase deficiency detectable by fluorescence *in situ* hybridization and biochemical analysis. Prenat Diagn 2002; 22: 1028–32

Zettersten E, Man M-Q, Sato J, et al. Recessive X-linked ichthyosis: role of cholesterol-sulfate accumulation in the barrier abnormality. J Invest Dermatol 1998; 111: 784–90

Lamellar ichthyosis

Major points

- Incidence: 1 per 300 000 persons
- Collodion membrane at birth
- Large, dark, plate-like scales (generalized) with fissuring between scales (Figure 20.4)
- Mild erythroderma
- Ectropion
- Eclabium
- Dystrophic nails
- Alopecia
- No abnormality of mucosa or teeth
- Decreased sweating
- Autosomal recessive

Pathogenesis

- Increased cell hyperplasia of the basal cells and increased transit rate through the epidermis
- Decreased transit time of epidermal cells with increased mitotic activity
- Alteration of scale lipids
- Gene defect in transglutaminase 1 (TGM1) that catalyzes cross-linking of proteins in the upper layers of the epidermis
- Gene locus: 14q11.2, 2q33-35, 19p12-q12

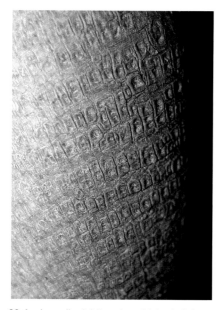

Figure 20.4   Lamellar ichthyosis – thick, dark brown, plate-like scales in an adult

Diagnosis

- Clinical diagnosis
- Histology: massive orthohyperkeratosis and mild/moderate acanthosis
- Genetic testing

Differential diagnosis

- Congenital ichthyosiform erythroderma (nonbullous)
- Sjögren–Larssen syndrome
- Netherton syndrome
- Other ichthyoses

Treatment

- Topical keratolytic agents
- Moisturize skin with emollients immediately after bathing and frequently through the day
- Oral retinoids (isotretinoin, acetretin)
- Increase ambient humidity

Prognosis

- Persistent life-long hyperkeratosis and peeling
- Secondary infection common

References

Akiyama M, Sawamura D, Shimizu H. The clinical spectrum of nonbullous congenital ichthyosiform erythroderma and lamellar ichthyosis. Clin Exp Dermatol 2003; 28: 235–40

Allen DM, Esterly NB. Significant systemic absorption of tacrolimus after topical application in a patient with lamellar ichthyosis. Arch Dermatol 2002; 138: 1259–60

DiGiovanna JJ, Robinson-Bostom L. Ichthyosis: etiology, diagnosis, and management. Am J Clin Dermatol 2003; 4: 81–95

Hennies HC, Kuster W, Wiebe V, et al. Genotype/phenotype correlation in autosomal recessive lamellar ichthyosis. Am J Hum Genet 1998; 62: 1052–61

Huber M, Rettler I, Bernasconi K, et al. Mutations of keratinocyte transglutaminase in lamellar ichthyosis. Science 1995; 267: 525–8

Congenital ichthyosiform erythroderma (nonbullous) (CIE)

Major points

- Born with collodion membrane
- Generalized scaling and erythroderma, not as severe as lamellar ichthyosis (Figure 20.5)

- Scales fine and white on face, trunk and scalp
- Scales large, plate-like and dark on legs
- Ectropion
- Corneal dystrophy
- Sparse hair
- Nail dystrophy
- Small stature (occasional)
- Mental retardation (occasional)

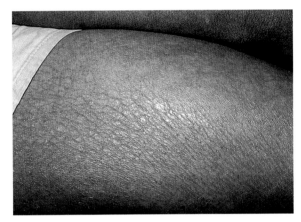

Figure 20.5 Congenital ichthyosiform erythroderma – with erythema and fine scales

Pathogenesis

- Epidermal cell turnover markedly increased; decrease in transit time of epidermal cells
- Autosomal recessive or dominant
- Gene locus: 14q11.2
- Gene: TGM1 (transglutaminase-1)

Diagnosis

- Clinical diagnosis
- Histology: nondiagnostic; focal or extensive parakeratosis and acanthosis

Differential diagnosis

- Lamellar ichthyosis
- Other ichthyoses

Treatment

- Topical keratolytic agents
- Moisturize skin with emollients immediately after bathing and frequently through the day
- Increase ambient humidity

Prognosis

- Persistent, life-long scaling and erythema (can be mild to severe)

References

Akiyama M, Sawamura D, Shimizu H. The clinical spectrum of nonbullous congenital ichthyosiform erythroderma and lamellar ichthyosis. Clin Exp Dermatol 2003; 28: 235–40

Laiho E, Ignatius J, Mikkola H, et al. Transglutaminase 1 mutations in autosomal recessive congenital ichthyosis: private and recurrent mutations in an isolated population. Am J Hum Genet 1997; 61: 529–38

Porter RM, Lane EB. Phenotypes, genotypes and their contribution to understanding keratin function. Trends Genet 2003; 19: 278–85

Williams ML, Elias PM. Enlightened therapy of the disorders of cornification. Clin Dermatol 2003; 21: 269–73

Epidermolytic hyperkeratosis

Synonym: bullous congenital ichthyosiform erythroderma

Major points

- Incidence is 1 per 300 000 births
- Blisters, erosions or erythema at birth
- Generalized scaling develops in later infancy
- Scales are warty, ridged and columnar (Figure 20.6)
- Spontaneous erosions throughout life where scales come off

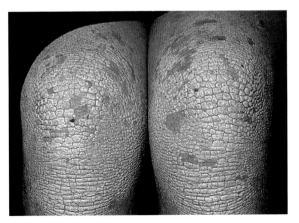

Figure 20.6 Epidermolytic hyperkeratosis with columnar thick odiferous scales

- Prominent keratoderma on the palms and soles
- No ectropion
- Heat intolerance
- Secondary infection common, resulting in malodor
- Autosomal dominant or sporadic

Pathogenesis

- Chromosomes 12q and 17q
- Gene: keratin 1 and 10
- Increased germinative cell hyperplasia of the basal cells and increased transit rate through the epidermis
- Increased transepidermal water loss

Diagnosis

- Clinical presentation
- Histology: characteristic intracellular vacuolar degeneration of upper spinous/granular cell layers and large clumped keratohyalin granules
- Prenatal diagnosis by fetal skin biopsy at 20–22 weeks' gestation

Differential diagnosis

- Lamellar ichthyosis
- Congenital ichthyosiform erythroderma (nonbullous)
- Epidermolysis bullosa at birth
- Incontinentia pigmenti at birth
- Staphylococcal scalded skin syndrome
- Ichthyosis hystrix
- Conradi–Hünermann syndrome
- Other ichthyoses

Treatment

- Increase ambient humidity
- Topical keratolytic agents
- Bathing, add antimicrobial agents to water (e.g. dilute sodium hypochlorite dilution to reduce odor) (See Chapter 21)
- Moisturize skin with emollients immediately after bathing
- Low-dose retinoids (e.g. isotretinoin)
- Support group

Prognosis

- Persistent, life-long scaling
- Malodor is a persistent problem
- Secondary infection is common

References

Nazzaro V, Ermacora E, Santucci B, Caputo R. Epidermolytic hyperkeratosis: generalized form in children from parents with systematized linear form. Br J Dermatol 1990; 122: 417–22

Porter RM, Lane EB. Phenotypes, genotypes and their contribution to understanding keratin function. Trends Genet 2003; 19: 278–85

Schmuth M, Yosipovitch G, Williams ML, et al. Pathogenesis of the permeability barrier abnormality in epidermolytic hyperkeratosis. J Invest Dermatol 2001; 117: 837–47

Siegel DH, Howard R. Molecular advances in genetic skin diseases. Curr Opin Pediatr 2002; 14: 419–25

Smith F. The molecular genetics of keratin disorders. Am J Clin Dermatol 2003; 4: 347–64

Virtanen M, Smith SK, Gedde-Dahl T Jr, et al. Splice site and deletion mutations in keratin (KRT1 and KRT10) genes: unusual phenotypic alterations in Scandinavian patients with epidermolytic hyperkeratosis. J Invest Dermatol 2003; 121: 1013–20

Harlequin ichthyosis

Major points

- Born with massive hyperkeratotic plates resembling the diamond pattern on a harlequin's costume (Figure 20.7)
- Distorted facial features with severe ectropion, eclabium, and rudimentary ears and nose
- Deformities of fingers/toes
- Premature delivery
- Autosomal recessive

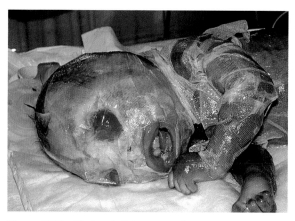

Figure 20.7   Harlequin fetus – massive plate-like scales

Pathogenesis

- Gene locus: 18q21.3
- Genetic heterogeneity and division into three subtypes: in types 1 and 2 profilaggrin is expressed but not processed to filaggrin; type 3 lacks profilaggrin; types 2 and 3 both have keratins 6 and 16 in addition to normal keratins 5/14 and 1/10 seen in all three subtypes

Diagnosis

- Clinical appearance
- Histology: compact orthohyperkeratosis
- Electron microscopy: absence of lamellar bodies
- Prenatal diagnosis by fetal skin biopsy at 20–22 weeks' gestation

Differential diagnosis

- Collodion membrane

Treatment

- Oral retinoids (e.g. isotretinoin, acetretin) within a few days of birth has increased survival in a few patients
- Topical keratolytic agents
- Moisturize skin with emollients immediately after bathing and frequently through the day
- Ophthalmology consultation – important to open eyes to prevent blindness
- Management of fluid and electrolytes

Prognosis

- Very poor, despite treatment
- Most die perinatally from sepsis or massive hyperkeratotic plaques interfering with respiration and feeding
- Survivors shed restrictive scale and develop severe congenital ichthyosiform erythroderma (CIE) phenotype

References

Chan Y-C, Tay Y-K, Tan L K-S, et al. Harlequin ichthyosis in association with hypothyroidism and juvenile rheumatoid arthritis. Pediatr Dermatol 2003; 20: 421–6

Culican SM, Custer PL. Repair of cicatricial ectropion in an infant with harlequin ichthyosis using engineered human skin. Am J Ophthalmol 2002; 134: 442–3

Fleckman P, Hager B, Dale BA. Harlequin ichthyosis keratinocytes in lifted culture differentiate poorly by morphologic and biochemical criteria. J Invest Dermatol 1997; 109: 36–8

Gunes T, Akcakus M, Kurtoglu S, et al. Harlequin baby with ecthyma gangrenosum. Pediatr Dermatol 2003; 20: 529–30

Prasad RS, Pejaver RK, Hassan A, et al. Management and follow-up of harlequin siblings. Br J Derm 1994: 130; 650–3

Singh S, Bhura M, Maheshwari A, et al. Successful treatment of harlequin ichthyosis with acetretin. Int J Dermatol 2001; 40: 472–3

Zeeuwen PL, Dale BA, de Jongh GJ, et al. The human cystatin M/E gene (CST6): exclusion candidate gene for harlequin ichthyosis. J Invest Dermatol 2003; 121: 65–8

Conradi–Hünermann–Happle syndrome

Synonym: X-linked dominant chondrodysplasia punctata

Major points

- Thick scaling in whorl-like pattern (early) following Blaschko lines which clears in 3–6 months, followed by follicular atrophoderma (Figure 20.8)
- Asymmetrical, calcific, epiphyseal stippling by X-ray in newborn
- Unusual facies: flat facies with depressed nasal bridge
- Joint contractures
- Kyphoscoliosis
- Patchy, scarring alopecia
- Dry, lusterless hair

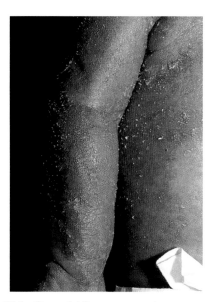

Figure 20.8 Conradi–Hünermann syndrome – hyperkeratotic streaks following Blaschko lines

- Shortening of humeri and femurs
- Asymmetrical skeletal deformities
- Lens opacities, other eye problems
- Normal mentation
- X-linked dominant (seen in girls), or autosomal dominant

Pathogenesis

- Gene locus: Xp11.22-p11.23
- Gene: delta (8)–delta (7) sterol isomerase (emopamil-binding protein)
- Mosaic disorder

Diagnosis

- Clinical presentation
- Genetic testing

Differential diagnosis

- Epidermolytic hyperkeratosis
- Goltz syndrome
- Other ichthyoses

Treatment

- Topical keratolytic agents
- Moisturize skin with emollients immediately after bathing and frequently through the day
- Increase ambient humidity

Prognosis

- Scaling resolves by 12 months, but other features persist

References

Braverman N, Lin P, Moebius FF, et al. Mutations in the gene encoding 3-beta-hydroxysteroid-delta(8),delta(7)-isomerase cause X-linked dominant Conradi–Hunermann syndrome. Nature Genet 1999; 22: 291–4

Bruch D, Megahed M, Majewski F, Ruzicka T. Ichthyotic and psoriasiform skin lesions along Blaschko's lines in a woman with X-linked dominant chondrodysplasia punctata. J Am Acad Dermatol 1995; 33: 356–60

Corbí MR, Conejo-Mir JS, Linares M, et al. Conradi–Hünermann syndrome with unilateral distribution. Pediatr Dermatol 1998; 15: 299–303

Milunsky JM, Maher TA, Metzenberg AB. Molecular, biochemical, and phenotypic analysis of a hemizygous male with a severe atypical phenotype for X-linked dominant Conradi–Hunermann–Happle syndrome and a mutation in EBP. Am J Med Genet 2003; 116A: 249–54

Offiah AC, Mansour S, Jeffrey I, et al. Greenberg dysplasia (HEM) and lethal X linked dominant Conradi–Hunermann chondrodysplasia punctata (CDPX2): presentation of two cases with overlapping phenotype. J Med Genet 2003; 40: 129

Wessels MW, Den Hollander NJ, De Krijger RR, et al. Fetus with an unusual form of nonrhizomelic chondrodysplasia punctata: case report and review. Am J Med Genet 2003; 120A: 97–104

Yanagihara M, Ueda K, Asano N, et al. Usefulness of histopathologic examination of thick scales in the diagnosis of X-linked dominant chondrodysplasia punctata (Happle). Pediatr Dermatol 1996; 13: 1–4

PALMOPLANTAR KERATODERMAS

Major points

- Characteristic thickening of the palms and soles (Figure 20.9)
- Three major patterns: diffuse, focal or punctuate (Figure 20.10)
- Can be inherited (autosomal or recessive) or acquired
- Can be associated with ichthyoses or other abnormalities
- Associated syndromes: Unna–Thost syndrome, Vohwinkel syndrome, pachyonychia congenita, tyrosinemia type II, epidermolytic hyperkeratosis, hidrotic ectodermal dysplasia, and other dermatoses such as psoriasis, atopic dermatitis, etc.

Pathogenesis

- Abnormalities of keratin 1, 9, 16, connexin 26, loricrin, desmoplakin, others

Diagnosis

- Clinical features

Treatment

- Salicylic acid 4–6% in petrolatum (watch for salicylism)
- Mechanical debridement
- Oral retinoids have variable effect

Prognosis

- Persistent, can be progressive

References

Kimyai-Asadi A, Kotcher LB, Jih MH. The molecular basis of hereditary palmoplantar keratodermas. J Am Acad Dermatol 2002; 47: 327–43

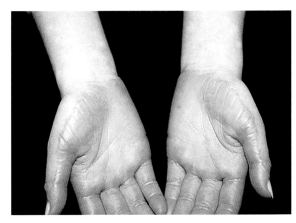

Figure 20.9 Palmoplantar keratoderma with yellow thickened plaques

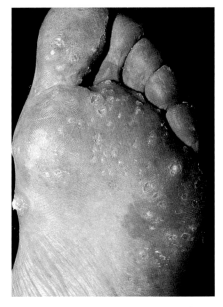

Figure 20.10 Punctate palmoplantar keratoderma

McGrath JA, Eady RA. Recent advances in the molecular basis of inherited skin diseases. Adv Genet 2001; 43: 1–32

McLean WH. Epithelial Genetics Group. Genetic disorders of palm skin and nail. J Anat 2003; 202: 133–41

Paller AS. The molecular basis for the palmoplantar keratodermas. Pediatr Dermatol 1999; 16: 483–5

Richard G. Connexin disorders of the skin. Adv Dermatol 2001; 17: 243–77

Smith F. The molecular genetics of keratin disorders. Am J Clin Dermatol 2003; 4: 347–64

Whittock NV, Ashton GHS, Dopping-Hepenstal PJC, Gratian MJ. Striate palmoplantar keratoderma resulting from desmoplakin haploinsufficiency. J Invest Deramtol 1999; 113: 940–6

Yan AC, Aasi SZ, Alms WJ, et al. Aquagenic palmoplantar keratoderma. J Am Acad Dermatol 2001; 44: 696–9

OTHER GENODERMATOSES

Neurofibromatosis

Major points

- Neurofibromatosis type 1 (von Recklinghausen disease)
  1. Incidence 1 : 3500 of the general population
  2. Characterized by multiple café au lait macules and neurofibromas in the skin, CNS, bones, muscles and endocrine system
  3. Diagnostic criteria (must have two for diagnosis)
     a. ≥6 café au lait macules which are >5 mm (before puberty) and >1.5 cm (after puberty) (Figure 20.11)
     b. Axillary freckling (Crowe sign) (Figure 20.12)
     c. ≥2 Lisch nodules (iris hamartomas)
     d. Distinctive osseous lesion such as sphenoid dysplasia or thinning of long bone cortex with or without pseudarthrosis
     e. Optic glioma
     f. ≥2 neurofibromas or a plexiform neurofibroma (large doughy mass with or without underlying limb hypertrophy which may be present at birth) (Figures 20.13 and 20.14)

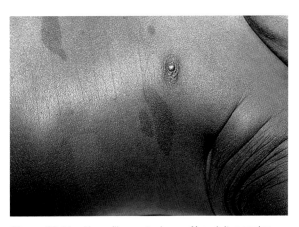

Figure 20.11 Neurofibromatosis – café au lait macules

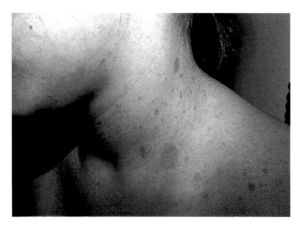

Figure 20.12 Neurofibromatosis – Crowe sign with freckling on neck or axillae

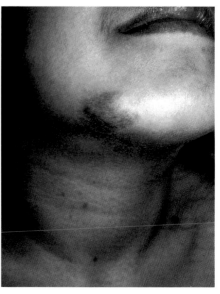

Figure 20.13 Neurofibromatosis – plexiform neurofibroma on chin; also note the café au lait macules on the neck

    g. First-degree relative with neurofibro-
       matosis type 1
  4. Neurologic: learning disorders, mental
    retardation, seizures, intracranial tumors
  5. Ophthalmic: Lisch nodules, proptosis, ptosis,
    optic gliomas, congenital glaucoma
  6. Skeletal: scoliosis, kyphosis, pseudarthrosis,
    macrocephaly, scalloping of vertebrae, short
    stature
  7. Endocrine abnormalities: sexual precocity
  8. Other associations: pheochromocytoma, Wilms
    tumor, leukemia and other malignancies
  9. Autosomal dominant with 50% spontaneous
    mutations
- Neurofibromatosis type 2
  1. Acoustic neuromas of the eighth cranial nerve
    (90% bilateral)
  2. Multiple CNS tumors (various types)
  3. Few café au lait macules or neurofibromas
  4. No axillary freckling
  5. No iris hamartomas (Lisch nodules)
  6. Autosomal dominant

Pathogenesis

- Neurofibromas are caused by loss of a tumor
  suppressor gene with uncontrolled growth of tissues
- Neurofibromatosis type 1
  1. Gene locus: chromosome 17q11.2
  2. Gene: neurofibromin, a protein that acts as a
    negative feedback control for the ras proto-
    oncogene (tumor suppressor gene)
- Neurofibromatosis type 2
  1. Gene locus: 22q12.2

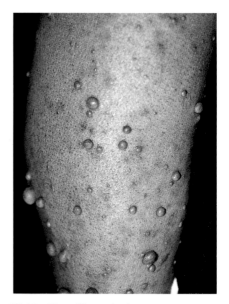

Figure 20.14 Neurofibromatosis – numerous neurofibromas in an adult

  2. Gene: NF2, merlin (Moesin, Ezrin, Radixin-
    Like proteIN)

Diagnosis

- See Major points

Differential diagnosis

- Neurofibromas:
  1. Lipomas
  2. Epidermal cysts
  3. Intradermal nevi
  4. Anetoderma
- Café au lait macules:
  1. McCune–Albright syndrome
  2. Watson syndrome
  3. Bannayan–Riley–Ruvalcaba syndrome
  4. Epidermal nevus syndrome
  5. Proteus syndrome

Treatment

- Annual visits (more frequent, as indicated) with a clinician familiar with neurofibromatosis type 1
- Patients should be followed for complications: optic glioma, neural tumors, developmental disabilities, vascular problems, elevated blood pressure, orthopedic problems, malignancy, psychological problems
- Surgical excision of neurofibromas that are rapidly growing or painful
- Genetic testing is not routine or necessary in the majority of patients
- Specific treatment geared to specific complications

Prognosis

- Type 1: progressive and variable; may be an increase in complications around puberty or pregnancy
- Type 2: deafness usually in adulthood

References

Ablon J. Parents' responses to their child's diagnosis of neurofibromatosis 1. Am J Med Genet 2000; 93: 136–42

Dasgupta B, Gutmann DH. Neurofibromatosis 1: closing the GAP between mice and men. Curr Opin Genet Dev 2003; 13: 20–7

DeBella K, Szudek J, Friedman JM. Use of the National Institutes of Health criteria for diagnosis of neurofibromatosis 1 in children. Pediatrics 2000; 105: 608–14

Dugoff L, Sujansky E. Neurofibromatosis type 1 and pregnancy. Am J Med Genet 1996; 66: 7–10

Drappier J-C, Khosrotehrani K, Zeller J, et al. Medical management of neurofibromatosis 1: a cross-sectional study of 383 patients. J Am Acad Dermatol 2003; 49: 440–4

Gutmann D, Aylsworth A, Carley J, et al. The diagnostic evaluation and multidisciplinary management of neurofibromatosis 1 and neurofibromatosis 2. J Am Med Assoc 1997; 278: 51–7

Evans DGR, Trueman L, Wallace A, et al. Genotype/phototype correlations in type 2 neurofibromatosis (NF2): evidence for more severe disease associated with truncating mutations. J Med Genet 1998; 35: 450–5

Goldberg Y, Dibbern K, Klein J, et al. Neurofibromatosis type 1 – an update and review for the primary pediatrician. Clin Pediatr 1996; 35: 545–61

Johnson NS, Saal HM, Lovell AM, Schorry EK. Social and emotional problems in children with neurofibromatosis type 1: evidence and proposed interventions. J Pediatr 1999; 134: 767–72

Kandt RS. Tuberous sclerosis complex and neurofibromatosis type 1: the two most common neurocutaneous diseases. Neurol Clin 2003; 21: 983–1004

McLaughlin ME, Jacks T. Neurofibromatosis type 1. Methods Mol Biol 2003; 222: 223–37

Task Force: Eichenfield LF, Levy ML, Paller AS, Riccardi VM. Guidelines of care for neurofibromatosis type 1. Academy guidelines. J Am Acad Dermatol 1997; 37: 625–30

Van Es S, North KN, McHugh K, De Silva M. MRI findings in children with neurofibromatosis type 1: a prospective study. Pediatr Radiol 1996; 26: 478–87

Tuberous sclerosis complex

Synonym: Bourneville disease

Major points

- Incidence: 5 per 100 000
- Characterized by a triad of features (commonly, only one or two of these classic features is present):
  1. Adenoma sebaceum (angiofibromas) (>50%)
     a. Begins at ages 2–5 years as pink/red small papules on the cheeks and nasolabial folds and they enlarge slowly over time
  2. Mental retardation in 30–65%; ranges from mild to severe
  3. Seizures or infantile spasms (80%)

Pathogenesis

- Gene locus/gene:
  1. TSC-1, 9q34/ hamartin (tumor suppressor gene)

2. TSC-2, 16p.13.3/ tuberin (GAP protein)
- 50–75% of cases are sporadic

Diagnosis

- Diagnostic criteria (see Table 20.1)
- Examination with a Wood's light can aid in the visualization of the hypopigmented macules in light-skinned individuals
- Examination of family members
- Histology (angiofibroma): dermal fibrosis and vasodilatation
- Histology (shagreen patch): increased collagen and elastin
- MRI can demonstrate CNS hamartomas

Differential diagnosis

- Facial lesions
  1. Acne
  2. Milia
  3. Trichoepitheliomas
  4. Molluscum contagiosum
  5. Seborrheic dermatitis
- Hypopigmented macules
  1. Vitiligo
  2. Nevus depigmentosus
  3. Pityriasis alba
  4. Hypomelanosis of Ito
  5. Nevus anemicus
  6. Postinflammatory hypopigmentation
  7. Tinea versicolor
- Periungual fibromas
  1. Warts
  2. Infantile digital fibromatosis

Treatment

- Hypopigmented macules – none needed
- Adenoma sebaceum: CO_2 laser or other destructive therapy
- Close follow-up by pediatrician and specialists as indicated

Prognosis

- Variable
- Some patients have severe CNS difficulties, some have severe development of angiofibromas, others have only minor stigmata of the disease and are only diagnosed when a family member is diagnosed
- Hypopigmented lesions are static, or become less obvious with time

Table 20.1   Diagnostic criteria for tuberous sclerosis (TSC)

Definite TSC: either one primary feature, two secondary features or one secondary plus two tertiary features

Probable TSC: either one secondary plus one tertiary feature or three tertiary features

Suspect TSC: either one secondary feature or two tertiary features

Primary features

Facial angiofibromas (adenoma sebaceum)
Multiple ungual fibromas
Cortical tuber (histologically confirmed)
Subependymal nodule or giant cell astrocytoma (histologically confirmed)
Multiple calcified subependymal nodules protruding into the ventricle (radiographic evidence)
Multiple retinal astrocytomas

Secondary features

Affected first-degree relative
Cardiac rhabdomyomas (histologic or radiographic confirmation), often multiple
Retinal hamartoma or achromic patch
Cerebral tubers (radiographic confirmation)
Noncalcified subependymal nodules (radiographic confirmation)
Shagreen patch (connective tissue nevus) – most common in lumbar area (Figure 20.15)
Forehead plaque (angiofibromas)
Renal angiomyolipoma (radiographic or histologic confirmation)
Renal cysts (histologic confirmation)
Pulmonary lymphangioleiomyomatosis (histology required)

Tertiary features

Hypomelanotic macules/poliosis (white patches of hair) (Figure 20.16)
Confetti skin lesions
Renal cysts (radiographic evidence)
Randomly distributed enamel pits in teeth
Hamartomatous rectal polyps (histologic confirmation)
Bone cysts (radiographic evidence)
Pulmonary lymphangioleiomyomatosis (radiographic evidence)
Cerebral white matter 'migration tracts' o heterotopias (radiographic evidence)
Gingival fibroma
Hamartoma of the other organs (histologic confirmation)
Infantile spasms

Continued...

Table 20.1   Continued
Other findings
Pneumothorax
Diffuse bronzing
Retinal gliomas
Optic atrophy
Mental retardation
Seizures

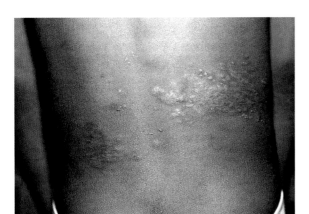

Figure 20.15   Tuberous sclerosis – shagreen patch on lower back

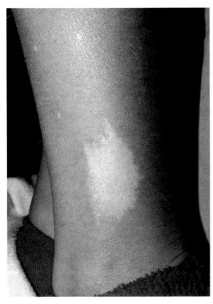

Figure 20.16   Tuberous sclerosis – hypopigmented macules

References

Dahan D, Fenichel GM, El-Said R. Neurocutaneous syndromes. Adolesc Med State Art Rev 2002; 13: 495–509

Kandt RS. Tuberous sclerosis complex and neurofibromatosis type 1: the two most common neurocutaneous diseases. Neurol Clin 2002; 20: 941–64

Kwiatkowski DJ. Tuberous sclerosis: from tubers to mTOR. Ann Hum Genet 2003; 67: 87–96

Narayanan V. Tuberous sclerosis complex: genetics to pathogenesis. Pediatr Neurol 2003; 29: 404–9

Tsao H. Update on familial cancer syndromes and the skin. J Am Acad Dermatol 2000; 42: 939–69

Vanderhooft SL, Francis JS, Pagon RA, et al. Prevalence of hypopigmented macules in a healthy population. J Pediatr 1996; 129: 355–61

Zuvlunov A, Esterly NB. Neurocutaneous syndromes associated with pigmentary skin lesions. J Am Acad Dermatol 1995; 32: 915–35

Basal cell nevus syndrome

Synonyms: nevoid basal cell carcinoma syndrome, Gorlin syndrome

Major points

- Multiple basal cell carcinomas at an early age (Figure 20.17)
- Palmoplantar pits
- Multiple jaw cysts (odontogenic keratocysts) with malignant potential
- Skeletal abnormalities
  1. Spina bifida occulta
  2. Rib anomalies (splayed, bifid, fused, missing, etc.)
  3. Scoliosis
  4. Short fourth metacarpals
  5. Mandibular prognathism
  6. Vertebral anomalies
  7. Pectus excavatum
- Hypertelorism
- Medulloblastoma
- Mental retardation
- Calcification of the falx cerebri
- Agenesis of the corpus callosum
- Frontal bossing
- Autosomal dominant

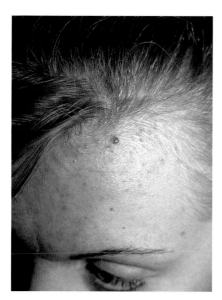

Figure 20.17 Basal cell nevus syndrome – with basal cell carcinoma resembling a nevus

Pathogenesis

- Gene locus: 9q22.3, 9q31
- Gene: PTC1 (patched gene) (PTC protein binds and inhibits transmembrane protein SMOOTHENED (SMO)
- Histology: similar to ordinary basal cell carcinomas

Diagnosis

- Clinical features
- X-rays looking for skeletal abnormalities and odontogenic keratocysts
- Biopsy of suspicious lesion

Differential diagnosis

- Melanocytic nevus
- See Table 17.2

Therapy

- Careful periodic evaluation to assess development of basal cell carcinoma and other abnormalities
- Radiotherapy should be avoided
- Removal of growing lesions
- Sun avoidance, sunscreens
- Genetic counseling

Prognosis

- Slow progression of basal cell carcinomas, jaw cysts
- Depends upon behavior of tumors

References

Barbagallo JS, Kolodzieh MS, Silverberg NB, Weinberg JM. Neurocutaneous disorders. Dermatol Clin 2002; 20: 547–60, viii

Boutet N, Bignon Y-J, Drouin-Garraud V, et al. Spectrum of PTCH1 mutations in French patients with Gorlin syndrome. J Invest Dermatol 2003; 121: 478–81

Kulkarni P, Brashear R, Chuang TY. Nevoid basal cell carcinoma syndrome in a person with dark skin. J Am Acad Dermatol 2003; 49: 332–5

LeSueur BW, Silvis NG, Hansen RC. Basal cell carcinoma in children: report of 3 cases. Arch Dermatol 2000; 136: 370–2

Turner MB, Mallory SB. Nevoid basal cell carcinoma syndrome. Curr Opin Dermatol 1997; 4: 162–7

EHLERS–DANLOS SYNDROME

Synonym: cutis hyperelastica

Major points

- Ehlers–Danlos syndrome I. Gravis type (classic, severe): skin fragility and hyperextensibility; soft, velvety skin; joint hypermobility; easily bruised skin; atrophic scars; varicose veins (Figure 20.18)
  1. Autosomal dominant
  2. Biochemical defect: COL5A1, or COL5A2, or COL1A1
  3. Gene locus: 2q31, 17q21.31-q22, 9q34.2-q34.3
- Ehlers–Danlos syndrome II. Mitis type (classic, mild): similar to type I, but less severe; easily bruised skin; floppy mitral valve; absence of inferior labial frenulum and lingual frenulum
  1. Autosomal dominant
  2. Biochemical defect: COL5A1, COL5A2
  3. Gene locus: 9q34.2-q34.3
- Ehlers–Danlos syndrome III. Hypermobile type: large and small joint hypermobility (marked) and dislocations; soft skin
  1. Autosomal dominant
  2. Biochemical defect: COL3A1 and tenascin-XB
  3. Gene locus: 2q31
- Ehlers–Danlos syndrome IV. Vascular type: arterial, bowel and uterine rupture; marked skin fragility with thin, translucent skin; easily bruised skin; absence of skin and joint extensibility; tendency to form keloids; characteristic facial

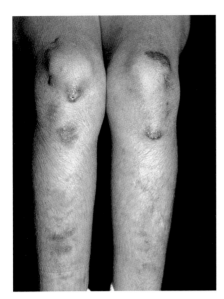

Figure 20.18 Ehlers–Danlos syndrome – pseudotumors from scars

appearance with parchment-like skin and very thin nose; reduced life expectancy
1. Autosomal dominant or autosomal recessive
2. Biochemical defect: abnormal type III collagen (COL 3A1)
3. Gene locus: 2q31
- Ehlers–Danlos syndrome V. X-linked type: similar to EDS type II
1. X-linked recessive
2. Biochemical defect unknown
- Ehlers–Danlos syndrome VI. Ocular-scoliotic type: marked joint and skin involvement; scleral and corneal fragility; keratoconus; intraocular hemorrhage; scoliosis; hypotonia; arterial rupture
1. Autosomal recessive
2. Biochemical defect: lysyl hydroxylase
3. Gene locus: 1p36.3-p36.2
- Ehlers–Danlos syndrome VII. Arthrochalsis multiplex congenita type: extreme joint hypermobility with congenital hip dislocation; short stature; excessive, soft skin particularly on the limbs; normal scarring; micrognathia
1. Autosomal recessive
2. Biochemical defect: COL1A1, COL1A2
3. Gene locus: 17q21.31-q22, 7q22.1
- Ehlers–Danlos syndrome VIII. Periodontal type; moderate joint and skin involvement; periodontitis, gingival regression, tooth loss

1. Autosomal dominant
2. Biochemical defect unknown
- Ehlers–Danlos syndrome X. Fibronectin type: similar to EDS type II; striae distensae; prominent bruising; abnormal clotting studies; normal skin texture
1. Autosomal recessive
2. Biochemical defect: fibronectin-1
3. Gene locus: 2q34

Diagnosis

- Clinical presentation
- Genetic testing
- Histology: large, irregular collagen fibrils in Ehlers–Danlos syndrome types I, II, III

Differential diagnosis

- Cutis laxa
- Normal hypermobility

Treatment

- Protection against injury to skin and joints
- Orthopedic management with physical therapy and braces if needed

Prognosis

- Depends upon type
- Stable or worsens with injury
- Vascular type (Ehlers–Danlos syndrome type IV) has a guarded prognosis, because of vascular or bowel rupture

References

Beighton P. The Ehlers–Danlos syndrome. McKusick's Heritable Disorders of Connective Tissue. Mosby–Year Book: St Louis. MO 1993: 189–251

Byers PH. Ehlers–Danlos syndrome: recent advances and current understanding of the clinical and genetic heterogeneity. J Invest Dermatol 1994; 103: 47S–52S

Byers PH. Ehlers–Danlos syndrome type IV: a genetic disorder in many guises. J Invest Dermatol 1995; 105: 311–13

Dahan D, Fenichel GM, El-Said R. Neurocutaneous syndromes. Adolesc Med State Art Rev 2002; 13: 495–509

Germain DP. Clinical and genetic features of vascular Ehlers–Danlos syndrome. Ann Vasc Surg 2002; 16: 391–7

Henry F, Goffin V, Piérard-Franchimont C, Piérard GE. Mechanical properties of skin in Ehlers–Danlos syndrome, types I, II, and III. Pediatr Dermatol 1996; 13: 464–7

Mao JR, Bristow J. The Ehlers–Danlos syndrome: on beyond collagens. J Clin Invest 2001; 107: 1063–9

Myllyharju J, Kivirikko KI. Collagens and collagen-related diseases. Ann Med 2001; 33: 7–21

Sidhu-Malik NK, Wenstrup RJ. The Ehlers–Danlos syndromes and Marfan syndrome: inherited diseases of connective tissue with overlapping clinical features. Semin Dermatol 1995; 14: 40–6

Cutis laxa

Major points

- Skin hangs in loose folds from birth or may develop during childhood or adolescence and becomes inelastic giving a 'hound dog' appearance
- Generalized elastic tissue abnormality predisposing to:
  1. Inguinal hernias
  2. Lax joints
  3. Bronchiectasis with pulmonary emphysema
  4. Mitral valve prolapse
  5. Aortic aneurysm
  6. Gastrointestinal diverticula
  7. Prolapse of the rectum or uterus
  8. Bladder or urinary tract diverticula

Pathogenesis

- Autosomal dominant (milder) – usually involves skin only
- Mutations in elastin (ELN) or fibulin-5 (FBLN5)
- Gene 14q32.1, 5q23.3-q31.2
- Autosomal recessive (severe): mutation in fibulin-5 (FBLN5) gene

Diagnosis

- Clinical presentation
- Histology: marked fragmentation or diminution of elastic fibers

Differential diagnosis

- Ehlers–Danlos syndrome
- Beare–Stevenson syndrome
- Costello syndrome
- Michelin tire baby syndrome
- Marfan syndrome
- Menkes kinky hair syndrome

Treatment

- None specific
- Surgery for cosmesis

Prognosis

- Slowly progressive

References

Andiran N, Sarikayalar F, Saraclar M, Caglar M. Autosomal recessive form of congenital cutis laxa: more than the clinical appearance. Pediatr Dermatol 2002; 19: 412–14

Baldwin L, Kumrah L, Thoppuram P, Bhattacharji S. Congenital cutis laxa (dermatochalasia) with cardiac valvular disease. Pediatr Dermatol 2001; 18: 365–6

Banks ND, Redett RJ, Mofid MZ, Manson PN. Cutis laxa: clinical experience and outcomes. Plast Reconstruct Surg 2003; 111: 2434–42

Hwang ST, Williams ML, McCalmont TH, Frieden IJ. Sweet's syndrome leading to acquired cutis laxa (Marshall's syndrome) in an infant with a1-antitrypsin deficiency. Arch Dermatol 1995; 131: 1175–7

Orlow SJ. Cutaneous findings in craniofacial malformation syndromes. Arch Dermatol 1992; 128: 1379–86

Sarkar R, Kaur C, Kanwar AJ, Basu S. Cutis laxa in seven members of a north-Indian family. Pediatr Dermatol 2002; 19: 229–31

Pseudoxanthoma elasticum

Major points

- Xanthoma-like papules ('plucked chicken' appearance) found in flexural areas and neck which thicken with age; other areas periumbilical, antecubital fossae, wrists, popliteal fossae
- Small (1–3 mm) yellowish papules in a linear or reticular pattern, may be in confluent plaques (Figure 20.19)
- Perforating lesions with hyperkeratosis (e.g. elastosis perforans serpiginosa)
- Abnormal elastic tissue in arteries
- Hyperextensible skin and joints
- Marfanoid features
- Hypertension
- Cerebrovascular accidents
- Gastrointestinal hemorrhages caused by cracking of calcified vessels
- Cardiovascular disease
- Arteriosclerosis
- Myocardial infarction (can be seen in teenagers)
- Ocular abnormalities:
  1. Angioid streaks in retina (breaks in Bruch membrane)

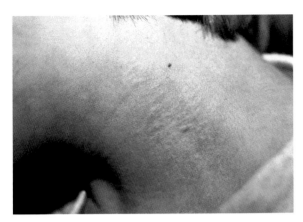

Figure 20.19   Pseudoxanthoma elasticum – firm, yellow papules on the sides of the neck as a presenting sign

2. Loss of vision, drusen, peau d'orange or maculopathy
- Autosomal dominant or recessive

Pathogenesis
- Aberrant calcification of elastic fibers
- Gene locus: 16p13.1
- Gene: ABCC6 (ATP-binding cassette)

Diagnosis
- Major criteria
  1. Characteristic skin involvement
  2. Histology: fragmented elastic tissue, clumped with calcium deposits demonstrated by von Kossa stain; calcification in vessels involving elastic media and intima
  3. Characteristic ocular disease
- Minor criteria
  1. Characteristic histologic features of nonlesional skin
  2. Family history of pseudoxanthoma elasticum in first-degree relative

Differential diagnosis
- Xanthomas
- Connective tissue nevus
- D-Penicillamine-induced skin lesions

Treatment
- Close observation for gastrointestinal hemorrhage and cardiovascular abnormalities
- Surgical excision of abnormal skin rarely indicated
- Possible restriction of calcium in childhood and adolescence

Prognosis
- Depends upon type of psudeoxanthoma elasticum; some have more severe internal involvement than others

References
Balus L, Amantea A, Donati P, et al. Fibroelastolytic papulosis of the neck: a report of 20 cases. Br J Dermatol 1997; 137: 461–6

Hacker SM, Ramos-Caro FA, Beers BB, Flowers FP. Juvenile pseudoxanthoma elasticum: recognition and management. Pediatr Dermatol 1993; 10: 19–25

Lebwohl M, Halperin J, Phelps RG. Brief report: occult pseudoxanthoma elasticum in patients with premature cardiovascular disease. N Engl J Med 1993; 329: 1237–9

Lebwohl M, Neldner K, Pope M, et al. Classification of pseudoxanthoma elasticum: report of a consensus conference. J Am Acad Dermatol 1994; 30: 103–7

Le Saux O, Urban Z, Tschuch C, et al. Mutations in a gene encoding an ABC transporter cause pseudoxanthoma elasticum. Nature Genet 2000; 25: 223–7

Ohtani T, Furukawa F. Pseudoxanthoma elasticum. J Dermatol 2002; 29: 615–20

Uitto J, Pulkkinen L, Ringpfeil F. Progress in molecular genetics of heritable skin diseases: the paradigms of epidermolysis bullosa and pseudoxanthoma elasticum. J Invest Dermatol Symp Proc 2002; 7: 6–16

Gardner syndrome

Major points
- Multiple gastrointestinal polyps (mainly colon) with 100% risk for adenocarcinoma (adolescence to adulthood)
- Osteomas - especially of mandible, maxilla and facial bones
- Epidermal cysts – typical, multiple or large
- Desmoid tumors – most often occur at sites of scars (25%)
- Fibromas (skin, subcutaneous tissues, mesentery)
- Congenital hypertrophy of retinal pigment epithelium – bilateral dark brown patches on fundoscopy
- Autosomal dominant with 100% penetrance

Pathogenesis
- Gene locus: chromosome 5q21-q22
- Gene: APC gene (adenomatous polyposis coli) – a tumor suppressor gene

Diagnosis

- Histology of polyps – adenomatous type
- Histology of epithelial cysts: lined with epithelial cells

Differential diagnosis

- Familial polyposis
- Peutz–Jeghers syndrome
- Cowden syndrome
- Common epidermal cysts
- Bannayan–Riley–Ruvalcaba syndrome

Treatment

- Screening should begin at age 5 years for polyps in family members
- Prophylactic colectomy in teens is recommended
- Surveillance for secondary findings by physician familiar with the disorder
- Desmoid tumors – suggest excision; 50% recurrence rate; sulindac has been reported to result in regression in some patients

Prognosis

1. Poor if colon not removed before cancer begins

References

Armstrong JG, Davies DR, Guy SP, et al. APC mutations in familial adenomatous polyposis families in the northwest of England. Hum Mutat 1997; 10: 376–80

Gregory B, Ho VC. Cutaneous manifestations of gastrointestinal disorders. Part I. J Am Acad Dermatol 1992; 26: 153–66

Herrmann SM, Adler YD, Schmidt-Petersen K, et al. The concomitant occurrence of multiple epidermal cysts, osteomas and thyroid gland nodules is not diagnostic for Gardner syndrome in the absence of intestinal polyposis: a clinical and genetic report. Br J Dermatol 2003; 149: 877–83

Parks ET, Caldemeyer KS, Mirowski GW. Gardner syndrome. J Am Acad Dermatol 2001; 45: 940–2

Quesnel S, Malkin D. Genetic predisposition to cancer and familial cancer syndromes. Pediatr Clin N Amer 1997; 44: 791–808

Rustigi AK. Hereditary gastrointestinal polyposis and nonpolyposis syndromes. N Engl J Med 1994; 331: 1694–702

Cowden disease

Synonym: multiple hamartoma syndrome

Major points

- Can present in childhood with craniomegaly
- Multiple hamartomas of ectodermal, endodermal, and mesodermal origin
- Trichilemmomas (especially facial)
- Facial papules, often grouped around the mouth, nose or ears, usually evident by age 20 years
- Oral papillomatosis (cobblestoning); can be seen in esophagus and duodenum
- Palmoplantar keratoses
- Other findings (seen in teens/adults)
  1. Strong association with malignancy of breast (33%) and thyroid (5%)
  2. Fibrocystic disease of the breast and follicular adenocarcinoma of the breast in women (75%)
  3. Thyroid adenoma or goiter (65%)
  4. Gastrointestinal polyps in both large and small bowel
  5. Ovarian, cervical and uterine cancer
- Autosomal dominant

Pathogenesis

- Gene locus: 10q23.3
- Gene: PTEN – a tumor suppressor gene

Diagnosis

- Clinical findings
- Histology: trichilemmomas which arise from outer root sheath; multiple biopsies may be necessary; keratoses show hyperkeratotic papillomas

Differential diagnosis

- Basal cell nevus syndrome
- Neurofibromatosis
- Gardner syndrome
- Tuberous sclerosis

Treatment

- Close observation for thyroid,breast and gynecologic cancer in females; bladder cancer in males
- Surgical removal of facial papules
- Close follow-up with physician familiar with disorder

Prognosis

- Depends upon complications

References

Eng C. PTEN: one gene, many syndromes. Hum Mutat 2003; 22: 183–98

Hanssen AMN, Fryns JP. Cowden syndrome. J Med Genet 1995; 32: 117–19

Hanssen AMN, Werquin H, Suys E, Fryns JP. Cowden syndrome: report of a large family with macrocephaly and increased severity of signs in subsequent generations. Clin Genet 1993; 44: 281–6

Lynch ED, Ostermeyer EA, Lee MK, et al. Inherited mutations in PTEN that are associated with breast cancer, Cowden disease, and juvenile polyposis. Am J Hum Genet 1997; 61: 1254–60

Marsh DJ, Kum JB, Lunetta KL, et al. PTEN mutation spectrum and genotype-phenotype correlations in Bannayan–Riley–Ruvalcaba syndrome suggest a single entity with Cowden syndrome. Hum Mol Genet 1999; 8: 1461–72

Marsh D, Zori R. Genetic insights into familial cancers–update and recent discoveries. Cancer Lett 2002; 181: 125–64

Tsao H. Update on familial cancer syndromes and the skin. J Am Acad Dermatol 2000; 42: 939–69

Waite KA, Eng C. From developmental disorder to heritable cancer: it's all in the BMP/TGF-beta family. Nature Rev Genet 2003; 4: 763–73

Waite KA, Eng C. Protean PTEN: form and function. Am J Hum Genet 2002; 70: 829–44

Ataxia–telangiectasia

Synomyn: Louis–Bar syndrome

Major points

- Progressive cerebellar ataxia beginning at age ~2 years
- Skin findings
    1. Telangiectasias begin on ears, conjunctiva and flexural folds of extremities usually at about 3–5 years, and progress to malar areas and the V of the chest (Figure 20.20)
    2. Granulomatous plaques (sterile)
    3. Vitiligo
    4. Poliosis
    5. Premature graying of hair
    6. Hypo- or hyperpigmentation
    7. Atrophy of the skin
    8. Chronic skin infections
    9. Acanthosis nigricans

- Frequent sinopulmonary infections: bronchitis, rhinitis, pneumonia, bronchiectasis
    1. Defective cell-mediated: lymphopenia, impaired lymphocyte transformation
    2. Humoral immunity: IgA and IgE deficiency
- Ocular findings
    1. Telangiectasias beginning about age 2–6 years on bulbar conjunctiva
    2. Nystagmus
    3. Strabismus
    4. Blepharitis
- Structural anomalies of thymus and lymph nodes
- Elevated α-fetoprotein
- Progressive mental and neurological deterioration
- Breaks and rearrangements of chromosomes particularly 7, 14
- High incidence of neoplastic disorders (e.g. lymphoma, leukemia, breast carcinomas, etc.) in patients and carriers
- Autosomal recessive; male/female ratio = 1

Pathogenesis

- Caused by a mutation in ATM gene which repairs chromosomal strand breakage
- Gene locus: 11q22
- Gene: ATM

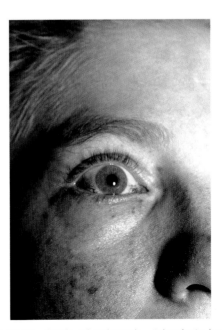

Figure 20.20 Ataxia–telangiectasia – telangiectasias on the conjunctivae

Diagnosis

- Clinical diagnosis with gene verification
- Histology: nonspecific; dilated blood vessels of subpapillary plexus

Differential diagnosis

- Hereditary hemorrhagic telangiectasia
- Angioma serpiginosum
- Generalized essential telangiectasia

Treatment

- Supportive, with antibiotics, respiratory therapy, physical therapy
- Genetic counseling

Prognosis

- Usually fatal in second decade from secondary infections, respiratory failure, or malignancies

References

Barbagallo JS, Kolodzieh MS, Silverberg NB, Weinberg JM. Neurocutaneous disorders. Dermatol Clin 2002; 20: 547–60, viii

De la Torre C, Pincheira J, Lopez-Saez JF. Human syndromes with genomic instability and multiprotein machines that repair DNA double-strand breaks. Histol Histopathol 2003; 18: 225–43

Koenig M. Rare forms of autosomal recessive neurodegenerative ataxia. Semin Pediatr Neurol 2003; 10: 183–92

Perlman S, Becker-Catania S, Gatti RA. Ataxia–telangiectasia: diagnosis and treatment. Semin Pediatr Neurol 2003; 10: 173–82

Swift M, Morrell D, Massey RB, Chase CL. Incidence of cancer in 161 families affected by ataxia – telangiectasia. N Engl J Med 1991; 325:1831–6

Darier disease

Synomyn: keratosis follicularis, Darier–White disease

Major points

- Firm greasy, yellow-brown, crusted papules which coalesce into plaques (Figure 20.21)
- Distribution: scalp, face, seborrheic and flexural areas, dorsa of hands and feet
- Palm and sole keratoses or minute pits
- Malodorous
- Onset usually between 8 and 15 years

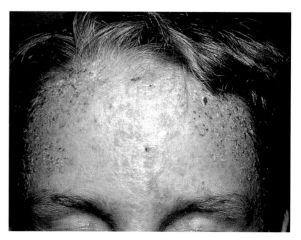

Figure 20.21   Darier disease – scaling on the face resembling seborrheic dermatitis

- Mucous membranes: white cobblestoning which coalesces into plaques; oropharynx, larynx and anorectal mucosa may be involved
- Nail changes: white or red longitudinal bands, V-shaped nicks at distal margin, subungual hyperkeratoses
- T-cell abnormalities in some patients
- Increased susceptibility to infections
- Mental disturbances or mild retardation
- Autosomal dominant, with male/female ratio >1

Pathogenesis

- Gene locus: 12q23-24.1
- Gene: SERCA 2 (ATP 2A2) – plays a role in cell adhesion

Diagnosis

- Clinical findings with classic histology of skin
- Histology: suprabasal acantholysis and dyskeratosis; characteristic corps ronds and corps grains in stratum corneum

Differential diagnosis

- Seborrhea
- Transient acantholytic dermatosis
- Pemphigus foliaceus
- Hailey–Hailey disease

Treatment

- Emollients
- Keratolytic agents

- Intermittent topical steroids for erythema or irritation
- Topical retinoids
- Systemic retinoids
- Antibiotics for secondary infection

Prognosis

- Persistent, chronic dermatosis with exacerbations and partial remissions
- Aggravated by sunlight and heat
- Responds to oral retinoids

References

Burge SM, Wilkinson JD. Darier–White disease: a review of the clinical features in 163 patients. J Am Acad Dermatol 1992; 27: 40–50

Cooper SM, Burge SM. Darier's disease: epidemiology, pathophysiology, and management. Am J Clin Dermatol 2003; 4: 97–105

Devries DT, Warren SJ. Recent advances in intraepidermal blistering diseases. Adv Dermatol 2002; 18: 203–45

Kennedy JL, Berg D, Bassett AS, et al. Genetic linkage for Darier disease (keratosis follicularis). Am J Med Genet 1995; 55: 307–10

Munro CS. The phenotype of Darier's disease: penetrance and expressivity in adults and children. Br J Dermatol 1992; 127: 126–30

O'Malley MP, Haake A, Goldsmith L, Berg D. Localized Darier disease. Implications for genetic studies. Arch Dermatol 1997; 133: 1134–8

Peacocke M, Christiano AM. Bumps and pumps, SERCA 1999. Nature Genet 1999; 21: 252–3

21

THERAPY

TOPICAL THERAPY

Major points

- Treatment should be simple
- Teach patients how to apply medications
- Write prescriptions for steroids in sizes of tubes (e.g. 15, 30, 45, 60, 90, 120 g), not just 'trade size'
  1. Patient may receive too little or too much medicine if not written correctly
  2. Include the diagnosis in addition to instructions so that there is no confusion (e.g. 'Apply at bedtime for acne')
- Thin application is desirable for most medicines except emollients, where thick application is preferred
- Apply moisturizers to damp skin to retain hydration
- Estimates of coverage of the skin can be made by using the 'Rule of Nines', in which the body surface is divided into 11 equal parts, each constituting ~9% of the total body surface area
  1. Head
  2. Arm (one)
  3. Chest (anterior)
  4. Back
  5. Abdomen
  6. Buttocks, lumbar area
  7. Leg (half each)
- Each area can be covered by ~2 g of cream or ointment (See Table 21.1)
- Factors which increase percutaneous absorption of a medication:
  1. Inflammation
  2. Hydration (after a bath)

3. Occlusion with plastic wraps, or diapers
4. Epidermal breakage or injury
5. Heat
6. Type of vehicle
- Topical agents are composed of: active medication and vehicle

VEHICLES

- Vehicles have a profound impact on the medication's delivery and stability

Table 21.1	Amount of medicine to dispense	
Area	One application in grams	BID application for 2 weeks in grams
Face	2	60
Hands	2	60
Head	2	60
Groin	2	60
One arm	3	80
Anterior chest	3	80
Back	3	80
One leg	4	120
Whole body	30–60	840–1680

Adapted from Weston WL, Lane AT, Morelli JG. Color Textbook of Pediatric Dermatology. Mosby: St Louis, 1996: 358

Ointments

- Simplest lubricating vehicle
- Ointments are oleaginous pure greases (e.g. petrolatum, lanolin) or greases with a small amount of water suspended in them
- Leave a greasy film on the skin, causing heat retention and water retention
- Indications:
  1. Dry, cracked skin (atopic dermatitis)
  2. Scaling (psoriasis)
  3. Lubrication
- Do not use (as a general rule of thumb):
  1. Moist skin areas (axillae, groin)
  2. Hot humid environments
- Disadvantages: messy, stains clothing (e.g. petrolatum)
- Advantages: fewest inactive ingredients (i.e. fewer sensitizing agents)

Creams

- Emulsion of water and oil plus chemical emulsifiers, preservatives and fragrances
- Creams require preservatives and stabilizers because of the addition of water
- Easier to use than ointments and cosmetically more acceptable
- Less occlusive than an ointment
- Indications:
  1. Dry skin in humid climates
  2. Semifold areas (antecubital area and neck)
  3. Face
- Do not use:
  1. Hairy scalp (in general)
  2. If allergic or sensitive to preservatives in a specific product

Emollient creams

- Generally more oily than nonemollient types
- Smooth application
- More moisturizing than creams

Solutions

- Solutions contain alcohol and propylene glycol with the active ingredient
- Completely evaporate, leaving the active medication on the skin

- Indications:
  1. Scalp
  2. Hairy areas
  3. Moist areas (toewebs)
- Do not use:
  1. Broken skin (causes stinging)
  2. Very dry skin

Lotions

- Lotions are mainly water with some lipids added
- Indications:
  1. Mild dry skin
  2. Moist folds
- Examples: Keri Lotion, Lubriderm, Eucerin Lotion, numerous others

Aerosols, sprays, and foams

- These products are solutions with a propellant system
- Indications:
  1. Scalp: with a small tubular applicator nozzle, aerosols are easy to use on the scalp
  2. Body: can cover large areas with a very fine coat of medication (e.g. insect repellents)
- Advantages
  1. Cosmetically elegant
  2. Convenient, easy to use
- Disadvantages: may be drying and irritating

Gels

- Gelled propylene glycol solutions which liquify on contact with skin
- Advantages:
  1. Permit good penetration of medications
  2. Leave little residue
- Disadvantage: very drying
- Indications:
  1. Facial dermatoses
  2. Scalp dermatoses
- Do not use on irritated or broken skin (causes stinging)
- Examples: tretinoin gel, steroid gels

Tape/plasters

- Tape impregnated with medicament
- Advantage

1. Stays in place
- Indications:
  1. Thickened, pruritic plaques of lichen simplex chronicus
  2. Warts
- Examples: Cordran tape, salicylic acid plasters

Shake lotions

- Liquid preparation to which powder has been added
- Must be shaken to suspend the powder in solution
- Antipruritics (menthol, camphor) often added
- Examples: calamine lotion
- Indications:
  1. Mild cooling and soothing effect
  2. Weeping, oozing dermatitis (e.g. poison ivy dermatitis)

Pastes

- Creams or ointments with powder added
- Disadvantages: thick and stiff in consistency
- Indications: barrier cream
- Example: zinc oxide paste

Powders

- Consist of fine particles of talc
- Indications:
  1. Increased surface area with a drying effect
  2. Moist sweaty areas (axillae, groin, feet)
  3. Reduce friction
- Examples: nystatin powder, Zeasorb AF
- Disadvantage: delivery of medication relatively poor

Oils

- Oily monophasic solution
- Examples: mineral oil, Dermasmoothe Oil

Oil-free products

- All avoid ingredients with the word 'oil'; however, may contain oils or fats which do not contain the word 'oil' (e.g. lanolin)
- May contain waxes or oily hydrocarbons
- Disadvantage: can be drying

- Borderline oil-free products, although not technically oils or fats, can contain oil-like emollient esters which may be comedogenic

PRODUCTS AND TREATMENT

Wet dressings

- Indications
  1. Useful for first 24–72 hours of an acute weeping dermatitis
  2. Evaporation of water is cooling, causing vasoconstriction
  3. Relief of pruritus by increasing humidity
  4. Helps remove crusts
- Examples: water, saline
- Examples:
  1. Burow's solution (aluminum acetate) for a more drying effect (e.g. Bluboro powder, Boropak powder, Domeboro powder or tablets)
  2. Dakin's solution (sodium hypochlorite) for antisepsis (strengths: 0.25%, 0.5%)
  3. Oatmeal bathing products (e.g. Aveeno)

Topical corticosteroids

- Potency of topical steroids (Table 21.2) based on vasocontriction assay, roughly corresponds to anti-inflammatory properties
- Indications: inflammatory skin disorders (steroids cause vasoconstriction and prevent inflammation)
  1. Low potency
     a. Ideal in infants
     b. Adults/teens – face, intertriginous, genitals
  2. Mid-potency
     a. Atopic dermatitis
     b. Psoriasis
  3. High potency/ultrapotency
     a. Palms and soles
     b. Psoriasis if thickened plaques
     c. Lichen simplex chronicus
     d. Acute contact dermatitis (e.g. poison ivy dermatitis)
  4. High-potency and ultrapotency topical steroids should not be used in children except in short courses for specific conditions
- Dose:
  1. Use a mid-strength steroid twice daily for 3–10 days until symptoms have subsided, then

Table 21.2 Potency of topical steroids	
Brand name	**Generic name**
Group I (ultrapotent)	
Cormax Ointment 0.05%	Clobetasol propionate
Cormax Scalp Solution 0.05%	Clobetasol propionate
Cordran Tape 4 µg/cm^2	Flurandrenolide
Diprolene Cream, Ointment, Gel 0.05%	Betamethasone dipropionate
Olux Foam 0.05%	Clobetasol propionate
Psorcon Ointment 0.05%	Diflorasone diacetate
Temovate Cream, Ointment, Gel,	Clobetasol propionate
E Emollient Cream 0.05%	
Ultravate Cream, Ointment 0.05%	Halobetasol propionate
Group II (potent)	
Cyclocort Ointment 0.1%	Amcinonide
Diprolene AF Cream 0.05%	Betamethasone dipropionate
Diprosone Ointment 0.05%	Betamethasone dipropionate
Elocon Ointment 0.1%	Mometasone furoate
Florone Ointment 0.05%	Diflorasone diacetate
Halog Cream, Oint., Sol., Emollient Cream 0.1%	Halcinonide
Kenalog Ointment 0.5%	Triamcinolone acetonide
Lidex Cream, Gel, Ointment, Gel 0.05%	Fluocinonide
Topicort Ointment, Cream 0.25%	Desoximetasone
Topicort Gel 0.05%	Desoximetasone
Group III (high mid-strength)	
Aristocort A Ointment 0.1%	Triamcinolone acetonide
Aristocort-HP Ointment	Triamcinolone acetonide
Cutivate Ointment 0.05%	Fluticasone propionate
Cyclocort Cream and Lotion 0.1%	Amcinonide
Florone Cream 0.05%	Diflorasone diacetate
Halog Ointment 0.1%	Halcinonide
Lidex E Cream 0.05%	Fluocinonide
Topicort LP Cream 0.05%	Desoximetasone
Valisone Ointment 0.1%	Betamethasone valerate
Group IV (middle mid-strength)	
Aristocort 0.1% Cream	Triamcinolone acetonide
Cordran Ointment 0.05%	Flurandrenolide
Dermatop Ointment 0.1%	Prednicarbate
Elocon Cream, Lotion 0.1%	Mometasone furoate
Kenalog Cream, Ointment 0.1%	Triamcinolone acetonide
Luxiq Foam 0.12%	Betamethasone valerate
Synalar Ointment 0.025%	Fluocinolone acetonide
Westcort Ointment 0.2%	Hydrocortisone valerate

Continued...

reduce to once daily, eventually weaning off medication; emollients are often helpful

2. Face and groin:
  a.   Only use low-potency steroids, class VI, VII (e.g. hydrocortisone 1–2.5%)

  b.   Prone to atrophy, striae and telangiectasias

3. Tachyphylaxis can occur with high-potency/ultrapotent steroids
  a.   Caused by intense vasoconstriction, followed by rebound vasodilatation

Table 21.2 Continued

Brand name	Generic name
Group V (low mid-strength)	
Aclovate Cream, Ointment 0.05%	Alclometasone dipropionate
Cordran Cream, Lotion 0.05%	Flurandrenolide
Cutivate Cream 0.05%	Fluticasone propionate
Dermatop Cream 0.1%	Prednicarbate
Kenolog Cream, Lotion 0.1%	Triamcinolone acetonide
Locoid Cream, Ointment, Solution 0.1%	Hydrocortisone butyrate
Synalar Cream 0.025%	Fluocinolone acetonide
Westcort Cream 0.2%	Hydrocortisone valerate
Dermatop Cream 0.1%	Prednicarbate
Group VI (low strength)	
Aclovate Cream, Ointment 0.05%	Alclometasone dipropionate
DesOwen Cream, Lotion, Ointment 0.05%	Desonide
Synalar Cream, Solution 0.01%	Fluocinolone acetonide
Tridesilon Cream 0.05%	Desonide
Group VII (lowest strength)	
Hytone 0.5%, 1%, 2.5%, dexamethasone	Hydrocortisone 0.5%, 1%, 2.5%

  b. Most commonly occurs on the face
      (causing perioral dermatitis or steroid
      rosacea)
- Monitor:
  1. Adrenal axis suppression can occur with
      long-term or overuse of mid- or high-potency,
      or ultrapotent topical steroids
  2. Limit total dosage to <50 g/week in adult/teen
  3. Steroid addiction
      a. Results from prolonged use of mid-strength
          or high-potency steroids, particularly on
          the face
      b. With discontinuation, rebound
          vasodilatation occurs, resulting in patients'
          continuing to apply steroid for relief
      c. With prolonged use, permanent redness,
          thinning and fine wrinkling, and acne can
          result
      d. Treatment – substitute a bland ointment
          and wean down to lower-potency steroids
          with eventual discontinuance
- Disadvantages/side-effects – accentuated with
  higher concentrations
  1. Atrophy manifestations
      a. Thinning of skin/wrinkling
      b. Translucency of skin

  c. Telangiectasias
  d. Striae
  e. Hypopigmentation
  f. Glaucoma when used on eyelids
  2. Occlusion increases penetration and increases
      potency

Oral corticosteroids

- Indications: inflammatory dermatoses, bullous
  dermatoses, urticaria, immunosuppressive therapy
- Types of oral corticosteroids:
  1. Prednisolone (Delta-Cortef, Prelone,
      Pediapred, others)
      a. Supplied: Prelone 15 mg/5 ml; Pediapred
          5 mg/5 ml; tabs: 5 mg
  2. Dexamethasone
      a. Supplied: tabs: 0.25, 0.5, 0.75, 1, 1.5, 2, 4,
          6 mg; liquid: 0.5 mg/5 ml; 0.1 mg/ml;
          1 mg/ml
      b. Dose: child: 0.08–0.3 mg/kg/24 hours
          given every 6–12 hours; adults:
          0.75–9 mg/24 hours
  3. Prednisone
      a. Supplied: Tabs: 1, 2.5, 5, 10, 20, 50 mg;
          liquid: 1 mg/ml, 5 mg/ml

b. Dose: 0.5–2 mg/kg per 24 hours given once daily to four times a day
4. Equivalents:
    a. Prednisone 5 mg = 0.75 mg dexamethasone
5. Stress dose (prednisolone/prednisone): 8–24 mg/m^2/24 hours (approximately 3 mg/day in a 6-month-old) divided BID, given during stressful event, fever, surgery

Intralesional corticosteroids

- Indications: keloids, alopecia areata
- Dose
  1. Keloids: 10–40 mg/ml
  2. Alopecia areata 2.5–5 mg/ml
- Supplied: triamcinolone 3 mg/ml, 10 mg/ml, 25 mg/ml, 40 mg/ml
- Monitor: atrophy, hypopigmentation (usually not permanent)

Anthralin

- Consists of tricyclic hydrocarbons made from the reduction of anthraquinone
- Indications:
  1. Antimitotic effect on epidermis
  2. Psoriasis
- Supplied: 0.1%, 0.25%, 0.5%, 1% cream (Drithocreme)
- Dose:
  1. Apply 1–2 times/day
  2. Short contact therapy
     a. Apply to affected area for 5–10 minutes once daily
     b. Wash off with a pH-neutral soap (e.g. Dove)
     c. Start with mid-strength cream and advance in strength and time of exposure as tolerated
- Disadvantages:
  1. Stains clothing and skin
  2. Difficult to use, especially over large areas
  3. Irritating
  4. Avoid mucosal contact

Tar

- Derived from distillation of coal
- Indications: anti-inflammatory, keratolytic, antipruritic, antimitotic

1. Psoriasis
2. Eczema
- Dose: apply BID, in direction of hair growth (not against, in order to avoid tar folliculitis)
- Supplied:
  1. Crude coal tar (CCT) 1–10% USP, compound in petrolatum or other base
  2. Tar gels (e.g. Estar 5%, Psorigel 17.5%)
     a. Clear and light brown
     b. Equivalent to CCT 5%
     c. Should be covered with an emollient (e.g. petrolatum) afterwards, as these products by themselves are drying
  3. Liquor carbonis detergens (LCD): an alcoholic extract of coal tar
     a. LCD 5%–10% equivalent to CCT 1%–2%
     b. Must be compounded
  4. Tar shampoos: apply to wet hair and leave on for 5–10 minutes; then rinse
  5. Tar oils
     a. Apply to skin 1–2 times/day
     b. Supplied (over the counter OTC): Cutar Emulsion 1.5%, Doak Tar Oil 2%
  6. Tar bath oils
     a. Add to bath water, soak for 10–20 minutes
     b. Supplied: Balnetar (2.5% coal tar)
- Disadvantages: stains skin and clothing, malodorous

Calcipotriene

- Calcipotriene is a synthetic analog of vitamin D$_3$
- Indications: psoriasis, morphea
- Dose: apply BID, thin application; do not use on face
- Examples: Dovonex 0.005% ointment, cream (30 g, 60 g, 100 g), scalp solution (60 ml)
- Disadvantages: burning and itching, expensive

Moisturizers with or without keratolytics

- Indications: dry skin (xerosis)
- Dose: apply 2–4 times/day as needed
- Disadvantages:
  1. Frequent application necessary
  2. Moisturizers contain water; preservatives are necessary to avoid contamination and contact dermatitis may occur
  3. Stinging

- Examples:
  1. Urea cream and lotions: cream 10% (AquaCare, Nutraplus), cream 20% (Carmol 20), lotion 10% (Nutraplus, AquaCare, Carmol 10)
  2. Lactic acid-containing lotions: 5% (Lacticare), 12% ammonium lactate (Lac-Hydrin – Rx), 6 % ammonium lactate (Lac-Hydrin – OTC)
  3. Lactic acid plus urea: Eucerin Plus Creme and Lotion (2.5% lactic acid plus 10% urea)
  4. α-Hydroxyacids (glycolic acid): Alpha Hydrox (7% glycolic acid), Curel Alpha Hydroxy Dry Skin Lotion, Aqua Glycolic (6% glycolic acid)
  5. Bath oils: RoBathol, Lubriderm Bath Oil, Alpha Keri Bath Oil, Neutrogena Sesame Seed Body Oil

Keratolytic agents

- Indications:
  1. Enhance stratum corneum desquamation
  2. Used to remove the superficial or thick scale in psoriasis, ichthyosis, keratosis pilaris or warts
- Disadvantages:
  1. Irritating; care should be used when applying them to the skin or scalp
  2. Systemic absorption of potentially toxic products may occur. Limit to <10% of skin surface area
- Examples:
  1. Scalp preparations:
     a. Massage into scalp and leave on overnight under a shower cap. As an alternative, leave on scalp for several hours before shampooing it out
     b. DermaSmoothe/FS (fluocinolone acetonide 0.01% in peanut oil, mineral oil)
     c. P&S Oil (< 1% phenol and saline solution)
     d. Mineral oil plus salicylic acid
  2. Topical keratolytic agents:
     a. Salicylic acid 0.5–6%. Can be compounded to preparations with creams or emollients. Keralyt Gel (salicylic acid 6%)
     b. Whitfield's Ointment USP (salicylic acid 3%, benzoic acid 6% in polyethylene glycol ointment) – OTC
     c. MG 217 Sal-Acid Ointment (3% salicylic acid) – OTC

     d. Salicylic acid preparations for warts: liquid or plasters: 14–40%, Mediplast 40%, Doctor Scholl's
     e. Acne washes 1–2% for acne preparations: Neutrogena Acne Wash
     f. Kerasal
  3. Lactic acid: see Moisturizers
  4. α-Hydroxyacids: see Moisturizers

Cleansers/soaps

- Indications:
  1. Help remove oil and dirt from skin
  2. Antibacterial or deodorant soaps help reduce bacteria concentrations on the skin
- Disadvantages:
  1. All soaps are irritating to broken skin
  2. Most soaps are drying and irritating
- Doses:
  1. In sensitive skin, neutral pH is preferred
  2. Examples of soap substitutes or mild soaps: Dove (unscented), Oil of Olay Bar, cetyl alcohol cleanser (Cetaphil, Aquanil), Purpose Gentle Cleansing Wash, Moisturel Sensitive Skin Cleanser, Cetaphil cleansing bar, Aveeno products (colloidal oatmeal)

Shampoos

- Shampoos contain water, sodium lauryl sulfate (emulsifier), dispersing agents and fragrance
- Indications:
  1. Helps remove oil, dirt and scale from the scalp
  2. Dandruff shampoos can be keratolytic and suppress inflammation and epidermal turnover
- Dose:
  1. Medicated shampoos: apply to scalp, leave on for 5–10 minutes, then rinse
- Disadvantages: all shampoos are irritating and drying
- Supplied:
  1. Examples of less irritating shampoos are: Free and Clear
  2. Medicated shampoos
     a. Selenium sulfide 1% (Selsun Blue - OTC), 2.5% (Selsun, Exsel- Rx)
     b. Zinc pyrithione (Head & Shoulders, Zincon, Denorex, DHS Zinc)

c. Ketaconazole (Nizoral 2% – Rx, 1% – OTC)
d. Tar shampoos 0.5–2% tar (Sebutone, TGel, DHS-T, Zetar, Ionil-T, Pentrax, Tegrin, Vanseb-T, X-SebT)
e. Keratolytic shampoos – help soften scales
   i   Salicylic acid 2% plus sulfur 2% (Sebulex, Ionil, Vanseb)
   ii P&S Shampoo
   iii TSal shampoo
f. Steroid shampoo (Rx) – Capex Shampoo

Antiperspirants

- Antiperspirants are liquid aluminum chloride hexahydrate in alcohol
- Indications: decrease sweating and odor; works by plugging sweat ducts
- Dose: apply at night; can cover with plastic wrap on hands and feet
- Examples: Drysol 20%, Xerac AC 6.25%

Sunscreens

- Important factors
  1. Sun protection factor (SPF) is the ratio of time it takes to develop erythema with the sunscreen applied compared to the time it takes to develop erythema without the sunscreen. For example, SPF 10 means a person can theoretically spend 10 times longer in the sun without developing a sunburn. People with skin that burns easily (type I) should use the most protection, SPF >15. For heavy sun exposure, SPF >30 is advised
  2. Vehicle: determines whether sunscreen is waterproof, or water resistant
  3. Reapply sunscreen especially after swimming or sweating
  4. With the regular use of an SPF 15 sunscreen during the first 18 years of life, the lifetime incidence of nonmelanoma skin cancers has been estimated to be reduced by 78%
  5. Contact dermatitis to sunscreens can be caused by either the chemical or the vehicle. Treat with topical steroids, or if severe, a short course of oral steroids (5–7 days)
- Ingredients in sunscreens:
  1. Para-aminobenzoic acid (PABA) and PABA esters – partial UVB and no UVA protection
  2. Cinnamates – full UVB protection
  3. Benzophenones – UVB and partial UVA protection
  4. Salicylates – full UVB, and no UVA
  5. Avobenzone (Parsol 1789) – UVA, no UVB
  6. Titanium dioxide and zinc oxide – physical sunblocks: entire UVB, UVA, visible light protection
- Types of sunscreen
  1. Physical barriers reflect and scatter UVB (e.g. titanium dioxide, zinc oxide; recommended especially for extremely sun-sensitive individuals
  2. UVB blockers (e.g. para-aminobenzoic acid (PABA) and its derivatives)
  3. UVA blockers (e.g. benzophenone)

COMMONLY USED DRUGS IN DERMATOLOGY

(Some of the indications are off-label – refer to Physician Desk Reference for indications)

Antihistamines

- Cetirizine (Zyrtec)
  1. Dose: 2–6 years: 2.5 mg daily; maximum 5 mg daily; >6 years: 5–10 mg daily
  2. Supplied: 5 mg/5ml; 5 mg, 10 mg
- Clemastine (Tavist-1)
  1. Dose: >6 years: 1–3 tsp BID
  2. Supplied: 0.67 mg/5 ml, 1.34 mg (OTC), 2.68 mg (Rx)
- Cyproheptadine (Periactin)
  1. Dose: 2–5 years: 2 mg BID–TID; 6–12 years: 4 mg BID–TID
  2. Supplied: 4 mg, 2 mg/5 ml
- Desloratadine (Clarinex)
  1. Dose: ≥12 years: 5 mg daily
  2. Supplied: 5 mg
- Diphenhydramine (Benadryl)
  1. Dose: 5 mg/kg per 24 hours PO, IV, IM given every 6–8 hours maximum 300 mg/24 hours
  2. Supplied: 12.5 mg/5 ml, 25 mg, 50 mg
- Fexofenadine (Allegra)
  1. Dose: 6–11 years: 30 mg BID; >12 years: 60 mg BID or 180 mg daily
  2. Supplied: 30 mg, 60 mg, 180 mg
- Hydroxyzine (Atarax, Vistaril)

1. Dose: <6 years, 2 mg/kg/24 hours divided every 6–8 hours >6 years 10–100 mg every 6 hours
2. Supplied: 10 mg/5 ml, 10 mg, 25 mg, 50 mg
- Loratadine (Claritin)
    1. Dose: >5 years: 5–10 mg daily
    2 Supplied: 5 mg/5 ml, 10 mg

Antibiotics

- Amoxicillin (Amoxil)
    1. Dose: child: 20–40 mg/kg per 24 hours divided TID; Adult 250 mg TID
    2. Supplied: 125 mg/5 ml, 250 mg/5 ml, 250 mg, 500 mg, 875 mg
- Ampicillin (Omnipen, Principen, Totacillin)
    1. Dose: child: 50–100 mg/kg per 24 hours, given every 6 hours; adult 250–500 mg PO, IM, IV given every 6 hours
    2. Supplied: 125 mg/5 ml, 250 mg/5 ml
- Augmentin (amoxicillin plus clavulanic acid)
    1. Dose: child: 20–40 mg/kg per 24 hours, divided TID; adult: 250–500 mg BID–TID
    2. Supplied: 200 mg/5 ml, 400 mg/5 ml, 250 mg, 500 mg
- Azithromycin (Zithromax)
    1. Dose: child (6 months–12 years) 5–12 mg/kg per 24 hours; adult 500 mg daily once; then 250 mg daily for 4 days
    2. Supplied: 100 mg/5 ml, 200 mg/5 ml, 100 mg, 250 mg; Z–Pak: 500 mg for 1 day, then 250 mg daily for 4 days; Tri-Pak: 500 mg daily for 3 days
    3. Comments: take on empty stomach; hepatic excretion
- Cefaclor (Ceclor)
    1. Dose: 20–40 mg/kg per 24 hours given TID, adult: 250–500 mg TID
    2. Supplied: 125 mg/5 ml, 250 mg/5 ml, 250 mg, 500 mg
- Cefadroxil (Duricef)
    1. Dose: child: 30 mg/kg per 24 hours; give BID; adult: 500 mg BID
    2. Supplied: 125 mg/5 ml, 250 mg/5 ml, 500 mg/5 ml, 500 mg, 1000 mg
- Cephalexin (Keflex)
    1. Dose: child: 25–50 mg/kg per 24 hours; adult: 250–500 mg every 6 hours or QID
    2. Supplied: 125 mg/5 ml, 250 mg/5 ml, 250 mg, 500 mg
- Ciprofloxacin (Cipro)
    1. Dose: 250–750 mg every 12 hours
    2. Supplied: 250 mg/5 ml, 500 mg/5 ml, 100 mg, 250 mg, 500 mg, 750 mg
    3. Interactions: antacids, sucralfate, Fe, Zn, theophylline, warfarin, cyclosporine
- Clarithromycin (Biaxin)
    1. Dose: child: 7.5–15 mg/kg every 12 hours; adult: 250–500 mg BID
    2. Supplied: 125 mg/5 ml, 250 mg/5 ml, 250 mg, 500 mg
- Clindamycin
    1. Dose: child: 8–25 mg/kg per 24 hours divided TID–QID; adult: 150–450 mg QID
    2. Supplied: 75 mg, 150 mg, 300 mg, 75 mg/5 ml
- Cloxacillin (Cloxapen)
    1. Dose: 50 mg/kg per 24 hours (given every 6 hours); adult: 250–500 mg every 6 hours
    2. Supplied: 125 mg/5 ml, 250 mg, 500 mg
- Diaminodiphenylsulfone (Dapsone)
    1. Dose: child:1–2 mg/kg per 24 hours given 1–2 times a day; adult: 25–150 mg per 24 hours
    2. Supplied: 25 mg, 100 mg
    3. Side-effects: methemoglobinemia, peripheral neuropathy, drug interactions, agranulocytosis
    4. Monitor:
        a. Baseline CBC, glucose-6-phosphate dehydrogenase (G6PD), complete metabolic panel, neurologic evaluation;
        b. CBC every week for 4 weeks, then once a month for 6 months, then every 6 months
        c. Complete metabolic panel and neurologic examination every 3–4 months
- Dicloxacillin (Dynapen)
    1. Dose:child: 12.5–50 mg/kg per 24 hours, given QID; adult: 125–500 mg QID
    2. Supplied: 62.5 mg/5 ml, 250 mg, 500 mg
- Doxycycline (Doryx, Monodox, Vibramycin, Vibr-Tabs)
    1. Dose: child: 3–5 mg/kg per 24 hours; given BID; adult: 50–200 mg/24 hours, given BID
    2. Supplied: 25 mg/5 ml, 50 mg/5 ml, 50 mg, 100 mg
    3. Side-effects: phototoxicity, dizziness, esophagitis
- Erythromycin
    1. Dose: child: 50 mg/kg per 24 hours divided QID; adult: 250–500 mg QID
    2. Supplied: Eryped (EES) 200 mg/5 ml, 400 mg/5 ml, 400 mg; E-mycin 250 mg, 333 mg, 500 mg

3. Side-effects: nausea
- Minocycline (Dynacin, Minocin, Vectrin)
  1. Dose: 2–4 mg/kg per 24 hours; 50–100 mg BID
  2. Supplied: 50 mg/5 ml, 50 mg, 100 mg
  3. Side-effects: discoloration of skin, teeth, pseudotumor cerebri
- Nafcillin (Unipen)
  1. Dose: 250–1000 mg every 4–6 hours IV or IM
  2. Supplied: 500 mg, 1000 mg powder for injection
  3. Side-effects: nephrotoxicity
- Oxacillin (Bactocill)
  1. Dose: child: 50–100 mg/kg per 24 hours divided 4–6 hours; adult: 500 mg every 4–6 hours
  2. Supplied: 250 mg/5 ml, 250 mg, 500 mg
- Penicillin V
  1. Dose: child: 25–50 mg/kg per 24 hours given every 6–8 hours; adult: 250–500 mg PO QID
  2. Supplied: 125 mg/5 ml, 250 mg/5 ml, 250 mg, 500 mg
- Rifampin
  1. Dose: 10–20 mg/kg per 24 hours, max 600 mg
  2. Supplied: 150 mg, 300 mg
  3. Warnings: interacts with antacids, Ca channel blockers, steroids, cyclosporine, digoxin, dapsone, quinolones, warfarin, L-thyroxine
- Sulfasalazine (Azulfidine)
  1. Dose: child: 30–60 mg/kg per 24 hours given every 4–6 hours; adult: 500 mg/24 hours for 1 week, then increase by 500 mg/24 hours for 1 week
  2. Max: 1–4 g/24 hours given QID
  3. Supplied: 500 mg/5 ml, 500 mg
  4. Monitor: CBC, liver enzymes every 2 weeks, monthly for 3 months, then every 3–6 months
  5. Warning: take with food
- Tetracycline (Panmycin, Sumycin)
  1. Dose: child: 25–50 mg/kg per 24 hours given QID; adult: 250–500 mg BID–QID, maximum 3 g/24hours
  2. Supplied: 250 mg, 500 mg
  3. Warning: do not use <8 years
- Trimethoprim–sulfamethoxazole (Septra, Bactrim)
  1. Dose: child: 0.5 mg/kg/dose, give BID; For child 10 kg – give 1 tsp BID; For child 20 kg – give 2 tsp BID; For child 30 kg – give 3 tsp BID; For child ≥40 kg – give 4 tsp BID or 1 double strength tab BID; for adult 1 tab (double strength) BID-QID

  2. Supplied: liquid: 200 mg/5 ml of sulfa, 40 mg/5 ml of TMP; tablet: 400 mg of sulfa, 80 mg of TMP; double strength: 800 mg of sulfa, 160 mg of TMP
  3. Warnings: white blood cell suppression, allergy

Preoperative endocarditis prophylaxis

- Amoxicillin: adults: 2 g, children 50 mg/kg; given orally 1 hour before procedure
- Allergic to penicillin:
  1. Clindamycin: adults: 600 mg, children 20 mg/kg; given orally 1 hour before procedure OR
  2. Cephalexin: adults: 2 g, children 50 mg/kg; given orally 1 hour before procedure OR
  3. Azithromycin or clarithromycin: adults: 500 mg, children 15 mg/kg; given orally 1 hour before procedure

Antibiotic agents (topical)

Indications: superficial folliculitis, impetigo
- See Table 21.3

Dakon solution

- Indications: antibiotic solution
- Dose: full strength (0.5%) 10 ml bleach, 20 ml $NaHCO_3$ in 1 liter of water; half strength (0.25%); quarter strength (0.125%)

Antifungal agents

Topicals

- Creams are best for dry areas
- Solutions are best for intertriginous areas
- Medicated powders help to dry the skin but are not very effective in treating fungus; helpful in prophylaxis
- Combination products with topical steroids can mask infections and are not recommended for most tinea or candidal infections
- See Table 21.4

Oral

- Griseofulvin (Grifulvin, Grisactin, Fulvicin)

Table 21.3   Topical antibiotic agents

Brand name	Generic name	Prescription/ OTC
Bactroban cream, ointment	mupirocin 2%	Rx
Bactitracin ointment	bacitracin (generic)	OTC
Betadine ointment	povidone 5–10%	OTC
Cortisporin ointment	polymyxin, neomycin, bacitracin, hydrocortisone (HC) 1%	Rx
Furacin cream, ointment	nitrofurazone 0.2%	Rx
Garamycin ointment, cream	gentamicin 0.1%	Rx
Mycitracin ointment	polymyxin, neomycin, bacitracin	OTC
Neosporin ointment	polymyxin, neomycin, bacitracin	OTC
Polysporin ointment	polymyxin, bacitracin	OTC
Silvadene cream	silver sulfadiazine 1%	Rx
Vioform-HC	clinoquinol 3% + 1% HC	Rx
Vytone cream	iodoquinol 1% + 1% HC	Rx

Table 21.4   Topical antifungal agents

Brand name	Generic name	Prescription or OTC
Exelderm	1% sulconazole	Rx
Lamisil (cream, solution, spray)	1% terbinafine	OTC
Lotrisone	1% clotrimazole + diprosone 0.05%	Rx
Loprox (cream, lotion)	1% ciclopirox	Rx
Lotrimin (cream, solution, lotion)	1% clotrimazole	OTC
Mentax	1% butenafine	Rx
Micatin	2% miconazole	OTC
Mycelex (cream, solution)	1% clotrimazole	OTC
Naftin (gel, cream)	1% naftifine	Rx
Nizoral (cream, shampoo	1% ketoconazole	OTC
	2% ketoconazole	Rx
Oxistat (cream)	1% oxiconazole	Rx
Spectazole	1% econazole	Rx

1. Dose (Microsize): child: 10–25 mg/kg per 24 hours; adult: 500–1000 mg/24 hours; max dose: 1 g/24 hours
2. Dose (Ultra Micro): child: 5–10 mg/kg per 24 hours given once daily or BID; adult: 375–750 mg/24 hours given once daily or BID; max dose 750 mg/24hours
3. Supplied: (equivalency: 250 mg Ultra Micro equals ~500 mg Micro). Micro (UF): 250, 500 mg tabs, 125 mg/5 ml syrup; Ultra Micro (PG): 125, 250, 330 tabs
4. Warning: take with food, drug interactions
5. Contraindications: pregnancy, liver failure, porphyria

- Fluconazole (Diflucan)
  1. Dose: child: 3–6 mg/kg per 24 hours; adult: 150–300 mg once weekly for nails for 3–12 months
  2. Supplied: 10 mg/ml, 40 mg/ml, 50 mg, 100 mg, 150 mg, 200 mg
  3. Monitor: liver enzymes, drug interactions
- Itraconazole (Sporanox)
  1. Dose: adult: 200–400 mg/24 hours; max dose: 400 mg/24 hours
  2. Dose: child:
     a Nails (pulse 1 week out of month): 10–20 kg: 1 cap every other day; 20–30 kg: 1 cap daily; 30–40 kg: 1 cap every other day

   alternating with 2 caps every other day;
   40–50 kg: 2 caps daily; >50 kg: 2 caps BID
   b. Hair (tinea capitis): 3–5 mg/kg per 24
      hours for 30 days, given once daily or BID;
      >60 lb: 100 mg/24 hours for 1 month;
      2-year-old: 100 mg every other day in apple
      sauce or Jello for 1 month
   c. Tinea versicolor: 200 mg once, repeat in 1
      week
   3. Supplied: 10 mg/ml, 100 mg
   4. Monitor: liver enzymes, drug interactions
- Ketoconazole (Nizoral)
   1. Dose: child ≥2 years: 3.3–6.6 mg/kg per 24
      hours given once daily; adult: 200–400 mg/24
      hours given once daily; max dose: 800 mg/24
      hours given BID
   2. Tinea versicolor: 400 mg once a week twice,
      week apart; or 200 mg daily for 5–10 days
   3. Supplied: 100 mg/5 ml compounded, 200 mg
   4. Monitor: liver enzymes in long-term use, drug
      interactions
- Nystatin
   1. Dose: child/adult: 4–6 ml swish and swallow
      QID
   2. Supplied: suspension 100 000 units/ml
- Terbinafine (Lamisil)
   1. Dose:
      a. Hair: 3–6 mg/kg per 24 hours for one
         month; <20 kg: one quarter tab/24 hours;
         20–40 kg: one half tab/24 hours; >40 kg:
         1 tab/24 hours
      b. Nails: 250 mg daily for 3 months or pulsed:
         250 mg BID for 1 week each month for 3
         months
      c. Adult: 250–500 mg/24 hours
   2. Supplied: 250 mg
   3. Monitor: CBC and liver enzymes before and
      monthly during continuous therapy, drug
      interactions

Antiparasitic agents

- Elimite cream (permethrin 5%)
   1. Apply for 8–14 hours (overnight); repeat in 1
      week
- Kwell (lotion, cream, shampoo) (lindane 1%)
   1. Apply for 8–14 hours; repeat in 1 week
- Nix Cream Rinse (permethrin 1%)
   1. Apply for 10 minutes to dry hair then wash out

- RID (pyrethrin 0.3% plus pipermylbutoxide)
   1. Apply for 10 minutes to dry hair then wash
      out
- Sulfur (precipitated) (5–10% ointment)
   1. Must compound in cream or petrolatum; apply
      daily for 3 days
- Ivermectin (0.2 mg/kg given in a single dose).
   15–24 kg: half tab (3 mg); 25–35 kg: 1 tab (6 mg);
   36–50 kg: 1 half tab (9 mg); 51–65 kg: 2 tab (12
   mg); 66–79 kg: 2 half tab (15 mg); ≥80 kg:
   0.2 mg/kg
   1. Supplied: 6 mg tab

Acne medicines (topicals)

Benzoyl peroxide (BP)

- Antibacterial/keratolytic
- Do not apply at same time with topical retinoid
- Water-based gels less irritating and less drying than
  acetone- or alcohol-based gels
- Concentrations of 2.5–5% are as effective as 10%
  gels and less irritating
- See Table 21.5

Topical antibiotics for acne

- Come as solutions, lotions, gels, creams and
  pads
- Kill *Propionibacterium acnes*
- Anti-inflammatory effects
- See Table 21.6

Keratolytics for acne

- See Table 21.7

Topical retinoids

- Available by prescription only
- Creams are less irritating than gels or solutions
- See Table 21.8

Sulfur products

- Broad-spectrum antimicrobial, keratolytic
- Treat: acne, rosacea, seborrheic dermatitis
- Do not use in sulfa-sensitive patients
- See Table 21.9

Other

- See Table 21.10

Table 21.5   Topical acne medicines

Medication	Prescription/OTC
Benzac AC (water emollient base) 2.5%, 5%, 10%	Rx
Benzac W (water) 2.5%, 5%, 10%	Rx
BenzaClin (BP 5% + 1% clindamycin)	Rx
Brevoxyl (water) 4%, 8%	Rx
Clear By Design 2.5%	OTC
Duac gel (clindamycin 1% + BP 5%)	Rx
Neutrogena Acne Mask 5%	OTC
Oxy 10% gel	OTC
Pan Oxyl 5%, 10% gel	Rx
Sulfoxyl (regular) 5% BP + 2% sulfur lotion	Rx
Sulfoxyl (strong) 10% BP + 2% sulfur lotion	Rx
Triaz 3%, 6%, 10% gel	Rx
Benzagel 5%, 10%	Rx
Desquam X 2.5%, 5%, 10% gel	Rx
Benzoyl peroxide wash	
Benzac AC Wash 2.5%, 5%, 10%	Rx
Brevoxyl Cleanser 4%, 8%	Rx
Brevoxyl Creamy Wash 4%, 8%	Rx

Table 21.6   Topical antibiotics for acne

Medication	Generic
Akne-Mycin (ointment or solution)	2% erythromycin
A/T/S (gel, solution)	2% erythromycin
Benzamycin	3% erythromycin + BP 5%
BenzaClin (gel)	1% clindamycin + BP 5%
Cleocin T (solution, gel, lotion, pledgets)	1% clindamycin
Clindets (pads)	1% clindamycin
Duac	1% clindamycin + BP 5%
Emgel (gel)	2% erythromycin
Erycette (swabs)	2% erythromycin
EryDerm (solution)	2% erythromycin
Erygel (gel)	2% erythromycin
Staticin solution	1.5% erythromycin
Theramycin Z (solution)	2% erythromycin + zinc acetate
Topicycline (solution)	tetracycline 2.2 mg/ml
T-Stat (solution, pads)	2% erythromycin

Table 21.7   Keratolytics for acne

Medication	Generic	Supplied
Clean & Clear	salicylic acid 0.5% or 2%	OTC
Oxy Night Watch	salicylic acid 1% or 2%	OTC
Stridex Clear Gel	salicylic gel 2%	OTC

Table 21.8   Topical retinoids for acne

Medication	Generic
Avita 0.025% cream, gel	tretinoin
Differin 0.1% cream, gel	adapalene
Retin-A Micro 0.1% gel	tretinoin
Retin A 0.025%, 0.05%, 0.1% cream	tretinoin
Retin A 0.01%, 0.025% gel	tretinoin
Tazorac 0.05%, 0.1% (cream, gel)	tazarotene

Table 21.9   Sulfur products for acne

Medication	Generic	Supplied
Clearasil	8% sulfur + 1% resorcinol	OTC
Fostril	2% sulfur	OTC
Klaron	10 % sodium sulfacetamide	Rx
Liquimat	5% sulfur	OTC
Novacet	5% sulfur + 10% sodium sulfacetamide	Rx
Sulfacet-R	5% sulfur +10% sodium sulfacetamide	Rx
Sulfoxyl (regular)	5% BP + 2% sulfur lotion	Rx
Sulfoxyl (strong)	10% BP + 2% sulfur lotion	Rx

Table 21.10   Other products for acne

Medication	Generic	Supplied
Azelex cream	20% azelaic acid	Rx
Finacea gel	15% azelaic acid	Rx

Rosacea medicines

- Anti-inflammatory
- Prescription only
- See Table 21.11

Antiviral agents

Topical

- Suppressive, not for primary treatment
- Prescription only
- See Table 21.12

Table 21.11   Rosacea medicines

Medication	Generic
Noritate (cream)	metronidazole 1%
MetroGel	metronidazole 0.75%
MetroCream	metronidazole 0.75%
MetroLotion	metronidazole 0.75%
Klaron (lotion)	sodium sulfacetamide 10%
Novacet Lotion sodium	sulfacetamide 10%/5% sulfur
Sulfacet-R sodium	sulfacetamide 10%/5% sulfur

Table 21.12   Antiviral agents

Medication	Generic
Zovirax ointment	acyclovir 5%
Viroptic solution	trifluridine 1%
Cidofovir gel	0.3, 1, 3% gel
Denavir cream	penciclovir 1% cream

Topical genital wart treatment

- Podocon-25 (podophyllin 25%)
  1. Apply in office; leave on 1–6 hours; then wash off
- Condylox (podofilox 0.5%)
  1. Dose: use BID for 3 days each week; reassess at 4 weeks
- Aldara (imiquimod 5%)
  1. Apply once daily 3 times per week at bedtime; wash in morning

Opioid analgesics

- Codeine
  1. Starting oral doses and intervals
     a. Child (<50 kg) 0.5–1.0 mg/kg per dose every 4–6 hours
     b. Max dose: 60 mg/dose
     c. Adult (>50 kg) 15–60 mg every 4–6 hours
  2. Supplied: 15 mg, 30 mg, 60 mg; 15 mg/ml, 60 mg/5 ml
     a. Acetaminophen with codeine: no. 2: 300 mg acetaminophen + 15 mg codeine; no. 3: 300 mg acetaminophen + 30 mg codeine; no. 4: 300 mg acetaminophen + 60 mg codeine
- Diazepam (Valium)
  1. Dose: child: 0.1–0.8 mg/kg per 24 hours given every 6–8 hours; adult: 2–10 mg/24 hours given every 6–12 hours
  2. Supplied: 5 mg/ml, 5 mg/5 ml, 1 mg, 2 mg, 5 mg, 10 mg
- Oxycodone (Oxycontin, Roxicodone)
  1. Starting oral doses and intervals
     a. Child (<50 kg) 0.05–0.15 mg/kg per dose every 4–6 hours
     b. Max dose: 10 mg/dose
     c. Adult (>50 kg) 5–10 mg every 4–6 hours
  2. Supplied: 1 mg/ml, 20 mg/ml, 5 mg
     a. Oxycontin controlled-release tabs: 10 mg, 20 mg, 40 mg; adults: 10–40 mg PO every 12 hours
     b. Percocet (oxycodone + acetaminophen); adult 1–2 tab every 4–6 hours
     c. Supplied: 500 mg acetaminophen + oxycodone 5 mg; 325 mg acetaminophen + oxycodone 5 mg; 325 mg acetaminophen + oxycodone 5 mg/5 ml
- Morphine
  1. Starting oral doses and intervals:
     a. Child (<50 kg) 0.2–0.5 mg/kg per dose every 3–4 hours
     b. Max dose: 15 mg/dose
     c. Adult (>50 kg) 10–30 mg every 4–6 hours
  2. Supplied: 10 mg/5 ml, 20 mg/5 ml, 100 mg/5 ml; 15 mg, 30 mg
  3. Controlled release tabs (given every 12 hours): 30 mg, 60 mg, 100 mg
- Midazolam (Versed)
  1. Dose (sedation/anxiolysis):
     a. Child (6 months to 5 years): 0.05–0.1 mg/kg per dose; can repeat in 2–3 minute intervals; max: 6 mg; 6–12 years: 0.025–0.05 mg/kg per dose; max: 10 mg; 12–16 years: 0.5–2 mg/dose; max: 10 mg; can repeat
     b. Adult: 5 mg or 0.07 mg/kg IM or 1 mg IV or 0.15 mg/kg IM
  2. Supplied: 2 mg/ml, 3 mg/ml

Nonopioid analgesics

- Acetaminophen (Tylenol)
  1. Dose:
     a. Child: 10–15 mg/kg per dose every 4–6 hours; 6 months to 5 years: 0.25–1 mg/kg per dose; 6–12 years: 0.25–0.5 mg/kg per dose
     b. Max daily dose: 75 mg/kg per 24 hours (not to exceed 4 g/24 hours)
     c. Adult: 325–650 mg every 4–6 hours
     d. Max daily dose (adults): 4 g/24 hours
  2. Supplied: 160, 325, 500, 650 mg
     a. Chewable tabs: 80, 160 mg
     b. Infant drops: 80 mg/ 0.8 ml
     c. Liquid: 80 mg/5 ml, 120 mg/5 ml, 160 mg/5 ml, 325 mg/5 ml
- Aspirin
  1. Dose:
     a. Child: 10–15 mg/kg per dose every 4–6 hours
     b. Adult dose 650–1000 mg every 4–6 hours
     c. Max daily dose: 4 g/24 hours
  2. Supplied: 325, 500 mg, others
     a. Chewable tabs: 81 mg
- Ibuprofen (Advil, Motrin)
  1. Dose:
     a. Child: 5–10 mg/kg per dose every 6–8 hours
     b. Max dose (child): 40 mg/kg per 24 hours
     c. Adult: 400–800 mg every 6–8 hours
     d. Max daily dose (adult): 3200 mg/24 hours
  2. Supplied: 100 mg/5 ml, 40 mg/ml
     a. Chewable tabs: 50 mg, 100 mg
     b. Tabs: 100, 200, 300, 400, 600, 800 mg
- Naproxen (Naprosyn, Aleve)
  1. Dose:
     a. Child >2 years: 5–7 mg/kg per dose every 8–12 hours
     b. Adult dose 250–500 mg every 12 hours
     c. Max daily dose (adult): 1000 mg

2. Supplied: 125 mg/5 ml, 220 mg, 250 mg, 375 mg, 500 mg

Topical anesthetics

- See Table 21.13

Table 21.13	Topical anesthetics
Medication	**Generic**
EMLA	2.5% lidocaine + 2.5% prilocaine
ELA-MAX	4% lidocaine
LMX	4% lidocaine
Pramosone	Pramoxine + 1% or 2.5% hydrocortisone
Lida-Mantle	3% Lidocaine + 0.13% benzalkonium Cl + 0.5% hydrocortisone

Local anesthetics

- Lidocaine (Xylocaine)
  1. Dose:
     a. Adults: max 4.5 mg/kg per dose without epinephrine; max 7 mg/kg per dose with epinephrine; max topical 3 mg/kg per dose, no more frequently than every 2 hours
  2. Supplied:
     a. Injection: 0.5%, 1%, 1.5%, 2%, 4%, 10%, 20%
     b. Injection with 1 : 50 000 epinephrine – 2% lidocaine
     c. Injection with 1 : 100 000 epinephrine – 1%, 2% lidocaine
     d. Injection with 1 : 200 000 epinephrine – 0.5%, 1%, 1.5%, 2% lidocaine; jelly: 2% lidocaine ; liquid (viscous): 2% lidocaine; solution: 2% lidocaine

Other medicines

- Acitretin (Soriatane)
  1. Indications: psoriasis, ichthyosis (off label)
  2. Dose: 0.5 mg/kg per 24 hours; adult: 25–50 mg/24 hours
  3. Supplied: 10 mg, 25 mg
  4. Monitor: CBC, electrolytes, blood urea nitrogen (BUN), creatinine, liver enzymes, lipids, urinalysis, fasting glucose, albumin, pregnancy tests
     a. Check baseline, then every 2 weeks for 2 weeks, then every month for 6 months, then every 3 months
  5. Contraindications: pregnancy, alcohol ingestion
  6. Warnings: see Physician's Desk Reference, avoid pregnancy for >3 years after cessation
  7. Side-effects: fetal abnormalities, pseudotumor cerebri, hepatotoxicity, decreased night vision, hyperostosis, lipid abnormalities
- Acyclovir (Zovirax)
  1. Dose:
     a. Primary herpes: child: 15–30 mg/kg per 24 hours every 8 hours; max dose in child: 80 mg/kg per 24 hours; adult: 400 mg TID or 200 mg 5 times daily for 7–10 days
     b. Recurrence: adult: 400 mg TID for 5 days, or 200 mg 5 times a day for 5 days
     c. Chronic suppression: adult: 800–1000 mg/24 hours given 2–5 times a day
     d. Varicella: child: 80 mg/kg per 24 hours given QID for 5 days; max dose: 3200 mg/24 hours
     e. Herpes zoster: 800 mg 5 times a day for 5–7 days
  2. Supplied: 200 mg/5 ml, 200 mg, 400 mg, 800 mg
- Chloral hydrate
  1. Indications: sedation for procedures, sedative
  2. Dose:
     a. Child: for anxiety: 5–15 mg/kg per dose (maximum 500 mg); for conscious sedation: 50–75 mg/kg per dose given every 6–8 hours; max: 1 g/dose
     b. Adult: 250–1000 mg/dose given TID; max: 2 g/24 hours
  3. Supplied: 250 mg/5 ml, 500 mg/5 ml, 250 mg, 500 mg
  4. Contraindications: hepatic or renal disease
- Cimetidine (Tagamet)
  1. Indications: histamine-2-antagonist
  2. Dose:
     a. Child: 20–40 mg/kg per 24 hours, given 3–4 times per day
     b. Adult 300 mg QID
     c. Max: 2400 mg/24 hours

3. Supplied: 100 mg (OTC), 200 mg tabs, 300 mg/5 ml, 300 mg, 400 mg, 800 mg
4. Warning: drug interactions

- Cyclosporine (Neoral)
  1. Indications: immunosuppressant, potent T-cell inhibitor, psoriasis
  2. Dose: 2.5–4 mg/kg per 24 hours divided BID for 4 weeks; increase every 2 weeks by 0.5 mg/kg per 24 hours
     a. Max: 5 mg/kg per 24 hours
  3. Monitor: CBC, liver enzymes, BUN, creatinine, Mg, K, uric acid, lipids, cyclosporine trough levels if >5 mg/kg per day
     a. Check blood pressure every 2 weeks for 3 months, decrease dose if creatinine is elevated >30%
     b. Check creatinine clearance every 6 months
  4. Contraindications: renal insufficiency, hypertension, infection
  5. Relative contraindications: malignancy, immunodeficiency, nephrotoxic drugs, hepatic disease, gout
  6. Side-effects: nephrotoxicity, hepatotoxicity, hypertension, tremor, gingival hyperplasia, long-term malignancy, hyperlipidemia, hypertrichosis, hyperkalemia, uricemia, hypomagnesemia
  7. Supplied: 100 mg/ml, 25 mg, 100 mg
- Doxepin
  1. Dose:
     a. Child: 1–3 mg/kg per 24 hours, given in single dose at bedtime
     b. Adult 25–100 mg PO at bedtime; start low and increase slowly; max 300 mg/24 hours
  2. Supplied: 10 mg/ml; 10 mg, 25 mg
  3. Topical - use in teens and adults only; use only in small areas; consider toxicity (drowsiness) if overused
- Epinephrine
  1. Indications: sympathomimetic, hypersensitivity reactions
  2. Dose:
     a. Child: 0.01 mg/kg per dose (maximum 0.3 mg)
     b. Adult: usually 0.1–0.25 mg of 1 : 1,000 solution subcutaneously
  3. Supplied: Epi Pen Jr 0.15 mg dose, Epi Pen 0.3 mg autoinjection

     a. For injection: 1 mg/ml, 5 mg/ml, 0.1 mg/ml, 0.01 mg/ml
  4. Warning: may produce arrhythmia, hypertension, nervousness, vomiting
- Famciclovir (Famvir)
  1. Dose: ages >18 years
     a. Primary herpes: 250 mg TID for 7–10 days
     b. Recurrence: 125–250 mg BID for 5 days
     c. Suppression: 250 mg BID
     d. Herpes zoster: 500 mg TID for 7 days
     e. Supplied: 125 mg, 250 mg, 500 mg
     f. Warning: do not give to HIV patients
- Folic acid
  1. Dose:
     a. Initial: child (1–10 years): 1 mg/24 hours or 5 mg per week; >11 years: 1–3 mg/dose divided daily to TID
     b. Maintenance: 0.1–0.5 mg/24 hours given QD; pregnant women 0.8 mg/24 hours
  2. Supplied: 0.4 mg, 0.8 mg, 1 mg; 1 mg/ml compounded
- Hydroquinone (HQ)
  1. Indications: bleaching agent
  2. Supplied: 1.5–2% OTC
     a. 4% by prescription
     b. Lustra (HQ, glycolic acid, no sunscreen)
     c. Lustra AF (HQ, sunscreen)
     d. Alustra (HQ, retinal, sunscreen)
  3. Warnings: do not use for prolonged periods (>3 months) because of risk of hyperpigmentation
- Hydroxychloroquine (Plaquenil)
  1. Dose: 200–400 mg/24 hours, given BID–TID
  2. Supplied: 200 mg
  3. Monitor:
     a. Initial G6PD (avoid if deficient), CBC, liver enzymes, eye examination
     b. Every 3 months: CBC, liver enzymes
     c. Every 6 months: eye examination
  4. Side-effects: retinal damage, myopathy, liver abnormalities, hemolysis, cutaneous eruptions or discoloration
- Isotretinoin (Accutane)
  1. Indications: severe recalcitrant or cystic acne, ichthyosis (off label)
  2. Dosage:
     a. Initial 0.5–2 mg/kg per 24 hours given BID for 15–20 weeks
     b. Max dose: 2 mg/kg per 24 hours

c. Adjust for side-effects and disease response
d. Repeat only if necessary after 2 months off drug
e. Take with food
3. Supplied: 10 mg, 20 mg, 30 mg, 40 mg
4. Contraindications: pregnancy, paraben sensitivity, concomitant vitamin A
5. Monitor: initial CBC; baseline and every month: liver enzymes, lipids, pregnancy tests
6. Warnings: see PDR; need special labels to prescribe

- Methotrexate (Rheumatrex)
  1. Indications: psoriasis, morphea, cutaneous T-cell lymphoma
  2. Dose: 2.5–25 mg given once a week either PO or IM
  3. Supplied: 2.5 mg
  4. Monitor: liver enzymes, creatinine, CBC, urinalysis every week for 4 weeks then once a month; chest X-ray as indicated; liver biopsy after 1–1.5 g total dose
  5. Contraindications: pregnancy, liver disease, alcohol ingestion, significant hematological abnormalities, active infectious disease, immunodeficiency
  6. Warning: multiple drug interactions, hepatoxicity, bone marrow depression, carcinogenesis, pulmonary fibrosis

- Minoxidil (Rogaine)
  1. Indications: androgenetic alopecia
  2. Dose: 2%, 5% solution, apply 1 ml to dry scalp BID
  3. Side-effects: hypertrichosis

- Mycophenolate mofetil (CellCept)
  1. Indications: immunosuppressive agent
  2. Dose: 2–4 g/24 hours given BID
     i. Child: 600 mg/m^2 per dose PO, BID
  3. Supplied: 250 mg, 500 mg
  4. Monitor: CBC (neutrophils) and liver enzymes once a week for 1 month, then once monthly
  5. Warning: drug interactions

- Oral contraceptive pills (with low androgenetic activity)
  1. Indications: acne, hirsutism
  2. Supplied: Ortho-Tricyclen (ethinyl estradiol–norgestimate), OrthoCyclen, Desogestrel, Ovulen, Demulen, Enovid, Orthocept, Desogen, OrthoCyclen, Desogen, Orthocept

3. Contraindications: pregnancy

- Pimecrolimus (Elidel)
  1. Ages >2 years: 1% pimecrolimus cream BID
  2. Supplied: 15 g, 30 g, 100 g
  3. Warnings: burning, stinging

- Robinul (glycopyrrolate)
  1. Indications: hyperhidrosis (anticholinergic)
  2. Dose:
     a. Child: 0.04–0.1 mg/kg per dose every 4–8 hours
     b. Adult: 1–2 mg BID–TID
  3. Supplied: 1 mg, 2 mg
  4. Warning: caution in liver or kidney disease; atropine-like side-effects

- SSKI (potassium iodide)
  1. Indications: larva migrans, erythema nodosum (off label), sporotrichosis
  2. Dose: 3–10 drops TID
     a. Adult: 300–650 mg TID–QID
     b. Child: 60–250 mg TID–QID
     c. Max: 4.5–9 g/24 hours
  3. Supplied: 1000 mg/ml, 325 mg/5 ml, 65 mg, 130 mg
  4. Monitor: thyroid tests
  5. Contraindications: pregnancy
  6. Warning: metallic taste, give with milk or meals

- Tacrolimus (Protopic)
  1. Ages 2–15 years: 0.03% tacrolimus ointment BID
  2. Ages >15 years: 0.1% tacrolimus ointment BID
  3. Supplied: 30 g, 60 g
  4. Warnings: burning, stinging

- Thalidomide
  1. Dose:
     a. Adult: 50–300 mg/24 hours given at night
  2. Supplied: 50 mg
  3. Side-effects: birth defects, peripheral neuropathy (sensory), sedation
  4. Monitor:
     a. Baseline human chorionic gonadotropin (hCG), neurological examination, sensory nerve action potential (SNAP)
     b. hCG every week for 4 weeks, then every 4 weeks
     c. Neurological examination every 3 months, and SNAP as indicated

- Valacyclovir (Valtrex)

1. Dose: ages: >18 years
   a. Primary herpes: 1–2 g BID for 7–10 days
   b. Recurrence: 500 mg BID for 5 days
   c. Suppression: 500 mg once daily
   d. Herpes zoster: 1 g TID for 7 days
2. Supplied: 500 mg, 1000 mg
3. Warning: do not prescribe to HIV patients

- Zinc
  1. Indications: zinc deficiency
  2. Dose:
     a. Child: 0.5–1 mg elemental zinc/kg per 24 hours, given daily to TID
     b. Adult: 25–50 mg elemental zinc/dose TID
  3. Supplied: 2 mg/ml
     a. Children >4 years: Centrum Jr + Fe (15 mg), Polyvisol + Fe Zn
     b. Tabs as sulfate with 23% elemental Zn: 110 mg (25 mg elemental Zn), 220 mg (50 mg elemental Zn)
     c. Tabs as gluconate with 14.3% elemental Zn
     d. Liquid as acetate: 5 mg, 10 mg elemental Zn/ml (compounded)
  4. Warning: GI upset

References

Archer JSM, Archer DF. Oral contraceptive efficacy and antibiotic interaction: a myth debunked. J Am Acad Dermatol 2002; 46: 917–23

Berde CB, Sethna NF. Analgesics for the treatment of pain in children. N Engl J Med 2002; 347: 1094–103

Brecher AR, Orlow SJ. Oral retinoid therapy for dermatologic conditions in children and adolescents. J Am Acad Dermatol 2003; 49: 171–82

Drake LA, Dinehart SM, Farmer ER, et al. Guidelines of care for the use of topical glucocorticosteroids. J Am Acad Dermatol 1996; 35: 615–19

Litt JZ. Pocketbook of Drug Eruptions. Parthenon Publishing: New York, 2001

Parker JF, Vats A, Bauer G. EMLA toxicity after application for allergy skin testing. Pediatrics 2004; 113: 410–11

Shapiro LE, Shear NH. Drug interactions: proteins, pumps, and P-450s. J Am Acad Dermatol 2002; 47: 467–84

Scheman AJ, Severson DL. Pocket Guide to Medication Used in Dermatology, 6th edn. Williams & Wilkins: Baltimore, 1999

INDEX